OXFORD MEDICAL PUBLICATIONS

Oxford Handbook of
Clinical and Laboratory Investigation

Second Edition

Oxford University Press makes no representation, express or implied, that the drug dosages in this book are correct. Readers must therefore always check the product information and clinical procedures with the most up-to-date published product information and data sheets provided by the manufacturers and the most recent codes of conduct and safety regulations. The authors and the publishers do not accept responsibility or legal liability for any errors in the text or for the misuse or misapplication of material in this work.

►Except where otherwise stated, drug doses and recommendations are for the non-pregnant adult who is not breast-feeding.

Oxford Handbook of
Clinical and
Laboratory
Investigation

Second Edition

Drew Provan

Senior Lecturer in Haematology,
St Bartholomew's and The Royal London Hospital
School of Medicine & Dentistry, London, UK

OXFORD
UNIVERSITY PRESS

OXFORD
UNIVERSITY PRESS

Great Clarendon Street, Oxford OX2 6DP

Oxford University Press is a department of the University of Oxford.
It furthers the University's objective of excellence in research, scholarship,
and education by publishing worldwide in

Oxford New York

Auckland Cape Town Dar es Salaam Hong Kong Karachi
Kuala Lumpur Madrid Melbourne Mexico City Nairobi
New Delhi Shanghai Taipei Toronto

With offices in

Argentina Austria Brazil Chile Czech Republic France Greece
Guatemala Hungary Italy Japan Poland Portugal Singapore
South Korea Switzerland Thailand Turkey Ukraine Vietnam

Oxford is a registered trade mark of Oxford University Press
in the UK and in certain other countries

Published in the United States
by Oxford University Press Inc., New York

British Library Cataloguing in Publication Data
Data available

Library of Congress Cataloging in Publication Data
Data available

Typeset by Drew Provan and Newgen Imaging Systems (P) Ltd., India
Printed in Italy
on acid-free paper by
LegoPrint, srl

ISBN 0-19-856663-8   9-780-19856663-2

10 9 8 7 6 5 4 3 2 1

Contents

Acknowledgements *vi*
Contributors *vii*
Preface to the first edition *ix*
Dedication *x*
Preface to the second edition *xi*
Foreword by Professor Sir George Alberti *xii*
Symbols & abbreviations *xiii*
Introduction: Approach to investigations *xxii*

Part 1 **The patient**

1	Symptoms & signs	3

Part 2 **Investigations**

2	Endocrinology & metabolism	107
3	Haematology	197
4	Immunology & allergy	287
5	Infectious & tropical diseases	327
6	Cardiology	379
7	Gastroenterology	439
8	Respiratory medicine	471
9	Neurology	517
10	Renal medicine	567
11	Poisoning & overdose	607
12	Rheumatology	639
13	Radiology	651
14	Nuclear medicine	727

Index *801*

Acknowledgements

Even small books such as this rely on the input of many people, besides the main editors and we are indebted to many of our colleagues for providing helpful suggestions and for proofreading the text. Dr Barbara Bain, St Mary's Hospital, London, kindly allowed us to peruse the proofs of *Practical Haematology*, 9th edition (Churchill Livingstone) to help make sure the haematology section was up to date. Dr Debbie Lillington, Department of Cytogenetics, Barts & The London NHS Trust, London, provided invaluable cytogenetic advice. Our registrars have had input into many sections and we thank the London registrars: Simon Stanworth, Jude Gaffan, Leon Clark and Nikki Curry, and the Southampton registrars: Fiona Clark, Michael Masding, Mayank Patel, Ruth Poole and Catherine Talbot. Thanks to Dr SJ Harris (Nottingham) for alerting me to some omissions in the book.

Dr Murray Longmore, the undisputed Oxford Handbook king, has provided invaluable wisdom and has very kindly allowed us to use his specially designed OHCM typeface (OUP) for many of the symbols in our text. Murray also provided page proofs of OHCM, which was invaluable for cross-referencing this handbook.

The team at Oxford University Press have, as ever, been a joy to work with and I extend my warmest thanks to my commissioning editor Catherine Barnes who always manages to stay calm despite being harassed by me. Georgia Pinteau, Catherine's administrative assistant, has worked wonders behind the scenes and miraculously has succeeded in keeping the workflow going. Kate Martin and Jonathan Coleclough have provided much needed help in the graphics and typography departments.

I am grateful to Dr Andrew Krentz, who co-edited the first edition of this book. Dr Krentz's sections on diabetes, hyperlipidaemias, and others remain a valuable component of the book, and have been updated by Dr Colin Dayan.

Contributors

Martyn Bracewell
Senior Lecturer and Senior
Consultant Neurologist,
University of Wales, Bangor
Neurology

Joanna Brown
Consultant Respiratory Physician,
Queen Alexandra Hospital,
Portsmouth
Respiratory medicine

Kuntal Chakravarty
Professor of Rheumatology (Hon),
London University of Southbank,
London
Rheumatology

Tanya Chawla
Assistant Professor,
University Health Network &
Mount Sinai,
Department of Medical Imaging,
Toronto, Canada
Radiology

Colin Dayan
Consultant Senior Lecturer
in Medicine,
Division of Medicine Laboratories,
Bristol Royal Infirmary,
Bristol BS2 8BX
Endocrinology & metabolism

James Dunbar
Specialist Registrar in Infectious
Diseases,
St James's Hospital, Leeds, UK
Infectious & tropical diseases

A Frew
Professor of Allergy and
Respiratory Medicine,
University of Southampton,
School of Medicine,
Southampton SO16 6YD
Respiratory medicine

David Gray
Reader in Medicine and
Consultant Cardiologist,
Queen's Medical Centre,
University Hospital NHS Trust
Nottingham
Cardiology

Stephen T. Green
Consultant Physician and Honorary
Senior Clinical Lecturer,
Department of Infection &
Tropical Medicine,
Royal Hallamshire Hospital,
Sheffield S10 2JF
Infectious & tropical diseases

Emma Greig
Consultant Gastroenterologist,
Taunton & Somerset NHS Trust
Taunton
Gastroenterology

Andrew R. Houghton
Consultant Cardiologist,
Grantham & District Hospital,
Grantham
Cardiology

Alison Jones
Consultant Physician and Clinical
Toxicologist,
Medical Toxicology Unit,
Guy's & St Thomas' Hospital,
London SE14 5ER
Poisoning & overdose

Val Lewington
Consultant Physician,
Nuclear Medicine,
Royal Marsden Hospital,
London, UK
Nuclear medicine

Drew Provan
Senior Lecturer,
Department of Haematology,
St Bartholomew's &
The Royal London School
of Medicine & Dentistry,
London E1 1BB
*Haematology, transfusion &
cytogenetics*

Rommel Ravanan
Specialist Registrar,
The Richard Bright Renal Unit,
Southmead Hospital,
Westbury-on-Trym,
Bristol BS10 5NB
Renal medicine

Dr Penelope Sensky
Department of Cardiology
King's Mill Hospital,
Suttan in Ashfield,
Cardiology

Dr Gavin Spickett
Consultant Clinical Immunologist
Regional Department of
Immunology,
Royal Victoria Infirmary,
Newcastle upon Tyne NE1 4LP
Immunology

Charlie Tomson
Consultant Nephrologist,
The Richard Bright Renal Unit,
Southmead Hospital,
Westbury-on-Trym,
Bristol BS10 5NB
Renal medicine

Ken Tung
Consultant Radiologist,
Department of Radiology,
Southampton University
Hospitals NHS Trust,
Southampton SO16 6YD
Radiology

Adrian Williams
Bloomer Professor of Clinical
Neurology,
Department of Neurology,
The Queen Elizabeth Hospital,
Birmingham B15 2TH
Neurology

Lorraine Wilson
Consultant in Nuclear Medicine,
The Royal Victoria Hospital,
Belfast, UK
Nuclear medicine

Our registrars
We are indebted to our juniors
for writing and checking various
sections, in particular
Symptoms & signs

Southampton University
Hospitals:
*Martin Taylor, Michael Masding,
Mayank Patel, Ruth Poole,
Tanay Sheth and Catherine Talbot*

St Bartholomew's & The Royal
London School of Medicine &
Dentistry:
*Simon Stanworth, Jude Gaffan, Leon
Clark and Nikki Curry*

My thanks, also, to those who contributed to the first edition: John Axford, Keith Dawkins, Praful Patel.

Preface to the first edition

With the increasing complexity of modern medicine, we now have literally thousands of possible investigative techniques at our disposal. We are able to examine our patient's serum and every other body fluid down to the level of individual nucleotides, as well as being able to perform precise imaging through CT, MRI and other imaging technologies. The problem we have all faced, especially as senior medical students or junior doctors is: which test should we use in a given setting? What hazards are associated with the tests? Are there any situations where specific tests should not be used or are likely to produce erroneous results? As medical complexity increases so too does cost; many assays available today are highly expensive and wherever possible we would ideally like to use a test which is cheap, reliable, reproducible and right for a given situation.

Such knowledge takes many years to acquire and it is a fact of life that senior doctors (who have attained such knowledge) are not usually those who request the investigations. In this small volume, we have attempted to distil all that is known about modern tests, from blood, urine and other body fluids, along with imaging and molecular tests. The book is divided into two principal parts: the first deals with symptoms and signs in *The patient* section, because that is how patients present. We have tried to cover as many topics as possible, discussing these in some detail and have provided differential diagnoses where possible. We also try to suggest tests that might be of value in determining the cause of the patient's symptom or sign. The second part of the book, *Investigations*, is specialty-specific, and is more relevant once you know roughly what type of disease the patient might have. For example, if the symptom section suggests a likely respiratory cause for the patient's symptoms, then the reader should look to the *Respiratory investigations* chapter in order to determine which tests to carry out, or how to interpret the results.

The entire book is written by active clinicians, rather than scientists, since we wanted to provide a strong clinical approach to investigation. We have tried, wherever possible, to cross-refer to the *Oxford Handbook of Clinical Medicine*, 5th edition, Oxford University Press, which provides the clinical detail omitted from this handbook. The symbol 📖 is used to highlight a cross-reference to OHCM, in addition to cross-referencing within this book.

We would value feedback from readers since there will doubtless be tests omitted, errors in the text and many other improvements we could, and will, make in future editions. All contributors will be acknowledged individually in the next edition. We would suggest you e-mail us directly: *a.provan@virgin.net*.

Drew Provan
Andrew Krentz
2002

Dedication

To Val and Fraser with much love.

Preface to the second edition

Modern medicine has advanced greatly even in the short time since the first edition of this handbook was published. The aim of the first edition was to provide a concise but readable account of most of the investigations used in medical practice, helping readers choose the correct test for a given situation. The book attempted to be both patient- and test-centred so that it could be used in the clinic when patients present with symptoms or signs. The majority of the book was devoted to the tests themselves, subcategorised by specialty. Rather than simply list the tests along with potential abnormal findings, we tried to provide information about interpretation of results, pitfalls associated with the tests, and the next steps in the investigative process.

This new edition has precisely the same ethos but has been improved greatly by the addition of new members to the writing team. We have enlisted the help of experts in cardiology, gastroenterology, rheumatology and immunology. The new authors have rewritten their respective chapters entirely and, as a result, the book is much enhanced. Other chapters have also seen major rewrites and the addition of many new graphics; in fact, the number of illustrations has almost doubled. This helps break up the text and also improves the readability of each chapter. With so much medical information available on the Internet, most chapters contain URLs for websites that provide full guidelines and other information which should be of value to the reader.

I am extremely grateful to all the contributors for writing such lucid and relevant chapters, and for submitting their work within the timelines set. This has allowed the book to be published without delay, thereby reducing any outdating of material which is all too common with textbooks.

As before, I take responsibility for errors or omissions in the book and welcome any comments readers may have. This book is meant to be used rather than kept on a bookshelf, and its usability relies on feedback from readers so please contact me at *a.provan@virgin.net* if there is anything you feel could be improved in the next edition.

Drew Provan
2005

Foreword

This book fills an obvious gap in the Handbook series and indeed a major lacuna in the medical literature. Too often investigations of a particular condition are lost in the welter of other text. Alternatively, they appear as specialist books in pathology and radiology. One unique feature of this book is the inclusion of all clinical investigative techniques, i.e. both truly clinical tests in the shape of symptoms and signs and then laboratory-based investigations. This stops what is often an artificial separation. Each section is clearly put together with the intent of easing rapid reference. This is essential if the book is to have (and I believe it does have) real usefulness for bedside medicine. There are many other useful aspects of the text. These include a comprehensive list of abbreviations—the bugbear of medicine, as well as reference ranges which some laboratories still do not append to results. Overall, the Handbook should be of benefit to not just clinical students and junior doctors in training, but all who have patient contact. With this in one pocket, and Longmore in the other, there should be little excuse for errors in diagnosis and investigation, with the added benefit that the balance between the two will allow the upright posture to be maintained.

Professor Sir George Alberti
President of The Royal College of Physicians of London
July 2002

Symbols & abbreviations

📖	Cross-reference to OHCM 6th edition, or section of this book
▶	Important
▶▶	very important
↓	Decreased
↑	Increased
↔	Normal
♂:♀	male:female ratio
1°	Primary
2°	Secondary
A&E	accident & emergency
AAFB	acid and alcohol fast bacilli
Ab	Antibody
ABGs	arterial blood gases
ACD	anaemia of chronic disease
ACE	angiotensin converting enzyme
ACh	acetylcholine
ACL	anticardiolipin antibody
ACR	acetylcholine receptor
ACS	acute coronary syndrome
ADA	American Diabetes Association
ADH	antidiuretic hormone
ADP	adenosine 5-diphosphate
AECG	ambulatory ECG
AF	atrial fibrillation
Ag	antigen
AIDS	acquired immunodeficiency syndrome
AIHA	autoimmune haemolytic anaemia
AKA	alcoholic ketoacidosis
ALL	acute lymphoblastic leukaemia
ALP	alkaline phosphatase
ALT	alanine aminotransferase
AMI	acute myocardial infarction
AML	acute myeloid leukaemia
ANA	antinuclear antibodies
ANAE	alpha naphthyl acetate esterase
ANCA	antineutrophil cytoplasmic antibody
ANF	antinuclear factor
APCR	activated protein C resistance
APL	antiphospholipid antibody

APML	acute promyelocytic leukaemia
APS	antiphospholipid syndrome
APTR	activated partial thromboplastin time ratio
APTT	activated partial thromboplastin time
ARF	acute renal failure
AT (ATIII)	antithrombin III
ATLL	adult T cell leukaemia/lymphoma
ATP	adenosine triphosphate
AXR	abdominal x-ray
BBB	blood–brain barrier
B-CLL	B-cell chronic lymphocytic leukaemia
Bd	*bis die* (twice daily)
BJP	Bence–Jones protein
BM	bone marrow
BMJ	*British Medical Journal*
BMT	bone marrow transplant(ation)
BP	blood pressure
Bx	biopsy
C1 INH	C1 esterase inhibitor
C3Nef	complement C3 nephritic factor
C&S	culture & sensitivity
Ca	carcinoma
Ca^{2+}	calcium
CABG	coronary artery bypass graft
CAH	congenital adrenal hyperplasia
cALL	common acute lymphoblastic leukaemia
CBC	complete blood count (American term for FBC)
CCF	congestive cardiac failure
CCK	cholecystokinin
CCU	coronary care unit
CD	cluster designation
cDNA	complementary DNA
CEA	carcinoembryonic antigen
CF	cystic fibrosis *or* complement fixation
cfu	colony-forming units
CGL	chronic granulocytic leukaemia
CHAD	cold haemagglutinin disease
CHD	coronary heart disease
CJD	Creutzfeldt–Jacob disease (v = new variant)
CK	creatine kinase
Cl^-	chloride
CLL	chronic lymphocytic ('lymphatic') leukaemia
CLO test	*Campylobacter*-like organism test
CML	chronic myeloid leukaemia
CMML	chronic myelomonocytic leukaemia

CMV	cytomegalovirus
CNS	central nervous system
CO_2	carbon dioxide
COPD	chronic obstructive pulmonary disease
CPAP	continuous positive airways pressure
CREST	calcinosis, Raynaud's syndrome, (o)esophageal motility dysfunction, sclerodactyly, and telangiectasia
CRF	chronic renal failure
CRP	C-reactive protein
CSF	cerebrospinal fluid
CT	computed tomography
CTLp	cytotoxic T lymphocyte precursor assay
CVA	cerebrovascular accident (stroke)
CVD	cardiovascular disease
CVS	cardiovascular system or chorionic villus sampling
CXR	chest x-ray
DAT	direct antiglobulin test
dATP	deoxy ATP
DCCT	Diabetes Control and Complications Trial
DCT	direct Coombs' test
DDAVP	desamino D-arginyl vasopressin
DE	evoked potential
DIC	disseminated intravascular coagulation
DIDMOAD	diabetes insipidus, diabetes mellitus, optic atrophy, and deafness
DKA	diabetic ketoacidosis
dL	decilitre
DM	diabetes mellitus
DNA	deoxyribonucleic acid
2,3-DPG	2,3-diphosphoglycerate
dRVVT	dilute Russell's viper venom test
DTT	dilute thromboplastin time
DU	duodenal ulcer
DVT	deep vein thrombosis
DXT	radiotherapy
EBV	Epstein–Barr virus
ECG	electrocardiograph
EDH	extradural haemorrhage
EDTA	ethylenediamine tetraacetic acid
EEG	electroencephalogram
ELISA	enzyme-linked immunosorbent assay
EMG	electromyogram
Epo	erythropoietin
ERCP	endoscopic retrograde cholangiopancreatography
ESR	erythrocyte sedimentation rate

ESREF	end-stage renal failure
ET	essential thrombocythaemia
etOH	ethanol
FAB	French–American–British
FACS	fluorescence-activated cell sorter
FBC	full blood count (*aka* complete blood count, CBC)
FDPs	fibrin degradation products
Fe	iron
$FeSO_4$	ferrous sulphate
FISH	fluorescence *in situ* hybridisation
FIX	factor IX
FL	femtolitres
FMRI	functional MRI
FOB	faecal occult blood
FPG	fasting plasma glucose
FUO	fever of unknown origin (like PUO)
FVIII	factor VIII
FVL	factor V Leiden
g	gram
G&S	group & save serum
GAD	glutamic acid decarboxylase
γGT	γ-glutamyl transpeptidase
GBM	glomerular basement membrane
GIT	gastrointestinal tract
GPC	gastric parietal cell
G6PD	glucose-6-phosphate dehydrogenase
GPI	general paralysis of the insane
GTN	glyceryl trinitrate
GU	gastric ulcer
GvHD	graft versus host disease
h	hour
HAV	hepatitis A virus
Hb	haemoglobin
HbA	haemoglobin A ($\alpha_2\beta_2$)
HbA$_{1c}$	haemoglobin A$_{1c}$
HbA$_2$	haemoglobin A$_2$ ($\alpha_2\delta_2$)
HbF	haemoglobin F (fetal Hb, $\alpha_2\gamma_2$)
HbH	haemoglobin H (β_4)
HBsAg	hepatitis B surface antigen
HBV	hepatitis B virus
HCG	human chorionic gonadotrophin
HCO_3^-	bicarbonate
Hct	haematocrit
HCV	hepatitis C virus
HDN	haemolytic disease of the newborn

HE	hereditary elliptocytosis
HELLP	haemolysis, elevated liver enzymes and low platelet count
HIV	human immunodeficiency virus
HLA	human leucocyte antigen
HNA	heparin neutralising activity
HONK	hyperosmolar non-ketotic syndrome
HPA	human platelet antigen
HPFH	hereditary persistence of fetal haemoglobin
HPLC	high-performance liquid chromatography
HPOA	hypertrophic pulmonary osteoarthropathy
HPP	hereditary pyropoikilocytosis
HTLV	human T-lymphotropic virus
IAGT or IAT	Indirect antiglobulin test
IBS	irritable bowel syndrome
ICA	islet cell antibodies
ICH	intracranial haemorrhage
IDA	iron deficiency anaemia
IDDM	insulin dependent (type 1) diabetes mellitus
IEF	isoelectric focusing
IFG	impaired fasting glucose
IFN-α	interferon alpha
IGT	impaired glucose tolerance
IHD	ischaemic heart disease
Ig	immunoglobulin
IgA	immunoglobulin A
IgD	immunoglobulin D
IgE	immunoglobulin E
IgG	immunoglobulin G
IgM	immunoglobulin M
IIF	indirect immunofluorescence
IM	intramuscular
INR	international normalized ratio
ITP	idiopathic thrombocytopenic purpura
ITT	Insulin tolerance test
ITU	intensive therapy unit
iu/IU	international units
IV	Intravenous
IVI	Intravenous infusion
IVU	Intravenous urogram
JCA	juvenile chronic arthritis
JVP	jugular venous pressure
K^+	Potassium
KCCT	kaolin cephalin clotting time ($\equiv$ APTT)
KDa	kiloDaltons

Kg	kilogram
KUB	kidney, ureter, bladder (x-ray)
L	litre or left
LA	lupus anticoagulant or lactic acidosis or local anaesthetic
LAP	leucocyte alkaline phosphatase (score)
LBBB	left bundle branch block
LCM	left costal margin
LDH	lactate dehydrogenase
LFTs	liver function tests
LIF	left iliac fossa
LKM	liver/kidney microsomal
LP	lumbar puncture
LUQ	left upper quadrant
LVF	left ventricular failure
LVH	left ventricular hypertrophy
MAG	myelin-associated glycoprotein
MAIPA	monoclonal antibody immobilisation of platelet antigens
MAOI	monoamine oxidase inhibitor
MC&S	microscopy, culture & sensitivity
MCH	mean cell haemoglobin
MCHC	mean corpuscular haemoglobin concentration
MCV	mean cell volume
MDS	myelodysplastic syndrome
MELAS	myelopathy, encephalopathy, lactic acidosis and stroke-like episodes
Mg	milligram (10^{-3} gram)
MGUS	monoclonal gammopathy of undetermined significance
MHC	major histocompatibility complex
MI	myocardial infarction
Min	minutes
MoAb	monoclonal antibody
MODY	maturity onset diabetes of the young
mOsm	milliosmole
MPD	myeloproliferative disease
MPV	mean platelet volume
MRI	magnetic resonance imaging
mRNA	messenger ribonucleic acid
MS	multiple sclerosis or mass spectroscopy
MSU	mid-stream urine
MTP	metatarsophalangeal
MUD	matched unrelated donor (transplant)
µg	microgram (10^{-6} gram)
Na^+	sodium
NaCl	sodium chloride
NADP	nicotinamide adenine diphosphate

NADPH	nicotinamide adenine diphosphate (reduced)
NAP	neutrophil alkaline phosphatase
NEJM	*New England Journal of Medicine*
NH_3	ammonia
NHL	non-Hodgkin's lymphoma
NRBC	nucleated red blood cells
NSAIDs	non-steroidal anti-inflammatory drugs
NSTEMI	non-ST-elevation myocardial infarction
OA	osteoarthritis
OCP	oral contraceptive pill
Od	*omni die* (once daily)
OGD	oesophagogastroduodenoscopy
OGTT	oral glucose tolerance test
OHCH	*Oxford Handbook of Clinical Haematology*
OHCM	*Oxford Handbook of Clinical Medicine*
PA	posteroanterior *or* pernicious anaemia *or* pulmonary artery
PACWP	pulmonary artery capillary wedge pressure
PAD	peripheral arterial disease
PAN	polyarteritis nodosa
PaO_2	partial pressure of O_2 in arterial blood
PAS	periodic acid-Schiff
PB	peripheral blood
PBC	primary biliary cirrhosis
PC	protein C *or* provocation concentration
PCH	paroxysmal cold haemoglobinuria
PCI	percutaneous coronary intervention
PCL	plasma cell leukaemia
PCP	*Pneumocystis carinii* pneumonia
PCR	polymerase chain reaction
PCT	proximal convoluted tubule *or* procalcitonin
PCV	packed cell volume
PDA	patent ductus arteriosus
PE	pulmonary embolism
PEFR	peak expiratory flow rate
PET	positron emission tomography
Ph	Philadelphia chromosome
PIFT	platelet immunofluorescence test
PK	pyruvate kinase
PO	*per os* (by mouth)
PO_4^{3-}	phosphate
PR	*per rectum*
PRL	Prolactin
PRV	Polycythaemia rubra vera
PS	protein S *or* Parkinson's syndrome
PSA	prostate-specific antigen

PT	prothrombin time
PV	plasma volume
Qds	*quater die sumendus* (to be taken 4 times a day)
RA	refractory anaemia *or* rheumatoid arthritis *or* right atrial
RAS	renal angiotensin system *or* renal artery stenosis
RBBB	right bundle branch block
RBCs	red blood cells
RCC	red blood cell count
RDW	red cell distribution width
Rh	Rhesus
RhF	rheumatoid factor
RIA	radioimmunoassay
RiCoF	ristocetin cofactor
RIF	right iliac fossa
RIPA	ristocetin-induced platelet aggregation
RNP	ribonucleoprotein
RPGN	rapidly progressive glomerulonephritis
RT-PCR	reverse transcriptase polymerase chain reaction
RUQ	right upper quadrant
S	seconds
SAECG	signal-averaged ECG
SAH	subarachnoid haemorrhage
SC	subcutaneous
SCA	sickle cell anaemia
SCD	sickle cell disease
SDH	subdural haemorrhage
SHBG	sex-hormone-binding globulin
SLE	systemic lupus erythematosus
SmIg	surface membrane immunoglobulin
SOB	short of breath
SOL	space-occupying lesion
SM	smooth muscle
SPECT	single photon emission computed tomography
stat	*statim* (immediate; as initial dose)
STEMI	ST-elevation myocardial infarction
STfR	soluble transferrin receptor assay
SVC	superior vena cava
SVCO	superior vena caval obstruction
SXR	skull x-ray
T°	temperature
T½	half-life
T4	thyroxine
TA	temporal arteritis
TB	tuberculosis
tds	*ter die sumendum* (to be taken 3 times a day)

TdT	terminal deoxynucleotidyl transferase
TENS	transcutaneous nerve stimulation
TFT	thyroid function test(s)
TIAs	transient ischaemic attacks
TIBC	total iron binding capacity
TN	trigeminal neuralgia
TNF	tumour necrosis factor
TOE	transoesophageal echocardiogram
TPA	tissue plasminogen activator
TPO	thyroid peroxidase
TRAB	thyrotropin receptor antibodies
TRALI	transfusion-related acute lung injury
TRAP	tartrate-resistant acid phosphatase
TSH	thyroid-stimulating hormone
TT	thrombin time
TTE	transthoracic echocardiography
TTP	thrombotic thrombocytopenic purpura
TXA	tranexamic acid
u/U	units
UC	ulcerative colitis
U&E	urea and electrolytes
UKPDS	United Kingdom Prospective Diabetes Study
URTI	upper respiratory tract infection
UTI	urinary tract infection
USS	ultrasound scan
VIII:C	factor VIII clotting activity
VIP	vasoactive intestinal peptide
Vit K	vitamin K
VSD	ventricular septal defect
VTE	venous thromboembolism
vWD	von Willebrand's disease
vWF	von Willebrand factor
vWFAg	von Willebrand factor antigen
WBC	white blood count *or* white blood cells
WHO	World Health Organisation
WM	Waldenström's macroglobulinaemia
XDPs	cross-linked fibrin degradation products

Approach to investigations

Why do tests?

Patients seldom present to their doctors with *diagnoses*—rather, they have symptoms or signs. The major challenge of medicine is being able to talk to the patient and obtain a history and then carry out a physical examination looking for pointers to their likely underlying problem. Our elders and, some would argue, betters in medicine had fewer tests available to them than we have today, and their diagnoses were often made solely from the history and examination. Of course, they would claim that their clinical acumen and skills were greater than ours and that we rely too heavily on the huge armoury of laboratory and other investigations available today. This, in part, is probably true, but we cannot ignore the fact that advances in science and technology have spawned a bewildering array of very useful and sophisticated tests that help us to confirm our diagnostic suspicions.

By 'test' we mean the measurement of a component of blood, marrow or other body fluid or physiological parameter to determine whether the patient's value falls within or outside the normal range, either suggesting the diagnosis or, in some cases, actually making the diagnosis for us.

Factors affecting variable parameters in health

Many measurable body constituents vary throughout life. For example, a newborn baby has an extremely high haemoglobin concentration which falls after delivery; this is completely normal and is *physiological* rather than pathological. A haemoglobin level this high in an adult would be pathological since it is far outside the normal range for the adult population.

Factors affecting measurable variables

- Age.
- Sex.
- Ethnicity.
- Altitude.
- Build.
- Physiological conditions (e.g. at rest, after exercise, standing, lying).
- Sampling methods (e.g. with or without using tourniquet).
- Storage and age of sample.
- Container used, e.g. for blood sample, as well as anticoagulant.
- Method of analysis.

Reference ranges (normal values)

These are published for most measurable components of blood and other tissue and we have included the normal ranges for most blood and CSF analytes at the end of the book.

What makes a test useful?

A really good test, and one which would make us appear to be out-standing doctors, would be one which would *always* be positive in the presence of a disease and would be *totally* specific for that disease alone; such a test would never be positive in patients who did not have the disorder. What we mean is that what we are looking for are *sensitive* tests that are *specific* for a given disease. Sadly, most tests are neither 100% sensitive nor 100% specific but some do come very close.

How to use tests and the laboratory

Rather than request tests in a shotgun or knee-jerk fashion, where every box on a request form is ticked, it is far better to use the laboratory selectively. Even with the major advances in automation where tests are batched and are cheaper, the hospital budget is finite and sloppy requesting should be discouraged.

Outline your differential diagnoses: what are the likeliest diseases given the patient's history, examination findings and population the patient comes from?

Decide which test(s) will help you make the diagnosis: request these and review the diagnosis in the light of the test results. Review the patient and arrange further investigations as necessary.

The downside of tests

It is important to remember that tests may often give 'normal' results even in the presence of disease. For example, a normal ECG in the presence of chest pain does *not* exclude the occurrence of myocardial infarction with 100% certainty. Conversely, the presence of an abnormality does not necessarily imply that a disease is present. This, of course, is where clinical experience comes into its own—the more experienced clinician will be able to balance the likelihood of disease with the results available even if some of the test results give unexpected answers.

Sensitivity & specificity	
Sensitivity	% of patients with the disease and in whom the test is positive
Specificity	% of people without the disease in whom the test is negative

Quick-fix clinical experience

This simply does not exist. Talking to patients and examining them for physical signs and assimilating knowledge gained in medical school are absolute requirements for attainment of sound clinical judgement. Those students and doctors who work from books alone do not survive effectively at the coal face! It is a constant source of irritation to medical students and junior doctors, when a senior doctor asks for the results of an investigation on the ward round and you find this test is the one that clinches the diagnosis. How *do* they do it? Like appreciating good wine—they develop a nose for it. You can learn a great deal by watching your registrar or consultant make decisions. This forms of basis of your *own* clinical experience.

Laboratory errors and how to avoid them

It is a fact of life that the sophisticated automated analysers in current use are not 100% accurate 100% of the time—but they come pretty close. In order to keep errors to a minimum, precautions need to be taken when sampling biological material, e.g. blood.

Minimising spurious results using blood samples

- Use correct bottle.
- Fill to line (if anticoagulant used). This is less of a worry when vacuum sample bottles are used since these should take in exactly the correct amount of blood, ensuring the correct blood:anticoagulant ratio. This is critical for coagulation tests.
- Try to get the sample to the lab as quickly as possible. Blood samples left lying around on warm windowsills, or even overnight at room temperature, will produce bizarre results, e.g. crenated RBCs and abnormal-looking WBCs in old EDTA samples.
- Try to avoid rupturing red cells when taking the sample (e.g. using narrow gauge needle, prolonged time to collect whole sample) otherwise a 'haemolysed' sample will be received by the lab. This may cause spurious results for some parameters (e.g. $[K^+]$).
- Remember to mix (not shake) samples containing anticoagulant.

Variations in normal ranges in health

As discussed earlier, most of the normal ranges for blood parameters discussed in this book are for non-pregnant adults. The reason for this is that blood values, e.g. Hb, RCC are high in the newborn and many FBC, coagulation and other parameters undergo changes in pregnancy.

Part 1

The patient

Abdominal distension 4
Abdominal pain 6
Alteration of behaviour 7
Alteration in bowel habit 8
Anaemia 9
Anaphylaxis 11
Angioedema 11
Anorexia 12
Anuria 13
Ataxia 14
Bradycardia 16
Breathlessness 17
Bruising 18
Calf swelling 19
Chest pain 20
Clubbing 23
Coma 24
Confusion 26
Constipation 27
Cyanosis 28
Diarrhoea 29
Dizziness & syncope 30
Dysarthria & dysphasia 32
Dysphagia 33
Facial pain 34
Fever of unknown origin (FUO or PUO) 35
First fit 36
Galactorrhoea 38
Gout 39
Gynaecomastia 40
Haematemesis 41
Haematuria 42
Haemoptysis 42
Headache 43
Heart sounds & murmurs 45
Hepatomegaly 50
Herpes zoster 51
Hyperlipidaemia 51
Hypertension 52
Incontinence: faecal 53
Incontinence: urinary 54
Indigestion 55
Infective endocarditis signs 56
Irregular pulse 57

Symptoms & signs

Jaundice 58
Joint pain/swelling 59
Jugular venous pulse 60
Loin pain 62
Lymphadenopathy 63
Nausea 64
Neck stiffness 66
Nystagmus 66
Obesity 68
Oliguria 70
Palpitations 71
Pancytopenia 72
Paraesthesiae 72
Peripheral neuropathy 74
Peripheral oedema 75
Petechiae & thrombocytopenia 76
Plethora 76
Polyuria 77
Pruritus 78
Ptosis 79
Pulmonary embolism 80
Pulse character 81
Purpura 82
Recurrent thrombosis 82
Retinal haemorrhage 83
Rigors 84
Short stature 84
Skin pigmentation 86
Splenomegaly 87
Steatorrhoea 88
Stridor 88
Suspected bleeding disorder 90
Suspected stroke 91
Sweating 92
Tachycardia 93
Tinnitus 94
Tiredness 95
Urgency of micturition 96
Urticaria 96
Vasculitis 97
Visual loss 98
Wasting of the small hand muscles 99
Weight loss 100
Wheeze 101

Abdominal distension

Patients may describe generalised abdominal swelling or localised fullness in a specific area of the abdomen.

In the history enquire specifically about
- Change in bowel habit.
- Weight loss.
- Associated pain.

Generalised swelling

Consider
- Fat.
- Fluid.
- Faeces.
- Flatus.
- Fetus.
- Full bladder.

Ascites

Fluid in the peritoneal cavity. Look for shifting dullness and fluid thrill on percussion, stigmata of chronic liver disease, lymphadenopathy, oedema and assess JVP.

Causes
- Malignancy.
- Cirrhosis/portal hypertension.
- Hypoproteinaemia.
- Right heart failure.

Investigations
- U&E.
- LFTs.
- Serum albumin.
- Ascitic tap for protein (transudate *vs.* exudate), cytology, M,C&S.
- USS abdomen.

See Fig. 1.1.

Flatus

Gaseous distension. Need to exclude bowel obstruction. Assess for colicky abdominal pain, bowel habit, flatus and vomiting. Look for resonant distension on percussion, altered or absent bowel sounds, focal tenderness with rebound and guarding. Always check for herniae and perform PR examination in suspected obstruction.

Causes
- *Intraluminal*: faecal impaction, gallstone ileus.
- *Luminal*: inflammatory stricture (e.g. Crohn's), tumour, abscess.
- *Extraluminal*: herniae, adhesions, pelvic mass, lymphadenopathy, volvulus, intussusception.
- *Paralytic ileus*: drug-induced, electrolyte disturbances.
- Age-related causes of obstruction.

- *Neonatal*: congenital atresia, imperforate anus, volvulus, Hirschsprung's disease, meconium ileus.
- *Infants*: intussusception, Hirschsprung's, herniae, Meckel's diverticulum.
- *Young/middle age adults*: herniae, adhesions, Crohn's.
- *Elderly*: herniae, carcinoma, diverticulitis, faecal impaction.

Investigations
- FBC.
- U&E.
- AXR (erect and supine).
- Consider barium enema, barium follow-through, sigmoidoscopy, surgical intervention for complete acute obstruction.

Localised swelling/masses: common causes according to site

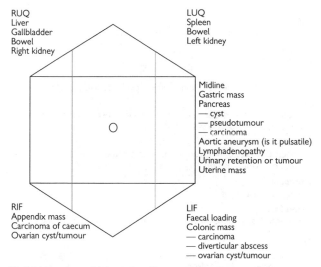

RUQ
Liver
Gallbladder
Bowel
Right kidney

LUQ
Spleen
Bowel
Left kidney

Midline
Gastric mass
Pancreas
— cyst
— pseudotumour
— carcinoma
Aortic aneurysm (is it pulsatile)
Lymphadenopathy
Urinary retention or tumour
Uterine mass

RIF
Appendix mass
Carcinoma of caecum
Ovarian cyst/tumour

LIF
Faecal loading
Colonic mass
— carcinoma
— diverticular abscess
— ovarian cyst/tumour

Fig.1.1 Main causes of abdominal swelling according to site.

Investigate according to site
- Consider USS abdomen and pelvis.
- CT scanning.
- Barium studies.
- IVU.

OHCM pp64, 518.

Abdominal pain

Abdominal pain may be acute or chronic. Severe, acute pain may indicate a surgical emergency including perforation, peritonitis or obstruction. Assess nature and radiation of pain, clinical status of patient including fever, tachycardia and hypotension.

Common causes of abdominal pain according to site

Epigastric pain
Peptic ulcer disease, gastritis or duodenal erosions, cholecystitis, pancreatitis.

Periumbilical
Pancreatitis, mesenteric artery ischaemia (older patient with vascular disease).

RUQ pain
Biliary colic, cholecystitis, hepatitis, peptic ulcer.

LUQ pain
Splenic, peptic ulcer.

Loin pain
Renal colic (colicky radiating loin → groin), pyelonephritis, renal pathology.

LIF pain
Constipation, diverticular disease, irritable bowel syndrome, pelvic referred pain, inflammatory bowel disease.

RIF pain
Appendicitis, pelvic referred pain, inflammatory bowel disease (e.g. Crohn's of terminal ileum).

Suprapubic
UTI, cystitis, salpingitis.

Generalised
Gastroenteritis, irritable bowel, constipation, generalised peritonitis.

Pitfalls

Metabolic causes—e.g. diabetic ketoacidosis, hypercalcaemia, Addison's disease, porphyria, lead poisoning.

Atypical referred pain—e.g. myocardial infarction, pneumonia.

Investigations

- FBC.
- U&E, e.g. deranged electrolytes following vomiting, diarrhoea or bowel obstruction.
- Plasma glucose.
- Serum amylase (↑ in pancreatitis and bowel obstruction).
- Urinanalysis and MSU, e.g. haematuria, proteinuria, glucose.
- LFTs (consider obstructive vs. hepatitic picture).
- Plain AXR (erect and supine to assess for perforation and bowel obstruction).

- KUB for renal tract calculi.
- USS abdomen, particularly for biliary tract, gallbladder and renal tract.
- IVU to assess for renal tract calculi/pathology.

📖OHCM pp64, 474.

Alteration of behaviour

This is usually reported by a relative or friend rather than by the patient. Often the patient will have little or no insight into the disease and taking a history can be difficult. In addition to a full general and neurological physical examination a mental state examination is required.

Find out if this is the first episode of altered behaviour or if the episodes are recurrent. Is there a gradual change in behaviour (and personality) over time?

Acute delirium

Causes
- Sepsis (common).
- Acute intracranial event, e.g. haemorrhage.
- Metabolic disturbance, e.g. uraemia, hypercalcaemia (common).
- Intracerebral tumour (including meningioma).
- Drugs—especially interactions in elderly.
- Alcohol (and withdrawal syndrome).
- Hypoxia (common).
- Hypoglycaemia (iatrogenic in diabetic patients receiving insulin treatment or oral insulin secretagogues or insulinoma and other causes).

Dementia

- Alzheimer's (common), Pick's (rare).
- Vascular, e.g. multi-infarct.
- Huntington's chorea.
- Vitamin B_{12} deficiency (severe).
- Hypothyroidism (severe).
- Wilson's disease.
- Alcoholism.
- Normal pressure hydrocephalus.

Note: 'Frontal lobe syndrome' from SOL, e.g. meningioma. Presents with disinhibition, impaired social functioning, primitive reflexes, e.g. grasp reflex.

Anxiety states

Usually psychogenic but consider organic possibilities such as
- Phaeochromocytoma (rare).
- Hyperthyroidism (common).
- Paroxysmal atrial tachycardia (fairly common).
- Alcohol withdrawal (usually history of excessive alcohol intake).

Psychosis
- Schizophrenia.
- Bipolar disorder or pseudo-dementia in
  - SLE.
  - Cushing's syndrome.
  - Multiple sclerosis.
  - Thyrotoxicosis ('apathetic' thyrotoxicosis in the elderly).

Temporal lobe epilepsy
- Temporary disturbance of content of consciousness.

Investigations: guided by history and examination
- U&E.
- Glucose (in non-diabetics take fasting venous plasma in fluoride oxalate tube with simultaneous serum or plasma for insulin concentration—e.g. suspected insulinoma).
- CXR.
- LFTs.
- TFTs.
- FBC.
- ESR.
- Urinalysis (protein, nitrites, glucose).
- Cranial CT scan.
- Serum vitamin B_{12}.
- Arterial blood gases (ABGs) ± carboxyhaemoglobin.
- Blood cultures.

Consider
- Syphilis serology.
- HIV test.
- Urine drug screen (📖Ch11).
- Blood ethanol level (may be low in withdrawal state).
- EEG.
- 24h ECG.
- Sleep study.

Alteration in bowel habit

A change in bowel habit in an adult should always alert you to the possibility of bowel cancer. Ask about associated features—PR bleeding, tenesmus, weight loss, mucus, abdominal pain or bloating.

Has the patient started any new medications, including 'over the counter'? Look for signs of systemic disease.

Consider
- Carcinoma of the colon.
- Diverticular disease.
- Irritable bowel syndrome (IBS).

- Constipation with overflow diarrhoea.
- All of the above may present with alternating diarrhoea and constipation.

Investigations
- Digital rectal examination.
- Proctoscopy.
- Sigmoidoscopy (rigid/flexible).
- Colonoscopy.
- Barium enema.

📖*Diarrhoea* (p29), *Constipation* (p27), *Incontinence: faecal* (p53).

Anaemia

Reduced Hb, no specific cause implied (and *not a diagnosis in itself, so don't be complacent*): ♂ <13.5g/dL, ♀ <11.5g/dL. Often associated with non-specific symptoms such as fatigue, poor concentration, shortness of breath and dizziness. Older patients may experience palpitations and exacerbation of angina, congestive cardiac failure or claudication.

Signs
Pallor of conjunctivae and skin creases, nail pallor and koilonychia (spoon-shaped nails, very rare finding in severe chronic iron deficiency), angular cheilitis and glossitis. Most of these signs are unreliable and it is difficult to gauge anaemia from skin signs alone.

Causes
Two common approaches to assess anaemia.

1. Red cell dynamics
- ↑ RBC loss/breakdown, e.g. haemolysis (congenital or acquired) or bleeding.
- ↓ RBC production, e.g. vitamin/mineral deficiency, marrow suppression/ infiltration, myelodysplasia, haemoglobin disorders (e.g. thalassaemia), chronic disease, renal failure.

2. Red cell indices

Table 1.1 Some causes of anaemia based on the MCV

Microcytic/hypochromic	↓ MCV, ↓ MCHC E.g. Fe deficiency Thalassaemia Anaemia of chronic disease
Macrocytic	↑ MCV Reticulocytosis (polychromasia on blood film) B_{12} or folate deficiency Chronic liver disease Hypothyroidism Alcohol Myelodysplasia
Normocytic, normochromic	↔ MCV & MCHC Anaemia of chronic disease e.g. – Chronic infection – Inflammation Inflammatory disease or malignancy Acute blood loss Renal failure Myeloma

Investigations

FBC and film

Assessment of RBC indices helps direct investigation as above.

Microcytic

- Check iron stores (ferritin or soluble transferrin receptor assay). *Note*: ferritin is ↑ in acute inflammation and may be misleading. Iron/TIBC no longer used for assessment of iron deficiency (□p210).
- Consider thalassaemia screening if not iron deficient (i.e. ↓ MCV ↔ ferritin).
- If iron deficient, assess dietary history (vegetarians) and look for risk factors for blood loss and increased demands.
- Premenopausal women—assess menstrual losses.
- Pregnancy/infants/adolescence consider physiological (↑ requirements).
- All others: look for source of blood loss. GI tract is most common source. Consider OGD and/or colonoscopy if clinically indicated by symptoms and barium studies.

Macrocytic

- Reticulocyte count.
- Serum B_{12} and red cell folate levels.
- If folate deficient: assess dietary history and physiological requirements.
- If B_{12} deficient: rarely dietary cause alone, usually an associated pathology. Pernicious anaemia is the most common cause: check parietal cell antibodies (90% patients with PA are +ve, but seen in other causes of gastric atrophy, especially in older individuals) and/or intrinsic

factor antibodies (+ve in only 50% with PA but specific). Consider ileal disease and malabsorption.
- LFTs.
- Thyroid function.

Normocytic
- Blood film.
- ESR.
- Renal function.
- Consider myeloma screen in older adults (Igs, protein electrophoresis, urine BJP. Skeletal survey of value if paraprotein or BJP).
- Autoimmune screen to exclude connective tissue disease.

Haemolysis screen
- FBC, MCV (↑ due to reticulocytosis—these are larger than RBCs).
- Blood film (spherocytes, polychromasia, bite cells and red cell fragmentation).
- Reticulocyte count.
- Serum bilirubin and serum LDH.
- Haptoglobins (absent in haemolysis).
- DAT (old term is direct Coombs' test).

Consider
- Congenital haemolytic anaemias: membrane defects, enzyme deficiencies (e.g. G6PD, pyruvate kinase).
- DIC/microangiopathic haemolysis—DIC screen.

Anaphylaxis

Defined as a systemic reaction (local oral angioedema is *not* anaphylaxis), with any or all of the following:
- Stridor (laryngeal obstruction).
- Wheeze (bronchospasm).
- Generalised urticaria and/or angioedema.
- Hypotension ± loss of consciousness.
- Abdominal pain/cramps, vomiting and diarrhoea.

Note: Not all patients have urticaria or rash—only 50% will do so.

Differentiate IgE-mediated reactions (*anaphylaxis*) from non-IgE mediated reactions (*anaphylactoid*)—due to direct mast cell degranulation).

Angioedema

Angioedema is deep tissue swelling which is non-itchy. May be premonitory tingling. May occur with or without urticaria. Caused by bradykinin not histamine.

Causes
- As for urticaria; also hereditary angioedema (rare).

- Also think of drugs—these are the commonest cause:
  - ACE-inhibitors (elevated bradykinin levels due to inhibition of breakdown).
  - AT-II receptor antagonists.
  - Statins.
  - Proton pump inhibitors.
  - NSAIDs.

May also be seen in patients with autoimmune disease such as lupus and RA (antibodies against C1q) and in older patients in association with paraproteins (myeloma, lymphoma).

Angioedema *with* urticaria is *not* due to hereditary angioedema.

Investigations

- Check drug history first! If suspect drugs, then stop drugs and wait! If no drugs then investigate.

Angioedema WITH urticaria

- Investigate as for urticaria.

Angioedema WITHOUT urticaria

- Complement C3 & C4.
- If C4 low check C1-esterase inhibitor (immunochemical and functional).
- Serum immunoglobulins and electrophoresis.
- Autoantibody screen.
- Full blood count and ESR.
- Thyroid function.
- Liver function.

Anorexia

This describes a loss of appetite for food, and is associated with a wide range of disorders. In fact, anorexia is a fairly common consequence of underlying disease, and represents a general undernourishment. Anorexia *per se* is associated with increased morbidity especially when present in patients undergoing surgery; post-operative infection is commoner, as is prolongation of the hospital stay.

The extent to which it will be investigated depends on the general status of the patient, presence and duration of any symptoms or signs. Clinical judgement will help!

Causes

- Anorexia nervosa.
- Depressive illness.
- Stress.
- Cancers: any, including carcinoma of stomach, oesophagus, metastatic, leukaemia or lymphoma.
- Drugs, including chemotherapy.
- Radiotherapy.
- Renal failure.
- Hypercalcaemia.
- Infections.
- Cigarette smoking.

Investigations
- Full history and examination.
- FBC—looking for anaemia or non-specific changes seen in underlying disease.
- ESR—may be elevated in inflammatory disorders.
- U&E.
- LFTs.
- Serum Ca^{2+}.
- CXR (e.g. lung cancer, TB, etc.).
- Cultures of blood, sputum, urine, stool if pyrexial and/or localising symptoms or signs.

Anuria

Anuria denotes absent urine production. Oliguria (<400mL urine/24h) is more common than anuria. A catheter must be passed to confirm an empty bladder.

Causes
- Urinary retention—prostatic hypertrophy, pelvic mass, drugs, e.g. tricyclic antidepressants, spinal cord lesions.
- Blocked indwelling urinary catheter.
- Obstruction of the ureters—tumour, stone, sloughed papillae (bilateral).
- Intrinsic renal failure—acute glomerulonephritis, acute interstitial nephritis, acute tubular necrosis, rhabdomyolysis.
- Pre-renal failure—dehydration, septic shock, cardiogenic shock.

An urgent ultrasound of the renal tract must be performed and any physical obstruction relieved as quickly as possible, directly (urethral catheter) or indirectly (nephrostomy). ►► *Renal function and serum electrolytes must be measured without delay.*

Further tests as clinically indicated
- FBC.
- Blood cultures.
- Arterial blood gases (ABGs).
- Uric acid.
- Autoimmune profile.
- ESR.
- CK.
- PSA (prostatic carcinoma).
- Serum Ca^{2+} & PO_4^{3-}
- 12-lead ECG.
- CXR.
- CVP measurement via central line (to guide IV fluids).
- MSU (UTI).
- Urine microscopy (for casts).
- Urine osmolality, sodium, creatinine, urea concentrations.

- IVU (📖p685).
- Urinary stone analysis, if available.
- CT pelvis.
- Renal biopsy (if intrinsic renal disease suspected, normal-sized kidneys).

📖OHCM p272.

Ataxia

Ataxia is an impaired ability to coordinate limb movements. There must be no motor paresis (e.g. monoparesis) or involuntary movements (e.g. the characteristic cog-wheel tremor in Parkinson's disease is not ataxia).

Ataxia may be
- Cerebellar.
- Vestibular.
- Sensory.

Note: Many forms of ataxia are hereditary (but are uncommon).

Hereditary causes
- Friedreich's ataxia.
- Ataxia telangiectasia.
- Spinocerebellar ataxia.
- Corticocerebellar atrophy.
- Olivopontocerebellar atrophy.
- Hereditary spastic paraplegia.
- Xeroderma pigmentosa.

Investigations
- Family studies.
- Genetic analysis (discuss with regional genetics laboratory—counselling may be required).

Vestibular ataxia
- Acute alcohol intoxication.
- Labyrinthitis.

Sensory ataxia
- Loss of proprioception—peripheral neuropathy, dorsal column disease.
- Visual disturbance.

Investigations
- Venous plasma glucose (diabetic neuropathy).
- Serum vitamin B_{12} (subacute combined degeneration of the cord—rare, but serious).
- LFTs.
- Cryoglobulins.

Cerebellar ataxia
- Demyelinating diseases, e.g. multiple sclerosis (MS).
- Cerebellar infarct or haemorrhage.

- Alcoholic cerebellar degeneration.
- Cerebellar tumour—primary in children, metastases in adults. *Note:* Von Hippel Lindau disease (OHCM section 19).
- Nutritional deficiency:
  - Vitamin B_{12}.
  - Thiamine.
- Cerebellar abscess.
- Drugs (supratherapeutic blood levels):
  - Carbamazepine.
  - Phenytoin.
- Tuberculoma.
- Paraneoplastic syndrome.
- Developmental.
- Arnold Chiari malformation.
- Dandy Walker syndrome.
- Paget's disease of skull.
- Wilson's disease (hepatolenticular degeneration).
- Hypothyroidism.
- Creutzfeldt–Jakob disease and other chronic infections.
- Miller Fisher syndrome.
- Normal pressure hydrocephalus.

Ataxia should be distinguished from movement disorders, e.g.

Chorea
- Huntington's, Sydenham's, thyrotoxicosis (very rare).

Athetosis

Hemiballismus
- Characteristic movement disorder; rare.

Tardive dyskinesia
- Chronic phenothiazine therapy.

Investigations
- Cranial CT.
- MRI brain (if demyelination suspected).
- CXR (cerebellar metastases from bronchogenic carcinoma; paraneoplastic syndrome).
- TFTs.
- Triple evoked potentials (demyelination).
- Lumbar puncture (p518).
- LFTs.
- Serum drug concentrations esp. anticonvulsants.
- Serum vitamin B_{12}.
- Erythrocyte transketolase (↓ in thiamine deficiency, e.g. alcoholism).
- Isotope bone scan (Paget's, metastases).
- Serum alkaline phosphatase (ALP)—bone isoenzyme (Paget's, metastases).
- Urine hydroxyproline (Paget's disease—reflects bone turnover).
- Caeruloplasmin (Wilson's disease).
- Serum and urine copper (Wilson's disease).

Consider whether the movement disorder is psychogenic (uncommon) rather than due to neuropathology. Uncommon and should not be confidently assumed.

📖OHCM p373.

Bradycardia

Bradycardia is defined as a heart rate <60 beats per minute. It is a normal physiological response to fitness training but should always be considered a marker of potential cardiac disease until proved otherwise.

Causes

A comprehensive history and thorough examination are important. A transient bradycardia can cause disabling symptoms of dizziness or blackouts in the elderly whilst persistent bradycardia often heralds systemic disease, e.g.:

- *Iatrogenic*: cardiac drugs e.g. β-blockers (including eye drops for glaucoma), amiodarone and calcium channel blockers, e.g. diltiazem and verapamil, cause sinus bradycardia; digoxin (atrioventricular block). The likelihood of extreme bradycardia or heart block is increased with combination therapy.
- *Cardiac causes*: acute myocardial infarction (often transient in inferior myocardial infarction); coronary artery disease; sick sinus syndrome; myocardial disease (amyloid, Chagas' disease, sarcoid, myocarditis).
- Increased vagal tone associated with nausea and vomiting.
- Diminished sympathetic activity.
- *Physiological*: bradycardia is normal in sleep and in athletes.
- *Hypothyroidism*: associated with characteristic symptoms and signs.
- ↑ intracranial pressure, e.g. cerebral tumour.
- *Hypothermia,* e.g. myxoedema coma.
- *Metabolic*: severe hyperkalaemia, anorexia.
- *Toxic*: severe jaundice.
- *Drug toxicity*: opiates.
- *Infective*: inappropriate bradycardia seen in diphtheria, typhoid.

Investigations

- 12-lead ECG to identify underlying rhythm.

If there are symptoms of chest pain
- Serum troponin and creatine kinase.
- Bedside ECG monitoring.
- Exercise ECG.

If there is a history of intermittent dizziness
- 24h ambulatory ECG monitoring, patient-activated event recorder or implantable loop recorder, depending on the frequency of symptoms.

If indicated by clinical presentation, consider
- Thyroid function tests (hypothyroidism).
- Low reading thermometer (hypothermia—check for J waves on ECG).
- CT brain scan (?intracranial pathology).

- U&E.
- LFTs (especially bilirubin).
- Toxicology screen.

📖OHCM pp88, 118.

Breathlessness

Breathlessness (dyspnoea) is the subjective awareness of difficulty in breathing. Almost universal during exercise, it is a common presenting symptom in a broad spectrum of disease. A comprehensive history and thorough examination are therefore essential. Speed of symptom onset, patient's age and occupation and local disease prevalence are particularly helpful in devising a differential diagnosis and a guide to investigations.

Causes
- *Acute pulmonary disease*: pneumonia, acute asthma, pulmonary embolus, inhaled foreign body, pneumothorax, acute respiratory distress.
- *Chronic pulmonary disease*: emphysema, chronic bronchitis, ruptured bulla; interstitial disease (sarcoid, fibrosing alveolitis, extrinsic alveolitis, pneumoconiosis).
- *Carcinoma*: bronchogenic carcinoma, lymphangitis carcinomatosis, secondary carcinoma.
- *Acute cardiac disease*: acute myocardial infarction (and associated complications of pulmonary oedema, ventricular septal defect, mitral valve chordal rupture and arrhythmias).
- *Chronic cardiac disease*: left ventricular dysfunction, valvular heart disease (mitral or aortic stenosis and regurgitation), ischaemic heart disease, pulmonary hypertension, pleural effusion, arrhythmias (especially atrial fibrillation).
- *Metabolic*: poisoning from salicylates, methanol and ethylene glycol, diabetic ketoacidosis, lactic acidosis, hepatic and renal failure.
- *Neuromuscular*: intercostal muscle/diaphragmatic weakness due to Guillain–Barré syndrome, muscular dystrophy.
- *Haematological*: anaemia.
- Anxiety and hyperventilation.
- *Morphological*: kyphoscoliosis, obesity.
- *Laryngeal obstruction*: extrinsic compression (retrosternal goitre), angio-oedema (often acute drug allergy), laryngeal spasm (hypocalcaemia).

Initial investigations
- FBC.
- U&E.
- Glucose.
- CXR.
- ABGs.
- Peak expiratory flow rate.
- 12-lead ECG.

Additional investigations (*as indicated*)

- Transthoracic echocardiography.
- 24-hour ambulatory ECG monitoring.
- Pulmonary function tests.
- CT chest.
- Bronchoscopy.
- V/Q scan/CTPA.
- LFTs.
- Ca^{2+}.
- ESR.
- Serum salicylate levels.
- Lactate.
- Lung biopsy.

📖OHCM pp5, 56, 768.

Bruising

Easy bruising is a common complaint and warrants careful assessment of onset and nature. Recent onset of spontaneous and unusual bruising or bleeding may suggest a serious acquired defect. A lifelong history of bruising and bleeding (e.g. post-tonsillectomy, dental extraction or surgery) may imply a congenital defect. Family history may be informative.

Examine: skin, mouth, dependent areas and fundi for mucocutaneous bleeding and purpura (non-blanching haemorrhages into the skin).

Platelet causes

- Thrombocytopenia or platelet dysfunction (e.g. aspirin).
- Marrow failure, infiltration, ITP, DIC, hypersplenism, drugs or alcohol.

Vascular causes

- Congenital, e.g. Osler–Weber–Rendu syndrome.
- Acquired, e.g. senile purpura, vasculitis (Henoch–Schönlein purpura, infection), diabetes, corticosteroid therapy, scurvy, connective tissue diseases.

Coagulopathy

- Congenital—mucocutaneous bruising is suggestive of a platelet-mediated defect (e.g. von Willebrand's disease, Glanzmann's thrombasthenia) rather than clotting factor deficiency (e.g. haemophilia A and B).
- Acquired, e.g. DIC, vitamin K deficiency.

Hyperviscosity

- Myeloma, Waldenström's macroglobulinaemia (low grade lymphoma associated with ↑ IgM and ↑ plasma viscosity), ↑↑ WBC in leukaemia.

Investigations

- FBC and film.
- Coagulation—INR and APTR.
- Bleeding time, measures platelet and vascular phase.
- DIC screen including fibrinogen, thrombin time, D-dimers or FDPs.

Consider further tests and referral to haematology for
- Factor assays.
- Platelet aggregation studies to assess platelet function.

OHCM p644.

Calf swelling

Assess whether swelling is bilateral or unilateral, precipitating factors and duration of onset. Careful examination of the affected leg should be extended to a full examination, particularly of abdominal and cardiovascular systems.

Causes

Venous and lymphatic
- Deep vein thrombosis (DVT).
- Superficial thrombophlebitis.
- Varicose veins.
- Post-phlebitic limb (post-DVT).

Soft tissue/musculoskeletal
- Calf haematoma or trauma.
- Ruptured Baker's cyst (synovial effusion in the popliteal fossa associated with rheumatoid disease).
- Cellulitis (associated fever, sepsis, tachycardia).

Systemic
- Congestive cardiac failure (bilateral limb oedema, ↑ JVP and signs of LVF).
- Hepatic failure.
- Hypoalbuminaemia.
- Nephrotic syndrome.
- Pregnancy: increased dependent oedema but note also an ↑ thrombotic risk and DVT should be excluded.

Deep vein thrombosis (DVT)

Usually affects lower limb and can extend proximally into iliofemoral veins and IVC with higher risk of associated PE and higher incidence of post-phlebitic limb. Occasionally seen affecting upper limb but this is atypical.

Risk factors for DVT
- Age >60 years.
- Previous DVT or PE.
- Recent major surgery, especially orthopaedic lower limb, abdo and pelvic.
- Marked immobility.
- Malignancy.
- Pregnancy and post-partum.
- High dose oestrogen oral contraceptive pill.
- Family history of VTE.

Investigation

USS Doppler studies, impedance plethysmography, venography, exclude PE. If any associated symptoms arrange V/Q scan, spiral CT, pulmonary angiography. Thrombophilia screening for younger patients (age <55), atypical site and extensive clots, spontaneous onset, family history.

Chest pain

Acute chest pain is a common symptom. A detailed history and a full physical examination should be performed in order to define the most likely cause and necessary investigation pathway.

History

Be sure to ask the following questions about the pain
- Site and radiation.
- Character.
- Onset and duration.
- Precipitating and relieving features.
- Associated symptoms.
- Response to pain relief, antacids or nitrates.

Most types of chest pain fall within one of these categories

Table 1.2

Pain source	Description of pain
Myocardial ischaemia	Retrosternal, heavy ache, can radiate → jaw, arms, precipitated by exertion and relieved by rest or nitrates
Aortic dissection	Severe central tearing pain, radiates to back
Gastro-oesophageal disease	Burning central pain, can radiate to shoulders, throat or abdomen, exacerbated by meals, eased with antacids/milk
Pleuritic pain	Focal sharp pain, exacerbated by inspiration
Pericardial pain	Sharp pain, radiates to left shoulder tip, worse on lying flat and during inspiration, eased by sitting forwards
Musculoskeletal pain	Sharp focal pain exacerbated by movement and palpation

Investigations

Table 1.3
Cardiovascular causes

All patients should have a 12-lead ECG and CXR

Suspected diagnosis	Investigations

Myocardial ischaemia/infarction
Consider:
   Coronary artery disease
   Aortic stenosis
   Hypertrophic obstructive cardiomyopathy
	Serial electrocardiograms
	Cardiac markers of necrosis
	FBC
	Thyroid function tests
	Echocardiogram
	Exercise electrocardiogram
	Stress cardiac imaging
	Coronary angiography

Thoracic aortic dissection Note: myocardial ischaemia may also be present if it involves the coronary arteries Syphilitic aortitis	FBC, U&E, X-match Echocardiogram (TTE or TOE) Computerized tomography Magnetic resonance imaging Syphilis serology
Mitral valve prolapse	Echocardiogram (TTE or TOE)
Acute pericarditis	FBC, viral titres, ESR Echocardiogram

Pulmonary causes

All patients should have CXR ± ABGs

Suspected diagnosis	Investigations
Pneumonia/pleurisy	FBC, CRP
Acute bronchitis	Sputum and blood cultures
Pulmonary tuberculosis (TB)	Aspiration if empyema suspected Early morning urine (TB) Mantoux test (TB)
Pneumothorax	CXR
Pulmonary embolus	D-dimers 12-lead ECG V/Q scan CT pulmonary angiography
Lung carcinoma	Sputum cytology
Pleural tumour e.g. mesothelioma	High resolution CT
Mediastinal tumour	Bronchoscopy Tissue biopsy

Table 1.3 Contd.

Gastro-oesophageal causes

Suspected diagnosis	Investigations
Oesophageal	FBC
Spasm	G&S
Oesophagitis	*Helicobacter pylori*
Candidiasis	Endoscopy
Reflux disease	Oesophageal manometry
Mallory–Weiss tear	Oesophageal biopsy
Peptic ulcer disease (perforation)	Erect CXR
	Endoscopy
	Gastrograffin swallow
Acute pancreatitis	Amylase
	Abdominal ultrasound scan
Cholecystitis/biliary colic	FBC, CRP, LFTs
	Urinalysis
	Abdominal ultrasound scan
	ERCP

Musculoskeletal & dermatological causes

Suspected diagnosis	Investigations
Muscular	
Bony structures	Chest x-ray
Chest wall bony metastases	Bone scan
Rib/sternal fractures	Spinal x-rays
Costochondritis (Tietze's syndrome)	CT scan
Ankylosing spondylitis	
Cervical/thoracic spine disease	
Thoracic outlet syndrome	
Skin/soft tissue	
Acute shingles	Herpetic serology/smear (rarely)
Post-herpetic neuralgia	

ACC/AHA 2002 Guideline Update for the Management of Patients with Chronic Stable Angina
⁀ʘ http://www.acc.org/clinical/guidelines/stable/stable_clean.pdf

📖OHCM pp92, 772.

Clubbing

Soft tissue hypertrophy under the nail bed distorts finger and toenail growth.

Characteristic features are
- Increased lateral and longitudinal nail curvature.
- The skin at the base of the nail becomes spongy.
- The angle between nail and skin is obliterated.
- In extreme cases, the terminal phalanx becomes bulbous like a drum-stick.

Clubbing can be an important visual indicator of major disease, although it can also be congenital. Rarely, clubbing may accompany swollen wrists and ankles as part of a proliferative periostitis seen in hypertrophic pulmonary osteoarthropathy (HPOA). This is associated with squamous carcinoma of the lung.

Major causes
- *Lung disease*: cystic fibrosis, bronchiectasis, empyema, lung abscess, asbestosis, mesothelioma, pulmonary sarcoid.
- *Carcinoma*: bronchogenic (especially squamous cell), mediastinal, pleural, oesophageal, gastric, colonic, thoracic lymphoma, familial polyposis coli.
- *Infection*: infective endocarditis, colonic amoebiasis.
- *Vascular disease*: cyanotic congenital heart disease, atrial myxoma, arteriovenous malformation.
- *Liver disease*: primary biliary cirrhosis, chronic active hepatitis.
- Ulcerative colitis and Crohn's disease, malabsorption.
- *Rare causes*: thyrotoxicosis, polycythaemia, SLE.

Investigations
As guided by differential diagnosis and clinical suspicion:
- FBC.
- ESR.
- CRP.
- LFTs.
- TFTs.
- Serum ACE.
- Autoantibodies.
- Blood cultures (at least 3 sets if infective endocarditis suspected).
- Faecal occult blood (3 samples).
- CXR.
- Echocardiography (TTE or TOE).
- OGD and biopsy.
- Colonoscopy and biopsy.
- Abdominal ultrasound scan.
- CT chest.
- Bronchoscopy, biopsy, washings.
- Liver biopsy.

OHCM pp39, 68.

Coma

The Glasgow Coma Scale (GCS) is used to assess level of consciousness. Minimum score is 3, maximum 15.

Assess level of consciousness and determine whether this is stable, fluctuating, improving or deteriorating on serial assessments.

Cerebral causes

- Intracranial haemorrhage (SAH, SDH, EDH, intracerebral bleed).
- Large cerebral infarct.
- Pontine haemorrhage (pinpoint pupils).
- Cerebral venous sinus thrombosis.
- Hypertensive encephalopathy.
- Cerebral tumour (associated local cerebral oedema may respond to dexamethasone).
- Head injury.
- Cerebral infection—encephalitis, meningitis, cerebral malaria, brain abscess.
- Post-ictal state.
- Sub-clinical status epilepticus (*Note*: this is an EEG diagnosis).
- Cerebral vasculitis, e.g. SLE.
- End-stage multiple sclerosis.
- Leucodystrophy.
- Creutzfeldt–Jakob disease (including variant CJD).

Table 1.4 Glasgow Coma Scale

Eye opening	1	Nil
	2	To pain
	3	To voice
	4	Spontaneously
Motor response	1	Nil
	2	Extension
	3	Flexion
	4	Withdrawal from pain
	5	Localising to pain
	6	Voluntary
Vocal response	1	Nil
	2	Groans
	3	Inappropriate words
	4	Disorientated speech
	5	Orientated speech

Metabolic causes

- Drugs (usually in deliberate overdose, ☐Ch11).
- Alcohol excess (*Note*: remember hypoglycaemia as a cause of coma in alcoholics, as well as extradural haematoma).

- Hypoglycaemia (iatrogenic, overdose of insulin or sulphonylureas, insulinoma, IGF-2-associated hypoglycaemia in certain tumours).
- Diabetic ketoacidosis (coma in ~10% of cases—adverse prognostic sign).
- Hyperosmolar non-ketotic coma (may present as severe dehydration ± coma).
- Uraemia.
- Late stages of hepatic encephalopathy.
- Severe hyponatraemia (relatively common—esp. inappropriate ADH syndrome).
- Hypothyroidism (myxoedema coma—rare).
- Hypercalcaemia.
- Inborn error of metabolism, e.g. porphyria, urea cycle disorders.
- Type 2 respiratory failure (CO_2 narcosis).
- Hypothermia (severe).
- Hyperpyrexia (neuroleptic malignant syndrome, NMS, after anaesthesia).
- Severe nutritional deficiency—thiamine, pyridoxine, vitamin B_{12}.

Investigations

- Venous plasma glucose (exclude hypoglycaemia with fingerstick + reflectance meter, confirm with venous plasma fluoride-oxalate sample).
- U&E.
- LFTs.
- Serum Ca^{2+}.
- Serum osmolality.
- Urine Na^+.
- Blood cultures.
- Clotting screen (📖pp244–246).
- ABGs.
- Drug screen (serum, urine).
- Cranial CT scan.
- Lumbar puncture (LP).
- CXR (bronchogenic carcinoma with cerebral metastases).
- 12-lead ECG.
- EEG.
- Erythrocyte transketolase (↓ in thiamine deficiency).
- Serum NH_3 (↑ in urea cycle disorders).
- Brain biopsy.

Always assess Airway, Breathing, Circulation before assessment of the cause of ↓ consciousness. Consider psychogenic unresponsiveness.

📖OHCM pp774, 776, 814.

Confusion

A reliable witness, family member or carer may be vital in assessing a patient with confusion, and care must be taken to discriminate between acute and chronic symptoms. Acute confusional states carry a very broad differential diagnosis and require careful initial evaluation. Any systemic illness can precipitate a confusional state.

Table 1.5 Causes of confusion

Hypoxaemia	Acute infection, asthma, COPD, etc.
Head injury	Cerebral trauma
Vascular	CVA, TIA, intracerebral, subdural haemorrhage
Infection	– Systemic
	– Meningitis or encephalitis
Endocrine/metabolic	Diabetic ketoacidosis, hypoglycaemia, thyrotoxicosis or myxoedema, uraemia, hypercalcaemia, hyponatraemia
Alcohol and drug abuse	Acute intoxification and withdrawal Also, consider overdose
Iatrogenic	Full and recent medication history (especially opiates, analgesia and sedatives)
Post-ictal state	
Cerebral tumour	
Psychiatric	
Wernicke's encephalopathy	

Investigations
- FBC, U&E, LFTs, serum Ca^{2+}, BM stix and blood glucose.
- ABGs.
- MSU, blood cultures, sputum culture.
- CXR.
- ECG.
- Thyroid function.
- Drug/toxicology screen—blood and urine.
- CT scan.
- Lumbar puncture.

▶▶Always look for MedicAlert™ bracelet, necklace or card.

📖OHCM pp372, 440, 452.

Constipation

Patients may use the term constipation to mean infrequent, hard, small volume or difficult to pass faeces. Patients vary enormously in their threshold to seek medical advice about bowel habit.

Ask about • associated pain • PR bleeding • tenesmus • weight loss.

Causes
- Carcinoma of the colon.
- Diverticular disease.
- Anorectal disease — fissure or haemorrhoid.
- Benign stricture.
- Rectocoele.
- Sigmoid volvulus.
- Hernia.
- Drugs, especially analgesics.
- Poor fluid intake.
- Low fibre diet.
- Change in diet.
- Immobility.
- Irritable bowel syndrome.
- Megarectum.
- Hirschsprung's disease.
- Spinal cord lesion.
- Stroke.
- Jejunal diverticulosis.
- Hypothyroidism.
- Diabetic neuropathy.
- Hypercalcaemia, hyperparathyroidism, hypokalaemia.
- Uraemia.
- Porphyria.
- Pregnancy.
- Multiple sclerosis.
- Parkinson's disease.
- Dermatomyositis.
- Myotonic dystrophy.
- Scleroderma.
- Psychological.

Investigations
- Digital rectal examination.
- Proctoscopy.
- Sigmoidoscopy.
- Colonoscopy.
- Barium enema.
- U&E.
- Ca^{2+}.
- TFTs.
- FBC.
- Bowel transit time studies.

- Anorectal manometry.
- Electrophysiological studies.
- Defaecating proctography.

▶▶Elderly patients are more prone to constipation.

📖OHCM p220.

Cyanosis

Cyanosis is a blue/purple dusky discolouration of tissue caused by a rise in blood deoxygenated haemoglobin content (>5g/dL). Rarely it may be caused by ↑ sulphaemoglobin, methaemoglobin or carboxyhaemoglobin. Cyanosis may be *peripheral*, affecting only cutaneous areas or *central*, when mucous membranes of the mouth and tongue are also discoloured.

Causes of peripheral cyanosis

- Central cyanosis.
- Shock.
- Hypothermia.
- Mitral stenosis.
- Raynaud's syndrome.
- Peripheral arterial disease.
- Patent ductus arteriosus (differential cyanosis, i.e. cyanosed toes but not fingers, is pathognomonic of this condition).

Causes of central cyanosis

Pulmonary disease with severely impaired oxygen transfer
- Pneumonia.
- Asthma.
- Chronic obstructive pulmonary disease.
- Pulmonary embolism.
- Fibrosing alveolitis.

Right to left shunt (Eisenmenger's syndrome)
- Atrial septal defect.
- Ventricular septal defect.
- Patent ductus arteriosus.
- Partial anomalous pulmonary venous drainage (APVD).
- Arteriovenous malformation.

Methaemoglobinaemia, sulphaemoglobinaemia, carboxyhaemoglobinaemia
- Congenital.
- Ingestion of oxidising agents, e.g. phenacetin, inorganic nitrates, local anaesthetic.

Cyanosis arising from pulmonary disease can be reversed by administration of oxygen to improve alveolar oxygen uptake. Oxygen has no effect where right to left shunts are the cause. Central cyanosis may be underestimated with significant anaemia and is more apparent in patients with polycythaemia. In methaemoglobinaemia, the arterial concentration of oxygen is normal. This condition can be treated with intravenous methylene blue (see Ch11).

Investigations
- FBC.
- ABGs.
- CXR.
- 12-lead ECG.
- Transthoracic echocardiogram (proceeding to transoesophageal echocardiogram if shunt is suspected).
- CT chest (if arteriovenous malformation is suspected).
- Cardiac MRI (if APVD suspected).

📖OHCM pp68, 136, 161, 192.

Diarrhoea

Patients may use the term diarrhoea to describe loose stools, increased frequency of defecation, increased volume of stool, steatorrhoea, melaena or faecal incontinence (📖p53).

Ask about
- Duration.
- Associated features (abdominal pain, vomiting, mucus or blood per rectum).
- Systemic symptoms.
- Recent foreign travel.
- Suspect food.
- Is anyone else in the household affected?

Causes
- Infection (including 'traveller's diarrhoea').
- Inflammatory bowel disease.
- Diverticular disease.
- Colonic carcinoma.
- Other tumour, especially villous adenoma.
- Coeliac disease.
- Tropical sprue.
- Irritable bowel syndrome (IBS).
- Ischaemic colitis/bowel infarction.
- Laxative use!
- Other drugs, e.g. metformin, orlistat.
- Over indulgence in fruit or vegetables.
- Overflow secondary to constipation.
- Carcinoid syndrome (uncommon).
- Gastrinoma (rare).
- VIPoma (rare).
- Glucagonoma (very rare).
- Hyperthyroidism (common).
- Medullary carcinoma of the thyroid (uncommon).

- Bile salt diarrhoea (previous ileal disease or surgery).
- Dumping syndrome (previous gastric surgery).
- Gut motility disorders.
- Malabsorption (cf. pancreatitis, lymphangiectasia, coeliac).
- Lactose intolerance.
- Scleroderma.
- Amyloidosis.
- Whipple's disease.

Investigations
- Stool culture, hot stool for parasites.
- *Clostridium difficile* toxin in stool.
- High rectal swab for parasites (*Note:* giardiasis is diagnosed on duodenal biopsy).
- Rectal examination, proctoscopy, sigmoidoscopy ± biopsy.
- Colonoscopy.
- AXR.
- Barium enema.
- Small bowel follow-through contrast studies.
- Upper GI endoscopy.
- Small bowel biopsy.
- FBC and blood film.
- ESR.
- CRP.
- Serum ferritin and folate.
- U&E (exclude haemolytic uraemic syndrome especially in children).
- Urine screen for laxatives.
- Antigliadin, antiendomysial antibodies and anti-tissue transglutaminase (coeliac disease).
- TFTs.
- Serum gut hormone profile (gastrin, VIP, glucagon—seek expert advice).
- 24h urine for 5HIAA (5-hydroxyindole acetic acid).
- Serum calcitonin (medullary carcinoma of thyroid).
- Lactose hydrogen breath test (for lactose intolerance).
- ^{14}C–xylose breath test (bacterial overgrowth in small bowel).
- CT abdomen.
- Mesenteric angiography (ischaemia).

Investigation must be guided by history and examination findings. If the patient is an inpatient they should be isolated until infection is excluded. Consider HIV and other immune disorders if an unusual bowel organism is found.

Dizziness & syncope

Dizziness is a term that may be used to describe a variety of symptoms, e.g. spinning (rotatory vertigo), light-headedness, muzzy feeling or un-steadiness on walking. It is therefore important to establish precisely what the patient means by dizziness.

Loss of consciousness or 'blackout' may not be reported by the patient and an eyewitness account is important. Enquire about any awareness of abnormal heart beat (rhythm-induced syncope), chest pain (ischaemia), neurological symptoms (cerebrovascular disease), preceding micturition, change of posture or unusual sensations (prodromal epileptic symptoms, e.g. strange taste or smell) prior to the collapse.

Causes of dizziness

- Rotatory sensation lasting >10 seconds and precipitated by movement or position—vestibular cause such as labyrinthitis, Menière's disease, cerebello-pontine angle tumour (acoustic neuroma).
- Rotatory sensation lasting 2 or 3 seconds and precipitated by movement—cervical spondylosis.
- Non-rotatory sensation lasting 2 or 3 seconds and precipitated by movement, position or standing up—cervical spondylosis, cerebro-vascular disease, postural hypotension, cardiac arrhythmia (usually back to normal in minutes), epilepsy (incontinence is common and return to normal may take hours).

Investigations
Suspected vestibular cause
- Hallpike manoeuvre.
- MRI or CT cerebello-pontine angle.
- Audiometry.

Suspected non-vestibular cause
- Blood glucose.
- 12-lead ECG.
- 24 hour ambulatory ECG monitoring.
- EEG.
- MRI or CT head.
- Tilt table test.

Causes of syncope
- Vasovagal: pain, fear, prolonged standing, excess heat, alcohol or food.
- Micturition (often elderly men standing up during night to urinate).
- Defecation (often elderly women with constipation).
- Coughing: chronic airways disease.
- Orthostatic hypotension:
  - Autonomic dysfunction (diabetic neuropathy, Shy–Drager syndrome).
  - Drugs (anti-hypertensives, diuretics, nitrates, tricyclics; dehydration and sodium depletion).
- Carotid sinus syndrome.
- Epilepsy.
- Drugs: alcohol, illicit drugs.
- Cardiac: arrhythmias, outflow obstruction (aortic stenosis, hyper-trophic obstructive cardiomyopathy, myxoma).
- Hyperventilation and anxiety.
- Acute cerebrovascular disease: transient ischaemic attack, stroke, subarachnoid haemorrhage.
- Acute vascular obstruction: pulmonary embolus, myocardial infarction.
- Hypoglycaemia: poorly-controlled diabetes.

Investigations
- 12-lead ECG.
- 24h Holter monitoring.
- Echocardiography.
- MRI or CT head.
- Tilt table test.
- Blood glucose, HbA_{1c}.
- U&E.
- Cardiac markers.
- ABG.
- Toxicology screen.
- V/Q scan.

Guidelines on Management (Diagnosis and Treatment) of Syncope. (2004) *Eur Heart J* **25**, 2054–2072.

▶**Driving and dizziness/syncope**
Guidance on driving in the UK
⌁ www.dvla.gov.uk

Dysarthria & dysphasia

Dysarthria is difficulty in articulating words. The patient may complain of 'slurred speech'. Dysphasia is a difficulty in the formation of speech due to interference with higher mental function. These disturbances often occur together, most commonly in the context of a stroke.

Damage to Wernicke's area causes a *receptive* dysphasia. Speech may be fluent but meaning is lost. Damage to Broca's area causes an *expressive* dyphasia. Speech is non-fluent and the patients are aware they are not using the right words.

Causes of dysphasia include stroke (usually with right hemiparesis, arm more affected than leg) or space-occupying lesion. Psychosis, especially schizophrenia, may cause a similar picture—so-called 'word salad'.

Causes of dysarthria
- Stroke (internal capsule or extensive lesion of motor cortex—acute).
- MND.
- Mid-brain or brainstem tumour.
- Parkinson's disease.
- Cerebellar disease (haemorrhage, infarct, multiple sclerosis, hereditary ataxia, alcoholic or paraneoplastic degeneration).
- Syringobulbia (chronic, progressive).
- Neuromuscular (myasthenia gravis, dermatomyositis, myotonic dystrophy).
- Acute alcohol or drug intoxication.

Dysarthria may be more obvious when the (English-speaking!) patient is invited to say '*Baby hippopotamus*', '*British constitution*', etc.

Investigations
- Cranial CT scan.
- Venous plasma glucose.
- ESR.
- Serum lipids.
- 12-lead ECG.
- Echocardiogram.
- Carotid Doppler studies (especially if bruit).
- CXR.
- LFTs.

Less commonly
- Serum muscle enzymes (polymyositis).
- Autoimmune profile.
- EMG.
- Skeletal muscle biopsy.

📖OHCM pp58, 68

Dysphagia

Dysphagia is difficulty in swallowing. The patient may have associated odynophagia (painful swallowing) or regurgitation of food (immediate or delayed?). Elicit whether the dysphagia is for liquid, solids or both. Is it intermittent or progressive? Are there associated symptoms?

A careful physical examination is mandatory. Pay special attention to the lower cranial nerves; search for lymph nodes in the supraclavicular fossae. Palpate the thyroid and percuss for retrosternal enlargement.

Causes
- Oesophageal carcinoma.
- Benign oesophageal stricture secondary to chronic acid reflux.
- Barrett's oesophagus.
- Achalasia or diffuse spasm.
- Stroke (bilateral internal capsule CVAs—pseudo-bulbar palsy).
- Oesophageal web (+iron deficiency anaemia = Plummer Vinson (Patterson Kelly Brown) syndrome).
- Pharyngeal pouch.
- Muscular problem (myasthenia gravis, dermatomyositis, myotonic dystrophy).
- Bulbar palsy (MS, MND, poliomyelitis).
- Scleroderma (including CREST syndrome—📖OHCM section 11).
- Infection (usually acute pain on swallowing).
- Mediastinal mass (goitre, carcinoma of the bronchus, enlarged left atrium, aortic aneurysm).

Investigations
- FBC.
- ESR.
- Upper GI endoscopy.
- Barium swallow.
- CXR.
- Oesophageal manometry studies (📖p459).
- Cranial CT or MRI (if neurological signs).
- Acetylcholine (ACh) receptor antibodies and Tensilon (edrophonium). test if myasthenia gravis suspected (📖p552).

Note: Consider HIV testing if there is oesophageal candida, herpes simplex or cytomegalovirus infection in the oesophagus.

📖OHCM pp212, 333, 394.

Facial pain

Is the pain unilateral or bilateral? Is it constant or intermittent? Precipitating factors or trigger points? A full examination of head and neck is required in addition to a detailed neurological and systemic examination.

Causes
- Trigeminal neuralgia (TN).
- Temporal arteritis (TA). ▶▶Risk of visual loss (📖OHCM section 11).
- Herpes zoster (shingles or post-herpetic neuralgia).
- Dental caries, sepsis.
- Sinusitis.
- Temporomandibular joint dysfunction.
- Cluster headache.
- Glaucoma.
- Angina pectoris.
- Tonsillitis.
- Syringobulbia.
- Atypical facial neuralgia.
- Migraine.

Investigations
- ESR—urgent in suspected TA.
- Temporal artery biopsy if TA strongly suspected. (▶▶Must be performed rapidly—*within days*—if steroid treatment is commenced. However, do not withhold corticosteroid therapy for this reason!). Because of 'skip' lesions, false −ve biopsies may be encountered. Be guided by the full clinical picture rather than reliance on a single test.
- Plain radiographs or CT imaging of frontal or maxillary sinuses.
- MRI to exclude MS, basilar aneurysm, trigeminal schwannoma, neuro-fibroma as causes of TN.
- MRI of cervical spinal cord to exclude syringobulbia if pain is accompanied by brainstem signs.

📖*Headache* (p43) & 📖OHCM pp72–73.

Fever of unknown origin (FUO or PUO)

Defined as T° >38.3°C on several occasions lasting 3 weeks or more. It is very important to take a full history and consider infectious contacts, recent travel abroad, recent surgery and dental treatment, sexual history and risk factors for HIV.

Signs

Examine for heart murmurs, splinter haemorrhages, splenomegaly, lymphadenopathy and rashes/pruritus.

Table 1.6 Causes

Infection	Abscesses (e.g. subphrenic, pelvic, lung), osteomyelitis, TB, endocarditis, parasites, rheumatic fever, brucellosis, toxoplasmosis, Lyme disease, histoplasmosis, viral (esp. EBV, CMV, hepatitis and HIV)
Malignancy	Lymphoma, leukaemia, hypernephroma, ovary, lung, hepatoma
Connective tissue	PAN, SLE, RA, Still's disease, temporal arteritis
Other	Sarcoidosis, atrial myxoma, drug fever, inflammatory bowel disease, factitious

Investigations

- Re-take the history and re-examine the patient (something might have been missed or new symptoms/signs may have developed).
- FBC, ESR.
- U&E, LFTs, Ca^{2+}.
- CXR.
- MSU, urinalysis.
- Serology for *Brucella* and *Toxoplasma*.
- All biopsy material should be sent for culture, including TB.
- Blood cultures (serial may be necessary).
- Monospot/Paul Bunnell.
- Autoimmune profile (ANA, RF, ANCA, etc.).
- Bone marrow aspirate/trephine/culture for TB with ZN stain.
- Abdominal USS (?masses).

Extend investigations as below according to symptoms and signs

- Consult microbiology or infectious disease consultant for advice.
- Stool cultures and fresh stool for ova, cysts and parasites.
- Repeat serological investigation for changing titres (2–3 weeks).
- Thick and thin blood film for malaria and parasites.
- Mantoux.
- Transthoracic or TOE to exclude endocarditic vegetations.
- CT chest, abdomen and pelvis.

▶▶Always re-examine the patient for evolving new signs if cause remains unknown.

📖OHCM p552.

First fit

▶▶A first fit in an adult requires careful evaluation since the probability of an underlying structural lesion increases with age.

Take a careful history, preferably from a witness as well as the patient. Most lay persons will recognise a generalised tonic-clonic fit. However, the occurrence of a few 'epileptiform' movements in patients with syncopal episodes (📖 Dizziness & syncope p31) may cause diagnostic uncertainty.

Be sure to ask about
- Aura preceding episode. ▶Temporal lobe epilepsy—olfactory or gustatory auras (not necessarily followed by convulsions).
- Loss of consciousness—how long? Often overestimated by witnesses!
- Tongue biting.
- Focal or generalised convulsive movements. *Note*: A clear history of a tonic-clonic fit commencing in a limb and progressing to a more gener-alised convulsion is highly suggestive of a structural intracerebral lesion; cranial imaging is mandatory.
- Central cyanosis (tonic phase).
- Urinary incontinence.
- Injuries.
- Post-ictal confusion.
- History of trauma.
- Alcohol intake. *Remember*: alcohol withdrawal fits as well as acute intoxication.
- Drug history—prescribed and recreational.
- History of insulin-treated diabetes or type 2 diabetes treated with oral secretagogues, i.e. sulphonylureas, repaglinide, nateglinide. *Note*: metformin and thiazolidinediones as monotherapy do not cause significant hypoglycaemia.

A full general and neurological examination is needed, specifically including
- Fever.
- Meningism, i.e. nuchal rigidity, +ve Kernig's sign (meningoencephalitis).
- Cutaneous rash or ecchymoses (?bleeding diathesis).
- Evidence of head trauma (preceding fit or as a consequence).
- Signs of chronic liver disease.
- Focal neurological deficit. ▶Third nerve palsy in intracranial space-occupying lesion (SOL), including aneurysm of the posterior communicat-ing artery. Sixth nerve lesion may act as a 'false localising sign' in ↑ ICP.
- MedicAlert™ bracelet (history of epilepsy or diabetes—search per-sonal belongings).

Bilateral extensor plantar reflexes can occur after a generalised fit with-out a structural brain lesion and there may be a transient hemiparesis (Todd's paresis).

Causes
- Epilepsy (📖OHCM section 10).
- Hypoglycaemia (acute, severe, history of diabetes?).

- Hyponatraemia (usually <110mmol/L or rapid development).
- Hypocalcaemia (📖OHCM section 17).
- Hypomagnesaemia (may accompany hypocalcaemia).
- Hypophosphataemia (rare).
- Alcohol withdrawal. ▶▶Risk of associated hypoglycaemia.
- Discontinuation of anticonvulsant medication.
- Infection—viral encephalitis or bacterial meningitis. ▶▶Consider intracerebral abscess, tuberculoma in predisposed patients.
- Encephalopathy—hepatic, uraemic, hypertensive, thyrotoxic (rare—'thyroid storm').
- Eclampsia.
- Porphyria.
- Cerebral SLE.
- Head injury.
- Hypoxia.
- Cerebral tumour.
- Stroke—cerebral infarct, haemorrhage.

Investigations
- Venous plasma glucose (fingerprick test at bedside useful as 'screen'—but can be unreliable).
- U&E.
- Serum Ca^{2+}, Mg^{2+}, PO_4^{3-}
- Cranial CT or MRI scan.
- EEG.
- LP (📖p518).
- CXR.
- Serum PRL (may be ↑ after generalised convulsions, but not pseudo-seizures).
- ABGs—remember transient lactic acidosis following generalised tonic-clonic convulsion.
- Blood ethanol (may be undetectable in withdrawal state).
- Serum or urine drug screen.

'Pseudo-seizures' may be encountered in patients with atypical recurrent fits (usually long history of epilepsy) and this is unlikely in an adult presenting with a first fit. ▶In UK, the National Driving License Authority prohibits driving for 12 months following a first fit.

📖OHCM p378.

Galactorrhoea

Denotes inappropriate breast milk production, i.e. in the absence of pregnancy. The most common cause is hyperprolactinaemia (↑ PRL) due to a pituitary microprolactinoma of <10mm diameter (📖p158). Prolactinomas (usually macroadenomas) may cause galactorrhoea in men.

Note: Other disease in the pituitary region, certain drugs and several systemic disorders may be associated with ↑ PRL (📖OHCM section 9).

Causes

Normoprolactinaemic galactorrhoea
- This has been described in pre-menopausal women occurring after the conclusion of:
  - Treatment with the combined contraceptive pill.
  - Breastfeeding (for >6 months afterwards).
- Increased sensitivity of lactogenic tissue prolactin (PRL) is postulated but the mechanism remains uncertain. In part, this may reflect difficulties that can arise in determining whether PRL is persistently elevated. Menstrual disturbances have been described.

Hyperprolactinaemia
- The differential diagnosis and investigation of hyperprolactinaemia is considered on p152.

Investigations

- Serum PRL (*Endocrinology & metabolism* 📖p152).
- Repeated measurements under controlled conditions may be required since PRL is a 'stress' hormone and may be increased by venepuncture.

Note: If ↑ PRL is confirmed, further investigations to exclude causes other than prolactinoma are required.

- Pituitary imaging (CT, or preferably, MRI) and visual field testing (Goldmann) may also be indicated if a macroprolactinoma is suspected (PRL concentrations usually very high).

Note: if there is doubt about the nature of the nipple discharge further specialised investigations may be required on the fluid, including:
- Casein.
- Lactose.
- Microscopy.

Clear fluid may result from benign breast disease.

Note: bloody discharge should prompt urgent specialist investigations to exclude carcinoma of the breast:
- Mammography.
- Biopsy.

📖OHCM p322.

Kleinberg DL *et al.* (1977) Galactorrhoea: a study of 235 cases, including 48 with pituitary tumors. *NEJM* **296**, 589–600.

Gout

Gout is a disease of deposition of monosodium urate monohydrate crystals in tissues and relates to hyperuricaemia. Hyperuricaemia is due to an imbalance between purine synthesis and uric acid excretion. Episodes of acute gout may be precipitated by alcohol, trauma, dietary changes, infection, chemotherapy or surgery. More common in men and very rare in pre-menopausal women.

Clinical features

- Inflammatory arthritis, classically a monoarthritis or oligoarthritis affecting 1st MTP joint of foot but can affect any joint including the spine.
- Tenosynovitis.
- Bursitis or cellulitis.
- Tophi—urate deposits in tendons, ear pinna and joints.
- Urolithiasis and renal disease.

Investigations

- ESR (may be ↑).
- Urate crystals demonstrated in synovial fluid or tissues—negatively birefringent on polarised light microscopy.
- Serum urate (not always ↑ in acute episode, and normal urate level does not exclude the diagnosis).
- X-ray—soft tissue swelling and punched out bony erosions.
- AIP (to exclude rheumatoid).
- Microscopy of synovial fluid (Gram stain and culture).

Treatment

Acute episode

- NSAIDs, colchicine, intra-articular steroids or oral steroids.
- Avoid precipitating factors and purine-rich foods.
- Urate lowering therapy indicated for tophi, recurrent attacks and urine/renal disease, e.g.
- Allopurinol (xanthine oxidase inhibitor).
- Probenecid (uricosuric).

Note: asymptomatic hyperuricaemia is more common than gout and a high serum urate with coexistent arthritis is not necessarily due to crystal deposition. Consider important other causes especially infective arthritis and pseudo-gout.

Pseudo-gout

Calcium pyrophosphate crystal deposition causing acute arthritis or chondrocalcinosis. Crystals are weakly +ve birefringent on polarised light microscopy. Associations include old age, dehydration, hyperparathyroidism, hypothyroidism, haemochromatosis, acromegaly, rheumatoid arthritis and osteoarthritis.

📖 OHCM p416.

Gynaecomastia

Gynaecomastia is benign bilateral hyperplasia of glandular and fatty breast tissue in the male. The balance between androgens and oestrogens is thought to be of importance in the pathogenesis; many conditions may influence this ratio. Most commonly, it appears transiently during normal puberty (detectable at some stage in ~50% cases). Gynaecomastia may also be caused by specific endocrine disease or be associated with certain chronic diseases. Treatment with certain drugs is a common cause (~30% of cases) and arises via several mechanisms. Investigations will be guided by the individual circumstances. A careful drug history and thorough physical examination are required, particularly in the post-adolescent period.

When indicated, and after excluding causes such as congenital syndrome and drug therapy, investigations are principally directed at

- Excluding endocrine carcinoma (rare).
- Identifying associated chronic diseases.

Note:

- Simple obesity is not usually a cause of true gynaecomastia, i.e. the glandular element is not increased.
- ↑ Serum prolactin (PRL) in isolation does not cause gynaecomastia.
- Unilateral, eccentric breast enlargement should prompt exclusion of breast carcinoma (rare).

Causes include

- Physiological states (transient):
  - Newborn.
  - Puberty.
  - Advanced age.
- Klinefelter's syndrome (47, XXY; mosaics).
- Secondary hypogonadism, e.g. mumps orchitis.
- Androgen resistance syndromes, e.g. testicular feminisation.
- ↑ Tissue aromatase activity (converts androgens to oestrogens).
- Oestrogen-producing tumours:
  - Leydig cell tumour.
  - Sertoli cell tumour.
  - Adrenal carcinoma.
- Chronic liver disease.
- Chronic renal failure.
- Panhypopituitarism.
- Tumours producing human chorionic gonadotrophin (hCG).
- Drugs: oestrogens (prostatic carcinoma, transsexuals), spironolactone, cimetidine, digoxin, cytotoxic agents, marijuana.
- Hyperthyroidism (↑ serum sex-hormone-binding globulin, SHBG).
- Primary hypothyroidism.
- Cushing's syndrome.
- Carcinoma of bronchus.
- Idiopathic.

Investigations
- Testosterone.
- FSH.
- LH.
- LFTs.
- TFTs.
- Oestradiol.
- β-hCG.
- PRL.
- SHBG (affinity of SHBG is higher for testosterone than for oestrogens, therefore ↑ SHBG causes disproportionate ↓ in free testosterone levels).
- Dehydroepiandrosterone sulphate (DHEAS).
- Androstenedione.
- Testicular USS.
- CXR.
- Abdominal CT or MRI imaging (for suspected adrenal tumours).
- Pituitary imaging.
- Karyotype.
- Urinary 17-oxo-steroids.

If carcinoma of breast is suspected
- Mammogram.
- Fine needle aspiration.

📖OHCM p316.

Braunstein GD. (1994) Gynecomastia. *NEJM* **328**, 490–495.

Haematemesis

This literally means vomiting blood, and is often associated with melaena (passage of black tarry stools).

Causes
- Chronic peptic ulceration (e.g. DU or GU) accounts for 50% of cases of bleeding from the upper GI tract.
- Acute gastric ulcers or erosions.
- Drugs (e.g. NSAIDs) or alcohol.
- Reflux oesophagitis.
- Mallory Weiss tear.
- Oesophageal varices.
- Gastric carcinoma (uncommon).

Investigations after admission and stabilisation of the patient
- Full history, including drugs, alcohol, past history, indigestion, etc.
- FBC (*Note*: Hb will take ~24h to fall; initially may be normal).
- U&E.
- Cross-match blood.
- Urgent upper GI tract endoscopy.
- Check *Helicobacter pylori* serology ± urea breath test.

📖OHCM pp224, 226, 804.

Haematuria

In health adults pass between 500,000 and 2,000,000 red cells over a 24h period. Haematuria implies the passage of excess blood that may be detectable using dipsticks (microscopic haematuria) or may be obvious to the naked eye (macroscopic haematuria).

Causes

- Many.
- Glomerular disease, e.g. 1° glomerulonephritis, 2° glomerulonephritis (SLE, vasculitis, infection).
- Vascular or interstitial disease due to hypersensitivity reactions, renal infarction, papillary necrosis or pyelonephritis.
- Trauma.
- Renal epithelial or vascular tumours.
- Lower renal tract disease, e.g. tumours, stones, infection, drug toxicity (e.g. cyclophosphamide), foreign bodies or parasites.
- Systemic coagulation abnormalities, e.g. platelet or coagulation factor abnormalities such as profound thrombocytopenia or DIC.

Investigations

- Urinalysis—dipstick, microscopic examination, culture.
- Radiology* e.g. KUB or IVU.
- Specialist investigation* e.g. angiography, CT or MRI scanning.
- Cystoscopy*.

*Ideally these tests should be arranged after discussion with either a nephrologist or urologist.

📖OHCM p258.

Haemoptysis

This describes coughing up blood or blood-stained sputum, and can vary from faint traces of blood to frank bleeding. Before embarking on investigation it is essential to ensure that the blood is coughed up from the respiratory tract and is not that of epistaxis or haematemesis (easily confused).

Causes

- Infective, e.g. acute respiratory infection, exacerbation of COPD.
- Pulmonary infarction, e.g. PE.
- Lung cancer.
- Tuberculosis.
- Pulmonary oedema.
- Bronchiectasis.
- Uncommon causes, e.g. idiopathic pulmonary haemosiderosis, Goodpasture's syndrome, microscopic vasculitis, trauma, haematological disease (e.g. ITP or DIC).

Investigations
- Colour of blood provides clues (pink frothy in pulmonary oedema, rust-coloured in pneumonia).
- Check O_2 saturation.
- FBC (? ↓ platelets).
- ESR.
- Coagulation screen.
- Sputum culture.
- CXR.
- Arrange bronchoscopy after discussion with respiratory team.

📖OHCM pp72–73.

Headache

📖*Facial pain* (p34).

Headache is an extremely common complaint. Most patients self-medicate and only a small proportion will seek medical advice. Headache may be acute or chronic, constant, recurrent or gradually progressive. It may arise from structures within the cranial vault or from external causes (📖OHCM section 7).

Causes differ according to age; temporal arteritis is very uncommon in patients under ~55 years, for example. Migraine may be associated with classic features (📖OHCM section 7). Remember to enquire about the combined oral contraceptive pill—may exacerbate migraine. 'Tension' headaches predominate.

Causes in adults include
- 'Tension' headache (very common; usually recurrent and stereotyped).
- Migraine. Although common, many patients who believe they have 'migraine' probably have 'tension' headaches. Classic migraine predominantly affects adolescents and young adults.
- Cluster headaches.
- As part of a generalised viral illness, e.g. 'flu'.
- Causes of ↑ ICP (📖OHCM section 7).
- Acute infective meningitis (bacterial, viral most commonly).
- Encephalitis (most commonly viral, e.g. herpes simplex).
- Intracerebral haemorrhage.
- Post-traumatic (common).
- Intracerebral tumour (primary or secondary, benign or malignant).
- Acute subarachnoid haemorrhage.
- Subdural haematoma.
- Acute glaucoma.
- Acute sinusitis.
- Rubeosis iridis (secondary glaucoma in patients with advanced diabetic eye disease).
- Trigeminal neuralgia.
- Referred pain, e.g. from dental caries or sepsis.

- Arterial hypertension; malignant or accelerated phase; essential hypertension is rarely the cause of headache.
- Temporal arteritis (TA). ►►Visual loss preventable with prompt corticosteroid therapy (🕮OHCM section 7).
- Venous sinus thrombosis.
- Benign intracranial hypertension (mimics intracerebral tumour).
- Pneumonia caused by *Mycoplasma pneumoniae* may be associated with headache (meningoencephalitis).
- Nocturnal hypoglycaemia (often unrecognised) may cause morning headaches in patients with insulin-treated DM.
- Analgesia-withdrawal headache (🕮OHCM section 7).
- Hangover following alcohol excess.
- Otitis media.
- Chronic hypercalcaemia (rare).

Investigations

- ESR (►►temporal arteritis—*exclude with urgency*).
- CRP.
- FBC.
- U&E.
- Throat swabs.
- Blood cultures (if febrile).
- Lumbar puncture (🕮p518).
- SXR ± cervical spine x-ray.
- Sinus x-rays (may be local tenderness in sinusitis).
- Cranial CT (🕮p530).
- CXR (cerebral metastases from bronchogenic carcinoma).
- Urinalysis.
- Intra-ocular pressure measurement and refraction.
- Cerebral angiography (if aneurysm or AV malformation).
- Serum Ca^{2+}.

🕮OHCM pp340, 768.

Heart sounds & murmurs

Auscultation of the heart should be conducted over several cardiac cycles. Heart sounds and murmurs are traditionally assessed at the apex, *lower left sternal edge*, *aortic area* and *pulmonary area* but may radiate into other regions such as the axilla or carotid arteries. The carotid pulse should be palpated simultaneously in order to time cardiac events. The following should be identified:

- First (S1) and second (S2) heart sounds.
- Added heart sounds such as third (S3) or fourth (S4) heart sounds, opening snaps, ejection clicks, prosthetic sounds.
- Murmurs, including location, intensity and characteristics.

The *first heart sound* is produced by closure of the mitral and tricuspid valves. It is best heard at the apex and is timed just prior to the carotid pulse. The *second heart sound* is caused by closure of the aortic (A2) and pulmonary (P2) valves and is heard just after carotid pulsation. Closure of the pulmonary valve is slightly delayed relative to the aortic valve and so the second heart sound is normally split. This split is exaggerated by inspiration (*see* Table 1.7).

Normal and abnormal heart sounds are shown in Table 1.7.

The *third heart sound* is heard just after S2 and arises as a consequence of rapid ventricular filling and volume overload. The *fourth heart sound* occurs just before S1 and is caused by atrial contraction against a stiff ventricle or pressure overload. Abnormal valves may cause extra heart sounds on opening, e.g. an opening snap or ejection click. The heart sounds generated by artificial valve closure are referred to as prosthetic heart sounds. These should be crisp, not muffled (*see* Table 1.8).

Murmurs may be graded according to the following criteria

1. Very soft (just audible in optimal conditions).
2. Soft.
3. Moderate (easily heard with a stethoscope).
4. Loud ± palpable thrill.
5. Very loud/palpable thrill.
6. Heard without stethoscope/palpable thrill.

Table 1.7

Description	Diagram	Differential diagnosis
Normal	S1 / A2 P2	Normal
Loud S1	S1 / A2 P2	Hyperdynamic circulation – anaemia, fever, thyrotoxicosis Mitral stenosis Left atrial myxoma
Soft S1	S1 / A2 P2	Low cardiac output Heart failure Tachycardia Mitral regurgitation Chronic obstructive pulmonary syndrome
Loud S2 (A2)	S1 / A2 P2	Systemic hypertension Dilated aortic root
Soft S2 (A2)	S1 / A2 P2	Aortic stenosis Cardiac failure
Soft S2 (P2)	S1 / A2 P2	Pulmonary stenosis
Loud S2 (P2)	S1 / A2 P2	Pulmonary hypertension
Normal split S2	Expiration / Inspiration / S1 / A2 P2	Normal Physiological splitting exaggerated in: right bundle branch block, pulmonary stenosis, pulmonary hypertension
Fixed splitting S2	Expiration / Inspiration / S1 / A2 P2	Atrial septal defect
Reversed splitting S2	Expiration / Inspiration / S1 / P2 A2	Left bundle branch block Systemic hypertension Aortic stenosis

Innocent murmurs are generated by turbulent flow such as in high cardiac output states, e.g. pregnancy, fever, anaemia and thyrotoxicosis. They have the following characteristics:
- No accompanying thrill.
- Never > grade 3.
- Systolic.
- Maximal at left sternal edge.
- Normal heart sounds.
- Normal pulses, ECG and CXR.

Systolic murmurs are synchronous with the carotid pulse and caused by
- Abnormal regurgitation through a structure that is normally closed in systole, e.g. atrioventricular valve, septum (pansystolic).
- Normal systolic flow through a narrowed or stenosed valve, e.g. aortic valve, pulmonary valve (ejection systolic).

Diastolic murmurs are audible after the carotid pulse and arise from
- Incompetence of the cardiac outflow valves, e.g. aortic or pulmonary valves.
- Narrowing of the cardiac inflow valves, e.g. mitral or tricuspid valves.

Mixed murmurs (systolic and diastolic) arise from
- Mixed valvular disease (stenosis and regurgitation).
- Patent ductus arteriosus.

Murmurs arising from the left heart structures are accentuated in expiration, whereas right heart murmurs are augmented in inspiration (see Table 1.9).

Table 1.8 Heart murmurs

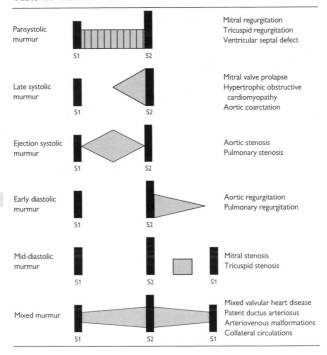

Pansystolic murmur	Mitral regurgitation Tricuspid regurgitation Ventricular septal defect
Late systolic murmur	Mitral valve prolapse Hypertrophic obstructive cardiomyopathy Aortic coarctation
Ejection systolic murmur	Aortic stenosis Pulmonary stenosis
Early diastolic murmur	Aortic regurgitation Pulmonary regurgitation
Mid-diastolic murmur	Mitral stenosis Tricuspid stenosis
Mixed murmur	Mixed valvular heart disease Patent ductus arteriosus Arteriovenous malformations Collateral circulations

Table 1.9 Added heart sounds

S3		Normal (young adult) Left ventricular failure Right ventricular failure Mitral regurgitation Constrictive pericarditis (pericardial 'knock')
	S1 A2 P2 S3	
S4		Normal (elderly) Left ventricular hypertrophy Left ventricular diastolic dysfunction Systemic hypertension Aortic stenosis Acute ischaemia
	S4 S1 A2 P2	
Opening snap		Mitral stenosis Tricuspid stenosis
	S1 A2 P2 OS	
Ejection click		Aortic stenosis Systemic hypertension Pulmonary stenosis Pulmonary hypertension
	S1 EC A2 P2	
Mid-systolic click		Mitral valve prolapse
	S1 MSC A2 P2	
Prosthetic heart sounds		Artificial valve replacement
	PS1 PS2 P2	

Hepatomegaly

Measure liver edge below the (R) costal margin after percussing out the upper and lower borders. Bruits may be heard in hepatoma and a friction rub may occur with malignant deposits. Other signs may suggest the underlying diagnosis (see below).

Common causes

- CCF.
- Malignant deposits.
- Hepatitis/cirrhosis (usually alcoholic or infectious, e.g. EBV, viral hepatitis).

Foreign residence?

If so, consider amoebic and hydatid cysts, schistosomiasis, malaria.

Investigations

- FBC, film, LDH (leukaemia, lymphoma).
- ESR.
- Virology (EBV, CMV, hepatitis A, B, C antibody serology).
- LFTs—transaminases.
- Serum albumin.
- Prothrombin time (hepatocellular damage).
- γ-glutamyl transpeptidase, MCV (alcohol).
- Alkaline phosphatase (obstructive causes; malignant deposits if isolated↑).
- Serum Igs may be polyclonal ↑ in IgG (autoimmune hepatitis), IgA (alcoholic liver disease) or IgM (PBC).
- Serum protein electrophoresis (myeloma, amyloid).
- Reticulocytes, bilirubin (if ↑ suggests haemolysis).
- Haemoglobinopathy screen (thalassaemia/sickle disorders).
- USS to assess liver texture, splenomegaly, lymphadenopathy.
- CXR and cardiac investigations (cardiomyopathies, sarcoid).
- α-fetoprotein (primary hepatocellular carcinoma).
- Serum ferritin, transferrin saturation, DNA analysis (haemochromatosis).
- Mitochondrial antibodies and autoimmune markers, e.g. ANA (autoimmune hepatitis), ANCA (primary sclerosing cholangitis).
- Caeruloplasmin, urinary copper (Wilson's disease).
- α1-antitrypsin (α1-antitrypsin deficiency).
- Porphyria screen.

Pitfalls

Hepatomegaly is a common sign but may not necessarily implicate liver pathology.

📖OHCM pp74, 518.

Herpes zoster

The pattern of the eruption varies from mild to dense with the involvement of several dermatomes. Complications may occur if involvement of the eye, motor nerves, autonomic nerves (bladder), or when disease presents as an encephalomyelitis or purpura fulminans.

▶▶In the immunocompromised host, zoster is both more likely to occur and to disseminate.

Investigations
- Confirm diagnosis by isolation of virus from vesicular fluid.
- Consider underlying disorders if recurrent or severe attacks.
- Look for lymphadenopathy (Hodgkin's or other lymphoma).
- FBC, blood film, LDH (↑ in lymphoma).
- Serum protein electrophoresis (myeloma, amyloid).
- Serology for HIV (zoster is common in adult HIV individuals).
- Immunodeficiency work-up.

Pitfalls
The rash is not always unilateral—it may be bilateral.

📖OHCM p568.

Hyperlipidaemia

Abnormalities of lipid metabolism are common in Western societies. Populations with high levels of cholesterol have high rates of vascular morbidity, especially cardiovascular disease, and premature death. Vascular risk can be estimated from published risk tables or calculators.

Various classifications of hyperlipidaemia exist, each with a characteristic lipid profile. Many patients with lipid disorders have cutaneous markers, which identify to a certain extent the type of lipid abnormality.

Clinical features

Lipid abnormalities may cause dermatological manifestations
- Grey-yellow plaques or xanthomata in tendons, especially forearm and Achilles. Usually indicative of elevated LDL-cholesterol.
- Corneal arcus, a thin white rim around the iris—whilst this is common in the elderly, it is not a sign of ↑ LDL except in the under 40s.
- Yellow, fatty deposits or xanthelasmata around the eyelids—associated with elevated LDL, these painless, non-tender plaques are common in the elderly.
- Yellow streaks in palmar creases—palmar xanthomata are associated with IDL-cholesterol.
- Plaques over the tibial tuberosities and elbows—tubero-eruptive xanthomata. Often seen with hepatosplenomegaly with elevated triglycerides.
- Eruptive xanthomata—in severe triglyceridaemia associated with pancreatitis, hepatomegaly.

Hyperlipidaemia may be secondary to drugs such as corticosteroids, oestrogens and progestagens as well as a range of conditions such as hypothyroidism, myeloma and alcoholism, each of which may be associated with specific clinical signs.

Hypertension

Blood pressure measurements are graded into a number of categories by the British Hypertension Society:

Optimal blood pressure	<120/80
Normal blood pressure	<130/85
High-normal blood pressure	130–139/85–89
Grade 1 hypertension (mild)	140–159/90–99
Grade 2 hypertension (moderate)	160–179/100–109
Grade 3 hypertension (severe)	≥180/110

Hypertension should not be diagnosed on the basis of a single blood pressure reading. Unless urgent treatment is required, e.g. malignant hypertension, blood pressure should be rechecked over a number of weeks to confirm the presence of sustained hypertension.

Causes

Remember that the cause of hypertension in most (95%) cases is unknown ('essential' hypertension). One of the following identifiable causes can be found in the remaining 5%:

- Renal disease, e.g. polycystic kidney disease.
- Renovascular disease, e.g. renal artery stenosis.
- Endocrine disease, e.g. Cushing's syndrome, Conn's syndrome, phaeochromocytoma, acromegaly.
- Coarctation of the aorta.
- Drugs, e.g. NSAIDs, oral contraceptive pill, steroids, erythropoietin, sympathomimetics, liquorice.
- Pregnancy, e.g. pre-eclampsia, eclampsia.

Routine investigation

The investigation of hypertensive patients has the following aims

- To confirm the presence and severity of hypertension.
- To assess overall cardiovascular risk.
- To identify target organ damage.
- To identify secondary causes (where present).

Routine investigations should include

- Urinalysis (protein, blood, glucose).
- U&E.
- Plasma glucose (ideally fasted).
- Lipid profile (ideally fasted).
- 12-lead ECG.

CXR, urine microscopy and culture and echocardiography are not required routinely but should be considered where indicated by your initial assessment and investigation of the patient. The use of 24h ambulatory blood pressure monitoring is often useful where clinic readings are thought to be unreliable because of 'white coat' hypertension.

Further investigation

Where more detailed assessment is required (for instance, to rule out a secondary cause or to identify end-organ damage), the following investigations may be appropriate:

Renal investigations
- Renal ultrasound scan (to assess overall renal morphology).
- Renal artery Doppler studies (for renal artery stenosis).
- Renal artery MR imaging (for renal artery stenosis).
- Captopril renogram (for renal artery stenosis).
- Renal angiography (for renal artery stenosis).
- Renal vein renin measurements (for Conn's syndrome).

Endocrine investigations
- Renin & aldosterone studies for Conn's syndrome (consult your local endocrine laboratory).
- Investigations for Cushing's syndrome.
- Investigations for acromegaly.
- Urinary catecholamine (& metabolite) excretion.

Williams B *et al.* (2004) Guidelines for management of hypertension: report of the fourth working party of the British Hypertension Society, 2004—BHS IV. *J Human Hypertension* **18**, 139–185.

Incontinence: faecal

📖 *Alteration of bowel habit, Constipation, Diarrhoea* (pp8, 27, 29).

Causes include
- Any cause of diarrhoea (📖OHCM section 7).
- Overflow diarrhoea from severe constipation.
- Inflammatory bowel disease (acute or chronic).
- Coeliac disease (diarrhoea is a variable feature).
- Infectious diarrhoea (📖OHCM section 1).
- Hyperthyroidism (may cause diarrhoea; rare cause of incontinence).
- Carcinoma of colon (stricture).
- Diverticular disease of colon (acute attack, chronic stricture).
- Neurological (multiple CVAs, MS, spina bifida, post-childbirth neuropathy) may often be associated with sphincter disturbances.
- Drugs, e.g. laxatives, orlistat (causes fat malabsorption).
- Causes of steatorrhoea (📖OHCM section 7).
- Intestinal hurry, e.g. post-gastrectomy (📖OHCM section 7).
- Diabetic diarrhoea (autonomic neuropathy—rare; diagnosis of exclusion but may cause nocturnal faecal incontinence).
- VIPoma (very rare).

Investigations

Non-invasive tests
- Stool cultures (ova cysts, parasites). *Note: Clostridium difficile*—relatively common in patients who have received recent antibiotic therapy.
- FBC (anaemia, especially iron deficiency).
- CRP.
- ESR.
- U&E.
- TFTs.

Imaging
- Pelvic/abdominal x-ray.
- Barium enema.
- CT abdomen.

Procedures
- Colonoscopy.
- Sigmoidoscopy ± biopsy.

OHCM pp72, 73, 209.

Incontinence: urinary

 Anuria (p13).

Consider
- Common causes of polyuria (OHCM section 4); these may present as, or aggravate, urinary incontinence.
- Acute or chronic confusional state (common; loss of voluntary sphincter control).
- Urinary tract infection (very common—always exclude).
- Drug-induced, e.g. thiazide or loop diuretics; α-adrenergic blockade, e.g. doxazosin (uncommon).
- Psychological, e.g. severe depression.
- Immobility, e.g. Parkinson's disease (Shy–Drager syndrome is uncommon).
- Other causes of autonomic neuropathy (OHCM section 10).
- Detrusor muscle instability.
- Urethral incompetence.
- Stool impaction.
- Spinal cord compression.
- Tabes dorsalis.

Investigations
- U&E.
- Urinalysis for blood, protein, glucose, nitrates, nitrites.
- MSU for C&S.
- Plasma glucose (if glycosuria).
- Serum Ca^{2+}.

In selected patients, consider referral to urology or gynaecology services for consideration of
- Bladder manometry studies.
- Post-voiding USS of bladder.
- Pelvic imaging, e.g. CT scan.

📖 OHCM p500.

Indigestion

This term is often loosely used by patients to describe a variety of symptoms. These are often regarded as representing relatively minor and usually intermittent pathology. However, serious pathology, e.g. carcinoma of the stomach, may present as a vague complaint of 'indigestion'. The symptoms may be retrosternal or abdominal. A detailed history is essential, focusing on features that raise the probability of serious pathology, e.g. dysphagia and weight loss.

Examination should include a search for the following signs, particularly in the middle-aged and elderly patients
- Anaemia (especially iron deficiency—common).
- Ascites.
- Troissier's sign (malignant involvement of left supraclavicular lymph nodes due to carcinoma of the stomach—rare).

Note: The presence of associated pathologies, e.g. pernicious anaemia (📖 OHCM section 7)—↑ risk of stomach cancer—will alter the threshold for more detailed, expert investigation. Carcinoma of stomach is more common in Japanese.

Peptic ulceration may have classic elements that point to the diagnosis. Non-ulcer dyspepsia is very common and is often treated empirically with antacids, H_2 receptor antagonists or H^+ pump inhibitor drugs. The clinical challenge is to identify the patient for whom more detailed, and often invasive, investigation is indicated.

Alternative causes, e.g. cardiac ischaemia, should be considered in the differential diagnosis; similarities of the symptoms between cardiac and upper gastrointestinal disorders are well recognised and sometimes pose considerable diagnostic difficulties.

Causes include
- Oesophageal acid reflux.
- Hiatus hernia.
- Inflammatory disease.
- Peptic ulcer disease of duodenum or stomach.
- Biliary colic (usually distinctive clinical features).
- Malignancy of oesophagus, stomach or rarely small intestine.
- Cardiac symptoms, usually ischaemia.
- Irritable bowel syndrome.
- Symptoms arising from other structures within the chest or abdomen.

Investigations
- FBC.
- U&E.
- ESR.
- Upper GI endoscopy ± tissue biopsy.
- LFTs.
- Creatine kinase (CK) if MI/ACS suspected.
- Troponin (T or I) if MI/ACS suspected.
- Serum amylase (normal in chronic pancreatitis; may be ↑ by duodenal ulcer eroding posterior wall).
- Barium swallow and meal (for oesophageal disease).
- CLO test for *Helicobacter pylori*.
- Urea ^{13}C breath test for *H. pylori*.
- USS of biliary tract (📖p690).
- Cholecystogram.

If diagnosis remains uncertain consider
- CT abdomen (discuss with radiologist).
- Serum gastrin (Zollinger–Ellison syndrome, 📖OHCM p740).
- 24h ambulatory oesophageal pH monitoring.
- Oesophageal manometry (oesophageal motility disorders).

Infective endocarditis signs

Infective endocarditis is characterised by infection of the endocardial surface of the heart. The left heart valves are the most commonly affected, but the right heart valves and congenital heart lesions such as ventricular septal defects may also become infected. Vegetations (composed of the organism, white cells, platelets and fibrous tissue) are formed at the site of infection. They give rise to periodic septicaemia and may embolize to other parts of the body. There is gradual destruction of the valve with increasing valvular dysfunction, regurgitation and heart failure.

Clinical features
- Pyrexia (low-grade or swinging).
- Pale conjunctivae suggestive of anaemia (of chronic disease).
- Clubbing (chronic low-grade infection).
- Cardiac murmur (new or changing).
- Left or right heart failure.
- Splenomegaly (friction rub if splenic infarction is present).
- Microscopic haematuria (on urinalysis).

Embolic phenomena
Embolic phenomena are common and produce clinical signs classically associated with infective endocarditis
- Splinter haemorrhages (>5, sited in the proximal finger and toenail beds).
- Janeway lesions (palmar macular spots).
- Osler's nodes (painful nodules on palmar surface of the fingers or toes).

- Roth spots (retinal haemorrhages).
- Conjunctival haemorrhages.
- Microvascular infarction (in the distal limbs).

Prendergast BD. (2004) Diagnostic criteria and problems in infective endocarditis. *Heart* **90**, 611–613; Task Force on Infective Endocarditis of the ESC. (2004) Guidelines on prevention, diagnosis and treatment of infective endocarditis. *Eur Heart J* **25**, 267–276.

Irregular pulse

In health, the pulse is usually regular although a minor degree of variation in heart rate with respiration (sinus arrhythmia) is common, particularly in children and young adults. In sinus arrhythmia, the heart rate increases with inspiration and decreases with expiration. This is a benign phenomenon.

An irregular pulse can present as a symptom (with the patient complaining of an awareness of irregular or 'missed'/'extra' heartbeats) or as a sign (incidental finding on clinical examination).

Pulse irregularities are traditionally classified into two groups
- Regular irregularities.
- Irregular irregularities.

A regularly irregular pulse
Most commonly the result of ventricular or supraventricular ectopic activity. Ectopic beats often occur after a certain number of sinus beats—thus in ventricular bigeminy, every other beat will be a ventricular ectopic beat and thus occur prematurely with reduced volume. In trigeminy, every third beat will be early.

A regularly irregular pulse
Can also be evident in 2nd degree atrioventricular block (Mobitz type I or II).

An irregularly irregular pulse is most commonly the result of
- Multiple ectopic beats (supraventricular or ventricular).
- Atrial fibrillation.
- Atrial flutter with variable atrioventricular block.

Investigations
The key to diagnosis is to record an ECG while the pulse irregularity is present. If the paroxysmal irregularity is infrequent, this can prove challenging. A 12-lead ECG is mandatory and may provide an immediate diagnosis. If not, a number of ambulatory ECG monitoring techniques are available:
- 24 hour ambulatory ECG monitoring.
- Cardiac event monitoring.
- Implantable loop recorder.

The choice of technique should be guided by how frequently the irregularity is thought to occur.

Additional investigations depend upon the nature of the suspected arrhythmia
- FBC.
- U&E.
- TFTs.

One may also consider
- CXR (to assess heart size and valvular calcification).
- Echocardiogram (if structural heart disease suspected).
- Exercise treadmill test (if IHD suspected, or to provoke arrhythmias thought to be exercise-related).

Jaundice

This defines the yellow discoloration of the sclerae, mucous membranes and skin that occurs when bilirubin accumulates. Bilirubin is the major bile pigment in humans, and is produced as an end-product of haem catabolism. Jaundice usually only becomes noticeable when the serum bilirubin >30–60µmol/L.

Causes
- Can be pre-hepatic, hepatic or post-hepatic.
- Haemolysis.
- Hepatitis (viral, drugs, alcohol).
- Pregnancy.
- Recurrent cholestasis.
- Hepatic infiltration.
- Stones in the common bile duct.
- Carcinoma of the bile duct, head of pancreas or ampulla.
- Biliary strictures.
- Sclerosing cholangitis.
- Pancreatitis.

Investigations (Fig. 1.2)
- FBC (?haemolysis).
- Clotting screen (often deranged in liver disease).
- LFTs.
- Viral serology for HAV, HBV and HCV.
- USS abdomen.
- Consider ERCP.
- Liver biopsy may be indicated depending on history, examination and laboratory findings. Discuss with gastroenterology team before embarking on this.

📖 OHCM pp222, 552.

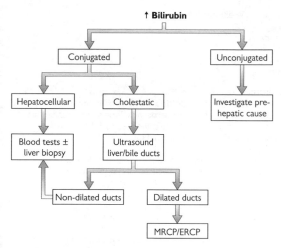

Fig. 1.2 Investigation of jaundice.

Joint pain/swelling

Covers a multitude of disorders including

- Osteoarthritis.
- Rheumatoid arthritis.
- Tendinitis.
- Bursitis.
- Trigger finger.
- Mechanical low back pain.
- Fibromyalgia.
- Other arthropathies.

History and examination

- Ask about affected joints, site of origin, mono- or polyarticular, oligo-articular (e.g. 2–4 joints involved), migratory features, arthralgia (joint pain without swelling).
- Is pain constant or intermittent?
- Aggravating or precipitating factors?
- Any associated neurological features?
- Is there swelling?
- Associated redness or excessive warmth?

- Drug history (e.g. diuretic induced).
- Race (e.g. sickle).
- Past history.
- Family history.
- Occupational history.
- Social history.

Investigations
- FBC—a normochromic normocytic anaemia is common in chronic inflammatory disorders. May be microcytic if long-standing inflammation or associated iron deficiency (e.g. induced by NSAIDs).
- ESR—non-specific marker of inflammation.
- CRP—as for ESR.
- Biochemistry screen, especially looking at bone profile and LFTs.
- Consider serum Igs and protein electrophoresis (myeloma).
- Uric acid levels (gout).
- X-ray affected joint(s).
- Consider USS, especially if soft-tissue swelling.
- MRI can be useful to help visualise intra-articular structures.
- CT scan.
- Bone scintigraphy (helps identify abnormal bone turnover).
- DEXA scan (useful for diagnosis and monitoring of osteoporosis).
- Arthroscopy may help in selected cases.
- Joint aspiration (allows culture and examination of fluid for crystals).

Jugular venous pulse

The height and waveform of the internal jugular venous pulse (JVP) reflect right atrial pressure and haemodynamics. The JVP should be inspected with the patient positioned at 45° to the horizontal. The JVP may be distinguished from the carotid pulse by the following features:
- Pulsation is not palpable.
- It may be compressed and obliterated by pressure.
- It rises on compression of the right upper quadrant (hepatojugular reflux).
- It varies with posture.
- Height decreases with inspiration.

The height of the JVP is measured as the vertical distance between the manubriosternal angle and the top of the venous pulsation. Elevation is defined as >3cm.

There are several components of the jugular venous pulsation waveform. The *a* wave is produced by atrial systole. This is followed by the *x* descent at the end of atrial contraction. The *x* descent is interrupted by a small barely perceptible deflection called a *c* wave. This deflection is caused by the rapid increase in right ventricular pressure just before the tricuspid valve closes. A subsequent *v* wave results from the rise in right atrial pressure as it fills with venous return during ventricular systole and whilst the tricuspid valve remains closed. At the end of ventricular systole, the tricuspid valve opens and the pressure in the right atrium falls leading to the *y* descent (see Table 1.10).

Table 1.10

Description Diagram	Diagnosis	Comment
Normal	Normal	
↑ JVP Normal waveform	Right heart failure Fluid overload Pulmonary embolus Cardiac tamponade	↑ right atrial pressure
Absent *a* wave	Atrial fibrillation	Poor atrial contraction fails to generate a wave
Large *a* waves	Tricuspid stenosis Right ventricular hypertrophy	Resistance to right atrial emptying causes ↑ right atrial pressure
Large *v* waves	Tricuspid regurgitation	Reflux of blood into the great veins with right ventricular contraction
Cannon (*a*) waves	Complete heart block Ventricular tachycardia	RA contracts against closed tricuspid valve creating a cannon wave
Rapid *y* descent	Constrictive pericarditis Cardiac tamponade Tricuspid regurgitation Right heart failure	A steep y descent is caused by RV diastolic collapse (Freidrich's sign)
Absent pulsation ↑ JVP	Superior vena caval obstruction	No right atrial pressure can be transmitted to the JVP

Loin pain

Definition: pain located in the renal angle.

Causes
- Ureteric colic.
- Renal or ureteric obstruction.
- Acute pyelonephritis.
- Renal infarction or papillary necrosis.
- Acute nephritis (uncommon).
- IgA nephropathy—pain caused by extension of the renal capsule.
- Musculoskeletal causes.
- Shingles at T10–12 (obvious if a rash is seen on examination or be suspected if pain is in a dermatomal distribution).
- Infection or bleeding into a cyst in polycystic kidneys.
- Vesico-ureteric reflux—pain occurs when the bladder is full, this worsens at the initiation of micturition and then is rapidly relieved on voiding.
- Loin pain-haematuria syndrome—this is recurrent pain which occurs in young women. Angiography reveals tortuous vessels.

Investigations
- U&E.
- Serum creatinine.
- Creatinine clearance (if renal impairment).
- FBC.
- ESR.
- Urine dipstick for protein, blood, nitrites, leucocytes.
- Urine microscopy (for casts).
- MSU for culture and sensitivity testing.
- Blood cultures (if bacteraemia suspected).
- Plain x-ray (KUB view).
- IVU (e.g. if +ve urine dipstick for haematuria).
- Renal USS (useful for rapid non-invasive exclusion of obstruction).
- CT of urinary tract.
- Angiogram (if suspicion of thrombus, embolus or loin pain-haematuria syndrome).
- Serum IgA concentration.
- Cystoscopy (specialist procedure).
- Retrograde pyelography.
- Renal biopsy (only after specialist advice).

Lymphadenopathy

Lymph node enlargement may be localised or generalised.

Localised cervical lymphadenopathy

- Local causes in mouth (pharyngitis, dental abscess).
- Scalp (skin malignancies or disease).
- Nose (nasopharyngeal carcinoma).

Enlargement of left supraclavicular nodes

- May suggest carcinoma of stomach.

Isolated posterior cervical node enlargement

- Is less often due to malignancy.

Other causes

- Sometimes drugs may be associated with lymph node enlargement (phenytoin, antithyroid).

Table 1.11

Infection	
Viral	Infectious hepatitis, EBV syndromes, HIV, rubella, varicella, herpes zoster
Bacterial	Streptococcal, staphylococcal, salmonella, brucellosis, *Listeria*, cat-scratch (*Bartonella*)
Fungal	Histoplasmosis, coccidioidomycosis
Chlamydial	
Mycobacterial	
Parasites	Trypanosomiasis, microfilaria, toxoplasmosis
Spirochaetes	Syphilis, yaws, leptospirosis
Connective tissue	Rheumatoid arthritis, SLE, dermatomyositis, serum sickness
Drugs	E.g. phenytoin
Malignancy	
Haematological	Hodgkin's lymphoma, non-Hodgkin's lymphoma, acute and chronic lymphoid malignancies (CLL, ALL), AML
Non-haematological	Metastases from carcinomas (breast, bowel, lung, prostate, kidney, head & neck)
Endocrine	Thyrotoxicosis
Miscellaneous	Sarcoidosis, amyloidosis

Investigations

- FBC, blood film, LDH (leukaemia, lymphoma, Hodgkin's).
- Serology/virology/microbiology/other antigen detection tests:
  - Viral (EBV, hepatitis, CMV, HIV).
  - Bacterial (tuberculosis, bacterial endocarditis, syphilis).

- Fungal (histoplasmosis).
- Protozoal (toxoplasmosis).
- ANA (collagen disorder, systemic lupus).
- TFTs (hyperthyroidism).
- CXR (sarcoid, tuberculosis).
- USS/CT scan (to assess intra-abdominal, mediastinal/hilar lymphadenopathy).
- LFTs/hepatomegaly (↑ alkaline phosphatase suggests malignant deposits).
- Lymph node biopsy (groin nodes should usually be avoided because commonly enlarged due to skin and infectious disorder).
- BM (may confirm haematological malignancy).

Note: Fine-needle aspiration, although easier to perform, may not be diagnostic and lymph node biopsy should be considered for microbiology and histology.

📖 OHCM p578.

Although we have provided a large list of possibilities common sense should be used in determining the cause. For example, an 80-year-old woman with axillary lymphadenopathy is unlikely to have cat-scratch disease! Common things are common.

Nausea

The so-called vomiting centre is located in the medulla oblongata and is stimulated by the chemoreceptor trigger zone in the 4th ventricle. There are many causes of acute and chronic nausea. These can be divided into gastrointestinal (GI) causes and non-GI causes.

GI causes of nausea

- Food poisoning (viral, bacterial—common).
- Acute and chronic gastritis (remember *Helicobacter pylori*).
- Peptic ulceration.
- Biliary and renal colic.
- Inflammatory bowel disease.
- Cholecystitis.
- Appendicitis.
- Pancreatitis.
- Gastric outflow obstruction.
- Post-gastrectomy syndrome.
- Acute liver failure.
- Pseudo-obstruction of bowel.

Investigations
- U&E.
- LFTs.
- ESR.
- CRP.
- Serum or urinary amylase.
- Abdominal x-ray (erect and supine—*beware* perforated viscus).
- Abdominal ultrasound.

Consider
- OGD.
- Barium swallow and meal.
- Isotopic gastric emptying studies.
- Oesophageal manometry.
- Oesophageal muscle biopsy (rarely indicated).

Non-GI causes
- Acute infections, e.g. UTI.
- Metabolic disorders including:
  - Hypercalcaemia.
  - Ketoacidosis (diabetic, alcoholic).
  - Uraemia.
- Pregnancy. *Note*: hyperemesis gravidarum may be associated with ↑ FT4, ↓ TSH.
- Many drugs, notably opiates and digoxin toxicity (check serum levels).
- MI (nausea common; exacerbated by opiates).
- Acute glaucoma.

Investigations
- FBC.
- ESR.
- Venous plasma glucose.
- Urine dipstick (UTI).
- Serum Ca^{2+}.
- Serum drug levels, e.g. digoxin, theophylline.
- 12-lead ECG.
- CK.
- Troponin I.

Neurological causes
- Acute migraine.
- ↑ intracranial pressure.
- Acute labyrinthine lesions.
- Menière's disease.
- Cerebellar lesions (e.g. infarct, haemorrhage, metastases, demyelination).

Investigations
- Cranial CT.
- MRI if cerebellar lesion suspected.
- Tilt table test (📖p436).
- Audiometry (specialist technique).

📖OHCM p438.

Neck stiffness

The main concern in a patient with neck stiffness is that s/he may have meningitis which may result from infection or may reflect infiltration by a disease such as acute leukaemia.

Causes
- Bacterial infection.
- Viral infection.
- Fungal infection.
- Tuberculosis.
- Infiltration by malignancy (e.g. acute lymphoblastic leukaemia, high grade lymphoma, or sometimes acute myeloid leukaemia).
- Drug-induced.
- Contrast media (myelogram).
- Blood (e.g. post-subarachnoid haemorrhage).
- Mechanical/trauma.
- Connective tissue disease, e.g. rheumatoid arthritis.

Investigations
- CT scan of brain ± contrast.
- Lumbar puncture if no ↑ intracranial pressure:
  - Glucose.
  - Protein.
  - MC&S ± TB culture.
  - Xanthochromia if SAH suspected.
- If patient immunocompromised consider:
  - PCR for viruses, e.g. HSV.
  - Toxoplasma serology.
  - India ink stain for *Cryptococcus*.
- If considering malignancy, send CSF for cytospin.

📖OHCM pp368, 370, 808.

Nystagmus

An involuntary oscillatory or (more commonly) rapid jerking movement of the eyes that is rhythmic and repetitive. It results from acute or chronic lesions of the eight cranial nerves, brainstem or cerebellum. The 'slow' phase is pathological, the rapid rhythmic jerking phase (used arbitrarily to define the direction of nystagmus) being a corrective response. Nystagmus 'to the right' describes the direction of the quick phase. Such 'saw tooth' nystagmus may be evident in the horizontal or vertical plane (including 'downbeat' nystagmus of foramen magnum lesions) or as oscillations around a central point (e.g. in albinism).

Jerk nystagmus may be graded in severity depending on whether it occurs
- Only in the direction of directed gaze.
- When eyes are in the midline *or*

• Is present even on looking in direction contralateral to the rapid movement.

Note: nystagmus (or more correctly, nystagmoid jerks) may be induced by inappropriate testing, often being present at the extremes of gaze. Do not ask patient to follow visual target beyond ~30° of midline when testing at the bedside.

In unilateral causes

Cerebellar nystagmus
Greatest when gaze directed towards the side of the destructive lesion.

Vestibular nystagmus
Greatest away from the side of the lesion.

Pathological nystagmus
May be due to labyrinthine and vestibular lesions—occurs in one direction only. If visual fixation is removed, nystagmus becomes worse.

Central lesions
Including brainstem lesions caused by e.g. tumour, MS; cerebellar lesions or medial longitudinal fasciculus lesions leading to internuclear ophthalmoplegia (OHCM section 10) with ataxic nystagmus.

Investigations

• Positional nystagmus may be investigated by using the Hallpike manoeuvre (OHCM section 10). Abrupt alteration of the spatial position of the head (from supine, with head below the bed, rapidly to a sitting position) will induce nystagmus. This will demonstrate benign positional vertigo (common), vestibular disorders or brainstem lesions.
• Audiometry (specialised investigation).
• Auditory and visual evoked potentials (VEPS) may be pathologically reduced in MS. Examination of CSF may reveal oligoclonal bands.
• MRI to include brainstem. (Upbeat nystagmus will suggest a midbrain lesion and downbeat nystagmus will suggest a foramen magnum lesion.) MRI is superior to CT for demonstrating cerebellopontine angle lesions. Gadolinium enhancement is used to investigate acoustic neuromas.
• Ototoxicity can be caused by some drugs such as gentamicin and phenytoin. Acute poisoning with alcohol or barbiturates may cause transient nystagmus. Chronic alcoholism can lead to permanent cerebellar damage. Excessive doses of anticonvulsant drugs, e.g. phenytoin, are a common cause—measure serum concentrations of drug.

OHCM p56.

Obesity

The World Health Organisation defines obesity as a body mass index (BMI) greater than 30kg/m^2.

Table 1.12

		BMI (kg/m^2)
Underweight		<18.5
Normal		18.5–24.9
Overweight		>25.0–29.9
Obesity	Class I	30.0–34.9
	II	35.0–39.3
	III	>40

Note: central (abdominal) fat distribution—commoner in men—is associated with greater health risks. Waist to hip ratio or simply waist girth can be used to identify levels at which long-term health risks warrant intervention:

| Men | >102cm |
| Women | >88cm |

Aetiology

The great majority of obese subjects have no identifiable metabolic or hormonal defects and detailed investigation is rarely indicated. A chronic imbalance of the equation with energy intake (dietary calories) on the one hand and expenditure (resting metabolic rate + physical activity) on the other is thought to be responsible. Reduced levels of habitual activity allied to an abundance of energy-dense foods appears to account for the current pandemic of obesity and related disorders:

- Impaired glucose regulation.
- Type 2 DM.
- Dyslipidaemia.
- Hypertension.
- CVD.
- Osteoarthritis.
- Impaired physical functioning.
- Gout.
- ↑ Surgical risk.
- Depression.
- Certain cancers, e.g. bowel, breast.

Weight gain tends to occur in middle age; ♀ are more at risk than ♂. Socioeconomic factors are also important.

Specific causes

Genetic

E.g. Prader–Willi syndrome, Laurence–Moon (Biedl–Bardet) syndrome.

Single gene defects
E.g. mutations of leptin (provides feedback from adipocytes to hypothalamus about body fat stores) or its hypothalamic receptor (very rare).

Hypothalamic lesions
Lesions which damage the ventromedial nucleus (the 'satiety' area) may lead to obesity.

Lesions include
- Trauma.
- Tumours—craniopharyngiomas and astrocytomas.
- Inflammation—such as TB and meningitis.
- Infiltration—histiocytosis and sarcoidosis.

Cushing's syndrome
With 'buffalo' hump and central obesity.

Hypothyroidism
Disputed unless severe myxoedema, but hyperthyroidism is associated with unphysiological weight loss.

Insulinoma
Often associated with moderate weight gain; rare.

Marked ↓ motor inactivity
E.g. severe mental retardation or physical disability.

Investigations
- Weight (calibrated scales).
- Height (stadiometer).
- Waist circumference (maximal).
- BP (large cuff required).
- Venous plasma glucose (or OGTT).
- TFTs.
- LFTs (↑ non-alcoholic steatohepatitis in obese subjects).
- Fasting lipid profile (📖p184).
- Serum urate.

Additional investigations
These may occasionally be indicated if clinical features give cause for suspicion of organic cause
- Cranial CT or MRI of pituitary and hypothalamus.
- Investigations for Cushing's syndrome (📖p126).
- Genetic testing (seek advice of genetics service).

Lean MEJ, Han TS, Seidell JC. (1998) Impairment of health and quality of life in men and women with a larger waist. *Lancet* **351**, 853–856.

Oliguria

Causes
Acute renal failure: distinguish pre-renal from renal and post-renal causes.

Pre-renal
- Severe sepsis.
- Hypovolaemia, e.g. GI haemorrhage, diuretics.
- Burn injury.
- CCF.
- Addison's disease.
- Acute pancreatitis.

Renal
- Acute tubular necrosis (ATN, e.g. $2°$ to nephrotoxins such as aminoglycosides and radiological contrast media).
- Acute cortical necrosis.
- Renal infarction.
- Accelerated hypertension.
- Salicylate overdose.
- Hepatorenal syndrome.

Post-renal
- Renal calculi.
- Retroperitoneal calcinosis.
- Papillary necrosis.
- Bladder, prostate and cervical tumours.
- Blocked urinary catheter (common!).

Investigations
- U&E.
- Serum creatinine.
- Creatinine clearance.
- FBC.
- ESR.
- Autoimmune profile.
- LFTs.
- Urinary Na^+ excretion (<20 pre-renal, >40 ATN).
- Urine osmolality (>500mOsmol/L = re-renal, <350mOsmol/L = ATN).
- Urine dipstick for blood, protein, nitrites, leucocytes.
- Urine microscopy for casts.
- Renal ultrasound ($\pm$ biopsy in selected cases).
- IV urogram.
- CT pelvis.
- Investigation of renal stones:
  - Serum calcium, phosphorus.
  - 24h excretion of oxalate, calcium, creatinine.

⊞OHCM pp78, 257, 272, 458.

Palpitations

Patients generally use the term palpitations to refer to an awareness of an abnormally fast, forceful or irregular heart rhythm. Palpitations can be physiological, as in the fast and/or forceful heart rhythm felt with exercise or anxiety, or pathological.

Common arrhythmias

Supraventricular arrhythmias

- Sinus tachycardia (☐see *Causes of sinus tachycardia*, p193).
- Atrial fibrillation.
- Atrial flutter.
- Atrial tachycardia.
- AV re-entry tachycardias.
- Supraventricular ectopics.

Ventricular arrhythmias

- Ventricular tachycardia.
- Torsades de pointes.
- Ventricular ectopics.

Investigations

The key to diagnosis is to record a 12-lead ECG while the palpitations are present. Although simple in principle, infrequent paroxysmal palpitations can make this very challenging. A 12-lead ECG is mandatory and may provide an immediate diagnosis if the patient is experiencing palpitations as it is performed. As well as assessing the heart rhythm, it is important to inspect the 12-lead ECG for evidence of abnormal atrioventricular conduction (short PR interval, pre-excitation) or abnormal repolarisation (long QT interval). Check also for evidence of underlying structural heart disease, e.g. pathological Q waves indicative of previous myocardial infarction.

If the patient's palpitations are paroxysmal, a number of ambulatory ECG monitoring techniques are available:

- 24 hour ambulatory ECG monitoring.
- Cardiac event monitoring.
- Implantable loop recorder.

The choice of technique should be guided by how frequently the palpitations occur.

Additional investigations depend upon the nature of the suspected arrhythmia. It is generally prudent to check

- FBC.
- U&E.
- TFTs.

One may also consider

- CXR (to assess heart size and valvular calcification).
- Echocardiogram (if structural heart disease suspected).
- Exercise treadmill test (if IHD suspected, or to provoke arrhythmias thought to be exercise-related).

☐OHCM p78.

Pancytopenia

Pancytopenia (↓Hb, ↓WBC and ↓platelets) may occur because of bone marrow failure (hypoplasia) or inefficient production (MDS) or peripheral destruction of cells or sequestration (splenomegaly/hypersplenism).

▶▶*Pancytopenia usually means something is seriously wrong.*

Bone marrow assessment is necessary to establish whether the marrow is hypocellular or hypercellular in the face of peripheral blood pancytopenia. If hypercellular, the cause may be an infiltrative process (due to leukaemia/carcinoma, granulomatous disease, fibrosis–myelofibrosis, osteosclerotic–osteopetrosis, increased macrophages–haemophagocytic syndromes due to viral infections). Causes of hypoplastic bone marrow failure may be hereditary (e.g. Fanconi's anaemia) or acquired (e.g. drugs). Critically ill patients may develop pancytopenia for multiple reasons (sepsis, haemorrhage, DIC).

Investigations

- FBC, film (aplastic anaemia usually presents with ↓ lymphocyte count but minor morphological changes).
- Reticulocytes (↓ if production failure).
- Serum vitamin B_{12}, folate (megaloblastic anaemia can be associated with pancytopenia).
- Serology for EBV, hepatitis A, B, C, HIV (associated with aplastic anaemia).
- Serology for parvovirus infection (if pure red cell aplasia also consider lymphoma, thymoma).
- ANA (lupus).
- NAP score (↑ in aplastic anaemia).
- Check for lymphadenopathy, hepatomegaly, splenomegaly.
- CXR (bronchial carcinoma, sarcoid, tuberculosis, lymphoma).
- USS/CT to assess lymphadenopathy/splenomegaly (pancytopenia may be due to hypersplenism and portal hypertension).
- Ham's test for paroxysmal nocturnal haemoglobinuria (PNH) or cell marker analysis of CD55 and CD59.
- BM aspirate and cytogenetics (myelodysplasia is a clonal disorder).

📖 OHCM p662.

Paraesthesiae

This may be described by the patient as an abnormal sensation of aching, pricking, tickling or tingling commonly in the extremities or face. Often described as feeling like 'pins and needles'.

The selection of investigations will be determined largely by the history (transient? chronic?), the surface anatomical site of the abnormal sensation and associated symptoms or precipitating factors (e.g. clear history of hyperventilation).

The common causes include the numbness or tingling associated with pressure on the peripheral nerves such as caused by sleeping awkwardly on an arm ('Saturday night palsy' of the radial nerve), or chronic or recurrent pressure, e.g. on the ulnar nerve at the elbow.

If paraesthesiae is persistent, consider the following conditions, depending on the distribution of the symptoms

- Carpal tunnel syndrome (with radiation proximally along forearm; worse at night).
- Peripheral neuropathy (DM, alcohol, drug-induced, 📖OHCM section 10).
- Sciatica (reduced straight leg raising).
- Meralgia paraesthetica (lateral cutaneous nerve of the thigh).
- Lateral popliteal palsy (common peroneal nerve).

Other less common causes include

Peripheral neuropathy due to
- DM.
- Vitamin B_1 or B_{12} deficiencies.
- Chronic renal failure.
- Chronic hepatic failure.
- Malignancy.
- Neurotoxic drugs:
  - Vinca alkaloids.
  - Metronidazole.
  - Nitrofurantoin.
  - Isoniazid (pyridoxine-dependent).
- Environmental toxins.
- Hypothyroidism.
- Guillain–Barré syndrome (acute).
- Certain porphyrias.
- Multiple sclerosis.

Acute hypocalcaemia causes a characteristic perioral paraesthesia and can be due to many causes including 1° and 2° hypoparathyroidism and alkalosis.

General investigations

- ABGs (acute or chronic acid–base disturbances leading to alterations in ionised Ca^{2+}).
- Serum calcium (not all laboratories measure ionised Ca^{2+}).
- Serum PTH (uncuffed sample).
- Serum magnesium (see *below*).
- Venous plasma glucose.
- Vitamin B_{12} (and other investigations in suspected chronic peripheral neuropathy).

If serum calcium or magnesium concentration is low, identify cause
- Chronic GI loss (fistula, excessive diarrhoea, bowel obstruction).
- Chronic renal loss (diuretic drugs, intrinsic renal disease).
- Diabetic ketoacidosis (DKA)—total body magnesium may be low but this very rarely causes symptoms.

Additional investigations
- Urinary $[Mg^{2+}]$.

Consider
- USS abdomen/renal tract and subsequent GI investigations.
- U&E.
- Nerve conduction studies.
- TFTs.
- IGF-1, GH response during 75g OGTT (if features of acromegaly present; 📖p122).

Peripheral neuropathy

The patient will complain of numbness in hands and feet that progresses proximally in a distribution classically termed 'glove and stocking'. Different aetiologies lead to motor, sensory or mixed sensorimotor picture.

Common causes
- Idiopathic (50%, most common).
- Diabetes mellitus.
- Vitamin B_{12} deficiency (may occur in absence of anaemia).
- Vitamin B deficiency (e.g. alcoholics).
- Vitamin E deficiency.
- Carcinomatous neuropathy.
- Drugs, e.g. isoniazid, vinca alkaloids, cisplatin, dapsone, gold, metronidazole.
- Paraproteinaemias (e.g. MGUS or myeloma).

Rarer causes
- Amyloidosis.
- Uraemia.
- Collagen vascular diseases, e.g. rheumatoid, SLE, PAN.
- Endocrine disease, e.g. myxoedema, acromegaly.
- Guillain–Barré syndrome.
- Infections, e.g. tetanus, leprosy, diphtheria, botulism.
- Sarcoidosis.
- Hereditary, e.g. Charcot–Marie–Tooth disease.
- Acute intermittent porphyria.
- Toxins, e.g. lead (predominantly motor), arsenic (mixed sensory and motor), mercury (sensory) and thallium (mixed sensory and motor).
- Chronic inflammatory demyelinating polyneuropathy.
- Hereditary motor and sensory neuropathy types I or II.

Investigations
- Nerve conduction studies to confirm the diagnosis.

Further investigations
- In order to determine the underlying cause.
- Discuss with neurology staff.

📖OHCM pp336, 390.

Peripheral oedema

Swelling of the legs or peripheral oedema is a common presenting symptom, which occurs when excess tissue fluid is redistributed by gravity. Severe oedema is usually pathological and swelling of the ankles may progress to ascites and even pleural and pericardial effusion.

Causes of generalised swelling
- Cardiac failure: congestive heart failure, dilated cardiomyopathy, constrictive pericarditis, cor pulmonale.
- Hypoalbuminaemia: liver failure (hepatic cirrhosis), renal failure (nephrotic syndrome), protein-losing enteropathy, malnutrition (malabsorption or starvation).

Causes of localised swelling
- Immobility: common in old age, long distance travel.
- Infection: cellulitis.
- Deep vein thrombosis and/or subsequent venous insufficiency.
- Drugs: calcium channel blockers (nifedipine, amlodipine), NSAIDs.
- Malignancy: compression of deep vein, enlarged lymph nodes or lymphatics.
- Lymphatic obstruction: congenital, infiltrative (filariasis).
- Milroy's disease.
- Pregnancy.
- Wet beri-beri.
- Idiopathic.

Patients at special risk
- Pregnancy.
- Prolonged bed rest.
- Following removal of lower limb plaster cast.
- Relative immobility: long-distance travel.
- Congestive cardiac failure.

Investigations
These should be guided by the history and examination.
- FBC.
- U&E.
- Albumin.
- ESR.
- Blood cultures.
- ECG.
- Echocardiography.
- Doppler studies of leg veins/contrast venography (according to local availability).
- Abdominal ultrasound.
- Malignancy screen for common cancers.
- Urine dipstick for proteinuria.
- 24h urinary protein excretion or urine protein/creatinine ratio.
- Small bowel biopsy.
- Xylose breath test.

Petechiae & thrombocytopenia

Spontaneous bleeding in the absence of trauma is uncommon with platelet counts >20 × 10^9/L. However, bleeding is much more likely if the thrombocytopenia is not immune in origin (e.g. aplastic anaemia, acute leukaemia, drug-induced, chemotherapy, myelodysplasia).

Thrombocytopenia may be inherited or acquired (e.g. DIC). As for pancytopenia, these may be classified as due to a failure of production, increased consumption in the peripheries (DIC, ITP) or due to abnormal tissue distribution (splenomegaly).

Idiopathic thrombocytopenic purpura (ITP) may be 1° or 2° (e.g. lymphoma, lupus, HIV).

Drugs (e.g. heparin) and blood transfusion (post-transfusion purpura) may cause severe thrombocytopenia.

Investigations

- FBC, film:
  - Inherited causes may be associated with giant platelets.
  - Morphological abnormalities may suggest MDS.
  - Red cell fragments suggest thrombotic microangiopathies, e.g. TTP.
- LDH (↑ in TTP and lymphoproliferative disorders).
- Serum vitamin B_{12}, folate (megaloblastic anaemia can be associated with ↓ platelets).
- ANA, autoimmune screen, immunoglobulins (lupus, hyperthyroidism).
- Virology (HIV, EBV, viral hepatitis, CMV).
- Clotting screen (DIC).
- Lupus anticoagulant, cardiolipin antibodies (antiphospholipid antibody syndromes).
- Platelet serology for drug- or transfusion-related causes.
- Bone marrow assessment to establish whether thrombocytopenia is due to a bone marrow production problem or due to peripheral consumption (discuss with haematology team: depending on degree of thrombocytopenia, other haematological findings and age of patient, a marrow may not be required).

Pitfalls

Thrombocytopenia due to HIV infection must be considered especially in all younger adults. Not worth checking platelet-associated IgG or IgM since these are elevated in thrombocytopenia caused by immune and non-immune mechanisms, so add no useful information.

Plethora

A plethoric appearance is typically seen in association with polycythaemia but may also be mistaken for a normal outdoors complexion or cyanosis. Patients with haematocrits above the normal reference range may or may not have an increased red cell mass (real or relative polycythaemia respectively).

Investigations
- FBC, film (repeat FBC as sampling errors can falsely cause elevations of Hb; PRV may be associated with neutrophilia, basophilia or ↑ platelets).
- Measurement of red cell mass may be necessary to confirm true polycythaemia.
  - Investigations are then aimed at establishing whether real poly-cythaemia, if documented, is due to a 1° bone marrow abnormality (PRV) or a 2° disorder (e.g. respiratory disease).
- Neutrophil alkaline phosphatase score (may be raised in PRV). Seldom used now (📖NAP score, p258).
- Vitamin B_{12} and urate (may be ↑ in PRV).
- ESR/CRP (acute phase reactants may suggest secondary causes).
- Blood gas analysis, oxygen saturation, carboxyhaemoglobin levels (2° polycythaemia due to respiratory disease, smoking).
- Biochemistry (urea, creatinine; renal disease).
- Erythropoietin (↑ in 2° causes).
- USS abdomen (renal cysts, liver disease, uterine fibroids and other malignancies may 'inappropriately' secrete erythropoietin; also check for splenomegaly in PRV).
- Sleep studies (obstructive sleep apnoea, supine desaturation).
- O_2-dissociation studies (polycythaemia due to abnormal, high affinity Hb variant).
- Bone marrow aspirate and chromosomal studies/cytogenetics (PRV is a clonal disorder).

Table 1.13 Polycythaemia

↑ red cell count	$>6.0 \times 10^{12}$/L	♂
	$>5.5 \times 10^{12}$/L	♀
↑ PCV	>50%	♂
	>45%	♀
↑ Hb	>18.0g/dL	♂
	>16.0g/dL	♀

Polyuria

Polyuria (the passage of an excessive volume of urine, which may be associated with frequency of micturition and nocturia) must be differenti-ated from urinary symptoms associated with prostatic disease and urinary infections. The latter are also characterised by frequency, urgency and nocturia, but usually small amounts of urine are passed at each void.

Causes include
- DM.
- Cranial DI (📖OHCM section 9):
  - Familial (autosomal dominant).
  - Secondary to posterior pituitary or hypothalamic disease, e.g. surgery, tumours, especially metastases, neurosarcoidosis.

- Nephrogenic DI:
    - Familial (X-linked recessive).
    - Chronic intrinsic renal disease, e.g. pyelonephritis.
    - Hypokalaemia.
    - Hypercalcaemia.
    - Sickle cell crisis.
    - Lithium, colchicine, amphotericin B.
    - Post-obstructive uropathy.
- Primary polydipsia (psychogenic).

Investigations
- 24h urinary volume.
- Venous plasma glucose.
- U&E.
- TFTs.
- LH.
- FSH (?panhypopituitarism).
- Serum calcium and PTH.
- Sickle cell test.
- CXR (?mediastinal lymphadenopathy in TB, sarcoidosis).

If no obvious cause found consider detailed investigations for cranial or nephrogenic DI (📖p118).

📖OHCM p80.

Pruritus

Implies generalised itching and may be associated with many disorders including
- Iron deficiency.
- Malignant disease, e.g. lymphoma.
- Diabetes mellitus.
- Chronic renal failure.
- Liver disease, e.g. primary biliary cirrhosis.
- Thyroid disease.
- Polycythaemia rubra vera.
- HIV infection.

Investigations
- Aim to exclude the above diseases.
- FBC.
- Biochemistry screen, including LFTs and renal function.
- Glucose.
- TFTs.

📖OHCM pp80, 438.

Ptosis

Ptosis can be unilateral and bilateral. Bilateral ptosis can be more difficult to recognise. Ptosis must be considered in association with other signs and symptoms. Ptosis may be long-standing, of recent onset, progressive or intermittent, especially at the end of the day—myasthenia gravis (MG).

Unilateral ptosis

Causes
- Constitutional (congenital).
- Oculomotor (III) nerve palsy—levator palpebrae. 'Down and out' pupil with loss of light reflex (e.g. DM, SOL, demyelination).
- Aneurysm (basilar or posterior communicating arteries).
- Cavernous sinus disease.
- Meningitis.
- Horner's syndrome—superior tarsal muscle (brainstem infarction, syringobulbia, SOL, MS).
- Encephalitis.

If abnormal (reduced) sweating on ipsilateral side face (damage to cervical sympathetic chain)
- Pancoast's tumour.
- Aortic arch aneurysm.
- Cervical injuries.

No disorder of sweating
- Cluster headache.
- Parasellar tumours.
- Carotid artery aneurysm or dissection.
- Nasopharyngeal tumours.

Investigations
- Venous plasma glucose.
- CXR (Pancoast's syndrome).
- Cranial CT or MRI.
- Cerebral angiography (aneurysm).

Bilateral ptosis

Causes
- Guillain–Barré syndrome (Miller–Fisher syndrome).
- Myotonic dystrophy (MD).
- Myasthenia gravis (MG).
- Neurosyphilis (bilateral; Argyll Robertson pupils).

Investigations
- Syphilis serology.
- EMG ('dive-bomber' in MD).
- Serum anti-acetylcholine receptor antibodies (MG).
- Intravenous edrophonium (Tensilon) test (MG, 📖p552).

📖OHCM p80.

Pulmonary embolism

Occurs when thrombus in systemic veins or the right side of the heart embolises into the pulmonary arterial system. Impaired gas exchange occurs because of a mismatch between ventilation and perfusion.

Investigations

- FBC (may be leucocytosis, neutrophilia most likely).
- ESR (often ↑).
- Plasma D-dimers: ↑ with fresh thrombus.
- ABGs: hypoxia and hypocapnia.
- ECG: look for AF. Usually sinus tachycardia, may be evidence of RV 'strain'. In massive PE there may be $S_1Q_3T_3$.
- CXR: often normal but may show signs of pulmonary infarction or effusion.
- V/Q scan (may be useful for detection of areas of the lungs that are being ventilated but not perfused).
- Spiral CT scan: useful for detection of medium-sized pulmonary emboli but does not exclude small PEs.

📖OHCM pp180, 802.

Pulse character

Rate and heart rhythm can be determined from palpation of the radial pulse. The arm should then be elevated to check for a collapsing pulse. Pulse volume and additional characteristics are assessed from palpation of the brachial or carotid pulse (see Table 1.14).

Table 1.14

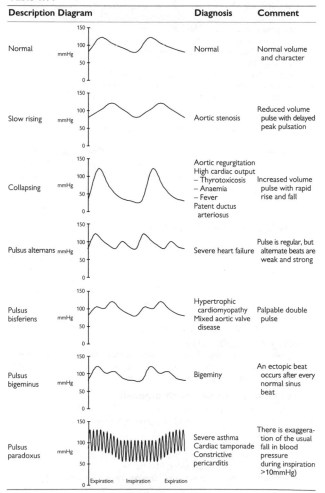

Description	Diagram	Diagnosis	Comment
Normal		Normal	Normal volume and character
Slow rising		Aortic stenosis	Reduced volume pulse with delayed peak pulsation
Collapsing		Aortic regurgitation High cardiac output – Thyrotoxicosis – Anaemia – Fever Patent ductus arteriosus	Increased volume pulse with rapid rise and fall
Pulsus alternans		Severe heart failure	Pulse is regular, but alternate beats are weak and strong
Pulsus bisferiens		Hypertrophic cardiomyopathy Mixed aortic valve disease	Palpable double pulse
Pulsus bigeminus		Bigeminy	An ectopic beat occurs after every normal sinus beat
Pulsus paradoxus		Severe asthma Cardiac tamponade Constrictive pericarditis	There is exaggeration of the usual fall in blood pressure during inspiration >10mmHg)

Purpura

Implies bleeding of varying degrees into the skin. Includes petechial haemorrhages (pinpoint) and ecchymoses (bruises). There are many causes including disorders of platelets and blood vessels.

Causes

- Congenital, e.g. Osler–Weber–Rendu syndrome (= hereditary haemorrhagic telangiectasia), connective tissue (Ehlers–Danlos), osteogenesis imperfecta, Marfan's.
- Severe infection (septic, meningococcal, measles, typhoid).
- Allergic, e.g. Henoch–Schönlein purpura.
- Drugs, e.g. steroids.
- Miscellaneous, e.g. senile purpura, scurvy, factitious.
- Thrombocytopenia—any cause (immune, marrow infiltration, deficiency of vitamin B_{12} or folate, myelofibrosis, DIC, TTP/HUS).

Investigations

- FBC (looking for platelet abnormalities and presence of leukaemic cells or other signs of infiltration).
- Coagulation screen (looking for clotting factor deficiencies, DIC, etc.).
- Bleeding time using template device (previously used as test of platelet function but largely abandoned now because of poor reproducibility).

📖 OHCM pp282, 644, 726.

Recurrent thrombosis

The pathogenesis (and hence causes) of thrombosis reflect abnormalities in the dynamics of the circulation, the blood vessel walls or the blood constituents (Virchow's triad). A hypercoagulable or thrombophilic risk factor is an inherited or acquired disorder of the haemostatic mechanisms, which may be associated with an increased likelihood of a thrombotic event (venous or arterial) or recurrent thrombosis. This concept of risk factors for thrombosis is analogous to that for heart disease, and similarly for most patients *multiple causal factors operate*.

Hereditary thrombotic disease may be suggested by a positive family history but should be tested for if the venous thrombotic events occur in the absence of acquired causes, at a younger age, at unusual sites (e.g. mesenteric) or as recurrent thromboses.

Investigations in recurrent thrombosis

Inherited thrombophilia screening

- Deficiency of factors, e.g. protein C, protein S or antithrombin.
- Abnormal protein (FVL).
- Increased procoagulant (PT, VIII); others (homocysteinuria).
- Consider occult malignancy (PSA in ♂, pelvic USS in ♀).
- FBC (myeloproliferative disorder, PNH).
- Biochemistry (cardiac disease, liver disease, nephrotic syndrome).

- ESR/CRP (ulcerative colitis).
- ANA/lupus anticoagulant/cardiolipin antibodies (antiphospholipid antibody syndromes, lupus).

Table 1.15 Thromboembolic risk factors

Acquired	
Cardiac disease	MI, AF, cardiomyopathy, CCF
Post-op	Especially abdominal, pelvic or orthopaedic surgery
Pregnancy	
Malignancy	Any
Polycythaemia	
Immobilisation	Prolonged
Fractures	Especially hip and pelvis
Obesity	
Varicose veins	
Drugs	E.g. oestrogen-containing oral contraceptive
Inherited	Activated protein C resistance e.g. factor V Leiden mutation Protein C or S deficiency Dysfibrinogenaemias

Pitfalls

Thrombophilia testing may be complicated if the patient is on warfarin/heparin: discuss with lab before sending samples.

📖OHCM p672.

Retinal haemorrhage

May be

- Flame-shaped (e.g. hypertension).
- Dot & blot (e.g. diabetes mellitus, vein occlusion or haematological disease).
- Pre-retinal haemorrhage, suggests new vessel formation, e.g. diabetes or post-retinal vascular occlusion.
- Hyperviscosity syndromes.
- Severe anaemia.
- Severe thrombocytopenia.
- Haemoglobinopathy, e.g. HbSC.

Investigations

- Check BP.
- Renal function.
- FBC (↑↑ Hb or platelets).

- ESR or plasma viscosity (hyperviscosity syndromes such as myeloma or Waldenström's macroglobulinaemia).
- Serum Igs and protein electrophoresis.
- Hb electrophoresis.

Rigors

Fever is due to a resetting of the anterior hypothalamic thermostat, is mediated by prostaglandins (hence aspirin is beneficial), and is most commonly caused by infection. Large variations in temperature may be accompanied by sweats, chills and rigors. An undulant fever may suggest Hodgkin's disease or brucellosis. 'B' symptoms define fever (>38°C), night sweats (drenching), weight loss (>10%) and suggest a diagnosis of lymphoma. (Fever is unusual in CLL in the absence of infection.)

Investigations
- FBC, film (Hodgkin's disease is associated with anaemia, neutrophilia, eosinophilia, lymphopenia).
- LDH (↑ in lymphoma, non-specific test).
- Microbiological tests, blood/urine cultures (also consider pyogenic infection and abscesses in more unusual sites, e.g. renal).
- Antigen detection tests for specific pathogens.
- CXR (tuberculosis, lymphoma).
- ANA (connective tissue disease).
- BM aspirate/trephine may be necessary as part of leukaemia and lymphoma work-up.

Pitfalls
Not all fever is caused by infection.

📖 OHCM pp82, 552, 554.

Short stature

The assessment of short stature can be a long and difficult process. Constitutional short stature is the most common cause. Psychosocial disease must be considered, but extensive investigation is required to rule out organic disease. If no cause is found, a period of observation may make the underlying cause apparent. Specialist evaluation should be undertaken in all cases.

Causes
Endocrine
- Growth hormone (GH) deficiency.
- GH resistance (very rare).
- Hypothyroidism (readily treatable).
- Cushing's syndrome (rare in children—*Note*: corticosteroid treatment for chronic asthma).
- Rickets.

- Pseudohypoparathyroidism.
- Type 1 DM—Mauriac's syndrome, now rare.

Non-endocrine
- Constitutional short stature (short parents).
- Emotional deprivation.
- Intrauterine growth retardation.
- Achondroplasia.
- Mucopolysaccharidoses (rare).
- Turner's syndrome (46 XO and variants).
- Noonan's syndrome (46 XY but features of Turner's in a male).
- Congenital cardiac disease, e.g. left-to-right shunt, cardiac failure.
- Cystic fibrosis.
- Other causes of malabsorption, e.g. coeliac disease, Crohn's colitis.
- Chronic liver disease.
- Haematological disease, e.g. sickle cell disease.
- Chronic renal disease.

Investigations
- Current height + weight (compare to any previous data available;
  plot on growth charts).
- Growth velocity—normal if prior problem, e.g. intrauterine growth
  retardation.
- Physical stigmata of physical disease. *Note*: CNS examination
  mandatory.
- FBC.
- ESR.
- U&E.
- LFTs.
- TFTs.
- Serum albumin (?nutritional status).
- Venous plasma glucose.
- Serum calcium.
- Serum alkaline phosphatase (bone isoenzyme).
- Serum phosphate (reduced in rickets).
- X-ray pelvis (Looser's zones), epiphyses (wide, irregular in rickets),
  ribs (multiple fractures).
- Serum antigliadin and antiendomysial antibodies (coeliac).
- Testosterone or oestradiol, LH, FSH, PRL (if puberty delayed—
  panhypopituitarism?).
- X-ray of wrist for bone age. If delayed, measure serum IGF-1 (if IGF-1
  normal, then GH deficiency unlikely; if IGF-1 low, consider nutritional
  and general health status before diagnosing GH deficiency—stimulation
  tests required, p158). If normal—constitutional short stature.
- Karyotype (Turner's and Noonan's syndromes).
- 24h urinary free cortisol (as screen for Cushing's syndrome, p126).
- CT or MRI of pituitary (if GH deficiency or panhypopituitarism).

Skin pigmentation

Skin pigmentation can be due to increased melanin deposition, e.g. racial differences in skin pigmentation or due to ↑ melanin deposition seen in sun exposure. Lentigines and freckles are common. Haemosiderin and other substances can ↑ skin pigmentation. Increased pigmentation can be seen in various dermatological conditions; chronic inflammation and fungal infection can result in increased skin pigmentation. Lichen planus and fixed drug eruptions are associated with increased pigmentation.

Increased pigmentation may also be found in association with chronic systemic disease

- Addison's disease (palmar creases, buccal pigmentation, recent scars).
- Porphyria cutanea tarda (especially exposed areas—dorsum of hands).
- Chronic malabsorption syndromes.
- Drugs, e.g. amiodarone, psoralens, mepacrine, minocycline, chloroquine.
- Chronic uraemia.
- Haemochromatosis (so-called 'bronzed diabetes').
- Primary biliary cirrhosis (deep green-yellow jaundice, chronic pruritus).
- Ectopic ACTH syndrome, e.g. bronchial carcinoma.
- Nelson's syndrome (excessive ACTH secretion from pituitary basophil adenoma in Cushing's disease treated by bilateral adrenalectomy).
- Carotenaemia (orange discoloration does not involve sclerae cf. jaundice).
- Chloasma (pregnancy, oestrogen-containing oral contraceptive pill).
- Acanthosis nigricans—most often a marker of insulin resistance in obese patients with type 2 DM. Rarely in association with underlying carcinoma.
- Peutz–Jegher's syndrome (fingers, lips in association with small intestine polyposis).

Contrast with hypopigmentation

- Localised acquired depigmentation (vitiligo) is a marker of auto-immune disease.
- Oculocutaneous albinism (autosomal recessive).
- Chronic hypopituitarism (🕮p112).
- Phenylketonuria.

Investigations

- FBC.
- U&E.
- Venous plasma glucose.
- Antigliadin and antiendomysial antibodies.
- Short synacthen test (if 1° hypoadrenalism suspected, 🕮p193).
- Urinary porphyrins.
- LFTs, serum albumin and prothrombin time (INR).
- Fe/TIBC/ferritin + genetic markers for haemochromatosis + liver biopsy.
- ESR and/or CRP.
- Autoimmune profile (🕮Ch4).
- Testosterone (or oestradiol) + LH, FSH.
- Antimitochondrial antibodies, liver Bx (1° biliary cirrhosis).
- Investigations for Cushing's syndrome (🕮p126).
- Investigations for causes of chronic renal failure.

Splenomegaly

A palpable spleen is at least twice its normal size, when its length >14cm. Enlargement may represent changes in the white pulp (lymphoid tissue expansion, inflammation), red pulp (blood congestion, extramedullary haemopoiesis) or occasionally supporting structures (cysts).

Cause in Western societies
- Leukaemias.
- Lymphomas.
- Myeloproliferative disorders.
- Haemolytic anaemias.
- Portal hypertension.
- Infections, e.g. infective endocarditis, typhoid, TB, brucellosis, viral (EBV, viral hepatitis).

Less common causes
- Storage disorders (e.g. Gaucher's).
- Collagen diseases.
- Sarcoid.
- Amyloid.

If foreign residence, consider infectious causes (malaria, leishmaniasis, schistosomiasis) and haemoglobinopathies (HbC, HbE, thalassaemia).

Massive splenomegaly (>8cm palpable below LCM)
- Myelofibrosis.
- CML.
- Gaucher's.
- Malaria.
- Leishmaniasis.

Investigations
Thorough history and physical examination.
- FBC, blood film, LDH (leukaemia, lymphoma, pernicious anaemia).
- Reticulocytes, bilirubin (if ↑ suggests haemolysis).
- Virology/microbiology (sepsis, bacterial endocarditis, EBV, CMV).
- Serum protein electrophoresis (myeloma, amyloid).
- Autoantibody screen, ANA (collagen disease, lupus, RA).
- Haemoglobinopathy screen.
- LFTs (splenomegaly may be associated with hepatomegaly, or due to portal hypertension).
- Peripheral blood cell markers (immunophenotype—may show leukaemia or lymphoma).
- BM aspirate/trephine/cell markers/cytogenetics.
- Leucocyte glucocerebrosidase activity (Gaucher's disease).
- USS to assess liver texture, splenomegaly, lymphadenopathy.

OHCM pp458, 671, 673.

Steatorrhoea

Implies that the patient is passing pale, bulky stools that are offensive (contain fat and tend to float) and are difficult to flush away.

Causes
- Any disorder that prevents absorption of micellar fat from the small bowel.
- Ileal disease.
- Ileal resection.
- Parenchymal liver disease.
- Obstructive jaundice.
- Pancreatic disease, including cystic fibrosis.
- ↓ bile salt concentration.
- Bile salt deconjugation by bacteria.
- Cholestyramine.
- β-lipoprotein deficiency.
- Lymphatic obstruction.

Investigations
Blood tests
- LFTs.
- Bone profile.
- Vitamin B_{12} and serum (or red cell) folate.
- Autoantibody profile.
- Serum amylase.

Pancreatic investigations
- Pancreatic function tests.
- CT scan.

Small bowel
- Small bowel follow-through.
- Jejunal biopsy (?villus atrophy).
- Bacterial overgrowth (^{14}C glycocholate breath test).

Parasites
- Stool culture (e.g. *Giardia*).

Ileal disease
- Consider Crohn's.

📖 OHCM pp218, 252.

Stridor

Stridor denotes a harsh respiratory added sound during inspiration. It may be a high-pitched musical sound similar to wheeze but arises from constriction of the larynx or trachea. Stridor may be aggravated by coughing.

▶▶Progressive breathlessness accompanied by indrawing of intercostal spaces and cyanosis indicates severe laryngeal obstruction with risk of sudden death.

In young children

Because of the smaller size of the larynx and trachea in children, stridor may occur in a variety of conditions.

- Postural stridor (laryngomalacia).
- Allergy, e.g. nut allergy, insect stings—common. Note: emergency Rx with IM or SC adrenaline (epinephrine)—self-administered or by parent, and parenteral hydrocortisone.
- Vocal cord palsy.
- Croup (acute laryngitis—often coryza).
- Acute epiglottitis.
- Inhaled foreign body, e.g. peanut (common—inhalation further down the respiratory tract, usually into the right main bronchus, may produce localised wheeze or distal collapse, 📖pp662–663).

Investigations
- Pulse oximetry (non-invasive measurement of PO_2).
- Plain lateral x-ray of neck (for radio-opaque foreign body).
- Endoscopic nasolaryngoscopy.

Adults

- Infection especially *Haemophilus influenzae*.
- Inflammatory or allergic laryngeal oedema, e.g. penicillin allergy (*see above*); may be accompanied by anaphylactic shock.
- Pharyngeal pouch (may be recurrent lower respiratory tract infection).
- Inhaled vomitus or blood in unconscious patient.
- Tetany (due to low serum calcium or alkalosis, 📖OHCM section 17).
- Large multinodular goitre, carcinoma or lymphoma of thyroid (uncommon).
- Laryngeal tumours.
- Bronchogenic tumour with bilateral cord paralysis (subcarinal and paratracheal gland involvement. Note: 'Bovine' cough of right recurrent laryngeal nerve palsy).
- Shy–Drager syndrome (of autonomic neuropathy).

Investigations
- CXR.
- Lateral x-ray of neck.
- Ultrasound of thyroid.
- Endoscopic nasolaryngoscopy.
- Bronchoscopy.
- Barium swallow (pharyngeal pouch).
- CT neck and mediastinum.

📖OHCM p84.

Suspected bleeding disorder

Bleeding problems present a considerable challenge. Patients may present with simple easy bruising—a common problem—or catastrophic post-traumatic bleeding. The best predictors of bleeding risk are found in taking an accurate history, focusing on past haemostatic challenges (e.g. tonsillectomy, teeth extraction, menses—especially at time of menarche) and current drug history (e.g. aspirin). The history may also help delineate the type of defect. Platelet bleeding (e.g. thrombocytopenia) starts at the time of the (even minor) haemostatic insult but if controlled by local pressure tends not to recur. Bleeding due to coagulation factor deficiency tends to be associated with internal/deep muscle haematomas as the bleeding typically occurs in a delayed fashion after initial trauma and then persists.

Inappropriate bleeding or bruising may be due to a local factor or an underlying systemic haemostatic abnormality.

▶Acquired causes of bleeding are much more common than inherited causes.

Causes of bleeding include
- Surgical.
- Trauma.
- Non-accidental injury.
- Coagulation disorders.
- Platelet dysfunction.
- Vascular disorders.

Clinical features
History and presenting complaint. Is this an isolated symptom? What type of bleeding does the patient have—e.g. mucocutaneous, easy bruising, spontaneous, post-traumatic. Duration and time of onset—?recent or present in childhood. Menstrual and obstetrical history are important.

Systemic enquiry
Do the patient's symptoms suggest a systemic disorder, bone marrow failure, infection, liver disease, renal disease?

Past medical history
Previous episodes of bleeding, recurrent—?ITP, congenital disorder. Exposure to trauma, surgery, dental extraction or pregnancies.

Family history
First degree relatives. Pattern of inheritance (e.g. autosomal, sex-linked). If family history is negative this could be a new mutation (one-third of new haemophilia is due to new mutations).

Drugs
All drugs cause some side effects in some patients. Bleeding may result from thrombocytopenia, platelet dysfunction. Don't forget to ask about aspirin and warfarin.

Physical examination

Signs of systemic disease

Is there any evidence of septicaemia, anaemia, lymphadenopathy ± hepatosplenomegaly?

Assess bleeding site

Check palate and fundi. Could this be self-inflicted? Check size—petechiae (pin head); purpura (larger ≤1cm); bruises (ecchymoses; ≥1cm).

Joints

Swelling or other signs of chronic arthritis.

Vascular lesions

Purpura—allergic, Henoch–Schönlein, senile, steroid-related, hypergamma-globulinaemic, HHT—capillary dilatations (blanches on pressure), vascu-litic lesions, autoimmune disorders, hypersensitivity reactions.

Investigations

- FBC, film, platelet count, biochemistry screen, ESR, coagulation screen.
- Special tests, e.g. BM for 1° haematological disorders; radiology, USS.
- Family studies.

Suspected stroke

A stroke denotes an acute neurological deficit. Strokes may vary in presentation, e.g. rapidly resolving neurological deficit to a severe perma-nent or progressive neurological defect (e.g. multi-infarct disease). Neu-rological deficits persisting >24h termed 'completed stroke' cf. transient ischaemic attack (TIA). With suspected stroke, a full history and general physical examination are mandatory. Risk factors for cerebrovascular disease should be sought, including a history of hypertension (common—major risk factor), DM (common—major risk factor) and dyslipidaemia. Ask about recent falls or trauma. Hemiparesis can occur as a post-ictal phenomenon or a result of migraine or hypoglycaemia (*see below*). Hys-terical or functional paralysis is also seen but should not be confidently assumed at presentation. Neuroanatomical localisation of the deficit and the nature of the lesion(s) requires appropriate imaging. *Note*: the post-ictal state may be associated with temporary (<24h) limb paresis (Todd's paralysis) in focal epilepsy (suggests structural lesion—cranial imaging is mandatory).

General investigations

- FBC (polycythaemia, anaemia).
- U&E.
- ESR.
- Protein electrophoresis (if hyperviscosity syndrome suspected, e.g. ↑↑ ESR).
- ECG (atrial fibrillation, IHD—statins reduce risk of stroke in patients with previous MI).
- CXR (cerebral metastases from bronchogenic carcinoma?).

Specific risk factors

- Venous plasma glucose. *Note:* severe hypoglycaemia, e.g. insulin-induced or 2° to sulphonylureas, may mimic acute stroke. Always check capillary fingerprick glucose concentration to exclude this possibility—even if there is no history of DM. Take venous sample in fluoride-oxalate tube (+serum for insulin concentration) if hypoglycaemia confirmed. (See 📖p172 for further details of investigation and treatment.) Hyperosmolar non-ketotic diabetic coma may also be misdiagnosed as stroke (plasma glucose usually >50mmol/L with pre-renal uraemia.
- Thrombophilia screen (if indicated by clinical or haematological features).
- Lipid profile (not an immediate investigation; secondary prevention, see *above*).
- Blood cultures (if SBE or other sepsis suspected. *Note:* cerebral abscess).

Imaging

- Cranial CT scan (± IV contrast).
- Echocardiogram (if mural thrombus, endocarditis suspected).
- Carotid Doppler studies—may not be indicated if surgical intervention (endarterectomy) is unlikely because of poor prognosis, e.g. dense hemiplegia or coma.

Consider alternative diagnoses including

- Primary or secondary brain tumour (may present as acute stroke—search for primary).
- Cerebral abscess (usually clear evidence of sepsis).
- Cerebral lupus (ESR, autoantibodies).

📖OHCM pp354, 356.

Sweating

Fairly non-specific symptom, but one which may indicate serious underlying disease.

Causes

- Excess heat (physiological).
- Exercise (physiological).
- Fever—any cause.
- Anxiety.
- Thyrotoxicosis.
- Acromegaly.
- Diabetes mellitus.
- Lymphoproliferative disease, e.g. lymphomas.
- Cancer (any).
- Hypoglycaemia.
- Alcohol.
- Nausea.
- Gustatory.
- Neurological disease, e.g. lesions of sympathetic nervous system, cortex, basal ganglia or spinal cord.

Investigations
- FBC.
- ESR.
- Biochemistry screen including LFTs.
- Glucose.
- TFTs.
- Urinalysis and culture.
- Blood cultures.
- CXR.
- Further investigation depending on results of above.

Tachycardia

Tachycardia is arbitrarily defined as a heart rate above 100 beats per minute. It is a normal physiological response to exercise and to emotional stress, but can also herald a cardiac rhythm disorder. One should always begin by assessing the nature of the tachycardia and identifying any underlying cause or contributing factor.

Assessment begins with a 12-lead ECG, performed whilst the patient is tachycardic. This will enable the immediate identification of the heart rhythm. One must then differentiate between sinus tachycardia (which may or may not have a pathological cause) and tachycardias due to other (abnormal) cardiac rhythms.

Causes of sinus tachycardia
- Sympathetic stimulation, e.g. anxiety, pain, fear, fever, exercise.
- Drugs, e.g. adrenaline, atropine, salbutamol.
- Stimulants, e.g. caffeine, alcohol, amphetamines.
- Thyrotoxicosis.
- Heart failure.
- Pulmonary embolism.
- IHD, acute myocardial infarction.
- Anaemia.
- Blood or fluid loss, e.g. post-operative.
- Inappropriate sinus tachycardia (a persistent resting sinus tachycardia, diagnosed when all other possible causes have been excluded).

In assessing abnormal heart rhythms causing tachycardia, it is helpful to divide them into narrow-complex tachycardia (QRS duration <120msec) and broad-complex tachycardia (QRS duration >120msec).

Narrow-complex tachycardias
- Sinus tachycardia (see *above*).
- Atrial tachycardia.
- Atrial flutter.
- Atrial fibrillation.
- AV re-entry tachycardias.

Broad-complex tachycardias
- Narrow-complex tachycardia with aberrant conduction.
- Ventricular tachycardia.
- Accelerated idioventricular rhythm.
- Torsades de pointes.

Investigations
- 12-lead ECG to identify the underlying rhythm.
- Consider bedside monitoring on CCU, particularly if the patient is compromised or ventricular arrhythmias are suspected.
- Other investigations depend upon the underlying cause, but may include:
  - FBC.
  - U&E.
  - TFTs.
  - Cardiac markers.
  - CXR.
  - ABGs.
  - V/Q scan/CTPA.
  - Echocardiogram.
  - Exercise treadmill test.
  - Cardiac catheter.
  - Electrophysiological studies.

It can be useful to perform carotid sinus massage (▶ Exclude carotid bruits first) or to give IV adenosine (▶ Do not use in asthma/COPD) while the patient is on a bedside ECG monitor. Supraventricular tachycardias will usually slow transiently, allowing clearer identification of underlying atrial activity, and re-entry tachycardias may terminate altogether. Ventricular tachycardias will be unaffected.

📖 OHCM pp96, 128, 129, 132, 133, 791–792.

Tinnitus

Tinnitus is a common symptom in which the patient perceives a sound, often chronic and distressing, in the absence of aural stimulation. It usually manifests as a 'ringing' or 'buzzing' in the ears. Tinnitus may occur as a symptom of nearly all disorders of the auditory apparatus. Psychological stresses may be relevant in some cases.

Causes include
- Acoustic trauma (prolonged exposure to loud noise, e.g. gun shots, amplified music).
- Barotrauma (blast injury, perforated tympanic membrane).
- Obstruction of the external auditory meatus (wax, foreign body, infection).
- Otosclerosis.
- Menière's disease.
- Drug-induced ototoxicity.

- Gentamicin—may be irreversible.
- Acute salicylate toxicity.
- Quinine toxicity.
- Acute alcohol poisoning.
- Hypothyroidism.
- Hypertension (rare symptom).
- Intra- or extracranial aneurysm (typically cause 'pulsatile' tinnitus).
- Glomus jugulare tumours.

Note: consider acoustic neuroma in unilateral tinnitus (OHCM section 10).

Investigations
- FBC.
- Serum concentrations of e.g. salicylates, gentamicin (▶mandatory during systemic therapy).
- TFTs.
- BP.

Audiological assessment
Specialist investigations include
- Assess air and bone conduction thresholds.
- Tympanometry and acoustic reflex testing.
- Speech perception thresholds.

Consider
- CT temporal bone (acoustic neuroma).
- Cranial MRI (following specialist advice).

OHCM p348.

Tiredness

Tiredness is a common presenting complaint in the endocrine clinic. Important diagnoses to exclude are hypo/hyperthyroidism, hypoadrenalism, hypercalaemia, diabetes mellitus. A U&E is useful to exclude hyponatraemia or hypokalaemia (muscle weakness) as well as renal failure.

Recommended investigations for tiredness in the absence of an obvious cause from history and examination
- TSH.
- FT4.
- Synacthen test.
- Serum Ca^{2+}.
- Glucose.
- U&E, creatinine.
- FBC.
- ESR (or CRP).
- LFTs.

Urgency of micturition

Urgency of micturition denotes a strong desire to void and the patient often has to rush to the toilet because of an acute call to micturate. Urinary incontinence may result, especially if physical mobility is impaired. Urgency forms part of a cluster of symptoms which include frequency of micturition (📖p77), nocturia and hesitancy of micturition.

Men

- Prostatic disease.
- Urinary tract infection.
- Bladder irritability.
- Urethritis.
- States of polyuria (📖p77); may lead to urinary incontinence (📖p54).

Investigations to consider

- Urinalysis—stick test for glucose, protein, blood, nitrites.
- MSU for microscopy and culture.
- FBC.
- U&E.
- Venous plasma glucose.
- ESR.
- Serum PSA.
- PSA is increased in 30–50% of patients with benign prostatic hyperplasia, and in 25–92% of those with prostate cancer (depending on tumour volume), i.e. a normal PSA does not exclude prostatic disease. Check reference range with local laboratory.
- Transrectal USS of prostate.
- Prostatic biopsy (specialist procedure).

Women

- Urinary tract infection.
- Gynaecological disease, e.g. pelvic floor instability, uterine prolapse.
- Bladder irritability.
- Urethritis.
- States of polyuria; may lead to urinary incontinence (📖p54).

Investigations to consider

- FBC.
- U&E.
- MSU for microscopy and culture.
- Urodynamic studies.

📖OHCM pp52, 500–501.

Urticaria

Itchy superficial wheals; may be giant. Distinguish acute from chronic: chronic is rarely allergic in origin. If persists >24h and fade with brown staining consider urticarial vasculitis (rare).

Causes

- Allergic: drugs, foods, additives, acute infection e.g. HBV, *Mycoplasma*.
- Physical: sunlight, heat, cold, pressure, vibration.
- Stress.
- Thyroid disease: hypo- or hyperthyroidism.
- Occult infection: gallbladder, dental, sinus.
- Vitamin deficiency: B_{12}, folic acid, iron.
- Autoimmune: antibodies against IgE receptor on mast cells—very rare.

Investigations

Based on history but should include as baseline
- FBC (with eosinophil count).
- Thyroid function.
- Infection marker (CRP).
- Liver function.

Further tests may include
- B_{12} and red cell folate.
- Serum ferritin.

Allergy tests are of little value unless there is a clearly identified trigger.

Vasculitis

Definition

Disease caused by inflammatory destructive changes of blood vessel walls.

Presentation

Wide variety of clinical presentations affecting one or more organ systems.

Skin: splinter haemorrhages, nail fold infarcts, petechiae, purpura, livedo reticularis.

Respiratory: cough, haemoptysis, breathlessness, pulmonary infiltration, sinusitis.

Renal: haematuria, proteinuria, hypertension, acute renal failure.

Neurological: mononeuritis multiplex, sensorimotor polyneuropathy, confusion, fits, hemiplegia, meningoencephalitis.

Musculoskeletal: arthralgia, arthritis, myalgia.

Generalised: pyrexia of unknown origin, weight loss, malaise.

Table 1.16 Causes of 1° vasculitis

	Granulomatous	**Non-granulomatous**
Large vessel	Giant cell arteritis	Takayasu's arteritis
Medium vessel	Churg–Strauss disease	Polyarteritis nodosa
Small vessel	Wegener's arteritis	Microscopic arteritis

Causes of secondary vasculitis
- Infective endocarditis.
- Meningococcal septicaemia.
- Malignancy.
- Rheumatoid arthritis.
- Henoch–Schönlein purpura.
- SLE.
- Cryoglobulinaemia.
- Drug reaction.

Investigations
- FBC.
- U&E.
- LFTs.
- ESR.
- CRP.
- Protein electrophoresis.
- ANA.
- Rheumatoid factor.
- ANCA.
- CXR.
- Biopsy of artery and/or skin lesions.
- Urine dipstick and microscopy.

OHCM pp412, 422, 424.

Visual loss

Total loss of vision may be bilateral or unilateral. Unilateral blindness is due to a lesion either of the eye itself or between the eye and the optic chiasm. Determine whether the visual loss is gradual or sudden. Gradual loss of vision occurs in conditions such as optic atrophy or glaucoma. In the elderly, cataract and macular degeneration are common. Remember tobacco amblyopia and methanol toxicity. Trachoma is a common cause worldwide.

Causes of sudden blindness include
- Optic neuritis, e.g. MS.
- Central retinal artery occlusion.
- Central retinal vein occlusion.
- Vitreous haemorrhage (*Note*: proliferative diabetic retinopathy).

- Acute glaucoma.
- Retinal detachment.
- Temporal (giant cell) cell arteritis (TA). *Note*: visual loss is potentially preventable with early high-dose corticosteroid therapy (◻OHCM section 11).
- Migraine (scotomata).
- Occipital cortex infarction.
- Acute severe quinine poisoning (consider stellate ganglion block).
- Hysteria (rare) e.g. is blindness:
  - *Complete*? No pupil response or optikokinetic nystagmus.
  - *Cortical*? Normal papillary light reflex, no optikokinetic nystagmus.
  - *Hysterical*? Normal papillary light reflex, normal optikokinetic nystagmus.
- HELLP syndrome (haemolysis, elevated liver enzymes and low platelet count syndrome) complicating pre-eclampsia—rare.

Investigations will be determined by history and examination findings; a specialist opinion should be sought without delay.

If TA suspected
- ESR/CRP.
- Autoimmune profile including cANCA/pANCA.
- Temporal artery biopsy (within days ▶▶do not withhold steroid therapy).

Investigations in sudden onset of visual loss
- Visual acuity (Snellen chart).
- Goldmann perimetry.
- Intraocular pressure measurement (tonometry).
- Fluorescein angiography (specialist investigation—may delineate diabetic retinopathy in more detail. ▶▶Risk of anaphylaxis).
- Cranial CT scan.
- Cranial MRI scan.
- LP (CSF protein and oligoclonal bands if MS suspected).

Screen for risk factors and causes of cerebrovascular thromboembolic disease
- Venous plasma glucose.
- Serum lipid profile.
- Carotid Doppler studies.
- 12-lead ECG.
- Echocardiogram.

Wasting of the small hand muscles

Wasting of the small muscles of the hand may be found in isolation or may be associated with other neurological signs. If found in isolation this suggests a spinal lesion at the level of C8/T1 or distally in the brachial plexus, or upper limb motor nerves.

Unilateral wasting of the small muscles of the hand may occur in association with
- Cervical rib.
- Brachial plexus trauma (Klumpke's palsy).
- Pancoast's tumour (may be associated with a Horner's syndrome).
- Cervical cord tumour.
- Malignant infiltration of brachial plexus.

Bilateral wasting of the small muscles of the hand occurs in
- Carpal tunnel syndrome (common).
- Rheumatoid arthritis (common).
- Cervical spondylosis (common).
- Bilateral cervical ribs.
- Motor neurone disease.
- Syringomyelia.
- Charcot–Marie–Tooth disease.
- Guillain–Barré syndrome.
- Combined median and ulnar nerve lesions.
- Cachexia.
- Advanced age.
- Peripheral neuropathies.

Investigations
- ESR.
- C-reactive protein.
- Rheumatoid factor.
- CXR.
- X-ray cervical spine.
- Nerve conduction studies (📖p534).
- Electromyography (📖p537).
- LP, CSF protein, etc. (📖p518).
- CT thorax.
- MRI of cervical cord/brachial plexus.

Weight loss

Causes
- Diet.
- Anorexia.
- Diabetes mellitus.
- Malnutrition.
- Small intestinal disease (coeliac, bacterial overgrowth).
- Malignant disease (carcinoma and haematological malignancies).
- HIV/AIDS.
- Chronic pancreatitis.
- Chronic respiratory failure.
- Cirrhosis.
- Diuretic therapy.

- Hyperthyroidism.
- Addison's disease.

Investigations
May well need extensive investigation before determining the cause but start with
- FBC.
- ESR or CRP.
- Biochemistry screen.
- TFTs.
- MSU including C&S.
- CXR.
- Stool culture (if appropriate).
- Blood culture.
- Other endocrine tests as appropriate.
- Consider HIV testing.

📖OHCM p88.

Wheeze

Wheezes (rhonchi) are continuous high-, medium- or low-pitched added sounds audible during respiration. Typically they are loudest on expiration in asthma and may on occasion be heard without a stethoscope. The implication is reversible or irreversible airway obstruction. If wheeze is audible only during inspiration this is termed stridor, implying upper respiratory obstruction. An important distinction must be made between monophonic and polyphonic wheezes and whether wheeze is localised to a single area or is heard throughout the thorax.

Polyphonic wheeze
Wheezes with multiple tones and pitch. The commonest causes of wheeze (usually recurrent) are:
- Asthma.
- Chronic obstructive pulmonary disease (COPD; often audible during both phases of respiration).

Fixed monophonic wheeze
A wheeze with a single constant pitch. Implies local bronchial obstruction, usually due to:
- Bronchogenic carcinoma.
- Foreign body.

Note: stridor is a harsh form of monophonic wheeze arising from upper airway obstruction (📖*Stridor* p88).

Investigations
- ABGs (*Note*: inspired O_2 concentration should be recorded).
- Pulse oximetry at bedside (does not provide information about PCO_2).

- Spirometry (PFR, pre- and post-bronchodilator therapy).
- Pulmonary function tests (FEV_1, FVC, total lung capacity; 📖p488).
- CXR (PA and lateral).
- Sputum cytology (if tumour suspected).
- CT thorax.
- Bronchoscopy and biopsy (specialist procedure—especially if foreign body or suspected tumour).

📖OHCM pp50, 88.

Part 2

Investigations

Endocrinology & metabolism

Guiding principles of endocrine investigation *108*
Hypothalamus/pituitary function *112*
Acromegaly (growth hormone excess) *116*
Polydipsia & polyuria: diabetes insipidus *118*
Hyponatraemia (including SIADH) *122*
Obesity/hypercortisolism *126*
Endocrine hypertension *132*
Hypokalaemia *140*
Hyperkalaemia *142*
Adrenal failure *144*
Amenorrhoea *148*
Infertility *150*
Hirsutism/virilisation (raised testosterone) *150*
Galactorrhoea (hyperprolactinaemia) *152*
Impotence/loss of libido/male hypogonadism *154*
Gynaecomastia *155*
Delayed puberty *156*
Short stature *158*
Precocious puberty *158*
Thyroid function testing—general *160*
Hyperthyroidism (thyrotoxicosis) *161*
Hypothyroidism *163*
Hyercalcaemia *166*
Hypocalcaemia/osteomalacia *168*
Diabetes mellitus *172*
Potential diagnostic difficulties of DM *177*
Monitoring diabetic control *179*
Laboratory assessment of glycaemic control *180*
▶▶Diabetic emergencies: diabetic ketoacidosis, hyperosmolar
    non-ketotic syndrome & lactic acidosis *182*
Investigation of hyperlipidaemia *184*
Test protocols *188*
Combined anterior pituitary function testing *189*
Water deprivation test *190*
Diagnostic trial of DDAVP *191*
Low dose dexamethasone suppression test *191*
High dose dexamethasone suppression test *192*
Short synacthen test *193*
Long (depot) ACTH test *193*

Guiding principles of endocrine investigation

Investigations for endocrine disease have caused a lot of confusion in the minds of clinicians (many still do!). Tests have come and gone over the years and have been adopted with varying degrees of enthusiasm by specialist centres. In particular, there is often confusion over which tests to do, what procedures to follow and how to interpret the results. In some areas (e.g. Cushing's syndrome), controversy persists among the experts. In others, a clear consensus approach exists.

Here are some useful general principles:

1. *Use dynamic tests*—rather than random (untimed) sampling where the hormone under investigation is secreted in infrequent pulses (e.g. growth hormone, GH) or levels are easily influenced by other factors (e.g. cortisol varies markedly with stress levels and has a marked circadian rhythm)—see Table 2.1.

In general

If you are suspecting a LOW level—do a **STIMULATION** test (*to see if it stays LOW*)

If you are suspecting a HIGH level—do a **SUPPRESSION** test (*to see if it stays HIGH*)

2. *Use the correct collection method*—e.g. ACTH or insulin levels require rapid separation of the sample and prompt freezing (−20°C); urinary catecholamines require a specific acid preservative in the collection container. Timing of sampling may also be critical. Label samples carefully, including time of collection! Check procedures with the local laboratory. Many units will have protocols for endocrine investigations.
3. *Do tests in the correct sequence*—e.g. ACTH levels can only be interpreted once the cortisol status is known. In many cases simultaneous samples are required for interpretation, e.g. PTH with calcium for hypo/hyperparathyroidism, glucose with insulin for insulinoma.
4. *'Normal' results may be 'abnormal'* depending on the activity of the hormone axis under investigation. Interpretation of the absolute levels of hormones in isolation may be highly misleading. For example, a serum PTH within the normal range in the presence of hypocalcaemia suggests hypoparathyroidism; 'normal' LH and FSH levels in the presence of a very low serum testosterone concentration suggest pituitary failure. In both instances, the regulatory hormone concentration is inappropriately low. Thus, the level of the regulatory hormone (or releasing factor) must be considered in the light of the simultaneous level of the 'target' hormone or metabolite.
5. *Results may vary according to the lab assay*—Reference ranges vary between labs—it is especially important with endocrine tests to interpret your results according to your lab's 'normal range'. Also, interfering factors may differ between assays, e.g. different prolactin assays

cross-react very differently with macroprolactin (📖*Galactorrhoea* p152). Some individuals have a heterophile interfering antibody that affects the results of many radioimmunoassays. Resist 'discarding clinical evidence in favour of a numerical value'.

6. *Beware of interfering medication*—e.g. inhaled beclomethasone can suppress serum cortisol levels, administered hydrocortisone (cortisol) is detected by the cortisol assay, synthetic androgens and oestrogens can appear to cause low serum testosterone/oestrogen (as they are not detected in the testosterone/oestrogen assay), some anti-emetics and antipsychotics can raise circulating prolactin levels, carbenoxolone or liquorice may cause hypokalaemia. Always ask patients for a full medication list (including herbal remedies and other self-medication).

7. *Take a family history*—familial forms of many common endocrine problems exist which require important changes in management approach, e.g. familial hypercalcaemia may suggest MEN-1 or MEN-2 requiring a different form of parathyroid surgery and a risk of phaeochromocytoma (MEN-2).

Endocrine tests are generally expensive and should not be performed unnecessarily or outside of standard protocols. Dynamic tests may have cautions and contraindications and *can be hazardous* if used inappropriately. A high degree of organisation and close liaison with the lab is required to perform these tests in a way that can be clearly interpreted. Dynamic tests should ideally be performed in an endocrine investigation unit. Chemical pathologists (clinical biochemists) and other lab staff generally have great experience with performing and interpreting endocrine tests—seek their advice wherever possible—*before* embarking on tests with which you are unfamiliar. Tests in children should be performed and interpreted under expert paediatric guidance.

American Association of Clinical Endocrinologists clinical guidelines

🖰www.aace.com/clin/guidelines/

National Academy of Clinical Biochemistry (USA) guidelines

🖰www.nacb.org/lmpg/main.stm

Royal College of Physicians guidelines (UK)

🖰www.rcplondon.ac.uk/college/ceeu/ceeu_guidelinesdb.asp

Ismail AAA, Bart JH. (2001) Wrong biochemistry results. *BMJ* **232**, 705–706.

Table 2.1 Random sampling *vs.* dynamic testing

Hormone	Random or dynamic sampling?
GH	Dynamic: Glucose tolerance test for excess; insulin stress test for deficiency
IGF-1	Random
LH, FSH	Random in ♂, post-menopausal ♀ Timed with menstrual cycle in pre-menopausal ♀ Random or stimulated in pre-pubertal children
Testosterone	Random
Oestrogen (oestradiol)	Random in ♂, post-menopausal ♀ Timed with menstrual cycle in pre-menopausal ♀
ACTH	Random
Cortisol	Dynamic: Dexamethasone suppression test for excess Synacthen stimulation test if suspect deficiency
TSH	Random
T4 & T3	Random
Prolactin	Random
ADH/vasopressin	Don't normally measure directly
Osmolality	Dynamic: Water deprivation test if suspect diabetes insipidus
Parathyroid hormone	Random, but need simultaneous calcium value
Insulin	Fasting, plus simultaneous glucose value
Calcitonin	Random
Renin/aldosterone	Upright usually, off medication
Catecholamines	Measure in urine, 24h sample
5HIAAs	Measure in urine, 24h sample

Hypothalamus/pituitary function

Hypothalamic dysfunction

Causes

- Familial syndromes (Laurence–Moon–Biedl, Prader–Willi).
- Tumours (esp. craniopharyngiomas, dysgerminomas, optic gliomas, meningioma—rarely pituitary tumours).
- Pituitary surgery.
- Infiltration (histiocytosis X, sarcoidosis).
- Trauma.
- Meningitis.
- Encephalitis.
- TB.

Symptoms & signs

- Obesity/hyperphagia.
- Somnolence.
- Thermodysregulation.
- Diabetes insipidus.
- Hypogonadism.
- Precocious puberty.

Investigations

- MRI.
- Water deprivation test for diabetes insipidus (Polydipsia & polyuria, p118, tests of pituitary function).

Hypopituitarism

Definition

- Failure of one or more pituitary hormones (usually multiple).

Causes

- Congenital.
- Pituitary tumour (including infarction of tumour 'apoplexy').
- Craniopharyngioma.
- Post-cranial irradiation.
- Following pituitary irradiation.
- Metastases to pituitary (especially breast).
- Post-surgery.
- Empty sella syndrome (occasionally).
- Sheehan's syndrome (infarction with post-partum haemorrhage).

Symptoms & signs

Often very vague, e.g. tiredness, normocytic anaemia (easily missed). Combined with impotence or amenorrhoea—very suggestive. Other clues include: loss of body hair (especially axilliary), reduced shaving, hyponatraemia, growth failure in children. Diabetes insipidus is not a feature (unless there is also hypothalamic damage) as ADH can be secreted directly from the hypothalamus. May also be signs of space-occupying lesion: bitemporal hemianopia (rarely optic nerve compression, homonymous hemianopia), headache (esp. following apoplexy), III, IV, V_1,

V_2 or VI cranial nerve lesions, CSF rhinorrhoea. Occasionally galactorrhoea following pituitary stalk compression by tumour ('disconnection'). *Note*: Generally GH is lost first, then LH/FSH, and ACTH/TSH last. With any degree of hypopituitarism, GH secretion is usually affected.

Investigations

See Fig. 2.1. Basal free T4 (not TSH which can be misleadingly normal), LH, FSH, prolactin and oestrogen/testosterone are usually sufficient to test the thyroid and gonadal axes. Adrenal and growth hormone testing require dynamic tests (ITT). Note that the short synacthen test (📖*Protocols*, p193) is only suitable for testing the hypothalamo-pituitary adrenal axis if pituitary failure is of long standing (>6 weeks) allowing time for adrenal atrophy to occur.

Alternative investigations

Alternative GH stimulation tests including GHRH administration, GHRH + synthetic GH-releasing peptides, IV arginine test, IV glucagon test (causes nausea), oral L-dopa test (also causes nausea) and IV/oral clonidine test in children. The reliability of these tests has not been confirmed and the ITT (📖*Protocols*, p188) remains the gold standard; however it seems likely that it will be replaced with the less demanding GHRH/arginine test in the future (see *reference at end of section*). Combined anterior pituitary testing—giving LHRH, TRH, ACTH and GHRH (📖*Protocols*, p189)—no clear advantage of this approach has been demonstrated and the results of the LHRH test in particular are difficult to interpret in prepubertal children. Long (depot) synacthen test—rarely required (📖*Hypoadrenalism*, p144).

Fig. 2.1 Investigation of suspected hypopituitarism.

Abs R. (2003) Update on the diagnosis of GH deficiency in adults. *Eur J Endocrinology* **148**, Suppl 2, S3–8; Bouloux P-MG, Rees LH. (1994) *Diagnostic Tests in Endocrinology and Diabetes*. Chapman & Hall Medical, London; Mahajan T, Lightman SL. (2000) A simple test for growth hormone deficiency in adults. *J Clin Endocrinol Metab* **85**, 1473–1476; Nieman LK. (2003) Dynamic evaluation of adrenal hypofunction. *J Endocrinol Invest* **26** (7 Suppl), 74–82; Valetto MR *et al.* (1996) Reproducibility of the growth hormone response to stimulation with growth hormone releasing hormone plus arginine during lifespan. *Eur J Endocrinol* **135**, 568–572.

Acromegaly (growth hormone excess)

For growth hormone deficiency—see *Hypopituitarism* (p112).

Clinical features

- Often insidious over many years.
- Enlarging hands and feet with rings having to be resized.
- Increase in shoe size.
- Coarsening of facial features especially enlargement and broadening of the nose.
- Sweating.
- Headache.
- Malocclusion (protuberance of lower jaw) and splaying of teeth.
- Skin tags.
- Hypertension.
- Cardiac failure.
- Renal stones.
- Arthritis.
- Colonic polyps.
- Sleep apnoea.
- Carpal tunnel syndrome.
- Diabetes mellitus.
- May be local symptoms from the pituitary tumour and symptoms/signs of loss of other pituitary hormones (📖*Hypopituitarism*, p112).
- Growth hormone excess commencing before puberty results in gigantism (tall stature).

Investigations

- A random growth hormone is not helpful—may be high in normal people.
- Perform a standard 75g oral GTT with glucose and growth hormone measurements at 0, 30, 60, 90 and 120min.
- If no growth hormone values are <2mU/L then the diagnosis of acromegaly is confirmed.
- A random insulin-like growth factor 1 (IGF-1) level should be measured and compared to laboratory normal ranges corrected for age. This can be used as a screening test but IGF-1 assays vary in reliability. IGF-1 levels should be raised in all cases of acromegaly but levels can be affected (reduced) by fasting and systemic illness.
- The vast majority (99%) of cases of acromegaly are due to pituitary tumours. If a pituitary tumour is not seen on MRI scanning yet acromegaly is confirmed, a GHRH level should be requested to exclude ectopic production of this polypeptide by non-pituitary tumours stimulating the release of growth hormone from the pituitary.
- For follow-up of treated cases of acromegaly, IGF-1 levels (more sensitive) and nadir of growth hormone in a series of 4 estimations over 2h is a reasonable approach.
- Life expectancy appears to return to normality when the nadir of GH values is <5mU/L.

Polydipsia & polyuria: diabetes insipidus

'First line tests'

It is relatively common for patients to report excess thirst or increased need to pass urine. Figure 2.2 and Table 2.2 summarise the causes. Prostatism and urge incontinence resulting in urinary frequency should be distinguished by history taking as the patients do not have thirst. Then the first step is to identify straightforward causes such as drugs (diuretics), diabetes mellitus, hypercalcaemia, hypokalaemia and chronic renal failure with U&E, creatinine, glucose and calcium. Measuring 24h urine volume is also useful as volumes over 3L are likely to be pathological and volumes under 2L do not require further investigation. A glucose tolerance test should not be required to diagnose diabetes mellitus as the renal threshold for glucose needs to be exceeded (~10mmol/L) to cause polyuria and there should be glucose in the urine.

Table 2.2 Causes of polyuria/polydipsia

- Diabetes mellitus
- Diabetes insipidus (cranial or nephrogenic)
- High Ca^{2+}
- Low K^+
- Chronic renal failure
- Primary polydipsia (including dry mouth, e.g. Sjögren's)

'Second line tests'

Once other diagnoses have been excluded, subsequent tests aim to distinguish diabetes insipidus from primary polydipsia (compulsive water drinking). A carefully supervised water deprivation test should be performed (□Protocols, p190). However, it is not always easy to arrive at a conclusive diagnosis. Serum sodium levels are helpful as diabetes insipidus is unlikely if Na^+ <140mmol/L. Morning spot urine osmolality after overnight water restriction (not shown on chart) is occasionally useful: values >600mOsmol/L make significant degrees of diabetes insipidus unlikely. Measuring 24h urine volume is also useful as volumes over 3L are likely to be pathological. However, obligate urine volumes as low as 2L could still cause the patient to complain of polyuria. In such borderline cases, the distinction between partial diabetes insipidus, normality and primary polydipsia can be very difficult. Guidance on interpretation of the second line tests including the water deprivation test is given in Table 2.3. Note that primary polydipsia may be a psychiatric condition but can also occur in patients with a dry mouth (e.g. Sjögren's syndrome, anticholinergic drugs) or who have been previously encouraged to drink regularly 'to help their kidneys'.

Distinction between partial cranial diabetes insipidus and habitual (psychogenic) water drinking is complicated by the fact that drinking very high volumes over time may 'wash out' the renal medullary concentrating gradient. In this situation a plasma vasopressin level at the end of the water deprivation test may be very helpful to distinguish lack of vasopressin from a lack of vasopressin action. 24h urine volume is also helpful as volumes of less than 3L/day are unlikely to cause renal 'wash-out'. Clues to primary polydipsia include an initial plasma osmolality (and serum Na^+) that is low, plasma osmolality rises to >295mOsmol/L and thirst is not abolished by DDAVP despite a rise in urine osmolality. Note that 'full blown' cranial diabetes insipidus results in urine volumes around 500mL/h (12L/day).

Fig. 2.2 Investigation of polydipsia/polyuria.

Interpretation of second line tests for polyuria/polydipsia

Table 2.3

	Normal	Partial diabetes insipidus: cranial (**C**) or nephrogenic (**N**)	Primary polydipsia
Random serum Na$^+$	Normal	>140mmol/L	<140mmol/L
Random serum osmolality**	Variable	>290	<290
Morning urine mOsm**	Variable	Unlikely if >600 (**C**) Excluded if >600 (**N**)	
End of water deprivation test **before** DDAVP**	Urine >600 Plasma 280–295	Urine <600 Plasma >295	Urine >600* Plasma 280–295
Urine osmolality after DDAVP SC**	>600	Rises to >600 or >50% increase (**C**) Rises to <600 or <50% increase (**N**)	Rises to >600 or >than 50% increase
Plasma vasopressin at end of water deprivation test	Normal for plasma osmolality	Low for plasma osmolality (**C**) Normal for plasma osmolality (**N**)	Normal for plasma osmolality

*With longstanding large volume polyuria (>3L/day), these values may not be achieved due to wash-out of the renal medullary concentrating gradient—if results equivocal, see text.

**Osmolalities are all expressed in mOsmol/L.

'If all else fails'

In cases of doubt, a carefully supervised therapeutic trial of DDAVP (desmopressin) can be useful to distinguish diabetes insipidus from primary polydipsia (💻Protocols, p191). This should be done as an inpatient as there is a risk of significant hyponatraemia in habitual water drinkers. The principle is that patients able to regulate water intake according to their thirst (diabetes insipidus) should not develop a hypo-osmolar plasma. In primary polydipsia, the urine volume will fall and the urine concentrating gradient will gradually recover. However, if the patient continues to drink due to their psychological drive rather than their thirst, they will become water overloaded and hypo-osmolar.

An additional valuable test to distinguish partial diabetes insipidus from primary polydipsia is hypertonic saline infusion testing, which usually requires access to a plasma vasopressin assay but has been used with urinary vasopressin levels (*see references*). MRI scanning typically shows an increased signal in the posterior pituitary which is lost in cranial diabetes insipidus. However, this sign is not helpful in distinguishing more subtle degree of diabetes insipidus from other causes.

Robertson GL. (1995) Diabetes insipidus. *Endocr Metab Clin N Am* **24**, 549–572; Thompson CJ, Edwards CR, Baylis PH. (1991) Osmotic and non-osmotic regulation of thirst and vasopressin secretion in patients with compulsive water drinking. *Clin Endocrinol (Oxf)* **35**, 221–228; Diederich S, Eckmanns T, Exner P et al. (2001) Differential diagnosis of polyuric/polydipsic syndromes with the aid of urinary vasopressin measurements in adults. *Clin Endocrinol (Oxf)* **54**, 665–671.

Hyponatraemia (including SIADH)

Hyponatraemia is a very common clinical problem. Figure 2.3 shows a flow chart for investigation. If patients are on diuretics, further evaluation is usually not possible. The diuretic will need to be discontinued. If this is not possible, the hyponatraemia is likely to be attributable to an underlying condition (cardiac, renal or liver failure). Pseudo- or dilutional hyponatraemia is important to exclude at an early stage (see Table 2.4). A careful clinical assessment should be made of volume status including identification of oedema, fluid loss (e.g. diarrhoea, fistula leakage) and signs of dehydration including postural drop in blood pressure. A urine sodium and TSH estimation is useful at this stage (see Fig. 2.3). Note that the most important diagnosis not to miss is hypoadrenalism as this can be fatal if untreated. Clinicians should have a low threshold for performing a short synacthen test (📖*Protocols*, p193). Hypoadrenalism due to pituitary failure may not be accompanied by hyperkalaemia, hypotension or hyperpigmentation and can easily be missed.

Table 2.4 Causes of pseudohyponatraemia

- With normal serum osmolality
  - Hyperproteinaemia (e.g. myeloma)
  - Hyperlipidaemia (hypertriglyceridaemia)
  - Glycine or sorbitol (from bladder irrigant)
- With ↑ serum osmolality
  - Hyperglycaemia
  - Mannitol
  - Glycerol

The syndrome of inappropriate ADH (SIADH) is a diagnosis of exclusion.

Table 2.5 Criteria for diagnosing SIADH

- Hyponatraemia present
- No diuretics
- No oedema
- Normal renal function
- Normal adrenal function
- Normal thyroid function
- Urine Na^+ >20mmol/L
- Euvolaemic

The diagnosis can be made if hyponatraemia persists in patients not on diuretics, without oedema who have normal renal, adrenal and thyroid function. Volume status should be normal and urine Na^+ is normally >20mmol/L. A specific cause is frequently not found or there may be a combination of precipitating factors (see Table 2.6). In the elderly, a state of chronic SIADH is relatively common and usually explains hyponatraemia persisting for many years without any other apparent cause. Affected individuals should be encouraged to drink less than a litre a day ('5 cups or less'), to only drink if they are thirsty and avoid exacerbating factors (see Table 2.6).

Table 2.6 Causes of SIADH

Cause	Examples
Drugs	Carbamazepine, chlorpropamide, opiates, psychotropics, cytotoxics
CNS disorders	Head trauma, post-pituitary surgery (transient), stroke, cerebral haemorrhage, Guillain Barré, meningitis, encephalitis, fits
Malignancy	Small-cell lung cancer, pancreas, prostate
Chest disease	Pneumonia, TB, abscess, aspergillosis
General stimuli	Nausea, pain, smoking
Other	Acute intermittent porphyria

The following features of SIADH/hyponatraemia are often underappreciated

1. Other than a chest x-ray, there is no requirement to search for an underlying malignant cause. If there is underlying malignancy it is usually extensive, very apparent and incurable (e.g. extensive small-cell carcinoma of the lung).

2. The urine osmolality does not have to be high. In individuals drinking large volumes of fluid, a urine osmolality as low as 250mOsmol/L (i.e. less than plasma) may be inappropriately concentrated reflecting true SIADH.

3. Conditions previously diagnosed as 'sick cell syndrome' are now thought to represent SIADH in ill patients.

4. 'Water intoxication' is usually the combination of SIADH and excessive fluid intake. Healthy patients drinking to excess can rarely exceed the renal capacity to excrete a water load (~12L/day) and hence do not become hyponatraemic. A degree of SIADH is required for potomaniacs (excess water drinkers) to become hyponatraemic.

5. The post-operative state contains many precipitants to SIADH (nausea, pain, opiates, pneumonia) and ADH secretion is promoted by hypovolaemia from blood loss. The administration of '3L of intravenous fluid a day' post-operatively therefore frequently results in hyponatraemia.

6. Symptoms of hyponatraemia such as drowsiness, coma or fits are dependent on the rate of fall of serum Na^+ not the absolute value. Patients who are alert with Na^+ <125mmol/L have clearly been chronically hyponatraemic and their serum sodium requires only gentle correction. However, a very rapid fall in serum Na^+ to <130mmol/L (typically due to massive infusion of hypotonic fluid into the bladder) may cause coma and needs to be corrected as a medical emergency with hypertonic saline.

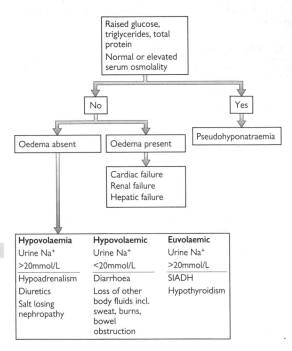

Fig. 2.3 Investigation of hyponatraemia.

Obesity/hypercortisolism

Endocrinologists are frequently asked to determine whether there is an underlying endocrine cause in patients who are obese. Secondary causes of obesity are listed in Table 2.7. A long history of obesity typically going back to childhood is characteristic of constitutional obesity and further investigation other than thyroid function is rarely necessary. However, simple obesity may result in effects suggestive of hypercortisolism, e.g. striae, bruising, central obesity, rounded facial features, mild hyperandrogenism in women, buffalo hump, hypertension and hyperglycaemia. Rapidly progressive obesity, marked hypertension, hypokalaemia, proximal muscle weakness, poor sleep, osteoporosis/vertebral collapse and marked hirsutism or acne are more suggestive of hypercortisolism and require further investigation. Hypothalamic damage is usually apparent from the history.

Table 2.7 Secondary causes of obesity

- Constitutional
- Hypothyroidism
- Cushing's syndrome
- Hypothalamic damage (extreme hyperphagia)
- Genetic, e.g. Prader–Willi
- Growth hormone deficiency
- Drugs, e.g. antidepressants

The optimal approach to the diagnosis of hypercortisolism (Cushing's syndrome) is probably the most controversial subject in endocrinology. Endocrinologists who have seen many cases of Cushing's syndrome have seen exceptions to every rule, and the episodic nature of ACTH and cortisol secretion means that low values can occur even in disease. True cyclical Cushing's disease also occurs but is rare.

Diagnosis consists of two phases

1. Does the patient have hypercortisolism or not?
2. What is the cause of the hypercortisolism? Phase 1 must be completed first as phase 2 tests can only be interpreted if hypercortisolism is present.

Investigation of hypercortisolism phase 1

Does the patient have hypercortisolism?
Patients being investigated for hypercortisolism should look Cushingoid. Depression and alcoholism may cause abnormal tests for hypercortisolism without representing a true hypercortisolaemic state and hence are termed 'pseudo-Cushing's syndrome'. Such depressed patients often do not appear Cushingoid and alcoholism should be identifiable clinically and biochemically. If there is a high degree of suspicion of hypercortisolism in a depressed patient, midnight cortisol levels <140nmol/L or a negative result on dexamethasone-CRH testing (▢*Protocols*, p191) may be helpful in excluding the diagnosis. *Note* that iatrogenic or factitious Cushing's syndrome is usually due to a steroid other than hydrocortisone

(not detected In the cortisol assay) and characteristically results in apparent suppression of the hypothalamo-pituitary-adrenal axis on testing.

Four tests are used to determine whether a patient does have hypercortisolism

1. 24h urinary free cortisol collections (UFC). Three collections with simultaneous creatinine excretion estimation are ideal. If the creatinine excretion varies >10% between collections, the samples are not true 24h collections and should be repeated. If two or more collections have a value >3 times the laboratory upper limit of normal (e.g. >800nmol/24h), then the diagnosis of hypercortisolism is secure. Patients with intermediate values should have repeat sampling after several weeks or additional tests. Steroids, adrenal enzyme inhibitors, statins and carbamazepine must be discontinued prior to testing. False positives can be caused by pregnancy, anorexia, exercise, psychoses, alcohol and alcohol withdrawal.

2. Low dose dexamethasone suppression test (LDST). This can be preformed overnight or over 2 days (📖*Protocols*, p191), the latter having less false-positives. Some authorities believe it adds little to UFCs as when cortisol secretion is high, the UFC is clearly raised, but in times when it is intermediate, the LDST may be normal. It is a useful out-patient screening test (📖*Overnight protocol*, p191) in individuals who cannot reliably collect 24h urine samples.

3. Midnight cortisol levels. High serum cortisol levels (>200nmol/L) measured between 2300 and 0100h indicate loss of diurnal rhythm and, although inconvenient, are one of the best tests of hypercortisolism. Samples should be taken via an indwelling cannula in as relaxed state as possibly, preferably during sleep. Values <140nmol/L make hypercortisolism very unlikely. Late evening salivary cortisol levels in an outpatient setting can be used where the assay is available.

4. Dexamethasone-suppressed CRH test (📖*Protocols*, p191). This is a modification of the LDST which has been said to have a specificity of 100% for hypercortisolism. Experience suggests that exceptions still occur.

Summary

In patients who appear Cushingoid, 3 x UFCs should be performed (note causes of false +ves). If these give equivocal results additional tests are required including further UFCs, midnight cortisols and a formal 2-day LDST followed by CRH.

Yanovski JA, Cutler GB, Chrousos G *et al.* (1993) Corticotrophin-releasing hormone stimulation following low-dose dexamethasone administration; a new test to distinguish Cushing's syndrome from pseudo-Cushing's syndrome from pseudo-Cushing's states. *JAMA* **269**, 2232–2238.

Investigation of hypercortisolism phase 2: what is the cause of the hypercortisolism?

The common and rare causes of hypercortisolism are summarised in Tables 2.8 and 2.9, along with useful clinical features. Approximately 65% of cases are due to a pituitary adenoma (Cushing's disease), 20% are due to an adrenal adenoma or carcinoma and 10% to ectopic ACTH production.

These are the 3 main causes to be distinguished using a combination of the tests shown below. Distinction between a pituitary adenoma (which may not be visualisable on MRI) and a small indolent tumour (typically lung carcinoid) represents the greatest challenge. Despite extensive investigation, the cause will remain uncertain in some of these cases. Investigations

1. *Plasma ACTH level* (separate and freeze immediately). Undetectable plasma ACTH levels are strongly suggestive of an adrenal tumour. However, ACTH secretion is intermittent and two suppressed values with simultaneous high cortisol levels (>400nmol/L) are preferable and should prompt adrenal CT scanning.
2. *High dose dexamethasone suppression test* (□Protocols, p192). Greater than 90% suppression of basal urine free cortisol levels is strongly suggestive of a pituitary adenoma. Lesser degrees of suppression are seen with ectopic ACTH.
3. *Inferior petrosal sinus sampling* (IPSS). This is an excellent diagnostic tool but requires expert radiological support and should only be performed in tertiary referral centres. 100mg IV of CRH is also given via a peripheral vein while sampling to ensure active secretion of ACTH during the test. ACTH levels are compared between the inferior petrosal sinus on both sides, and a peripheral vein. Sampling is performed at −15, 0, +15 and +30min after CRH injection. Ratios >2 (ideally >3) post-CRH are strongly suggestive of pituitary-dependent disease. Risks include failure to enter the sinus, and sinus thrombosis.
4. *Imaging.* Pituitary and adrenal imaging should not be performed without biochemical testing as non-functioning tumours of the pituitary and adrenal are common (false +ves) and, conversely, functioning pituitary tumours are often be too small to be visualised by MRI (false −ve). However, if the findings are consistent with the biochemical tests this is useful supportive evidence. Patients with findings suggestive of ectopic ACTH production should have thin-slice CTs of the chest looking for a bronchial adenoma and MRI scanning of the pancreas for an islet tumour. [111]Indium-labelled octreotide scanning may also be useful in locating small tumours.
5. *Plasma CRH levels.* Very rarely 'ectopic ACTH' syndrome is actually due to ectopic CRH production stimulating ACTH from the pituitary (see Table 2.9). Raised plasma CRH levels may be diagnostic in this condition.

Additional tests include

- Metyrapone test. Here the adrenal enzyme blocker metyrapone is used to lower cortisol levels. Pituitary adenomas respond by increasing

ACTH production but ectopic sources of ACTH do not. The test can also be used to confirm that ACTH levels are truly suppressed in adrenal tumours (rarely necessary).

• Peripheral CRH test. ACTH levels are measured before (−30, −15min) and +15 and +30min after injection of 100mg IV of CRH into a peripheral vein. A rise in ACTH levels of >34% is suggestive of a pituitary adenoma. The addition of 5μg IV of desmopressin improves the response rate and reduces false negatives.

Table 2.8 Common causes of hypercortisolism (Cushing's syndrome)

Cause	Pathology	Characteristic features
ACTH-secreting pituitary adenoma (Cushing's disease)—65%	Pituitary adenoma	Typical features of hyper-cortisolism with little virilisation
Ectopic ACTH secretion—10%	Malignant: small cell lung cancer, thymic carcinoid, medullary thyroid cancer	Malignant: rapid progression marked hypokalaemia, proximal muscle weakness, ↑BP, tumour clinically apparent, few Cushingoid signs
	Indolent/benign: bronchial/pancreatic carcinoids, phaeo-chromocytoma	Indolent: indistinguishable from Cushing's disease, tumour not easily detected
Adrenal tumour—20%	Adrenal adenoma	Adenomas: typical Cushingoid signs, some-times virilisation
	Adrenal carcinoma	Carcinomas: rapid progres-sion (months) with virilisa-tion, poor prognosis

Summary
See Fig. 2.4.

Fig. 2.4 Hypercortisolism. Flow chart for diagnosing the cause once hypercortisolism is established.

Table 2.9 Rare causes of hypercortisolism (Cushing's syndrome)

Cause	Pathology	Characteristic features
Ectopic CRH secretion	Variety of tumours, mostly carcinoids	Clinical features indistinguishable from Cushing's disease but no pituitary tumour, ↑serum CRH and may fail to suppress with high dose dexamethasone
Ectopic gastrin-releasing peptide secretion	Medullary thyroid cancer	Very rare, resembles ectopic CRH
Factitious ACTH administration	Injections of ACTH	Very difficult to distinguish from ectopic CRH secretion or Cushing's disease, but if isolated from their ACTH source, become adrenally insufficient in days
Cyclical Cushing's disease	Cyclical secretion from pituitary adenoma	Cushing's disease with intermittently negative tests
Pseudo-Cushing's syndromes	Depression or alcoholism	Clinical evidence of Cushing's disease may be limited; evidence of depression or alcoholism
Bilateral micronodular adrenal hyperplasia	Often associated with Carney complex	Investigation suggestive of adrenal tumour (ACTH suppressed) but adrenals normal or slightly enlarged and contain pigmented nodules
Bilateral macronodular adrenal hyperplasia	Sporadic or familial	Investigation suggestive of adrenal tumour (ACTH suppressed) but marked or very marked bilateral nodular enlargement of adrenals on CT Scanning

Armadli G et al. (2003) Diagnosis and complications of Cushing's syndrome: a consensus statement. *J Clin Endocrinol Metab* **88**, 5593–5602; Boscaro M, Barzon L, Fallo F, Sonino N. (2001) Cushing's syndrome. *Lancet* **357**, 783–791; Findling JW, Raff H. (2001) Diagnosis and differential diagnosis of Cushing's syndrome. *Endocrinol Metab Clin North Am* **30**, 729–747.

Endocrine hypertension

95% of cases of hypertension are 'essential hypertension' with no specific underlying cause. If hypertension is very marked, occurring in younger patients, difficult to control with drugs, episodic/fluctuating, recent-onset, familial, associated with recurrent hypokalaemia or has associated features (see Table 2.10) then an underlying cause should be excluded.

History and examination should include features of conditions in Table 2.10, with particular attention to paroxysmal attacks, drugs (e.g. liquorice) and family history.

Table 2.10 Secondary causes of hypertension

Physical features absent	*Notes*
Phaeochromocytoma	May be familial, e.g. in MEN-2 (may have mucosal neuromas), von Hippel–Lindau syndrome, neurofibromatosis; paroxysmal ↑ BP in only 60% cases with headache, sweating and palpitations
Hyperaldosteronism	Multiple syndromes including Conn's syndrome (see Table 2.11)
Renal artery stenosis	Congenital or acquired (atheroma)
Renal disease	Any cause, including polycystic kidneys
Hyper/hypothyroidism	Diastolic hypertension with hypothyroidism, systolic hypertension with hyperthyroidism
Hyperparathyroidism	Does not usually improve after surgical cure
Drugs	Erythropoietin, cyclosporin, cocaine, amphetamines, steroids, liquorice, oestrogens and androgens
Physical features present	
Coarctation of the aorta	
Cushing's syndrome	
Acromegaly	
Pregnancy-induced	

Figure 2.5 provides a flow chart for further investigation. At least 3 separate blood pressure readings should be obtained—24h BP monitoring may be useful where 'white coat hypertension' is suspected.

The majority of secondary causes of hypertension can be rapidly excluded by the investigations shown in the first box of Fig. 2.5. If the results are normal or the only abnormality is a low potassium, then the possibilities of hyperaldosteronism or renal artery stenosis remain to be distinguished from essential hypertension. Further investigation should be driven by the severity of the hypertension, the (young) age of the patient and the difficulty in obtaining control with drugs.

Investigation of renal artery stenosis/high renin levels

Selective renal angiography remains the gold standard for diagnosing renal artery stenosis—other imaging methods can miss the diagnosis. Renal duplex scanning in experienced hands is a useful non-invasive test. Isotope renography (± captopril) and digital subtraction angiography can generate false negatives. 3D MR angiography is a promising non-invasive alternative. High renin levels associated with hypertension (off drugs) in the absence of renal artery stenosis should prompt a search for juxtaglomerular cell tumour of one kidney. Note that the presence of hypertension is essential, as many conditions associated with low or normal blood pressure can result in 'appropriate' hyper-reninaemia (e.g. diuretics, cardiac, renal or liver failure, hypocortisolism, hypovolaemia). High renin levels can also occur in essential hypertension.

Investigation of hyperaldosteronism

Hypertension with persistent hypokalaemia, raises the possibility of hyper-aldosteronism which may be due to a variety of causes (see Table 2.11). Note that investigation for hyperaldosteronism is also appropriate with K^+ levels in the normal range, if other investigations are negative and hypertension is marked, difficult to control or in a younger patient. The optimal approach to investigation remains controversial and equivocal cases frequently occur. If there is marked hypokalaemia of recent onset, a 24h urinary free cortisol (and review of medication) is indicated to exclude recent-onset hypercortisolism (usually due to ectopic ACTH production) in which Cushingoid features have not yet become apparent. True hyperaldosteronism is never due to a malignant lesion, so that if hypertension can be medically controlled, it is not always necessary to establish a definitive diagnosis of aetiology. Published guidelines for investigation are often ambiguous. A detailed practical scheme is therefore provided here (Fig. 2.6).

Establishing hyperaldosteronism

The initial investigation is an upright renin/aldosterone ratio, performed when the patient has been upright or sitting (not lying) for at least 2h. The sample needs to be taken to the laboratory and frozen immediately. Ideally, the patient should be on no antihypertensives other than α-blockers (e.g. doxazosin) as most drugs can affect interpretation of the test results (see Table 2.12). This is difficult to achieve in subjects with very marked hypertension. Combination antihypertensive therapy and spironolactone cause most confusion. An undetectable renin with an unequivocally high aldosterone level makes the diagnosis very likely. A normal or raised upright renin excludes hyperaldosteronism. Borderline results should be repeated off interfering medication and after potassium replacement (hypokalaemia can inappropriately lower aldosterone). A low renin with a normal aldosterone can be seen in essential ('low renin') hypertension. Refer to the laboratory for normal and diagnostic ranges. Additional tests (e.g. renin after sodium restriction/frusemide, aldosterone after captopril, sodium loading or IV saline) are used in specialist centres but their exact role in testing remains unresolved.

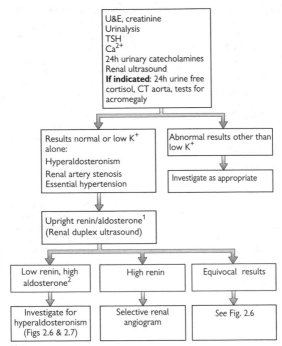

U&E, creatinine
Urinalysis
TSH
Ca^{2+}
24h urinary catecholamines
Renal ultrasound
If indicated: 24h urine free
cortisol, CT aorta, tests for
acromegaly

Results normal or low K^+
alone:
Hyperaldosteronism
Renal artery stenosis
Essential hypertension

Abnormal results other than
low K^+

Investigate as appropriate

Upright renin/aldosterone[1]
(Renal duplex ultrasound)

Low renin, high
aldosterone[2]

High renin

Equivocal results

Investigate for
hyperaldosteronism
(Figs 2.6 & 2.7)

Selective renal
angiogram

See Fig. 2.6

Notes
1 Ideally, this test should be performed off all antihypertensive drugs for
  2 weeks (6weeks for spironolactone) except alpha blockers.
2 Low renin and very low aldosterone should prompt investigations for
  'apparent mineralocorticoid excess'.

Fig. 2.5 Investigation of cause of hypertension.

Table 2.11 Investigating established primary hyperaldosteronism

	Change in aldosterone with posture	CT findings	Adrenal venous sampling (ratio of aldosterone between sides)	Response to glucocorticoids*	Treatment of choice	Notes
Adenoma (Conn's)	None/fall	Unilateral nodule	>10:1	Absent	Surgery	
Renin-responsive adenoma	Rise	Unilateral	10:1	Absent	Surgery	
Unilateral hyperplasia	None/fall	"Normal"	10:1	Absent	Surgery	
Bilateral hyperplasia	Rise	"Normal"	No difference	Absent	Medical	
Glucocorticoid "remediable aldos-teronism (GRA)"	None/fall	Normal	No difference	Present	Steroids	Very raised 18-oxo cortisols. Positive genetic screening**

* Dexamethasone 0.5mg 6-hourly for 2–4 days resulting in suppression of aldosterone levels to nearly undetectable levels (usually associated with a fall in blood pressure also).

** Positive for chimeric CYP11B1/CYP11B2 gene.

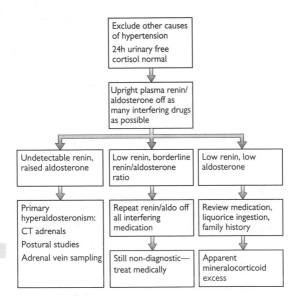

Fig. 2.6 Investigation of hyperaldosteronism/mineralocorticoid excess in patients with hypertension.

Table 2.12 Renin/aldosterone testing and drugs

Drug	Effect on PRA	Effect on aldosterone
Drugs that ↑ PRA		
Spironolactone	↑	Variable
Ca^{2+} channel blockers	May ↑	↓
ACE inhibitors*	↑	↓
Diuretics	↑	↑
Vasodilators	↑	↑
Drugs that ↓ PRA		
β-blockers	↓	↓
NSAIDs	↓	↓

PRA, plasma renin activity; *angiotensin II receptor antagonists are likely to have same effects.

Investigating the cause of established primary hyperaldosteronism

There are 5 causes of established primary hyperaldosteronism with suppressed renin and high aldosterone (see Table 2.13). Surgery (unilateral adrenalectomy) is indicated for adenoma (65% of cases), the unusual renin-responsive adenoma and the rare cases of unilateral hyperplasia but not for bilateral hyperplasia (idiopathic hyperaldosteronism, 30% of cases) or the rare, familial glucocorticoid-remediable aldosteronism (GRA). Tests to distinguish these are summarised in the table and Fig. 2.7.

📖OHCM p314

*See footnote table p135 for suppression protocol.

Fig. 2.7 Identifying the cause of established primary hyperaldosteronism.

Table 2.13 Causes of hyperaldosteronism/apparent mineralocorticoid excess

Primary hyperaldosteronism (↓ renin ↑ aldosterone)
- Aldosterone-producing adenoma (Conn's syndrome)
- Renin-responsive adenoma
- Idiopathic unilateral hyperplasia
- Idiopathic bilateral hyperplasia
- Glucocorticoid-remediable hyperaldosteronism

Apparent mineralocorticoid excess (↓ rennin ↓ aldosterone)
- Liquorice ingestion, carbenoxolone, fludrocortisone
- Congenital 11β hydroxysteroid dehydrogenase deficiency
- Liddle's syndrome
- Congenital adrenal hyperplasia (11β hydroxylase or 17α hydroxylase def.)
- Hypercortisolism

If hyperaldosteronism is established and a nodule is visible on CT/MRI imaging, it is reasonable to proceed to unilateral adrenalectomy/excision of the nodule. If no nodule or bilateral nodules are seen, then adrenal vein sampling is the most useful test to determine whether surgery should be performed. Aldosterone levels after glucocorticoid administration or genetic testing for the chimeric CYP11B1/CYP11B2 gene should be performed beforehand to exclude GRA (see Table 2.11, p135—family members may be only mildly hypertensive, making family histories unreliable). Unfortunately, the right adrenal vein cannot be catheterised in up to 25% of cases and there is a risk of precipitating adrenal haemorrhage. Postural studies identifying a >50% rise in aldosterone comparing recumbent and 2–4h of standing/walking suggest idiopathic hyperplasia, but a small renin-responsive adenoma not visible on CT could give similar results.

Investigating the cause of apparent mineralocorticoid excess

Rarely, investigation reveals low renin and low aldosterone levels in the presence of hypertension, hypokalaemia and alkalosis. There are 5 causes of this (see Table 2.13). A 24h urinary free cortisol estimation will rapidly exclude recent-onset, aggressive hypercortisolism. Repeated enquiry should be made for drug and liquorice product ingestion. The remaining causes may be diagnosed by urinary cortisol/cortisone ratio (11β OH steroid dehydrogenase deficiency—often referred to alone as 'apparent mineralocorticoid excess') or other appropriate changes in urinary and plasma cortisol metabolites (e.g. raised DOC levels—11 hydroxylase or 17α hydroxylase deficiency) or responsiveness to amiloride (Liddle's syndrome).

Phaeochromocytoma

Phaeochromocytoma is rare but an important diagnosis not to miss—can result in fatal hypertensive crisis especially during surgery or after inadvertent adrenoreceptor blockade without blockade. It can be sporadic (90%) or be the first clue to a familial syndrome (see Table 2.10). Approximately 10% of cases are extra-adrenal, 10% multiple and 10% malignant ('tumour of 10%'). 90% of cases have sustained or paroxysmal hypertension but paroxysmal attacks of some nature are a feature of only 55% of cases. Pure adrenaline-secreting lesions can occasionally cause hypotension. They are always intra-adrenal. Phaeochromocytoma needs to be excluded in cases of incidentally found adrenal masses.

24h urinary catecholamine estimations (collect into an acidified container) have now replaced measures of catecholamine metabolites (VMAS, metanephrines) as they are more sensitive and specific. A single clearly positive estimation in the presence of hypertension is usually sufficient. If non-diagnostic, sampling initiated immediately after an 'attack' should provide the answer. Mild ↑ can be seen in anxiety states, and with very small lesions detected in the follow-up of familial, recurrent disease. Causes of false positive results include methyldopa, levodopa, labetalol, clonidine withdrawal, intracranial events (e.g. subarachnoid haemorrhage, posterior fossa tumour) or metabolic stress (e.g. hypoglycaemia, myocardial infarction). Measurement of plasma catecholamines and stimulation tests are now largely obsolete. Measurement of plasma metanephrines is valuable but not widely available.

Once the diagnosis is established, blockade (typically with increasing bd doses of phenoxybenzamine) should be established before invasive investigation. The tumours are usually large (>2cm) and bright on T2-weighted images. CT/MRI scanning therefore identifies virtually all adrenal lesions. Radionuclide scanning with ^{131}I MIBG is useful to confirm activity if more than one adrenal nodule is present and to identify extra-adrenal lesions where no adrenal lesion is seen. Note that extra-adrenal phaeo-chromocytomas (paraganglionomas) are usually in the chest or abdomen but can occur in the neck (including chemodoctomas of the carotid body), pelvis and bladder. Biopsy of suspected phaeochromocytoma lesions is contraindicated.

📖OHCM p314.

Thakker RB, Oparil S. (2001) Primary aldosteronism: a practical approach to diagnosis and treatment. *J Clin Hypertens (Greenwich)* **3**, 189–195; Stewart PM. (1999) Mineralocorticoid hypertension. *Lancet* **353**, 1341–1347; Dluhy RG, Lifton RP. (1999) Glucocorticoid-remediable hyperaldosteronism. *J Clin Endocrinol Metab* **84**, 4341–4344; Gordon RD. (2004) The challenge of more robust and reproducible methodology in screening for primary aldosteronism. *J Hypertens* **22**, 251–255; Stewart PM. (1999) Mineralocorticoid hypertension. *Lancet* **353**, 1341–1347.

Hypokalaemia

Persistent hypokalaemia (<2.5mmol/L) can cause muscle weakness, cramps, tetany, polyuria, exacerbate digoxin toxicity and predispose to cardiac arrhythmias. The majority of cases are due to the common causes (see Table 2.14) and are relatively easy to diagnose. However, puzzling cases where none of these features are present occur and prompt further investigation. A flow chart is shown Fig. 2.8.

Table 2.14 Common causes of hypokalaemia*

- Diuretics
- Vomiting/diarrhoea
- Intestinal fistula
- Laxative or diuretic abuse
- Steroids (including fludrocortisone), liquorice, ACTH therapy

*See text for investigation of rare causes.

Note in Fig. 2.8 the importance of identifying the presence of acidosis and hypertension. Occult diuretic and purgative use should always be borne in mind. The commonest cause of persistent hypokalaemia with no other cause presenting in adulthood is Gitelman's syndrome, an asymptomatic congenital disorder which can usually be separated from the rare, more severe Bartter's syndrome (which usually presents neonatally or in early childhood) by low serum Mg^{2+} levels.

OHCM p692.

Fig. 2.8 Investigation of hypokalaemia.

Schurman SJ, Shoemaker LR. (2000) Bartter and Gitelman syndromes. *Adv Pediatr* **47**, 223–248.

Hyperkalaemia

Artefactual and common causes need to be excluded of which renal failure is the most important (see Table 2.15). If these fail to reveal a cause, then hypoadrenalism (which can be life-threatening), isolated mineralocorticoid deficiency and type IV renal tubular acidosis (RTA) need to be excluded.

Table 2.15 Causes of hyperkalaemia

Artefactual	Other	Rare but important
Sample left unseparated overnight	Excess K^+ replacement	Hypoadrenalism
Sample haemolysed	K^+-sparing diuretics, ACE inhibitors	Type IV RTA
Myeloproliferative disease (leakage of K^+ from high cell counts)	Renal impairment, esp. acute and after trauma or surgery	Isolated mineralocorticoid deficiency
	Metabolic acidosis (esp. DKA), rhabdomyolysis, burns, massive blood transfusion	

Hypoadrenalism is suggested by concomitant hyponatraemia, hypotension (including postural), malaise and skin pigmentation. Diagnosis is by short synacthen testing (▢▢*Adrenal failure*, p144). Note that hyperkalaemia is not a feature of secondary (pituitary) hypoadrenalism since aldosterone production is maintained by the renin–angiotensin system. Type IV renal tubular acidosis is common in patients with diabetes. It is associated with a renal tubular dysfunction as well as mildly impaired glomerular function. Serum creatinine is usually at or above the upper limit of normal. It is a state of hyporeninaemic hypoaldosteronism. Renin/aldosterone testing is suggestive but there is no definitive test. Isolated mineralocorticoid deficiency is usually congenital (e.g. due to aldosterone synthase deficiency), but can be acquired (e.g. HIV disease). High renin and low aldosterone levels would be expected. Aldosterone resistance (pseudohypoaldosteronism with high aldosterone levels but biochemical mineralocorticoid deficiency) has been described.

▢▢OHCM pp274, 692.

Schurman SJ, Shoemaker LR. (2000) Bartter and Gitelman syndromes. *Adv Pediatr* **47**, 223–248.

Adrenal failure

Hypoadrenalism is often insidious in clinical onset. However, it is an important diagnosis to make as it can be life-threatening especially at times of stress. The key is to have a high index of suspicion. Primary adrenal failure is suggested by hyperkalaemia, hyponatraemia, hypotension (including postural), malaise, weight loss, nausea, abdominal pain and skin pigmentation. In pituitary (secondary) adrenal failure, hyperkalaemia, hypotension and pigmentation are absent and malaise may be the only feature. Signs/symptoms of gonadal failure (e.g. loss of libido, reduced shaving or amenorrhoea) are often associated features with pituitary failure. Random cortisol levels can be misleading as they may be high in the morning and low in the evening. Nonetheless, a random cortisol level >550nmol/L excludes the diagnosis and is a useful test in patients undergoing severe stress/illness (e.g. in ITU).

►Where there is a strong suspicion of adrenal failure, treatment must not be delayed pending investigation. A short synacthen test or random cortisol should be performed immediately and treatment commenced with steroids awaiting results. Alternatively, treatment with dexamethasone, 0.5mg daily (which does not cross-react in the cortisol assay) can be used and then discontinued for the day of testing. Patients on other forms of glucocorticoid therapy should discontinue treatment on the morning of the test and ideally 24h beforehand (12h for hydrocortisone or cortisone acetate). Mineralocorticoid replacement need not be discontinued.

Short ACTH (synacthen) test

The standard test for adrenal failure is the short ACTH test (□□*Protocols*, p193). In recent years there has been interest in the low dose (1µg or 0.5µg) test. Although this appears to detect more minor cases of hypoadrenalism, the clinical significance of defining these differences remains uncertain.

For secondary (pituitary) adrenal failure, alternative tests include the insulin stress test (□□*Protocols*, p188) and the metyrapone test (p128). However, these tests involve applying a stress and carry a risk in patients who are profoundly hypoadrenal. They are only indicated in patients within 6 weeks of pituitary surgery or a pituitary insult, where hypotrophy of the adrenal cortices has yet to develop.

Test to distinguish primary vs. secondary adrenal failure

In the context of known pituitary disease and with failure of other pituitary hormones, adrenal failure can be assumed to be secondary (pituitary) in origin. Where isolated adrenal failure is identified, primary adrenal failure is most likely and suggested by increased skin pigmentation and hyperkalaemia.

Table 2.16 Causes of primary adrenal failure

Cause	Associated features	Diagnostic tests/notes
Autoimmune adrenalitis (>90% cases in developed countries)	Autoimmune damage may be associated with polyglandular failure types 1 and 2	Anti-adrenal (21-OH-ase) antibodies
Drugs	Ketoconazole, mitotane, etomidate, rifampicin, phenytoin	Exacerbate pre-existing adrenal impairment
Tuberculosis	Extra-adrenal TB	Calcified or enlarged adrenals, extra-adrenal TB, but may only show shrunken glands
Other infections, e.g. histoplasmosis, syphilis	Seen in N and S America	Adrenal glands enlarged
Metastatic malignancy	Common with breast, lung, melanoma or GI cancer though does not always cause adrenal failure	Enlargement/deposits in adrenal glands on CT
Bilateral adrenal haemorrhage	Anticoagulation, adrenal vein sampling	Signs of haemorrhage on CT
AIDS	CMV/TB, cryptococcus adrenalitis	
Adrenaleukodystrophy	Especially in ♂ <15 years, dementia, quadriplegia	
Adrenomyeloneuropathy	Neuropathy, blindness—may appear after adrenal failure	
Familial glucocorticoid deficiency	Defective melanocortin 2 receptors including Allgrove's syndrome, hypoadrenalism associated with seizures, achalasia and alacrima from childhood	
Defective cholesterol metabolism		
Congenital adrenal hypoplasia	Mutation on DAX1 or related genes causing failure of adrenal to develop. Adrenal insufficiency from birth	

Three additional tests can be used to confirm the level of adrenal failure

1. *Basal plasma ACTH.* This is usually the only additional test required. High levels are seen in primary adrenal failure, 'normal' or low levels are be seen in secondary adrenal insufficiency. Note that the sample must be taken and separated immediately at least 24h after the last dose of a short-acting glucocorticoid (e.g. hydrocortisone) to avoid pharmacological suppression. Patients on longer acting steroid, may have to have the test repeated more than 24h after cessation of the steroid if the result is equivocal.

2. *Anti-adrenal antibodies* (anti-21 hydroxylase antibodies). These antibodies are present in around 70% of patients with autoimmune adrenalitis (Addison's disease), the commonest cause of primary adrenal insufficiency. However, they can also be present without adrenal failure in patients with other autoimmune conditions.

3. *Long (depot) ACTH test.* Chronic stimulation with ACTH can recover function in adrenal glands that have failed because of lack of pituitary ACTH but not in primary adrenal failure. This is given in the form of ACTH in oil on 2 consecutive days (Protocols, p193), or as an infusion over 48h. With the advent of reliable ACTH assays, this test is rarely indicated.

Additional diagnostic tests

While the majority of cases of primary hypoadrenalism are due in developed countries to autoimmune disease, there are multiple other rare causes. These should particularly be considered where adrenal failure occurs in childhood and/or is associated with neurological disease or hypogonadism (see Table 2.16).

Ten S, New M, Maclaren N. (2001) Clinical review 130: Addison's disease 2001. *J Clin Endocrinol Metab* **86**, 2909–2922; Streeten DH. (1999) Shortcomings in the low-dose (1 microg) ACTH test for the diagnosis of ACTH deficiency states. *J Clin Endocrinol Metab* **84**, 835–837; Vaidya B, Pearce S, Kendall-Taylor P. (2000) Recent advances in the molecular genetics of congenital and acquired primary adrenocortical failure. *Clin Endocrinol (Oxf)* **53**, 403–418.

Amenorrhoea

Amenorrhoea is often separated into primary (never menstruated) and secondary (cessation of periods after menarche) amenorrhoea, but many causes are shared between the two categories. Structural assessment of the genital tract should be performed earlier in investigation of primary amenorrhoea. Investigation of oligomenorrhoea is similar to secondary amenorrhoea. Menorrhagia and intermenstrual bleeding are due to different causes, often gynaecological in origin. 'Irregular periods' can fall into either category, depending on whether it actually refers to intermenstrual bleeding or variably spaced (anovulatory) periods. A plan of investigation is shown in Fig. 2.9.

In secondary amenorrhoea, it is helpful early on to identify primary ovarian failure (e.g. due to Turner's syndrome, premature ovarian failure, radiation, mumps orchitis, radiation, chemotherapy or non-45XO gonadal dysgenesis) characterised by high gonadotrophins (LH, FSH). Where the gonadotrophins are equivocal or low, amenorrhoea due to hyperprolactinaemia or thyrotoxicosis should be excluded but the commonest diagnosis is chronic anovulation due to polycystic ovarian syndrome. In this condition, the ovaries still produce oestrogen resulting in a positive progesterone withdrawal test: 10mg of medroxyprogesterone is given daily for 5 days and the test is positive if any menstrual bleeding occurs in the following week. If the test is negative, a pituitary (e.g. pituitary tumour) or hypothalamic (e.g. stress, anorexia nervosa, systemic illness or weight loss) cause resulting in profound oestrogen deficiency must be considered.

Azziz, R. (2003) The evaluation and management of hirsutism. *Obstet Gynecol* **101** (5 Pt 1), 995–1007.

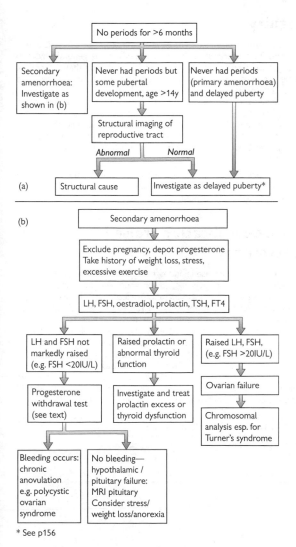

Fig. 2.9 Investigation of amenorrhoea: (a) primary and (b) secondary.

Infertility

Detailed assessment of infertility is beyond the scope of this text and is best referred to a specialist in this area. However, the general physician can take the following basic steps, always remembering that the couple should be assessed together as the problem may lie with the man, the woman or a combination of both:

1. Semen analysis of the male and where possible a post-coital test to confirm that live semen are delivered to the vaginal tract.
2. If amenorrhoea is present in the female, investigate as in Fig. 2.9.
3. If female is menstruating, determine if the cycles are ovulatory, e.g. by day 21 progesterone levels or home measurement urinary dipstick of the LH surge.

If live semen are delivered and ovulation is occurring, then structural damage or chlamydial infection in the female genital tract is likely and will require gynaecological assessment.

Hirsutism/virilisation (raised testosterone)

Hirsutism refers to an increase in androgen-dependent terminal hairs in the female, typically over the face/chin, lower abdomen, arms and legs and around the areola of the breast. Virilisation reflects much higher androgen levels and comprises the features shown in Table 2.17. Over 20% of women have more androgen-dependent hair than they consider to be normal. In >95% of cases, this is associated with androgen levels in the female normal range or slightly elevated in association with polycystic ovarian syndrome. Some drugs such as cyclosporin, diazoxide, minoxidil and androgenic steroids can also cause hirsutism. A history of recent onset (<6 months), rapidly progressive hirsutism, particularly when associated with features of virilisation and a testosterone level of >5nmol/L, should prompt a search for alternative adrenal or ovarian causes (Fig. 2.10).

Table 2.17 Features of female virilisation

- Clitoral enlargement
- Temporal hair loss
- Breast atrophy
- Deepening of voice

📖 OHCM p316.

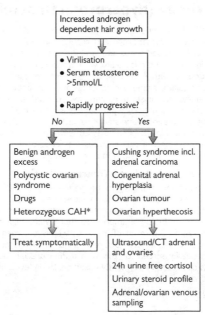

*CAH, congenital adrenal hyperpalsia

Fig. 2.10 Investigation of hirsutism.

Galactorrhoea (hyperprolactinaemia)

Galactorrhoea is always due to prolactin. Rarely, it can occur with prolactin levels in the normal range and regular menses, but usually is associated with mildly raised levels and amenorrhoea in females or very elevated levels in males. There is no link with breast size—gynaecomastia in males is associated with excess oestrogen. Once dopamine-blocking drugs (major tranquillisers and anti-emetics but not antidepressants), depot progesterone administration and hypothyroidism have been excluded, all patients should have pituitary imaging to exclude a large tumour pressing on the pituitary stalk (Fig. 2.11). Very high prolactin levels (>10,000IU/L) are invariably associated with prolactinomas. Nipple manipulation (e.g. to check if galactorrhoea has ceased) and chest wall trauma (including shingles) can also stimulate prolactin levels.

Asymptomatic raised prolactin (macroprolactin)

If prolactin is found (accidentally) to be persistently (>1000IU/L) but menstruation is normal and there is no galactorrhoea, consider the possibility of macroprolactin. This is a circulating complex of prolactin and immunoglobulins of no biological importance but gives a high reading in the prolactin assay and the result often varies widely between assays. If the lab is alerted to a mismatch between prolactin levels and clinical picture, they can easily screen for this with a PEG precipitation. Stress and epileptic fits can result in transiently raised prolactin levels insufficient to cause galactorrhoea.

📖OHCM p322.

Fig. 2.11 Investigation of galactorrhoea.

Fahie-Wilson MN, Ahlquist JA. (2003) Hyperprolactinaemia due to macroprolactins: some progress but still a problem. *Clin Endocrinol (Oxf)* **58**, 683–685; Leslie H, Courtney CH, Bell PM *et al.* (2001) Laboratory and clinical experience in 55 patients with macroprolactinemia identified by a simple polyethylene glycol precipitation method. *J Clin Endocrinol Metab* **86**, 2743–2746.

Impotence/loss of libido/male hypogonadism

Symptoms and signs of hypogonadism in men (low testosterone levels)

- Reduced shaving.
- Loss of libido.
- Impotence.
- Reduced energy/aggression levels.
- Loss of pubic, chest and axilliary hair.
- Gynaecomastia often results due to a lower testosterone/oestrogen ratio.

Note that very low levels of testosterone (at least <5nmol/L, typical normal range 10–30nmol/L) are required to result in symptoms. Mild reductions are common especially in the elderly and are rarely of importance. Impotence alone (without loss of libido) can also be caused by neurovascular and psychological causes (e.g. diabetes, spinal damage, urological surgery, atheroslerosis of the aorta, drugs, stress and psychosexual dysfunction).

After history taking for conditions described above, investigation of suspected male hypogonadism requires

- Prolactin.
- Thyroid function.
- LH & FSH.
- Testosterone.

Hyperprolactinaemia or thyrotoxicosis if present need to be treated on their own merits. If the testosterone level is clearly low, high gonadotrophins point to testicular failure (e.g. testicular surgery, irradiation or trauma, chemotherapy, crypto-orchidism, previous orchitis, gonadal dysgenesis including Klinefelter's syndrome XXY). Low gonadotrophin levels with a clearly low testosterone point to a hypothalamic or pituitary cause (systemic illness, pituitary tumour). If no cause is found for hypogonadotrophic hypogonadism, the likely cause is Kallman's syndrome, especially if associated with anosmia.

📖OHCM p316.

Sato N et al. (2004) Clinical assessment and mutation analysis of Kallmann syndrome 1 (KAL1) and fibroblast growth factor receptor 1 (FGFR1, or KAL2) in five families and 18 sporadic patients. *J Clin Endocrinol Metab* **89**, 1079–1088.

Gynaecomastia

Gynaecomastia results from an excessive effect of oestrogens or a raised oestrogen/testosterone ratio. Causes are summarised in Table 2.18. True gynaecomastia should be associated with palpable breast tissue and distinguished from apparent breast enlargement due to obesity. Though very rare, the most important diagnoses to exclude are hypogonadism, testicular and lung tumours.

Table 2.18 Causes of gynaecomastia

Physiological	Newborn, adolescent, elderly
Hypogonadism	e.g. Klinefelter's syndrome, testicular failure
Increased oestrogen	Testicular tumours, lung Ca producing hCG, liver disease, thyrotoxicosis
Drugs	Including oestrogens, spironolactone, cimetidine, digoxin, testosterone administration

Investigations should include

- LFTs.
- Thyroid function.
- LH & FSH.
- Testosterone.
- Oestradiol.
- hCG.
- AFP.
- Chest x-ray.
- Testicular ultrasound.
- Further review of drug history.

Physiological gynaecomastia should only be diagnosed if other causes have been excluded.

📖OHCM p316.

Delayed puberty

Definition

Puberty is considered delayed in girls if there is no breast development by age 13 (or menses by age 15) and in boys if there is no testicular enlargement by age 14. Note that 3% of normal children will fall into these categories.

Clinical features & initial investigations

A detailed history and examination is required for overt systemic disease, psychosocial stress, anorexia nervosa and to assess the child's height, pubertal features (pubic hair, testicular size, breast growth, menses) and any dysmorphic features (e.g. features of Turner's syndrome). Where possible growth rate should be calculated from sequential height measurements over at least 6 months.

If no obvious cause is identified, baseline investigations should include

- LH & FSH.
- TSH, FT4, prolactin.
- FBC, U&E, HCO$_3$, CRP, and antigliadin/endomysial antibodies for occult systemic disease.
- Bone age.

This should enable the child to be placed in one of 5 categories

1. Raised LH/FSH (primary gonadal failure).
   Causes: Turner's syndrome, Kleinfelter's syndrome, ovarian/testicular injury. Proceed to karyotyping (should be performed in all girls with delayed puberty as Turner's syndrome may not be apparent).
2. Short, low LH/FSH, overt systemic disease.
   Causes: asthma, anorexia nervosa, social deprivation, generalised illness, treatment for cancer including cranial irradiation, dysmorphic (Noonan's syndrome and others).
3. Short, low LH/FSH, occult systemic disease.
   Causes: hypothyroidism, hyperprolactinaemia, renal failure, renal tubular acidosis, coeliac disease, Crohn's disease.
4. Short, low LH/FSH, no systemic disease.
   Causes: constitutional delay of puberty, hypothalamic/pituitary disease.
5. Not short, low LH/FSH.
   Causes: Kallman's syndrome (if anosmia present) or isolated gonadotrophin deficiency. Cannot reliably distinguish from constitutional delay of puberty. Observe.

The investigation of children who fall into the commonest category, 'short, low LH/FSH, no systemic disease', is summarised in Fig. 2.12. The onset of puberty after a period of observation is reassuring but continued observation is required to ensure the process proceeds to completion including a growth spurt. If not, further investigation for disorders of steroidogenesis, androgen insensitivity, skeletal dysplasia, premature gonadal failure and, in the female, genital tract abnormalities and polycystic ovarian syndrome are indicated.

Notes

[1] Including normal thyroid function and prolactin.

[2] If develops headache, vomiting or visual symptoms proceed immediately to MRI.

[3] Refer to paediatric endocrinologist. Tests used vary, e.g. gonadotrophin respose to LHRH after androgenic priming and insulin tolerence test for growth hormone response.

Fig. 2.12 Investigation of delayed puberty in children who are short, with no evidence of systemic disease[1] and low LH/FSH levels.

Short stature

Evaluation of children who are below the 3rd growth centile for age or particularly small for their family should include
- Height for age (percentile).
- Mid-parental height (for girls mean of father's height minus 12.6cm + mother's; for boys add 12.6cm to mother's height).
- Bone age (to assess growth potential/height prediction).
- Observation over 3–6 months to determine growth velocity.

Children of short (but normal) parents who are growing normally can be observed. Dysmorphic children require further evaluation/specialist assessment. Children who are short for their parental heights (low predicted height), particularly if growing slowly, and short children of pubertal age who have not entered puberty should be investigated as for 'delayed puberty'. Referral for paediatric endocrinological assessment is advised.

Precocious puberty

Definition
Puberty is considered premature if multiple signs including accelerated growth rate and bone age appear by age 8 in girls or age 9 in boys. Note that isolated breast development (premature thelarche) or pubic hair (premature adrenarche) are benign conditions if no other evidence of puberty appears. True precocious puberty requires urgent investigation to determine the cause and avoid irreparable loss of final adult height. In girls, it is often idiopathic but not in boys.

Table 2.19 Causes of precocious puberty

Central	Gonadotrophin independent
Idiopathic (especially girls)	CAH (♂)
CNS hamartoma (esp. pinealoma)	Adrenal/ovarian/hCG-secreting tumour
Other CNS diseases, e.g. hydrocephalus, trauma	McCune–Albright syndrome, hypothyroidism, follicular cyst (♀) familial testitoxicosis (♂)

Investigations
Precocious puberty is confirmed by pubertal levels of sex steroids (oestradiol, testosterone). Testicular enlargement (or ovarian enlargement on ultrasound) and detectable LH/FSH levels suggest central precocious puberty and CT/MRI scan of the brain is indicated. Gonadal enlargement can also be seen with testitoxicosis, hCG-producing tumours, hypothyroidism and McCune–Albright syndrome. Further investigation should be performed in combination with a paediatric endocrinologist.

Thyroid function testing—general

In the majority of cases, thyroid function testing and interpretation are straightforward (see Fig. 2.14). However, the following points should be borne in mind.

Which first line test?—TSH

TSH levels are the most sensitive indicator of thyroid dysfunction but cannot be used in patients with pituitary disease. TSH used alone as a first line test will miss (levels 'normal') unsuspected cases of secondary hypothyroidism and some laboratories therefore combine TSH and T4 as first line tests.

Which tests?—T4/T3

Free T3 and T4 tests (FT3, FT4) are now more reliable and preferred (though more expensive) to total T3 or T4 measurements. Interference in the assays does occur but is increasingly rare. Total thyroid hormone levels are markedly influenced by changes in binding proteins (e.g. due to pregnancy, oestrogen-containing contraceptives).

Thyroid autoantibodies

These are markers of autoimmune thyroid disease. Antithyroid microsomal antibodies have been identified as antithyroid peroxidase (anti-TPO) antibodies. Antimicrosomal antibodies are much more sensitive than antithyroglobulin antibodies and are present in around 45–80% of Graves' disease and 80–95% of Hashimoto's disease/atrophic thyroiditis. Increasingly, labs are measuring anti-TPO directly as their only antibody test. Note that anti-TSH receptor antibodies—the cause of Graves' disease—are difficult to measure and not routinely assayed. Although they are the most reliable test for diagnosing Graves' disease, currently their only definite indications are to determine the cause of thyroid disease in pregnancy and the post-partum period and assess the risk of neonatal thyrotoxicosis.

Tests should agree

To confirm thyroid dysfunction at least two thyroid function tests and in cases of doubt all three (TSH, FT3, FT4) should be performed. The results of the tests should be in agreement—if not, assay interference (heterophile antibodies, anti-T4 or anti-T3 antibodies present in the serum) or unusual causes should be suspected.

Avoid thyroid function testing in systemically unwell patients

In very ill patients, especially in intensive care, a pattern of 'sick euthyroidism' is often seen, with low TSH levels, low free T3 levels and sometimes low free T4 levels. Accurate interpretation of true thyroid status is impossible. A raised free T3 level in a very ill patient suggests significant hyperthyroidism and a very raised TSH (>20mU/L) with undetectable free T4 levels suggests profound hypothyroidism. Other changes should be interpreted with extreme caution and the tests repeated after recovery.

ꆤOHCM pp302, 304.

Dayan CM. (2001) Interpretation of thyroid function tests. *Lancet* **357**, 619–624.

Hyperthyroidism (thyrotoxicosis)

Clinical features

Hyperthyroidism is rare in childhood but affects all adult age groups. Classic features include weight loss despite increased appetite, palpitations, atrial fibrillation, heat intolerance, anxiety, agitation, tremor and proximal weakness. Lid-retraction and lid-lag can be seen in any cause of hyperthyroidism but proptosis, periorbital oedema, chemosis, diplopia and optic nerve compression only occur in association with Graves' disease (thyroid eye disease), occasionally associated with pretibial myxoedema and thyroid acropachy. In the elderly, presentation with isolated weight loss or atrial fibrillation is common. Raised alkaline phosphatase and sex hormone-binding globulin, leucopenia and rarely hypercalcaemia are recognised associations.

Thyroid function testing

An undetectable TSH level and a ↑ free T3 level are required to diagnose hyperthyroidism. In milder cases, T4 levels may be in the normal range ('T3 toxicosis'). Normal TSH levels with ↑ T4 and T3 are seen in TSH-secreting pituitary tumours (very rare) or in patients with thyroid hormone resistance (also very rare).

Investigation of cause (see Fig. 2.13)

Under the age of 40, Graves' disease is the commonest cause. After this age, Graves' disease, toxic nodular goitre and toxic nodule all occur. However, a short history (≤1 month) of symptoms raises the possibility of self-resolving (transient) thyroiditis, a diagnosis supported by neck pain and raised ESR (viral/subacute/De Quervain's) or occurrence in the first 9 months post-partum (post-partum thyroiditis—painless). Transient thyrotoxicosis can also occur in patients with subclinical autoimmune thyroiditis ('silent thyroiditis'—painless) especially during cytokine therapy (e.g. interferon for hepatitis C). When thyroid eye disease is present, no further tests are required to diagnose Graves' disease. If not, antithyroid antibodies (e.g. anti-TPO antibodies) and isotope thyroid scanning can be useful to distinguish possible causes (see Fig. 2.13 and □Nuclear medicine). No uptake is seen in transient thyroiditis. Excess thyroid hormone ingestion rarely causes very marked thyrotoxicosis unless the active form (T3) is taken (T3 tablets or desiccated thyroid extract).

Iodine

Iodine has multiple and conflicting effects on the thyroid. Potassium iodide inhibits release of thyroid hormones from the gland and thyroid hormone biosynthesis (Wolff–Chaikoff effect) promoting hypothyroidism. However, escape from these effects occurs in most individuals in a few weeks. In patients with a multinodular goitre, excess iodine (e.g. in amiodarone or radiographic contrast media) can result in thyrotoxicosis by excess provision of substrate (Jod–Basedow effect).

Amiodarone

Has 3 main effects on the thyroid hormone axis: (1) inhibits T4 →T3 conversion, which in the pituitary can result in a mild rise in TSH (reduced thyroid hormone action), (2) can induce hypothyroidism, usually in the first year of treatment, (3) can induce hyperthyroidism either via the Jod–Basedow effect in patients with multinodular goitre or by a destructive thyroiditis in healthy glands. Thyrotoxicosis can occur at any time after commencing therapy and can be very difficult to treat.

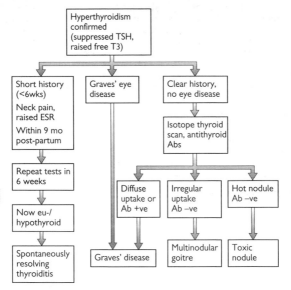

Fig. 2.13 Investigation of the cause of hyperthyroidism.

Hyperthyroidism in pregnancy

Significant hyperthyroidism in pregnancy is generally due to Graves' disease. Mild hyperthyroidism, particularly in association with hyperemesis gravidarum in the first trimester, is often due to a cross-reaction by the very high hCG levels with the TSH receptor ('gestational thyrotoxicosis'). In the post-partum period, thyrotoxicosis may be due to post-partum thyroiditis (self-resolving) or a recurrence of Graves' disease (requires treatment). Measurement of anti-TSH receptor antibody levels may be indicated to distinguish these possibilities.

Thyroid storm

This is defined as severe thyrotoxicosis with confusion/delirium not explained by other factors. There is no definitive test and levels of thyroid hormone are not higher than in other individuals with no features of storm. Severe agitation, tachycardia and hyperpyrexia are usually seen. Usually precipitated by infection, trauma or surgery, especially to the thyroid gland. Very rare but tends to occur in individuals who have been poorly compliant in the first few weeks of drug therapy for thyrotoxicosis.

Anti-TSH receptor antibody testing

This test is not routinely available in most labs. Although it is positive in >90% of cases of Graves' disease, in most cases it does not alter clinical management. Indications include distinguishing gestational thyrotoxicosis or post-partum thyroiditis from Graves' disease, indicating the risk of neonatal thyrotoxicosis and (controversial) predicting recurrence after a course of thionamide drug therapy.

📖OHCM p304.

National Academy of Clinical Biochemistry guidelines

🖑www.nacb.org/lmpg/thyroid_lmpg_pub.stm

Hypothyroidism

Clinical features

Classic clinical features of hypothyroidism include weight gain, cold intolerance, dry skin, constipation, memory loss, lethargy/slow thought/'slowing up', menorrhagia, periorbital/facial oedema, loss of outer two-thirds of eye brows, deafness, chest pain and coma. Rarely seen nowadays as thyroid function tests are easy to perform and detect the disease usually at an earlier stage. Weight gain, dry skin and lethargy are frequently reported, but even in biochemically hypothyroid individuals can only confidently be ascribed to thyroid status if they reverse on treatment.

Biochemical diagnosis

↑TSH with T4 in the normal range is referred to as subclinical hypothyroidism. ↑TSH with ↓T4 is overt hypothyroidism. ↓T4 with TSH in the normal range may be due to pituitary failure (2° hypothyroidism) and if persistent requires pituitary function testing. See Fig. 2.14 for other patterns of thyroid function tests.

Differential diagnosis (causes)

In iodine sufficient countries, most spontaneous hypothyroidism is due to autoimmune thyroiditis (Hashimoto's disease if goitre present, atrophic thyroiditis if goitre absent)—antithyroid antibodies present in 80–90% of cases. Other common causes are post-thyroidectomy, post-radioiodine therapy and side effects of amiodarone or lithium. Rarer causes include treatment with cytokines (e.g. interferons, GM-CSF, interleukin-2), vast excess iodine intake (iodine drops, water purifying tablets), congenital hypothyroidism (caused by a variety of genetic defects, should be detected by neonatal screening programme), iodine deficiency (urinary iodide excretion <45µg/day, commonest cause worldwide esp. mountainous areas, S. Germany, Greece, Paraguay—'endemic goitre'), thyroid-blocking substances in the indigenous diet (goitrogens esp. in brassicas and cassava, e.g. in Sheffield, Spain, Bohemia, Kentucky, Virginia, Tasmania—'endogenous goitre' without iodine deficiency), Pendred's syndrome (mild hypothyroidism with sensorineural deafness due to Mondini cochlear defect, positive perchlorate discharge test). For transient hypothyroidism—see *below*.

▶▶Diagnostic catches ↑TSH and ↓T4 always represents hypothyroidism. If the TSH alone is ↑ and the T4 is not even slightly low, a heterophile antibody interfering in the TSH assay may be present in the patient's serum. This is especially likely if there is no change in TSH level after thyroxine treatment but the T4 level rises (confirming compliance with tablets). For unusual patterns of thyroid function tests, see Fig. 2.14. Note that, within the first 1–3 months (or longer) after treatment of hyperthyroidism, profound hypothyroidism may develop with a ↓T4 but the TSH may still be suppressed or only mildly raised due to the long period of TSH suppression prior to treatment. Raised TSH alone with disproportionate symptoms of lethargy may be seen in hypoadrenalism.

Transient hypothyroidism

Transient/self-resolving hypothyroidism, often preceded by hyperthyroidism, is seen in viral thyroiditis, after pregnancy (post-partum thyroiditis) and in some individuals with autoimmune thyroiditis. Treatment temporarily with thyroxine only required if patient is very symptomatic. Thyroid function should return to normal within 6 months.

Subclinical hypothyroidism

A raised TSH (<20mU/L) with normal T4/T3 is very common and seen in 5–10% of women and ~2% of males. It is usually due to subclinical autoimmune thyroid disease and is frequently discovered on routine testing. In randomised trials, ~20% of patients obtain psychological benefit from beginning T4 therapy, in many others it is probably truly asymptomatic. If antithyroid antibodies are detectable, the rate of progression to overt hypothyroidism is ~50% at 20 years, but higher than this with higher initial TSH levels. If the TSH alone is raised with negative antibodies (or the TSH is normal with raised antibodies alone), overt hypothyroidism develops in 25% at 20 years. A reasonable approach is a trial of thyroxine for 6 months in symptomatic patients with subclinical hypothyroidism or TSH >10mU/L, and observing the TSH level at 6–12-monthly intervals in asymptomatic patients with TSH <10mU/L.

Hypothyroidism and pregnancy

Overt hypothyroidism is associated with poor obstetric outcomes. Recent evidence suggests that subclinical hypothyroidism is associated with a slight reduction in the baby's IQ and should be treated. Some authorities advocate screening for hypothyroidism in all antenatal patients as early as possible in pregnancy. Patients on T4 need to increase their dose by 25–50µg from the first trimester of pregnancy. Maternal thyroxine can compensate for fetal thyroid failure *in utero* but congenital hypothyroidism must be detected at birth (screening test) to avoid mental retardation developing. Where the mother and fetus are both hypothyroid—most commonly due to iodine deficiency—mental retardation can develop *in utero* (cretinism). Note that mothers with positive antithyroid antibodies and/or subclinical hypothyroidism have a 50% chance of developing (transient) post-partum thyroiditis.

📖OHCM p306.

National Academy of Clinical Biochemistry guidelines

🔗www.nacb.org/lmpg/thyroid_lmpg_pub.stm

Surks MI *et al.* (2004) Subclinical thyroid disease: scientific review and guidelines for diagnosis and management. *JAMA* **291**, 228–238.

	Low TSH	Normal TSH	Raised TSH
Raised FT4/FT3	**Thyrotoxicosis**	TSH-secreting pituitary tumour Thyroid hormone resistance (receptor defect) Intermittent T4 therapy/acute overdose Interfering anti-T4/T3 antibody Familial dysalbuminaemic hyperthyroxinaemia Acute psychiatric illness	
Normal FT4/FT3	Subclinical thyrotoxicosis Thyroxine ingestion Steroid therapy Non-thyroidal illness Dopamine infusion	Normal	Subclinical hypothyroidism Poor compliance with T4 therapy Interfering (heterophile) antibody Recovery from non-thyroidal illness Hypoadrenalism
Low FT4/FT3	Non-thyroidal illness Pituitary failure Recent (excessive) treatment for hyperthyroidism		**Hypothyroidism**

Note: free thyroid hormone assays are assumed—effects of changes in binding proteins on total thyroid hormone assays are not included.
(Adapted from Dayan CM. (2001) Interpretation of thyroid function tests. *Lancet*, **357**, 619–624)

Fig. 2.14 Patterns of thyroid function tests.

Hypercalcaemia

Clinical features

(Usually asymptomatic if Ca^{2+} <3.0mmol/L). polydipsia/polyuria, constipation, indigestion, pancreatitis, hypertension, tiredness, drowsiness/ confusion, abdominal pains, kidney stones. Renal failure can occur due to dehydration (reversible), nephrocalcinosis and/or staghorn calculi. Osteitis fibrosa cystica in cases of hyperparathyroidism (with subperiosteal resorption of bone, particularly of the distal phalanges and bone cysts—brown tumours) is now rare other than in renal failure but can be associated with bone pain.

Investigation of the cause (Fig. 2.15)

95% of persistent hypercalcaemia is due to either hyperparathyroidism or malignancy. Asymptomatic primary hyperparathyroidism is common in 50–70yr old women and a parathyroid hormone level (PTH, sampled simultaneously with the ↑ calcium and measured in a highly sensitive assay) which is raised or in the upper normal range in the presence of hypercalcaemia confirms the diagnosis. Low normal or low levels of PTH should prompt a search for malignancy, especially breast, prostate, bronchus, kidney, thyroid or myeloma. Bone-derived alkaline phosphatase levels may be raised in both malignancy and hyperparathyroidism. Bone scan may be useful in disseminated malignancy, but can be negative in cancers releasing PTH-related peptide (NOT detected in routine PTH assays) and in myeloma. If malignancy is not found, the conditions shown in Fig. 2.15 need to be considered. Markedly abnormal renal function is seen in milk-alkali syndrome, myeloma and tertiary hyperparathyroidism. Sarcoid may be difficult to diagnose but is suggested by a raised serum angiotensin converting enzyme level (ACE—not invariable), a dramatic response to steroids and a positive liver or other biopsy for granulomata.

Investigation of established hyperparathyroidism.

Familial benign hypocalciuric hypercalcaemia (FBHH or FHH) is a very rare condition caused by an inactivating mutation of the calcium-sensing receptor. This results in stable, lifelong hypercalcaemia with a raised PTH which rarely causes complications. It is inherited in autosomal dominant fashion.

The hallmark is hypocalciuria—defined as:

Urine $[Ca^{2+}]$ × plasma creatinine/plasma $[Ca^{2+}]$ × urine creat <0.01
(all in units of mmol/L)

Though rare, it is important to recognise as parathyroidectomy is not required.

Further investigation of primary hyperparathyroidism should include serum creatinine, kidney-ureters-bladder plain abdominal x-ray (KUB) to exclude renal stones and a spot urine Ca^{2+}/creatinine to rule out FBHH.

In >80% of cases, primary hyperparathyroidism is due to adenomatous change in one of the four parathyroid glands. In a minority of cases, and in familial hyperparathyroidism associated with multiple endocrine neoplasia type 1 (pituitary tumours, endocrine pancreatic tumours and hyperparathyroidism) or type 2 (medullary carcinoma of the thyroid, phaeochromocytoma and hyperparathyroidism) 4 gland hyperplasia occurs requiring resection of at least 3½ glands for treatment. Very rarely (<1% of cases) parathyroid carcinoma is the cause. Lithium therapy may also be associated with (mild) hyperparathyroidism. Imaging is rarely required for new cases of primary hyperparathyroidism—experienced surgical exploration for the parathyroid adenoma is more reliable. Following unsuccessful exploration a [99m]technetium-sestamibi radionucleotide scan or local venous sampling are the most reliable techniques for localising a parathyroid adenoma, especially if it is outside the neck.

Tertiary hyperparathyroidism

Refers to acquired autonomy of the parathyroid glands leading to hypercalcaemia following chronic vitamin D deficiency as seen in renal failure or with malabsorption. Secondary hyperparathyroidism is associated with hypocalcaemia and is the appropriate response to vitamin D deficiency.

Investigation of hypercalcaemia

Fig. 2.15 Investigation of hypercalcaemia.

Hypocalcaemia/osteomalacia

Clinical features

Chronic hypocalcaemia is often surprisingly asymptomatic. Symptoms and signs, when present, include muscle spasms, parasthesiae especially around the mouth and in fingers, tetany, fits, positive Chvostek's (VIIth nerve hyperexcitability) and Trousseau's signs (tetany of the hand when BP cuff inflated). Chronic hypocalcaemia is also associated with papilloedema, abnormal dentition (if begins in childhood), cataract and intracranial calcification (of no clinical consequence). Hypocalcaemia due to vitamin D deficiency is associated with muscle pains, proximal myopathy and osteomalacia. In some cases of pseudohypoparathyroidism (type 1a) there are phenotypic abnormalities including short 4th metacarpal, bone changes (Albright's hereditary osteodystrophy), mental retardation, short stature, obesity and resistance to other hormones, e.g. TSH, glucagon, gonadotrophins (see *below*).

Investigation of cause

Persistent hypocalcaemia with a normal serum creatinine is almost always due to either hypoparathyroidism or vitamin D deficiency (osteomalacia). Other causes and distinguishing features are shown in Table 2.20 and a scheme for diagnosis is shown in Fig. 2.16. In failure of PTH action, the calcium is very low (<1.8mmol/L), the phosphate is raised but the alkaline phosphatase is not raised and there is no osteomalacia. If the PTH is found to be raised, then pseudohypoparathyroidism can be diagnosed which is subclassified as type 1a (paternally inherited Gs-alpha defect with somatic features), type 1b ('renally selective' maternally inherited Gs alpha defect—no somatic features) or type II. The classic test is the Elsworth-Howard test—measuring the urine cAMP response to infused PTH (1–34) analogue—but PTH is currently difficult to obtain and this test is rarely required. Families with type 1a may also include patients with pseudopseudohypoparathyroidism, characterised by normocalcaemia but somatic changes of pseudohypoparathyroidism. The mutations are in the same gene. The aetiology of type II pseudohypoparathyroidism (normal renal Ca^{2+} excretion and no other somatic features) remains unclear.

A low or normal PTH in the presence of a Ca^{2+} level <1.8mmol/L makes hypoparathyroidism the likely diagnosis (see Table 2.20 *for possible causes*) but an attempt to rule out an activating calcium sensing receptor (CaSR) mutation with a urine Ca^{2+}/Creat ratio (see Fig. 2.15) should be made. In this rare genetic condition, Ca^{2+} levels are generally higher (around 1.75mmol/L). Importantly calcium or vitamin D replacement has a high likelihood of causing nephrocalcinosis and is best avoided. Autoimmune hypoparathyroidism in children or young people is particularly seen in association with autoimmune polyglandular syndrome type 1 (chronic candidiasis, coeliac disease, adrenal insufficiency).

In failure of vitamin D action (Fig. 2.16, Table 2.20), there is a compensatory PTH rise which partly corrects the calcium level but causes a raised alkaline phosphatase. In addition there is osteomalacia. In the presence of a significantly raised creatinine, renal osteodystrophy (impaired 25-OH vitamin D generation) is the most likely diagnosis, otherwise dietary vitamin D deficiency (low 25-OH vitamin D), or vitamin D resistance must be distinguished (Table 2.20).

Osteomalacia

Osteomalacia is strictly a histological diagnosis but is suggested by Looser's zones and pseudo fractures on x-ray (esp. pelvis and upper femur). If osteomalacia with muscle weakness occurs in the absence of hypocalcaemia or a raised alkaline phosphatase, hypophosphataemia ('vitamin D resistant rickets') is likely. Causes of a low phosphate include intrinsic renal disease, congenital phosphate leak, acquired phosphate leak and oncogenic osteomalacia. This last condition is associated with very difficult to find tumours, often benign, typically haemangiopericytomas of the naso/oropharynx that may take years to become manifest. It is believed to be due to raised levels of a circulating phosphaturic substance. Treatment is phosphate replacement until the tumour can be resected.

Investigation of hypocalcaemia

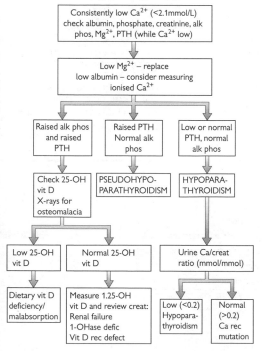

Fig. 2.16

Table 2.20 Causes of hypocalcaemia

Cause	Features
Lack of parathyroid hormone action:	*Very low Ca^{2+}, high PO_4^{3-}, normal alkaline phosphatase*
Hypoparathyroidism	Autoimmune, post-neck surgery (may be transient), radioiodine, congenital (e.g. DiGeorge)
Pseudohypoparathyroidism	Type Ia (paternally inherited Gs alpha mutation plus somatic features), Type Ib (maternally inherited, no somatic features 'renally selective'), Type II (no somatic features, normal Ca^{2+} excretion
Hypomagnesaemia	Inhibits PTH release
Activating Ca^{2+} sensing rec mutation	Indistinguishable from 1° hypoparathyroidism except present from childhood and urinary Ca^{2+}/creatinine ratio not ↓
Failure of vitamin D action:	*Ca^{2+} not v. low (>1.8mmol/L), ↑ alkaline phosphatase, ↓ PO_4^{3-} ↑ PTH, osteomalacia*
Vitamin D deficiency	Dietary/↓ sunlight, malabsorption, ↑ metabolism (phenytoin, rifamicin)
Renal failure	Failure of 1-hydroxylation of vitamin D
Inherited failure of 1-α hydroxylase (Vitamin D-dependent rickets type I)	Normal 25-OH vit D, ↓ 1,25OH
Vitamin D receptor defect (Vitamin D-dependent rickets type 2*)	Normal 25-OH vitamin D levels
Other:	
Acute pancreatitis	Transient
Hungry bone syndrome – immediately post-parathyroidectomy	Transient
Drugs e.g. foscarnet, bisphosphonates EDTA, citrate in blood	Transient
Neonatal (with prematurity)	Transient

*'Vitamin D resistant rickets' is rickets with a normal Ca^{2+} and vitamin D due to X-linked hypophosphataemia.

Diabetes mellitus

Glycosuria

Urine testing is a valuable pointer to diabetes mellitus (DM) but is insufficient to establish the diagnosis. Although modern glucose oxidase test strips are free from interference by other reducing substances, glycosuria does not always indicate DM; the converse also pertains. Thus, glycosuria has low sensitivity and specificity.

Causes of glycosuria

- DM.
- Impaired glucose tolerance (IGT).
- Lowered renal threshold for glucose (esp. pregnancy, children).

Note: Fluid intake, urine concentration and certain drugs may influence results.

The diagnosis of DM relies on the demonstration of unequivocally elevated blood glucose levels that can be

- Casual (random)—usually the first line investigation.
- Fasting plasma glucose (FPG)—an alternative to a casual reading.
- 75g oral glucose challenge—if necessary.

▶Neither the confirmation nor exclusion of DM should rest on measurement of longer term indicators of glycaemia such as glycated haemoglobin or fructosamine. Although of high specificity, these tests are not sufficiently standardised nor do they have sufficient sensitivity. False negative results are particularly likely with less marked degrees of hyperglycaemia, especially in subjects with IGT or IFG.

Blood glucose

A blood glucose measurement is the essential investigation in the diagnosis of DM. A glucose-specific assay is required. An appropriate sample must be collected, usually venous plasma and (in a tube containing fluoride oxalate as an inhibitor of glycolysis) and the sample tested without undue delay in an accredited laboratory. Serum or plasma glucose once separated from erythrocytes remains stable at room temperature up to 8h, or for up to 72h at 4°C. In the post-prandial state or during glucose load (OGTT) capillary blood glucose levels are approximately 1.0mmol/L (approximately 0.20g/L) higher than in whole venous blood. In whole blood as opposed to plasma/serum, glycolysis decreases the glucose concentration by 10–15% per hour at room temperature. When collecting and transporting blood for glucose analysis it is important either to separate the sample promptly into plasma/serum or to inhibit enzymatic degradation of blood glucose if whole blood is to be analysed using sodium fluoride (6g/L blood) or maleinimide (0.1g/L blood). As anticoagulant for plasma samples, EDTA (1.2–2g/L blood) is used.

Reagent test strips

Although convenient and readily available, reagent test strips for monitoring of capillary glucose (even when used in conjunction with a calibrated reflectance meter) are unsuitable for diagnosing DM; a confirmatory laboratory measurement must therefore always be performed.

In the absence of typical symptoms the diagnosis should be confirmed by a repeat measurement on a separate day; this may be either a casual or FPG sample.

▶Confirmation of the diagnosis is especially important in asymptomatic individuals.

An oral glucose tolerance test (OGTT) is rarely required to confirm the diagnosis and should not be regarded as a first line investigation. The OGTT is time consuming, requires trained staff and is less reproducible than FPG.

Table 2.21

	American Diabetes Association (2005)	WHO (2002)
Normoglycaemia	Fasting plasma glucose <5.6mmol/L (100mg/dL)* **OR** 2hr post 75g load plasma glucose <7.8mmol/l (140mg/dL)	Fasting plasma glucose <6.1mmol/L (110mg/dL)* **OR** 2h post 75g load plasma glucose <7.8mmol/L (140mg/dL)
Diabetes	Casual plasma glucose >11.1mmol/L (200mg/dL)[1] **OR** Fasting plasma glucose >7.0mmol/L (126mg/dL)[1] **OR** 2hr post 75g load plasma glucose >11.1mmol/l (200mg/dL)[2]	Casual plasma glucose >11.1mmol/L 200mg/dL)[1] **OR** Fasting plasma glucose ≥7.0mmol/L (126mg/dL)[1] **OR** 2hr post 75g load plasma glucose >11.1mmol/L (200mg/dL)
Impaired fasting glucose ('pre-diabetes)	Fasting plasma glucose 5.6–6.9mmol/L*	Fasting plasma glucose 6.1–7.0mmol/L (126mg/dL) BUT not officially recognised—recommend progress to 2h 75g GTT*
Impaired glucose tolerance	Not routinely measured 2h post 75g load plasma glucose 7.8–11.1mmol/L (140–199mg/dL)	2h post 75g glucose 7.8–11.1mmol/L (140–199mg/dL)
Gestational diabetes	Casual plasma glucose >11.1mmol/L (200mg/dL) **OR** fasting plasma glucose ≥7.0mmol/L (126mg/dL)* **OR** 2 or more of the following plasma glucose values after 75g glucose load: fasting >5.3mmol/L; 1h >10mmol/L; 2h >8.6mmol/L (155mg/dL)*	Casual plasma glucose 11.1mmol/L **OR** fasting plasma glucose ≥6.0mmol/L* **OR** 2h post 75g load plasma glucose >7.8mmol/L*

*ADA and WHO criteria differ.
[1] If patient does not have classic symptoms (polyuria, polydypsia, unexplained weight loss) then this test should be repeated on a different day.
[2] Not recommended by the ADA for routine clinical use.

False +ve diagnoses may arise if the subject has prepared inadequately (see Table 2.22). This possibility is more likely following the reduction in the diagnostic threshold for diabetes based on FPG in the recently revised criteria (see Table 2.21).

Table 2.22 Preparation for a fasting blood test

Refrain from any food or drink from midnight before the morning of the test

Water only is permitted

Regular medication can generally be deferred until blood sample has been taken

The appropriate sample is taken between 0800–0900h the following morning

---

This preparation is also required for a 75g oral OGTT or for measurement of fasting blood lipids. Fasting blood tests should be avoided in insulin-treated patients—risk of hypoglycaemia. Fasting is defined by the ADA as no caloric intake for at least 8h.

Normoglycaemic

The diagnostic criteria for normoglycaemia are given in Table 2.21 (note the difference between ADA and WHO for fasting plasma glucose cut-off). Note that there is NO defined random plasma glucose that confirms normoglycaemia, and this complicates the development of screening strategies for diabetes. However, if a random value is <5.6mmol/L, diabetes is extremely unlikely.

Impaired glucose tolerance

This is the preferred diagnostic category for pre-diabetes used by the WHO. The diagnosis of IGT can only be made using a 75g oral glucose tolerance test; a random blood glucose measurement will often point to the diagnosis when other results are non-diagnostic.

This category denotes a stage intermediate between normal glucose levels and DM (📖OHCM, section 9). By definition, plasma glucose levels are not raised to DM levels so typical osmotic symptoms are absent. Although subjects with IGT are not at direct risk of developing chronic microvascular tissue complications, the incidence of macrovascular complications (i.e. CHD, CVD, PAD) is increased. Presentation with one of these conditions should therefore alert the clinician to the possibility of undiagnosed IGT (or type 2 DM). Note that a proportion of individuals who are diagnosed by an OGTT may revert to normal on re-testing.

Impaired fasting glucose

This is the diagnostic category for pre-diabetes preferred by the American Diabetes Association and depends on the fasting plasma glucose. Instructions for fasting blood test are shown in Table 2.22. Recent criteria (2005) have lowered the lower limit for diagnosing IFG so the range according to the ADA is 5.6–7.0mmol/L. This category is also usually asymptomatic. To date, cross-sectional studies suggest that IGT and IFG may not be synonymous in terms of pathophysiology and long-term implications and a proportion of patients will fall into one category but not the other.

Oral glucose tolerance test

The OGTT (see Table 2.23) continues to be regarded as the most robust means for establishing the diagnosis of diabetes in equivocal cases. The WHO suggests that only when an OGTT cannot be performed should the diagnosis rely on FPG. OGTTs should be carried out under controlled conditions after an overnight fast.

The interpretation of the 75g glucose tolerance test is shown in Table 2.24. These results apply to venous plasma. Marked carbohydrate depletion can impair glucose tolerance; the subject should have received adequate nutrition in the days preceding the test.

Table 2.23 Oral glucose tolerance test

Preparation: 3d unrestricted, CHO-rich, and activity. No medication on day of test. 8–14h fast. No smoking
75g[1] of anhydrous glucose is dissolved in 250mL water; flavouring with sugar-free lemon and chilling increase palatibility and may reduce nausea. The subject sits quietly throughout the test
Blood glucose is sampled before (time 0) and at 120min after ingestion of the drink, which should be completed within 5min
Urinalysis may also be performed every 30min although is only of interest if a significant alteration in renal threshold for glucose is suspected

[1] In children 1.75g/kg, up to 75g.

Effect of intercurrent illness on glycaemia

Patients under the physical stress associated with surgery, trauma, acute MI, acute pulmonary oedema or stroke may have transient ↑ of plasma glucose—often settles rapidly without antidiabetic therapy. However, the hormonal stress response in such clinical situations is liable to unmask pre-existing DM or to precipitate DM in predisposed individuals. Blood glucose should be carefully monitored and urine tested for ketones. Sustained hyperglycaemia, particularly with ketonuria, demands vigorous treatment with insulin in an acutely ill patient. Re-testing is usually indicated following resolution of the acute illness—an OGTT at a 4–6-week interval is recommended if glucose levels are equivocal.

Table 2.24 Interpretation of the 75g oral glucose tolerance test (WHO)

	Venous plasma glucose (mmol/L)		
	Fasting		120min post-glucose load
Normal	<6.0		<7.8
IFG	6.1–6.9		<7.8
IGT	6.1–6.9	and/or	7.8–11.0
DM	>7.0		>11.1

1. In the absence of symptoms a diagnosis of diabetes must be confirmed by a second diagnostic test on a separate day. 2. For capillary whole blood, the diagnostic cutoffs for diabetes are >6.1mmol/L (fasting) and 11.1mmol/L (120min). The range for impaired fasting glucose based on capillary whole blood is >5.6 and <6.1mmol/L. In the diagnosis of diabetes, the 2h post blood value predominates if values do not agree.

Acute myocardial infarction (□OHCM section 5)

Hyperglycaemia at presentation is associated with a higher mortality—even in subjects with previously undiagnosed DM; tight metabolic control using an intravenous insulin-dextrose infusion (followed by subcutaneous insulin) significantly reduced mortality in a multicentre Swedish study.

Stroke (□OHCM section 10)

Hyperglycaemia on admission may be associated with a poorer outcome; however, there is no clinical trial evidence to date that intensive control of hyperglycaemia improves prognosis.

Re-testing is usually indicated following resolution of the acute illness—an OGTT at a 4–6-week interval is recommended if glucose levels are equivocal.

□OHCM p292.

Diabetes websites

American Diabetes Association
⌀www.diabetes.org

Diabetes UK (formerly British Diabetic Association)
⌀www.diabetes.org.uk

WHO
⌀www.who.int/bct/Main_areas_of_work/DIL/Lab_Tech/PDF_Documents/diabetes.pdf

American Diabetes Association (2005) Diagnosis and classification of diabetes mellitus. *Diabetes Care* **28**, S37–42; Gabir M et al. (2000) The 1997 ADA and 1999 WHO criteria for hyperglycaemia in the diagnosis and prediction of diabetes. *Diabetes Care* **23**, 1108–1112.

Potential diagnostic difficulties of DM

Table 2.25

Type of diabetes*	Comment
Type 1	Beta-cell destruction usually leading to absolute insulin deficiency: 1A—immune mediated; 1B—idiopathic (formerly known as juvenile onset or IDDM)
Type 2	Predominantly insulin resistant with relative insulin deficiency (formerly known as maturity-onset or NIDDM)
Gestational diabetes	Diabetes during pregnancy that resolves after post-partum. Often an early manifestation of type 2 diabetes
Other specific types	Includes genetic (MODY, mitochondrial, insulin resistance syndromes), pancreatic disease, drug-induced, occurrence in other genetic syndromes, endocrinopathies (e.g. acromegaly)

*Abbreviated from the American Diabetes Association classification.

- Type 1 DM: This is diagnosed principally on clinical and biochemical features (□OHCM section 12). The presence of serum islet cell antibodies (ICA, in ~30–60% of patients) at diagnosis may confirm the diagnosis. The proportion of patients testing positive for ICA ↓ with increasing duration of type 1 DM. If there is doubt, treat with insulin if indicated on clinical and biochemical criteria; the need for insulin can be reconsidered at a later date. However, discontinuation of insulin can be disastrous in patients with type 1 DM. The decision to stop insulin should be made only by an experienced diabetologist. ▶A –ve test for ICA does not necessarily exclude type 1 DM.
- Other humoral markers of autoimmunity, e.g. anti-GAD65, antibodies, anti-IA2, anti-insulin antibodies, are generally only available in research laboratories.
- Stiff man syndrome: rare condition presenting as a progressive spastic paraparesis with polyglandular endocrine involvement (p313). Anti-GAD65 antibodies are present; approximately 30% of patients develop insulin-requiring DM.
- MODY (maturity onset diabetes of the young): a small percentage of young patients with relatively minor hyperglycaemia and no ketonuria, will prove to have relatively uncommon inherited forms of DM, e.g. MODY. Such patients often receive insulin therapy from diagnosis, the assumption being that they have type 1 DM. Prerequisites for the diagnosis include:
  - A family history with an autosomal dominant inheritance.
  - Diagnosis under the age of 25 years.

Table 2.26 Genetically inherited forms of diabetes including MODY

Gene	% of MODY cases	Comments
Glucokinase	20	MODY 2 'mild' complications rare
HNF-1a	60	MODY 3 diagnosed later ~35yrs, progressive beta cell failure but very sensitive to sulphonylureas
HNF-4a	1	MODY 1
HNF-1b	1	MODY 5
IPF-1	1	MODY 4
NeuroD1	?<1	MODY 6
Unknown	15	'MODY X'
SUR1	<1%??	Hyperinsulinism in infancy and beta cell failure as adult
Mitochondrial	Not MODY	Maternally inherited. May be associated with nerve deafness, lactic acidosis or syndromes such as DIDMOAD
Lipodystrophy	Not MODY Lamin a/c and others	Associated with localised fat loss

In some subtypes of MODY (glucokinase mutations; MODY 2), good glycaemic control may be maintained life-long without insulin or even oral antidiabetic agents. The exception is pregnancy; insulin may be required temporarily in order to ensure optimal control—oral antidiabetic agents should be avoided. The diagnosis of MODY may be confirmed by molecular genetic testing although presently this is not widely available. Appropriate counselling is required. Seek expert advice through your local hospital diabetes unit.

• 'Flatbush' diabetes. Some young Afro-Caribbean patients present in diabetic ketoacidosis but subsequently have a disease course that is more like type 2 diabetes.
• Early-onset type 2 diabetes—In recent years there has been a dramatic increase in the incidence of type 2 diabetes in younger patients (children and adolescents) from non-white ethnic minorities. This may present diagnostic difficulties but some pointers suggest the diagnosis:
  • Obesity is usually a prominent feature.
  • Serum autoantibody tests for type 1 DM are negative.
  • A skin marker of insulin resistance (acanthosis nigricans) may be present.
  • Ethnic origin associated with early onset diabetes (e.g. S. Asian, Afro-Caribbean, Native American, Pacific Islander)

If in doubt, it is usually safer to treat younger patients with insulin; this is especially true if ketosis is present.

www.diabetesgenes.org

Monitoring diabetic control

Self-testing by diabetic patients

Self-testing of urine and/or capillary blood glucose testing can readily be performed by the majority of patients. Measurements of longer term glycaemic control are laboratory-based or require specialised techniques generally suitable only for use in a hospital clinic.

Urine testing

Glycosuria: Semiquantitative testing for glucose using reagent-impregnated test strips by patients is of limited value. Urinalysis provides retrospective information over a limited period of time. Other limitations:

- The renal threshold for the reabsorption of glucose in the PCT proximal convoluted tubule is ~10mmol/L on average but varies between individuals. Subjects with a low threshold will tend to show glycosuria more readily, even with normal glucose tolerance ('renal glycosuria'). Children are particularly liable to test positive for glucose. The renal threshold is effectively lowered in pregnancy. Conversely, a high threshold, common among the elderly, may give a misleadingly reassuring impression of satisfactory control. Fluid intake and urine concentration may affect glycosuria. Renal impairment may elevate the threshold for glucose reabsorption.
- Delayed bladder emptying, e.g. due to diabetic autonomic neuropathy (OHCM section 9), will reduce the accuracy of the measurements through dilution.
- Hypoglycaemia cannot be detected by urinalysis.

Ketonuria: Semiquantitative test strips for acetoacetate (e.g. Ketostix®) are available for patients with type 1 DM. Useful when intercurrent illness leads to disturbance of metabolic control. The presence of ketonuria on dipstick testing in association with hyperglycaemia indicates marked insulin deficiency (absolute, or more commonly, relative). Increased doses of insulin are indicated in such circumstances to avert more severe metabolic decompensation (DKA, *see below* and OHCM section 21). Occasionally, patients with type 2 DM develop ketosis during severe intercurrent illness, e.g. major sepsis. Neither Ketostix® nor Acetest® tablets detect 3-hydroxybutyrate (although acetone is detected by Acetest®). Occasional underestimation of the degree of ketonaemia using these tests is a well-recognised, albeit uncommon caveat of alcoholic ketoacidosis (OHCM section 9). Testing for blood ketones is possible with some newer reagent strips and in some laboratories.

Self-testing of blood glucose

Self-testing of capillary blood glucose obtained by fingerprick has become an established method for monitoring glycaemic control. Frequent testing is a prerequisite for adjusting insulin doses and for safe intensive insulin therapy such as that employed in the DCCT. Use in type 2 diabetes treated by diet or tablets only is controversial. Enzyme-impregnated dry strip methods are available which can be used in conjunction with meter devices to improve accuracy. Most are based on the glucose oxidase reaction:

$$\text{Glucose} + O_2 \xrightarrow{\hspace{2cm}} \text{Gluconic acid} + H_2O_2$$
$$\textit{Glucose oxidase}$$

The hydrogen peroxide generated by the reaction reacts with a reduced dye in the test strip producing an oxidised colour or electronic signal proportional to the amount of H_2O_2 formed. This reflects the amount of glucose that was oxidised. In most strips, blood cells are excluded by a layer within the strip. Thus, the glucose concentration in capillary plasma is measured. Adequate training and a system of quality control are important; even when trained health professionals use such systems in clinics or hospitals misleading results are possible, particularly in the lower range of blood glucose results. Where there is doubt, an appropriate sample (in a tube containing the glycolysis inhibitor fluoride oxalate) should be collected immediately for analysis by the clinical chemistry laboratory. However, acute treatment of hypoglycaemia, where indicated, should not be delayed.

Laboratory assessment of glycaemic control

Glycated haemoglobin

HbA_{1c} (comprises 60–80% total glycated haemoglobin, HbA_1) is formed by the slow, irreversible, post-translational non-enzymatic glycation of the N-terminal valine residue of the β chain of haemoglobin. In retina and renal glomerulus this process is implicated in the pathogenesis of the long-term complications of diabetes (🔲OHCM section 9). The proportion of HbA1c:total haemoglobin (normal non-diabetic reference range approximately 4–6%) provides a useful index of average glycaemia over the preceding 6–8 weeks. The result is disproportionately affected by the blood glucose levels during the final month before the test (~50% of value). Average HbA_{1c} levels collected over a longer period (i.e. years) provide an estimate of the risk of microvascular complications. Sustained high concentrations identify patients in whom efforts should be made to improve long-term glycaemic control.

In patients with type 1 DM, a landmark randomised, controlled clinical trial (the DCCT) confirmed a causal link between degree of metabolic control and the development and progression of microvascular complications of diabetes (especially retinopathy) and neuropathy. Consensus panels in the USA and Europe have suggested targets for HbA_{1c} of approximately 7–7.5% for most patients (if circumstances and frequency of hypoglycaemia allow). By contrast, tight glycaemic control may be contraindicated by advanced complications, e.g. clinical nephropathy with renal impairment. It is recommended that HbA_{1c} should be measured every 6 months in younger patients with type 1 DM. Pregnancy requires monthly monitoring of HbA_{1c} concentrations (although other measures may be preferable in pregnancy—see *below*: fructosamine). Blood can be collected by venesection ahead of the clinic visit (in primary care, by the hospital phlebotomy service or even by a nurse in the community if necessary). Alternatives include rapid assays for use in the clinic, or self-collection in advance of a fingerprick sample (in a capillary tube or on filter paper) which is mailed to the laboratory.

American Diabetes Association position statement: tests of glycaemia in diabetes (2004) *Diabetes Care* **27**, S91–S93.

Limitations of HbA₁c measurements

Although glycated haemoglobin levels are a reliable indicator of recent average glycaemic control they do not provide information about the daily pattern of blood glucose levels or the frequency of hypoglycaemic episodes; this supplementary information required for logical adjustment of insulin doses is derived from home blood glucose monitoring (see *below*). More recent changes in glycaemia (i.e. within the preceding 4 weeks or so) will influence HbA$_{1c}$ level more than glucose levels 12 or more weeks ago.

Spurious HbA$_{1c}$ levels may arise in states of
- Blood loss/haemolysis/reduced red cell survival (low HbA$_{1c}$).
- Haemoglobinopathy (□OHCM section 16).
- ↑ levels of HbS.
- ↑ levels of HbF (high HbA$_{1c}$).

Uraemia due to advanced diabetic nephropathy is associated with anaemia and ↓ RBC survival thereby falsely lowering HbA$_{1c}$ levels.

Fructosamine: refers to protein-ketoamine products resulting from the glycation of plasma proteins. The fructosamine assay measures glycated plasma proteins (mainly albumin) reflecting average glycaemia over the preceding 2–3 weeks. This is a shorter period than that assessed using glycated haemoglobin measurements and may be particularly useful when rapid changes in control need to be assessed, e.g. during pregnancy. Levels can be misleading in hypoalbuminaemic states, e.g. nephrotic syndrome (□OHCM section 8). Some fructosamine assays are subject to interference by hyperuricaemia or hyperlipidaemia.

Measurements of fructosamine are less expensive than glycated haemoglobin assays; this may be an important consideration for some laboratory services. The methodology is suitable for automation and rapid results can be obtained for use within a clinic attendance obviating the requirement for a prior blood test.

Goldstein DE, Little RR, Lorenz RA et al. (1995) Tests of glycemia in diabetes. *Diabetes Care* **18**, 896–909.

▶▶Diabetic emergencies: diabetic keto-acidosis, hyperosmolar non-ketotic syndrome & lactic acidosis

Diabetic keto-acidosis (DKA) should be considered in any unconscious or hyperventilating patient. The hyperosmolar non-ketotic (HONK) syndrome is characterised by marked hyperglycaemia (>30mmol/L) and dehydration in the absence of significant ketosis or acidosis. Lactic acidosis (LA) associated with metformin is uncommon. A rapid clinical examination and bedside blood and urine tests should allow the diagnosis to be made (ॼOHCM, section 12). Treatment (IV rehydration, insulin, electrolyte replacement) of these metabolic emergencies should be commenced without delay (see reference for details).

Confirm diagnosis by bedside measurement of
- Capillary blood glucose (glucose-oxidase reagent test strip; p172).
- Urinary dipstick for glucose and ketones (e.g. Ketostix®). *Note*: nitro-prusside tests detect acetoacetate, but not 3-hydroxybutyrate. This may be relevant in some circumstances, e.g. alcoholic ketoacidosis (see *below*). Venous plasma may also be tested for ketones.
- Urine for nitrites and leucocytes (UTI).

Venous blood for urgent laboratory measurement of
- Plasma glucose (fluoride-oxalate; ▶true 'euglycaemic' DKA is rare).
- U&E (arterial K^+ can be measured by some gas analysers). Plasma Na^+ may be depressed as a consequence of hyperglycaemia or marked hyperlipidaemia.
- Plasma creatinine (▶may be falsely elevated in some assays by DKA).
- Plasma lactate (if indicated—can also be measured by some gas analysers). Indicated if acidosis without heavy ketonuria is present. LA is a complication of tissue hypoxia (type A) and is a rare complication of metformin treatment in patients with type 2 DM (type B).
- Plasma osmolality in HONK—either by freezing point depression or calculated: $2 \times$ [plasma Na^+] + [plasma K^+] + [plasma glucose] + [plasma urea].
- FBC (non-specific leucocytosis is common in DKA).
- Blood cultures (signs of infection, e.g. fever, may be absent in DKA).
- ABGs (corrected for hypothermia) for:
  - Arterial pH, bicarbonate, PCO_2 and PO_2 (if shock or hypotension).

Repeat laboratory measurement of blood glucose, electrolytes, urea at 2, 4 and 6h and as indicated thereafter. Electrolyte disturbances, renal impairment or oliguria should prompt more frequent (1–2 hourly) measurements of plasma K^+. Capillary blood glucose is monitored hourly at the bedside. ▶Avoidance of hypokalaemia and hypoglycaemia is most important during therapy.

Other investigations, as indicated
- CXR.
- Microbial culture of urine, sputum, etc.
- ECG (acute MI may precipitate metabolic decompensation; note that serum transaminases and CK may be non-specifically elevated in DKA).

- Sickle cell test (in selected patients; 📖OHCM section 13).
- Venous plasma PO_4^{3-} (if there is respiratory depression).

▶Performance of investigations should not delay initiation of treatment and transfer to a high-dependency or intensive care unit.

A severe metabolic acidosis in the absence of hyperglycaemia (or other obvious cause of acidosis such as renal failure) raises the possibility of
- Lactic acidosis (LA).
- Alcoholic ketoacidosis—this occurs in alcoholics following a binge. Alterations in hepatic redox state may result in a misleading negative or 'trace' Ketostix® reaction. A similar caveat may occasionally be encountered when significant LA coexists with DKA. Venous plasma glucose may be normal or ↑.

Table 2.27 Causes of an anion gap acidosis

Ketoacidosis	Diabetic ketoacidosis
	Alcoholic ketoacidosis
	Lactic acidosis (▶metformin)
Chronic renal failure	
Drug toxicity	Methanol (metabolised → formic acid)
	Ethylene glycol (metabolised → oxalic acid)
	Salicylate poisoning

▶Anion gap (p432) >15mmol/L. Normally, the anion gap (<10mmol/L) results from plasma proteins, SO_4^{2-}, PO_4^{3-} and lactate ions. When the anion gap is increased, measurement of plasma ketones, lactate, etc. usually confirms the aetiology.

Krentz AJ, Nattrass M. (1997) Acute metabolic complications of diabetes: diabetic ketoacidosis, hyperosmolar non-ketotic syndrome and lactic acidosis, in *Textbook of Diabetes*, eds Pickup J, Williams G, Oxford, Blackwell Science.

Investigation of hyperlipidaemia

Primary dyslipidaemias are relatively common and contribute to an individual's risk of developing atheroma (e.g. CHD, CVD). Prominent examples include familial combined hyperlipidaemia (FCHL, ~2–3% of UK population) and heterozygous familial hypercholesterolaemia (FH, UK incidence 1 in 500). Major hypertriglyceridaemia also predisposes to pancreatitis. The key features of familial FH, FCHL and diabetic dyslipidaemia are considered later.

Investigations

Although many subtle alterations in plasma lipids have been described, therapeutic decisions rest on measurement of some or all of the following in serum or plasma (plasma being preferred since it can be cooled rapidly):

- Total cholesterol (may be measured in non-fasting state in first instance since levels are not greatly influenced by meals).
- Triglycerides (after 12h fast).
- Low-density lipoprotein (LDL)-cholesterol (calculated using the Friedewald formula when triglycerides are <4.5mmol/L):

$$\text{LDL-cholesterol} = [(\text{Total cholesterol} - \text{HDL-cholesterol}) - \text{Triglycerides}] \div 2.19$$

- HDL-cholesterol (regarded as the 'cardioprotective' subfraction)— HDL particles are synthesised in the gut and liver and thought to be involved in 'reverse transport' of cholesterol from peripheral tissues to the liver where it can be excreted as bile salts.

Notes on sampling in relation to lipoprotein metabolism
- Triglycerides (triacylglycerols) are measured after a ~12h overnight fast in order to clear diet-derived chylomicrons.
- Alcohol should be avoided the evening prior to measurement of triglycerides (can exacerbate hypertriglyceridaemia).
- A weight-maintaining diet is recommended for 2–3 weeks before testing.
- Lipid measurements should be deferred for 2–3 weeks after minor illness and 2–3 months after major illness, surgery or trauma since cholesterol may be temporarily ↓ and triglycerides ↑. Following acute myocardial infarction it is generally accepted that plasma cholesterol is reliable if measured within 24h of the onset of symptoms.
- The effects of certain drugs on lipids should be considered (see Table 2.28).
- Glycaemic control should be optimised wherever possible before measuring plasma lipids in patients with diabetes.

Important additional considerations are
- Day-to-day variability—generally, decisions to treat hyperlipidaemia should be based on more than one measurement over a period of 1–2 weeks. This is especially true for patients with mixed hyperlipidaemia (i.e. including hypertriglyceridaemia).
- Exclusion of secondary hyperlipidaemia—many common conditions, drugs and dietary factors can influence plasma lipids (see Table 2.28).

- Family members should also have their plasma lipids measured if a familial hyperlipidaemia is suspected in a proband.

Both cholesterol and triglycerides may be affected to some degree by these factors, but one often predominates. Pre-existing primary hyperlipidaemias may be exacerbated.

Clinical features

E.g. xanthelasma, tendon xanthomas, etc. should always be sought. A detailed family history, drug history and medical history (for diabetes and other cardiovascular risk factors such as hypertension) should always be obtained. Certain endocrine disorders, impaired hepatic or renal function can influence circulating lipid composition and cardiovascular risk. A classification of the major familial dyslipidaemias is presented in Table 2.29.

Table 2.28 Causes of secondary hyperlipidaemia

Hypercholesterolaemia

- Hypothyroidism (even minor degrees of 1° hypothyroidism)
- Cholestasis (*note*: lipoprotein X)
- Nephrotic syndrome
- Anorexia nervosa
- Diuretics
- Immunosuppressive agents
- Hepatoma
- Dysglobulinaemias

Hypertriglyceridaemia

- Obesity
- Diabetes (esp. type 2 DM)
- Lipodytrophic syndromes (of diabetes and HIV-associated)
- Alcohol excess (moderate alcohol consumption may raise HDL-cholesterol)
- Renal failure
- Antiretroviral agents
- Oestrogens (esp. oral preparations in some women)
- Corticosteroids
- Beta-adrenergic blockers
- Retinoids

Recommended investigation for exclusion of 2° hyperlipidaemia: • U&E • plasma creatinine • fasting venous glucose •LFTs •TFTs. For patients on statins check •LFTs •CK periodically (▶measure urgently if myositis occurs—a rare but potentially fatal complication).

▶Specialist advice should be sought in the management of major or resistant hyperlipidaemias.

Table 2.29 Familial hyperlipoproteinaemias

Genetic disorder	Defect	Presentation	Cholesterol	Triglycerides	Phenotype
Familial LPL deficiency	Absence of LPL activity	Eruptive xanthomata hepatosplenomegaly	↑	↑↑↑	I
Familial apo C-II deficiency	Absence of apo C-II	Pancreatitis	↑	↑↑↑	I or V
Familial hypercholesterolaemia	LDL receptor deficiency	Tendon xanthomata premature atheroma	↑↑↑	↑ or N	IIa or IIb
Familial dysbeta-lipoproteinaemia	Abnormal apo E and defect in TG metabolism	Tubo-eruptive and palmar xanthoma; premature atheroma	↑↑↑	↑↑↑	III
Familial combined hyperlipidaemia	Uncertain	Premature atheroma	↑ or N	↑ or N	IIa, IIb or IV
Familial hypertriglyceridaemia	Uncertain Eruptive xanthomata hepatosplenomegaly; pancreatitis		N ↑	↑, ↑↑↑	IV V

↑, ↑↑ and ↑↑↑, mildly, moderately or severely raised; cholesterol and triglycerides refers to concentrations in plasma; phenotype refers to Fredrickson classification (I to V, see table below); apo, apoprotein; LPL, lipoprotein lipase; n, normal; TG, triglycerides.

National Cholesterol Education Programme Guidelines
www.nhlbi.nih.gov/guidelines/cholesterol/

Table 2.30 Phenotypic (Fredrickson) classification of hyperlipidaemias

Type	Cholesterol	Triglycerides	Particle excess	Usual underlying cause
I	↑	↑↑↑	Chylomicrons	LPL or apo C-II deficiency
IIa	↑↑	N	LDL	LDL receptor defect LDL overproduction
IIb	↑↑	↑↑	VLDL, LDL	VLDL or LDL overproduction or ↓ clearance
III	↑	↑↑↑	Chlyomicron and VLDL remnants	Impaired remnant removal may be due to certain apo E phenotypes or apo E deficiency
IV	N or ↑	↑↑	VLDL	VLDL overproduction or ↓ clearance
V	↑	↑↑↑	Chylomicrons	LPL defect; apo C-II deficiency VLDL remnants

↑, ↑↑ and ↑↑↑, mildly, moderately or severely raised; LDL, low-density lipoprotein; VLDL, very-low-density lipoprotein; LPL, lipoprotein lipase; apo, apoprotein.

Jialal I. (1994) Dyslipidaemias and their investigation, in Diagnostic Tests in *Endocrinology and Diabetes*, eds Bouloux P-MG, Ree LH, Chapman & Hall Medical, London; Frayn KN. (1996) *Metabolic Regulation—a Human Perspective*, Portland Press, London; (1998) Joint British recommendations on prevention of coronary heart disease in clinical practice. *Heart* **80** (suppl 2), S1–S29; National Cholesterol Education Program (NCEP) expert panel on detection, evaluation and treatment of high blood cholesterol in adults (adult treatment panel III). (2001) Executive summary of the 3rd report. *JAMA* **285**, 2486–2497.

Test protocols

Insulin tolerance test (insulin stress test)

Indication: suspected ACTH or GH deficiency.

Contraindications: patients with epilepsy, coronary heart disease (check ECG).

Children: use no more than 0.1U/kg. Considerable care should be exercised; the test should only be performed in a centre with expertise.

Alternatives: short synacthen test for hypocortisolism; stimulation tests for growth hormone deficiency e.g. GHRH-arginine test (see *Hypopituitarism* p114).

Preparation: patient fasting overnight. Bed required (though day case procedure). Patient must be accompanied home and may not drive. OMIT morning hydrocortisone or other steroid hormone replacement if patient is taking this and previous day's growth hormone. Physician must be present throughout the test. Requires written consent.

Procedure: early morning outpatient test in fasting patient. Indwelling venous cannula and constant medical supervision required throughout. Cannula is kept patent by running saline infusion with three-way tap for sampling. Discard initial 2–3mL when each sample is taken. Label all samples clearly with time and patient details. Near-patient testing glucometer required.

1. Take baseline blood for glucose, cortisol and GH. Check IV access working well. Review test with the patient and explain symptoms s/he is likely to experience (see 5. below).
2. Draw up 25mL of 50% dextrose for immediate administration IF REQUIRED.
3. Give soluble (regular) insulin as an intravenous bolus in a dose of 0.15U/kg after an overnight fast. Consider 0.1U/kg (lower dose) if suspected profound hypocortisolism. ▶This appears a very small dose, e.g. typically around 10 units. CHECK DOSE CALCULATION CAREFULLY. Usually an insulin syringe is used to draw it up and then transfer it to a 2mL syringe containing saline.
4. Take blood at 15min intervals (0, 15, 30, 45, 60min) for glucose, cortisol and GH.
5. Observe for symptoms and signs of hypoglycaemia. First sign is usually profuse sweating. Patient may then be aware of symptoms such as palpitations, hunger, paraesthesiae. This typically occurs 30–45min into the test. Check near-patient glucose to confirm <3.5mmol/L. Continue to talk to and reassure patient. If patient becomes very drowsy or unrousable then give 25mL of 50% glucose. This does not invalidate the test as the hypoglycaemic stimulus has already occurred. Continue blood sampling at standard times.
6. If patient has not experienced hypoglycaemia by 45min and near-patient glucose is >4mmol/L, give a further intravenous bolus of 0.15U/kg or 0.3U/kg if patient known to be very insulin resistant (e.g. acromegalic). Repeat sampling at 15min intervals for 60min after this second bolus.

7. At end of procedure (usually 60min), give IV 25mL 50% dextrose if patient still has symptoms of hypoglycaemia.
8. Give patient a meal including complex carbohydrate (e.g. sandwiches or lunch) and observe for a minimum of 1h further before accompanied discharge.

Unwanted effects: severe hypoglycaemia with depressed level of consciousness or convulsion requires immediate termination of test with 25mL of 50% dextrose IV. Repeat if necessary and follow with 5 or 10% dextrose infusion. Continue to collect samples for hormone and glucose measurements.

Interpretation: test is only interpretable if adequate hypoglycaemia is achieved (<2.2mmol/L). Normal maximal cortisol response >550nmol/L. Normal GH response >20mU/L. Impaired responses (if hypoglycaemic stimulus adequate) denote corticotrophin (assuming adrenal glands are normal) or GH deficiency or both. Peak GH response <10mU/L is sufficient to consider GH replacement; peak GH response <5mU/L is severe growth hormone deficiency.

Combined anterior pituitary function testing

Indication: assessment for anterior pituitary hypofunction.

Contraindications: previous reaction to stimulatory hormones.

Alternatives: insulin tolerance testing for GH and adrenal axis; metyrapone test for adrenal axis. Other stimulation tests for GH, e.g. GHRH-arginine test.

Preparation: test usually performed in morning for basal sampling.

Procedure: IV cannula inserted. Basal blood samples taken for cortisol, oestradiol (♀) or testosterone (♂), free T4 and IGF-1. Hypothalamic hormones are given sequentially intravenously each as a bolus over around 20s: LHRH 100µg, TRH 200µg and ACTH 250µg. Additionally GHRH (1µg/kg body weight) may be given. (Reduce doses in children.) Samples are drawn at 0, 20, 30, 60 and 120min for LH, FSH, TSH cortisol and prolactin. If GHRH is given, samples are drawn at the same time points for GH.

Interpretation: normal values as follows:

TRH:	Suspect secondary hypothyroidism if peak response (at 20min) <20mU/L (Note: low levels also seen in hyperthyroidism—ensure free T4 or total T4 not raised).
ACTH:	Peak cortisol response >550nmol/L at 30 or 60min.
LHRH:	Peak LH/FSH response 2–5 × basal value. LH: Peak at 20min, FSH later.
GHRH:	Normal GH peak response >15mU/L.

Water deprivation test

Indication: diagnosis of diabetes insipidus (DI) and to distinguish cranial and nephrogenic diabetes insipidus.

Contraindications: none if carefully supervised. For correct interpretation, thyroid and adrenal deficiency should be replaced first. Interpretation in the presence of diabetes mellitus and uraemia can be difficult.

Alternatives: morning urine osmolality of >600mOsmol excludes significant degrees of DI. No other definitive test for diabetes insipidus.

Patient preparation: usually an outpatient procedure. Correct thyroid and adrenal insufficiency in advance. Renal function and blood glucose should have been checked in advance. Steroid and thyroid hormone replacement should be taken as normal on the day of the test. If the patient is on DDAVP, omit the dose on the evening before the test (or if not possible, halve this dose). Free fluids, but not to excess, up to 0730h on the day of the test. No alcohol on the night before the test or in the morning of the test. Light breakfast but no tea, coffee or smoking on the morning of the test. Empty bladder before attending for the test.

If urine volume is <3L/day ('mild cases'), ask patient to have no fluids or food from 1800h on the evening before the test ('prolonged water deprivation test').

Requirements for test: accurate weighing scales. Supervision for the whole test (up to 8h). DDAVP for injection (2µg). Immediate access to serum electrolyte, plasma and urinary osmolality assays. Access to a plasma AVP (ADH) assay desirable.

Procedure: 0730h
1. Weigh patient and calculate 97% of body weight.
2. Mark this target on the chart.
3. No food or fluid for next 8h.
4. Insert cannula for repeated blood sampling and flush.

0800h
5. Obtain plasma for Na^+ and osmolality and urine for osmolality.
6. Then collect urine hourly for volume and osmolality and plasma every 2h for Na^+ and osmolarity.
7. Weigh patient before and after passing urine if unobserved.
8. If patient loses 3% body weight, order urgent plasma osmolality and Na^+.
9. If plasma osmolality >300mOsmol (Na^+ >140mmol/L) stop test, allow patient to drink and give DDAVP (see *below*).
10. If plasma osmolality <300mOsmol, patient may have been fluid overloaded before test and water deprivation can continue.
11. Stop test at 8h (4pm) and take final recordings of urine and plasma.
12. Save an aliquot of plasma for vasopressin levels in case of difficulties in test interpretation.
13. Ideally urine osmolalities will have reached a plateau (<30mOsmol rise between samples).

14. Now give 2µg DDAVP IM (or 20µg intranasally) and collect urine samples only for a further 2h. Allow free fluids at this stage.

Interpretation: normal response: plasma osmolality remains in the range 280–295mmol, urine osmolality rises to >2x plasma (>600mOsmol). If urine volumes during water deprivation do not reduce and yet the plasma does not become more concentrated (rising osmolality) and weight does not fall, suspect surreptitious drinking during test. For interpretation of abnormal results see Table 2.3 (p120).

Diagnostic trial of DDAVP

Indication: distinction of partial diabetes insipidus from primary polydipsia.

Contraindications: cardiac failure. Current diuretic use (test uninterpretable). Note that this test may precipitate severe hyponatraemia in primary polydipsia and should be preformed in an inpatient unit with clinical and biochemical regular review.

Preparation: admission to assessment unit. First line tests for polydipsia/polyuria should have been performed (*see text*).

Procedure:

1. 24h urine volume, morning urine osmolality, weight, fluid intake (as far as possible), serum osmolality, Na^+, urea and creatinine should all be performed daily and the results reviewed the same day.
2. Subjects should have access to fluid *ad libitum* but should be reminded that they should only drink if they are thirsty.
3. After an initial 24h period of observation, desmopressin (DDAVP) is administered at a dose of 2µg bd SC for 3 days.
4. Stop test if serum Na^+ falls to <130mmol/L.

Interpretation: reduction in urine volume to <2L/day, ↑ in urine osmolality to >600mOsmol/L without fall in serum Na^+ to <140mmol/L suggests central diabetes insipidus. Reduction in urine volume with no increase in urine osmolality >600mOsmol/L and without a fall in serum Na^+ suggests partial nephrogenic diabetes insipidus. Limited reduction in urine volume, with some increase in urine osmolarity but a fall in serum Na^+ suggests primary polydipsia.

Low dose dexamethasone suppression test

Indication: to distinguish hypercortisolism from normality. The dexamethasone suppressed CRH test is believed to have less false positives in cases of alcoholic or depressive pseudo-Cushing's syndrome.

Patient preparation: patients should not be on oral steroids or drugs that increase steroid metabolism.

Overnight dexamethasone suppression test: 1mg dexamethasone is taken PO at midnight. Serum sample for cortisol is taken the following morning between 0800 and 0900h.

Interpretation: serum cortisol should suppress to <140nmol/L (usually <50nmol/L). Values 140–175nmol/L are equivocal and suggest a 2-day test should be performed. 10–15% false +ve rate.

2-day low dose dexamethasone suppression test (preferred)
Dexamethasone 0.5mg is given PO every 6h for 8 doses (2 days) starting in the early morning. Ideally tablets are taken strictly at 6-hourly intervals (0600, 1200, 1800, 0000h) which may necessitate an inpatient stay. A 24h collection for urine free cortisol is taken on the second day of the test and serum cortisol is measured at 0600h on the 3rd day, 6h after the last dose. IV administration of dexamethasone can be used if there are concerns over absorption or compliance.

Interpretation: serum cortisol 6h after the last dose should be <140nmol/L, usually <50nmol/L. Urinary free cortisol on the second day should be <70nmol/L, normally <30nmol/L. The 2-day test strictly performed has less false +ves than the overnight test.

Dexamethasone suppressed CRH test: dexamethasone 0.5mg is given PO every 6h for 9 doses (2 days) but starting at midnight and ending at 0600h. Tablets are taken strictly at 6-hourly intervals (0000, 0600, 1200, 1800h) which may necessitate an inpatient stay. Last dose is taken at 0600h and an injection of CRH (100µg IV or 1µg/kg) is given at 0800h. A blood sample for cortisol is taken at 0815h (i.e. 15min later).

Interpretation: serum cortisol level should be <38nmol/L (normal).

Yanovski JA, Cutler GB, Chrousos G et al. (1993) Corticotrophin-releasing hormone stimulation following low-dose dexamethasone administration: a new test to distinguish Cushing's syndrome from pseudo-Cushing's states. *JAMA* **269**, 2232–2238.

High dose dexamethasone suppression test

Indication: to distinguish between patients with Cushing's disease (ACTH-secreting pituitary tumour) and ectopic ACTH production in patients with established hypercortisolism.

Patient preparation: as low dose test except that the test can be performed immediately following the 2-day low dose test.

Procedure
1. 2 x 24h urine free cortisol collections are made to calculate the mean basal 24h urine free cortisol.
2. Baseline serum cortisol measurement is also taken before the first dexamethasone dose, ideally at 0600h. If the low dose test is performed first, the baseline values (urine and blood) must be taken prior to the low dose test (i.e. any doses of dexamethasone).

3. Dexamethasone 2mg is given PO every 6h for 8 doses (2 days) starting in the early morning. Ideally tablets are taken strictly at 6-hourly intervals (0600, 1200, 1800, 0000h) which may necessitate an inpatient stay.
4. A 24h urine collection for urinary free cortisol (final) is taken on day 2 and a blood sample is taken for (final) cortisol 6h after the last dexamethasone dose (0600h on day 3). Creatinine excretion should be measured and compared between urine samples to confirm true 24h collections.

Interpretation: % suppression of basal cortisol is calculated as:

(basal cortisol − final cortisol)/basal cortisol × 100

The same calculation is made for basal and day 2 urine free cortisol. 50% suppression is suggestive of pituitary-dependent disease. 90% suppression increases the likelihood (strict criteria). Thymic carcinoids and phaeochromocytomas releasing ACTH are source of false positives.

Short synacthen test

Indication: suspected adrenal insufficiency. Will not detect recent-onset secondary adrenal insufficiency.

Contraindication: asthma/allergy to ACTH—risk of allergic reaction (can be performed with careful medication supervision of patient).

Preparation: patient must not take hydrocortisone on the morning of the test as this will be detected in the cortisol assay. The test can be performed on low dose dexamethasone but the morning dose should be omitted until after the test. May have some value in patients on higher dose steroid therapy to indicate the degree of suppression of adrenocortical function.

Procedure: 250µg of synthetic ACTH (synacthen) given IM or IV. Blood taken at times 0, 30 and 60min for serum cortisol.

Low dose test: the test can be performed with a very low dose of ACTH (e.g. 1µg). This may detect more subtle degrees of hypoadrenalism but the clinical significance of these findings remains uncertain.

Interpretation: a value at any time >550nmol/L makes the diagnosis very unlikely.

Long (depot) ACTH test

Indication: distinguishing 1° and 2° adrenal failure.

Patient preparation: a short synacthen test should be performed prior to the test to diagnose adrenal failure. If patient is on steroid replacement, change to dexamethasone 0.5mg/day.

Procedure: blood is taken at 0900h for basal cortisol. 1mg of depot synthetic ACTH (synacthen) is then given IM on 2 consecutive days and blood collected 5h after each dose (1400h). A final cortisol sample is taken at 0900h on the 3rd day.

Interpretation: serum cortisol should rise to >1000nmol/L on the last day and, if adrenal failure previously indicated by a short synacthen test, such a rise indicates secondary adrenal failure (pituitary/hypothalamic cause incl. suppressive drugs).

Full blood count (FBC) *198*
Red cell parameters *199*
White cells *201*
Platelet count *201*
Peripheral blood film *202*
Red cell morphology *204*
Parasites on the blood film & marrow *206*
White blood cell morphology *208*
Assessment of iron status *210*
Assessment of vitamin B_{12} & folate status *213*
Erythrocyte sedimentation rate (ESR) *216*
Plasma viscosity *217*
Tests for glandular fever *218*
Investigation of haemolytic anaemia *220*
General tests of haemolysis *220*
Reticulocytes *222*
Serum haptoglobins *223*
Serum bilirubin *224*
Urobilin & urobilinogen *224*
Urinary haemosiderin *224*
Plasma haemoglobin *226*
Schumm's test *226*
Hereditary haemolytic anaemias *228*
Red cell membrane disorders *228*
Red cell enzyme assays *230*
Haemoglobin abnormalities *231*
Haemoglobin analysis *231*
Investigation of possible thalassaemia *234*
Investigation of sickle haemoglobin *234*
Estimation of haemoglobin A_2 ($\alpha_2\beta_2$) *235*
Estimation of fetal haemoglobin (HbF) *236*
Haemoglobin H bodies (β_4) *236*
Heinz bodies *236*
Testing for unstable haemoglobins *237*

Haematology

Molecular tests for diagnosis of thalassaemia 238
Acquired haemolytic anaemias 240
Ham's acid lysis test 241
Bleeding time 242
Prothrombin time (PT) 244
Activated partial thromboplastin time (APTT) 245
Thrombin clotting time (TCT) 246
D-dimers 246
▶▶Disseminated intravascular coagulation (DIC) 248
Platelet function tests 250
Thrombophilia screening 252
Antithrombin, proteins C&S 253
Bone marrow examination 254
Cytochemistry tests (leukaemia diagnosis) 256
Neutrophil alkaline phosphatase 258
Blood transfusion 260
▶▶Transfusion reactions 261
▶▶Immediate transfusion reaction 261
Urgent investigations 262
Febrile transfusion reactions 263
Delayed transfusion reaction 263
Bacterial contamination of blood products 264
Antiglobulin test 264
Kleihauer test 265
Erythropoietin assay 266
Immunohaematology 268
Immunophenotyping 269
Cytogenetics 270
Cytogenetics: prenatal diagnosis 272
Cytogenetics: haematological malignancies 274
HLA (tissue) typing 276
Southern blotting 278
PCR amplification of DNA 280
In situ hybridisation & FISH 282
Specialised haematology assays 284

Full blood count (FBC)

Called *complete blood count* (CBC) in the USA.

Before the advent of modern haematology blood analysers the blood count consisted of a Hb concentration (estimated using a manual colorimetric technique), a white cell count and manual platelet count. Other parameters such as MCV had to be mathematically calculated (*derived*) using the measured variables Hb, RCC and PCV.

Modern analysers use a variety of methods to provide a huge range of FBC variables including electronic impedance, laser light scatter, light absorbance and staining characteristics. The resultant FBC provides measured variables such as Hb, PCV and RCC along with derived (mathematically) MCV, MCH and MCHC. These machines also provide automated platelet counts and a 5-part differential WBC.

Sample: peripheral blood EDTA; the sample should be analysed in the laboratory within 4h, if possible.

Main parameters measured

1. Hb concentration.
2. Red cell count (RCC).
3. MCV.
4. MCH.
5. MCHC.
6. Haematocrit (Hct) or PCV.
7. Red cell distribution width (RDW).
8. White cell count.
9. WBC differential.
10. Platelet count.

Some machines are even more sophisticated and will measure *reticulocyte counts* in addition to determination of reticulocyte Hb and MCV.

Role of the FBC

Why ask for a FBC? How will this aid the diagnosis or management of the patient? The FBC assesses several different parameters and can provide a great deal of information. The red cell variables will determine whether or not the patient is anaemic. If anaemia is present the MCV is likely to provide clues as to the cause of the anaemia. The white cells are often raised in infection—neutrophilia in bacterial infections and lymphocytosis in viral (but not always so). Platelets (size or number) may be abnormal either as a direct effect of underlying blood disease or may simply reflect the presence of some other underlying pathology. Most of us take a somewhat cursory glance at the FBC when the report arrives on the ward or in clinic, but a more detailed look may reveal a great deal more!

⊕ http://www.bbc.co.uk/health/talking/tests/blood_full_blood_count.shtml
⊕http://www.rcpa.edu.au/pathman/full_blo.htm

Red cell parameters

Haemoglobin concentration (Hb)

Units: g/dL or g/L (Europe uses SI units; the USA still uses g/dL or grams%).

Defines anaemia (Hb <lower limit of normal adjusted for age and sex). Values differ between ♂ and ♀ since androgens drive RBC production and hence adult ♂ has higher Hb, PCV and RCC than adult ♀.

Red cell count (RCC)

Unit: $\times 10^{12}$/L.

Most clinicians pay little attention to the red cell count but this parameter is useful in the diagnosis of polycythaemic disorders and thalassaemias (the latter results in the increased production of red cells that are smaller than usual and contain low quantities of haemoglobin, i.e. are microcytic and hypochromic).

Causes of a low red cell count include
- Hypoproliferative anaemias, e.g. iron, vitamin B_{12} and folate deficiencies.
- Aplasias, e.g. idiopathic or drug-induced (don't forget chemotherapy).
- Parvovirus B_{19} infection-induced red cell aplasia resulting in transient marked anaemia.

Causes of high red cell count
- PRV.
- Thalassaemia.

Mean cell volume (MCV)

Unit: femtolitre (fL), 10^{-15}L.

Provided as part of the derived variables or can be calculated if you know the PCV and RCC (PCV ÷ RCC, e.g. if PCV 0.45 and RCC 5×10^{12}/L then MCV is 90fL).

Irrespective of the method used to determine the MCV, this index provides a useful starting point for the evaluation of anaemia (see Table 3.1).

Table 3.1

MCV ↓	MCV normal	MCV ↑
Iron deficiency	Blood loss	B_{12} or folate deficiency
β thalassaemia trait	Myelodysplasia	Myelodysplasia
Sideroblastic anaemia	Anaemia of chronic disease	

Mean cell haemoglobin (MCH)

Unit: pg.

High
- Macrocytosis.

Low
- Microcytosis, e.g. iron deficiency anaemia.

Mean cell haemoglobin concentration (MCHC)

Unit: g/dL or g/L.
Of value in evaluation of microcytic anaemias.

High
- Severe prolonged dehydration.
- Hereditary spherocytosis.
- Cold agglutinin disease.

Low
- Iron deficiency anaemia.
- Thalassaemia.

Haematocrit or PCV

These are not entirely synonymous terms (but they are, more-or-less). If blood is placed in a microcapillary tube and centrifuged the red cells are spun down to the bottom, leaving the plasma above. The RBCs will occupy about 40% of the blood in the tube—the blood will have a PCV of 0.4 (or 40%). The Hct is similar, but derived, using automated blood counters.

PCV unit: litres/litre (although the units are seldom cited on reports).

High PCV
- Polycythaemia (any cause).

Low PCV
- Anaemia (any cause).

Red cell distribution width (RDW)

Measures the *range* of red cell size in a sample of blood, providing information about the degree of red cell anisocytosis, i.e. how much variation there is between the size of the red cells. Of value in some anaemias:

e.g.   ↓ MCV with normal RDW suggests β thalassaemia trait.
    ↓ MCV with high RDW suggests iron deficiency.

(Probably noticed more by haematology staff than those in general medicine!)

White cells

The automated differential white cell count is provided as part of the FBC. The RBCs in the sample are lysed before WBCs are counted. A typical FBC will show the *total* WBC and the *5-part differential white cell count*, broken down into the 5 main white cell subtypes in peripheral blood which include:

- Neutrophils.
- Lymphocytes.
- Monocytes.
- Eosinophils.
- Basophils.

The printed FBC usually shows the % of each type of white cell but unless the absolute WBC (as $\times 10^9$/L) is known this % count is of little value.

▶As a general rule ignore the % count—you cannot detect abnormalities such as neutropenia unless you have the absolute values.

Abnormalities of the WBC, e.g. neutrophilia, neutropenia, etc., are discussed in 📖OHCM p630.

Platelet count

Unit: $\times 10^9$/L.

Normal: 150–400×10^9/L.

Platelets (*thrombocytes* in the USA) are the smallest cells in peripheral blood. Traditional counting methods with microscope and counting chamber now replaced by automated counting with haematology analysers.

Platelet distribution width (PDW)

This is analogous to the red cell distribution width (RDW) and provides information about the range of platelet size in a blood sample.

- The PDW will be high if there are giant platelets in the presence of normal sized platelets, e.g. essential thrombocythaemia (one of the myeloproliferative disorders).
- The PDW will be normal in a reactive thrombocytosis (where the platelet count is increased but they are all of normal size).

Platelet clumping

This is an *in vitro* artefact in some individuals. Platelets clump in EDTA and the blood analyser will report spurious thrombocytopenia. The actual *in vivo* count is normal, and the platelets function normally. Taking the blood into citrate or heparin will show the patient's platelet count to be normal. The presence of even a small blood clot in an EDTA sample may also reduce the platelet count (the haematology technical staff will usually check to see whether the sample contains a small clot before sending out the report).

Peripheral blood film

Examining a stained peripheral blood smear under the microscope allows the examination of red cells, white cells, and platelets. In addition the blood film will help detect parasites (e.g. malaria, trypanosomes) or abnormal cells in the blood.

When to request a blood film examination

The haematology lab will usually examine a peripheral blood film if the patient's indices are abnormal (unless there has been no major change from previous FBCs). If you suspect an underlying blood disorder you should request a film. *Note*: the lab staff may not make a film if the indices are completely normal.

Method

A fingerprick blood sample may be spread onto a glass slide (the phlebotomists may do this for you), air-dried, fixed and stained. Alternatively, a drop of EDTA blood may be treated in the same manner (the haematology lab staff will make the film). *Beware*: old EDTA samples produce strange artefacts such as extreme red cell crenation—for this reason, if a film is required it should be made from a fresh blood sample.

Sample: EDTA (as fresh as possible).

Information from the blood film

Red cells
- Size.
- Shape.
- Membrane changes (e.g. oxidative membrane damage).
- Colour.
- Basophilic stippling.
- Inclusions, e.g. Howell–Jolly bodies, malarial parasites, HbC crystals, etc.

White cells
- Number.
- Morphology.
- Abnormalities such as toxic granulation, dysplastic changes.
- Presence of abnormal cells, e.g. leukaemic blasts or lymphoma cells.

Platelets
- Number.
- Size.
- Shape.

Other features on the film
- Parasites.
- Red cell rouleaux (stacking effect, seen e.g. when ESR is ↑).
- Nucleated red cells.
- Plasma cells.
- Occasionally see circulating carcinoma cells.

📖 OHCM p628.

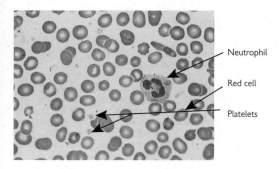

Neutrophil

Red cell

Platelets

Fig. 3.1 Normal peripheral blood film showing a neutrophil with its typical lobulated nucleus, numerous red cells and a few platelets.

Red cell morphology

In health the normal RBC is a pink biconcave disc-shaped cell, and most red cells are roughly the same size, shape and colour in health. They should be roughly the size of a small lymphocyte nucleus. Many disease and deficiency disorders alter the RBC appearance by either reducing its haemoglobin content, or altering the membrane such that characteristic morphological abnormalities are produced. Examples include target cells, sickle cells, bite cells, burr cells and many others (see Table 3.2). Most of the morphological features are *not* absolutely specific for one particular disorder, but rather they suggest a range of conditions which may be associated with the RBC feature. This should prompt you to look for conditions which might account for the abnormality.

▶Pay attention to the peripheral blood film comment (inserted on the report by the haematology lab staff, or automated blood counter)—it should help you decide which tests to carry out next. Conversely, cryptic lab comments like 'anisopoikilocytosis noted' do not help the clinician much. (*Note: aniso* = unequal, *poikilo* = varied.)

Stippled red cells in haemolysis.

Marked rouleaux in myeloma.

Single nucleated red cell (on left).

Crenated red cells.

Fig. 3.2 Red cell abnormalities in various disease states.

Table 3.2

Microcytic RBCs	Fe deficiency, thalassaemia trait & syndromes, congenital sidero-blastic anaemia, anaemia of chronic disorders (if longstanding)
Macrocytic RBCs	Alcohol/liver disease (round macrocytes), MDS, pregnancy and newborn, compensated haemolysis, B_{12} or folate def., hydroxyurea and antimetabolites (oval macrocytes), acquired sideroblastic anaemia, hypothyroidism, chronic respiratory failure, aplastic anaemia
Dimorphic RBCs	Two populations, e.g. Fe deficiency responding to iron, mixed Fe and B_{12}/folate deficiency, sideroblastic anaemia, post red cell transfusion
Hypochromic RBCs	Reduced Hb synthesis, e.g. iron deficiency, thalassaemia, sideroblastic anaemia
Polychromatic RBCs	Blood loss or haematinic treatment, haemolysis, marrow infiltration
Spherocytes	Hereditary spherocytosis, haemolysis e.g. warm AIHA, delayed transfusion reaction, ABO HDN, DIC and MAHA, post-splenectomy
Pencil/rod cells	Fe deficiency anaemia, thalassaemia trait & syndromes, PK deficiency
Elliptocytes	Hereditary elliptocytosis, MPD and MDS
Fragmented RBCs	MAHA, DIC, renal failure, HUS, TTP
Teardrop RBCs	Myelofibrosis, metastatic marrow infiltration, MDS
Sickle cells	Sickle cell anaemia, other sickle syndromes (*not* sickle trait)
Target cells	Liver disease, Fe deficiency, thalassaemia, HbC syndromes
Crenated RBCs	Usually storage or EDTA artefact. Genuine RBC crenation may be seen post-splenectomy and in renal failure (→ burr cells)
Burr cells	Renal failure
Acanthocytes	Hereditary acanthocytosis, a-β-lipoproteinaemia, McLeod red cell phenotype, PK deficiency, chronic liver disease (esp. Zieve's syndrome)
Bite cells	G6PD deficiency, oxidative haemolysis
Basophilic stippling	Megaloblastic anaemia, lead poisoning, MDS, liver disease, haemoglobinopathies, e.g. thalassaemia
Rouleaux	Chronic inflammation, paraproteinaemia, myeloma
↑ reticulocytes	Bleeding, haemolysis, marrow infiltration, severe hypoxia, response to haematinic therapy
Heinz bodies	Not seen in normals (removed by spleen), small numbers seen post-splenectomy, oxidant drugs, G6PD deficiency, sulphonamides, unstable Hb (Hb Zurich, Köln)
Howell–Jolly bodies	Composed of DNA, removed by the spleen, seen in dyserythropoietic states e.g. B_{12} deficiency, MDS, post-splenectomy, hyposplenism
H bodies	HbH inclusions, denatured HbH (β₄ tetramer), stain with methylene blue, seen in HbH disease (– –/-α), less prominent in α thalassaemia trait, not present in normal subjects
Hyposplenic film	Howell–Jolly bodies, target cells, occasional nucleated RBCs, lymphocytosis, macrocytosis, acanthocytes. Infectious mononucleosis, any viral infection, toxoplasmosis, drug reactions

Parasites on the blood film & marrow

Blood film

Although there are now highly sensitive monoclonal antibody kits for the diagnosis of diseases such as malaria, a well-stained blood film can often make the diagnosis more easily. Blood films are useful for confirming a diagnosis of:

- Malaria.
- Trypanosomiasis.
- Microfilaria.

Parasites in bone marrow

Some diseases such as Leishmaniasis require bone marrow aspiration and staining (in fact there are many infections that can be diagnosed using a bone marrow):

- *Leishmania donovani.*
- Tuberculosis.
- *Tropheryma whippelii* (Whipple's disease).
- *Cryptococcus neoformans.*
- *Penicillium.*
- *Histoplasma capsulatum.*
- *Candida albicans.*
- *Toxoplasma gondii.*

http://health.allrefer.com/health/bone-marrow-transplant-formed-elements-of-blood.html
http://www.nlm.nih.gov/medlineplus/ency/article/003642.htm
http://www.bcshguidelines.com/pdf/CLH165.pdf

Falciparum malaria (blood film)

Loa loa (bone marrow)

Trypanosome (blood film)

Fig. 3.3 Parasites such as malaria, loa loa and trypanosomes may be seen on a stained blood film.

White blood cell morphology

In much the same way as RBC morphology provides clues about underlying disease, so too does microscopical examination of stained peripheral blood WBCs. Modern counters enumerate WBCs and our greater reliance on modern technology means that visual inspection of blood films is becoming a dying art. A well-stained blood film may provide the diagnosis much more cheaply.

Blood film when WBC is ↓

- Sometimes difficult to determine diagnosis since so few WBCs.
- May suggest B_{12} or folate deficiency (are the RBCs normal or large?).
- Aplastic anaemia—are the platelets and Hb normal?
- Underlying leukaemia—are there any leukaemic blasts* present?
- Overwhelming infection—may see toxic granulation (large dark granules in the cytoplasm—not diagnostic but suggestive).
- May be immune or post-viral—atypical lymphocytes may be seen; other indices usually normal.

Blood film when WBC is ↑

What cell predominates?

- Lymphocytes? suggests viral, CLL, acute leukaemia (lymphoblastic).
- Granulocytic? (neutrophils, eosinophils, basophils)—may be reactive or CML.
- Abnormal looking WBC? Look for Auer rods (≡ AML), smear cells (CLL), bilobed neutrophils (pseudo-Pelger cells seen in MDS).

Diagnosis must be made in context

How old is the patient?

- Viral illnesses often produce bizarre films in children but beware of complacency (acute leukaemia may be the cause).
- MDS and malignancies like CLL and CML are diseases of older individuals.

Is the patient well?

- May be worth repeating FBC and film to see if abnormalities have resolved.
- If patient unwell or has lymphadenopathy or hepatosplenomegaly then underlying disease must be excluded.

---

*A blast is a primitive cell seen in the marrow in large numbers in leukaemia. We all have some blasts in our marrows but these should be <5% of the total nucleated bone marrow cells in health.

Some WBC abnormalities seen on FBC reports

Table 3.3

Atypical lymphocytes	Infectious mononucleosis, any viral infection, toxoplasmosis, drug reactions
Auer rods	Seen in myeloblasts; pathognomonic of AML Prominent in AML M3 subtype (acute promyelocytic leukaemia)
Pelger–Huët anomaly	Bilobed neutrophils. May be hereditary (neutrophils are functionally normal) or acquired, e.g. MDS (pseudo-Pelger cells)
Left shifted	Immature WBCs seen in peripheral blood. Seen in severe infections, inflammatory disorders, DKA, marrow 'stress', MPD, CML
Right shifted	Hypermature WBCs seen in e.g. megaloblastic anaemia and iron deficiency
Toxic granulation	Coarse granules in neutrophils. Seen in severe infection, post-operatively and inflammatory disorders
Smear cells	Lymphocytes in which the cell membrane has ruptured when making the blood film—there are no smear cells *in vivo*! Seen in CLL

Fig. 3.4 Blood film: atypical white blood cells (this was from a patient with glandular fever, but these cells may be seen in any viral illness).

Atlas of haematology slides

http://pathy.med.nagoya-u.ac.jp/atlas/doc/atlas.html

Assessment of iron status

The anaemia of iron deficiency is caused by defective synthesis of haemoglobin resulting in red cells that are smaller than normal (microcytic) and contain reduced amounts of haemoglobin (*hypochromic*). The diagnosis of iron deficiency anaemia is generally straightforward but it may be confused with that due to the anaemia of chronic disease (ACD) or other hypochromic anaemias (see Table 3.4).

Iron plays a pivotal role in many metabolic processes and the average adult contains between 3 and 5g of iron of which two-thirds is present in the O_2-carrying molecule, haemoglobin. Somewhat surprisingly, there is no specific excretion mechanism in humans. Iron balance is controlled at the level of gut absorption, and relies on two iron-sequestering proteins, *transferrin* (iron transport and recycling of iron) and *ferritin* (safeguards iron entry into the body, and maintains surplus iron in a safe and readily accessible form).

Ferritin

This is the primary iron-storage protein consisting of 24 apoferritin subunits forming a hollow sphere (each can hold up to 4500 Fe atoms).

Haemosiderin

Haemosiderin, located predominantly in macrophages, is a water-soluble protein–iron complex with an amorphous structure.

Transferrin and its receptor

Transferrin contains only 4mg iron and is the principal iron transport protein with more than 30mg iron transported round the body daily. Synthesis of transferrin is inversely proportional to the body iron stores, with increased transferrin concentration when iron stores are reduced.

The transferrin receptor (TfR) is a disulphide-linked dimer composed of two identical 85kDa subunits. The serum TfR concentration is elevated in iron deficiency. However, sTfR may also increase in any condition in which there is increased erythropoiesis, e.g. haemolytic anaemias, thalassaemia, polycythaemia vera and other myeloproliferative disorders.

Assessment of iron status

Several parameters are available
- Haemoglobin concentration.
- Serum ferritin.
- Serum iron and transferrin (as total iron binding capacity, TIBC).
- % hypochromic cells in peripheral blood.
- Red cell protoporphyrin assay (not widely available).
- Bone marrow aspirate (stained for iron)—the 'gold standard'.
- Soluble transferrin receptor assay (sTfR).

Remember, iron deficiency is not an 'all-or-nothing' phenomenon. In progressive deficiency there is a gradual loss of iron with subtle alterations of iron-related parameters during which the red cells may look entirely normal. In the initial stages of developing iron deficiency macrophages become depleted of iron and the serum ferritin ↓ to the lower end of the normal range; during this 'latency' period the Hb is normal. As the deficiency progresses plasma iron levels ↓ and TIBC ↑. Free RBC protoporphyrin levels ↑ as it accumulates, and eventually hypochromic RBCs appear in the peripheral blood. At this stage a full blood count will usually show ↓ Hb, MCV, MCH and MCHC, and the peripheral blood film will show microcytic hypochromic red cells.

Confirmation of simple iron deficiency anaemia

- Hb ↓.
- Serum ferritin will be ↓.

> **Beware**: serum ferritin is an acute phase protein and may be normal or even ↑ in inflammatory, malignant or liver disease. During the inflammatory response the iron/TIBC are unlikely to be of any value (iron ↓ and TIBC will be ↓). If an inflammatory process is suspected, an alternative test is required, e.g. sTfR, which is not affected by inflammatory disorders.

- Serum iron ↓ and TIBC ↑ (generally unhelpful and little used today).
- sTfR ↑.
- MCV ↓.
- MCH & MCHC ↓.
- Microcytic & hypochromic RBCs on blood film.
- Absent marrow iron.

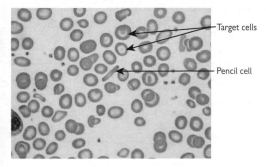

Target cells

Pencil cell

Fig. 3.5   Blood film of iron deficiency anaemia. Note the variation in cell size and shape.

Additional routine parameters

% Blasts:	1.2
% Hyper:	0.0
% Hypo:	86.8 ←
% Macro:	0.0
% Micro:	62.9
RBC fragments:	0.09

RBC volume

RBC V/HC

RBC HC

Fig. 3.6 The % hypochromic red cells (provided by some automated counters) helps in the diagnosis of iron deficiency. Notice that the RBC volume and haemoglobin content (HC) are both shifted to the LEFT (=small pale red cells).

Table 3.4 Hypochromic anaemias—may be confused with iron deficiency

Disorder	Example
Disorders of Fe metabolism	Iron deficiency anaemia –Blood loss –Reduced iron intake –Impaired iron transport
Anaemia of chronic disorders	Chronic inflammatory diseases Malignant disease
Disorders of haem synthesis	Sideroblastic anaemias *Hereditary* *Idiopathic* *Secondary* –Drugs –Alcohol –Lead poisoning
Globin synthesis disorders	Thalassaemias –β thalassaemia –α thalassaemia

📖OHCM p628.

🖰http://www.ironpanel.org.au/AIS/AISdocs/adultdocs/Acontents.html
🖰http://www.irondisorders.org/disorders/ida/

Provan D, Weatherall D. (2000) Acquired anaemias and polycythaemia. *Lancet* **355**, 1260–1268.

Assessment of vitamin B₁₂ & folate status

Measurement of the serum B_{12} and red cell folate levels is necessary in the investigation of macrocytic anaemia and certain other situations (see *below*). Serum folate levels are an unreliable measurement of body stores of folate—the red cell folate level is probably more meaningful.

B_{12} unit: ng/L.

Serum & red cell folate units: µg/L.

Sample: clotted blood sample (serum B_{12} and folate) and peripheral blood EDTA (red cell folate).

Deficiency of either vitamin leads to megaloblastic anaemia where there is disruption of cell division in all actively dividing cells (includes the bone marrow and gut). In the marrow there is nuclear:cytoplasmic asynchrony where the nuclei are immature despite a mature well-haemoglobinised cytoplasm. In the peripheral blood there may be anaemia, often with pancytopenia; the red cells show oval macrocytic changes with basophilic stippling and occasionally nucleated red cells. Neutrophils typically become hypersegmented (they have >5 lobes).

Until recently, B_{12} and folate assays were tedious microbiological assays but these have now been replaced by automated techniques using radio-isotopic methods which allow large numbers of samples to be batched and tested fairly cheaply.

Deficiencies of B_{12} or folate do not always cause macrocytic anaemia

In the past, deficiency of either B_{12} or folate was synonymous with macrocytic anaemia but deficiency of either vitamin may present without anaemia or macrocytosis—*remember*, these are *late* features of the disease. However, in most cases of deficiency the marrow will show characteristic megaloblastic change (nuclear asynchrony with giant metamyelocytes). ▶*Deficiency of B_{12} may cause neurological problems in the absence of anaemia.*

Whom should you test?

- Patients with GIT disease, glossitis, abnormalities of taste, previous surgery or radiotherapy to stomach or small bowel.
- Neurological disease, e.g. peripheral neuropathy, demyelination.
- Psychiatric disturbance, e.g. confusion, dementia.
- Malnutrition, e.g. growth impairment in children; vegans.
- Alcohol abuse.
- Autoimmune disease of thyroid, parathyroid or adrenals.
- Patients with family history of pernicious anaemia.
- Others, e.g. drugs that interfere with vitamin absorption or metabolism such as nitrous oxide, phenytoin, etc.

Look for blood film abnormalities

▶B_{12} & folate deficiencies produce similar clinical and laboratory features.

- Oval macrocytes.
- Hypersegmented neutrophils (also seen in renal failure, iron deficiency and MDS).

Fig. 3.7 Blood film of megaloblastic anaemia. There are large oval macrocytes and two hypersegmented neutrophils (the nucleus has >5 lobes).

Which test next?

Make sure you have the following
- FBC.
- Blood film.
- Serum B$_{12}$ level.
- Serum and red cell folate level.
- Intrinsic factor antibodies (IFA), +ve in 50–75% patients with PA.
- Consider bone marrow (helps exclude MDS, myeloma and other pathologies that give rise to macrocytic anaemia, but seldom performed today since it is easy to get a B$_{12}$ and folate result back quickly).

Interpretation of results: vitamin B$_{12}$

Normal ranges are based on 2 standard deviations either side of the mean, so there will be 'normal' people who have 'abnormal' B$_{12}$ (or folate) levels.

B$_{12}$ <normal   – deficiency
                               – altered metabolism
                               – 'normal'

The *lowest levels are seen in those most deficient*. What matters is whether there is *tissue deficiency* (leads to marrow and neurological changes).

Mild ↓ in B$_{12}$ level?

Difficult, but common! Probably worth repeating the test and reviewing the patient and other results. If no evidence of tissue deficiency, can probably observe the patient. If there is evidence of tissue deficiency then the patient will require treatment.

Detecting tissue deficiency
The most reliable method is probably the measurement of serum homocysteine (accumulates in vitamin B_{12} and folate deficiency).

Beware B_{12} not associated with tissue deficiency
- Folate deficiency.
- Pregnancy.
- Myeloma.
- Transcobalamin I deficiency (very rare).

Folate
↓ level seen in hospitalised patients due to negative folate balance.

The B_{12} level is low—what next?
Available tests for the cause of B_{12} deficiency include
- Parietal cell (+ve in serum of 90% patients with PA but also found in other disorders and 15% of the normal elderly) and intrinsic factor antibodies (IFA better—if +ve confirms diagnosis of PA).
- Schilling test (urinary excretion method where addition of if restores B_{12} absorption in PA but not in intestinal, e.g. ileal, disease) or
- Whole body B_{12} counting.
- Endoscopy with duodenal biopsy.
- Other gastroenterology tests for malabsorption (📖Ch 7).

The folate level is low—what next?
- Check dietary history.
- Endoscopy with duodenal biopsy.
- Other gastroenterology tests for malabsorption (📖Ch 7).

📖OHCM p632.

http://www.hlth.gov.bc.ca/msp/protoguides/gps/b12.pdf
http://www.med.utah.edu/healthinfo/adult/Hemat/folate.htm

Provan D, Weatherall D. (2000) Acquired anaemias and polycythaemia. *Lancet* **355**, 1260–1268.

Erythrocyte sedimentation rate (ESR)

This simple but very useful qualitative test measures how fast a patient's red cells fall through a column of blood. It is a sensitive but non-specific index of plasma protein changes which result from inflammation or tissue damage. The ESR is affected by haematocrit variations, red cell abnormalities (e.g. poikilocytosis, sickle cells) and delay in analysis, and is therefore less reliable than measurement of the plasma viscosity. The ESR is affected by age, sex, menstrual cycle, pregnancy and drugs (e.g. OCP, steroids).

The ESR is widely used in clinical medicine and despite attempts (by haematology departments) to replace the ESR with the plasma viscosity the ESR has remained in use and appears to retain a valuable place in the armoury of disease diagnosis and monitoring.

Sample: peripheral blood EDTA; the sample should be analysed in the laboratory within 4h.

Normal ranges (upper limits)

Table 3.5

Age	Men	Women
17–50 years	10mm/h	12mm/h
51–60	12	19
>60	14	20

There are many factors which influence the ESR causing a high or low result:

High ESR (significant*—look for a cause)
- Any inflammatory disorder, e.g. infection, rheumatoid, TB.
- Myocardial infarction (the ESR ↑ as an early response).
- Anaemia.

*Depends exactly *how high*. An ESR of 30 probably means little but if >100 is *highly significant* and indicates something seriously wrong.

Low ESR (rarely important, but useful for exams)
- Polycythaemia.
- Hypofibrinogenaemia.
- CCF.
- Poikilocytosis.
- Spherocytosis.
- Sickled cells.
- ▶▶A normal ESR does not exclude organic disease.
- 📖OHCM p670.

🔗http://www.aafp.org/afp/991001ap/1443.html

Harris GJ. (1972) Plasma viscometry and ESR in the elderly. *Med Lab Technol* **29**, 405–410; Lewis SM. (1980) Erythrocyte sedimentation rate and plasma viscosity. *Ass Clin Pathol Broadsheet* **94**, 1–6.

Plasma viscosity

This test is a sensitive but non-specific index of plasma protein changes which result from inflammation or tissue damage. Provides much the same information as the ESR. The ESR and PV tend to rise in parallel but the PV is *unaffected* by haematocrit variations (e.g. severe anaemia or polycythaemia) and delay in analysis up to 24h, and is therefore more reliable than the ESR. It is not affected by sex but is affected by age, exercise and pregnancy. It is constant in health and shows no diurnal variation. There is a suggestion that the PV may be a more sensitive indicator of disease severity than the ESR.

Sample: peripheral blood EDTA. The sample is centrifuged and the plasma removed.

Normal range: 1.50–1.72CP (or MPA/s at 25°C).

High and low plasma viscosity

High PV generally signifies some underlying pathology; low PV can be ignored.

Note: Despite the advantages outlined the PV has not been adopted by all medical staff (who still prefer the ESR as a measure of inflammation). The PV is better for monitoring hyperviscosity syndromes, e.g. Waldenström's macroglobulinaemia. The fact that both tests are still used shows that there is a role for both.

📖OHCM p670.

Cooke BM, Stuart J. (1988) Automated measurement of plasma viscosity by capillary viscometer. *J Clin Pathol* **41**, 1213–1216.

Tests for glandular fever

This infection is caused by Epstein–Barr virus (EBV). Infected cells produce so-called heterophile antibodies (these are IgM molecules that agglutinate horse and sheep RBCs but do not agglutinate ox RBCs and do not react at all with guinea-pig RBCs).

There are various kits available that can detect the presence of heterophile antibodies and in the right clinical context will confirm a diagnosis of EBV infection. The Monospot test is probably the commonest in current use. The Paul–Bunnell test was the first to demonstrate the presence of heterophile antibodies in patients with EBV infection.

Clinical features
Glandular fever often affects young adults (12–25 years) and results in malaise, fever, tonsillitis, petechial haemorrhages on palate and lymphadenopathy. Splenomegaly is fairly common. A similar clinical picture is seen in CMV, *Toxoplasma* and early HIV infections.

Sample: EDTA.

Positive Monospot
- EBV infection.

False positives
- Toxoplasmosis.
- CMV infection.
- Rheumatoid.
- Malaria.

Hoff G, Bauer S. (1965) A new rapid slide test for infectious mononucleosis. *JAMA* **194**, 351–353.

Investigation of haemolytic anaemia

The normal red cell has a lifespan of ~120 days. Anaemia resulting from ↓ RBC lifespan is termed *haemolytic*. May be inherited or acquired and the basic underlying mechanisms may involve abnormalities of the RBC *membrane*, RBC *enzymes* or *haemoglobin*.

Extravascular vs. intravascular

Extravascular haemolysis implies RBC breakdown by the RES (e.g. liver, spleen, and macrophages at other sites) while intravascular haemolysis describes RBC breakdown in the circulation itself. There are many investigations available which will help determine the predominant site of destruction, which in turn will help define the underlying cause of haemolysis, which is why we do the tests in the first place.

Detection of haemolysis itself

The main question is whether the patient's anaemia is due to haemolysis or some other underlying mechanism such as blood loss, marrow infiltration, etc.

📖 OHCM p638.

General tests of haemolysis

Is haemolysis actually occurring? Suggestive features are

- Evidence of ↑ red cell destruction.
- Evidence of ↑ red cell production (to compensate for red cell loss).
- Evidence of autoantibody in the patient's serum.

Evidence of RBC destruction

- ↑ serum bilirubin.
- ↑ serum LDH (reflecting ↑ RBC turnover).
- Spherocytes or other abnormal RBCs, e.g. fragments on blood film.
- Plasma haptoglobins may be ↓ or absent.
- ↑ Faecal & urinary urobilinogen (faecal not measured).
- ↓ RBC lifespan (seldom measured nowadays).

Evidence of ↑ RBC production

- ↑ Reticulocytes (on film, manual or automated count). Not absolutely specific, will ↑ in brisk acute bleed, e.g. GIT.
- ↑ MCV (reticulocytes are larger than mature RBCs, and don't forget folate deficiency which occurs in haemolytic disorders).

Is it mainly intravascular?

- ↑ Plasma Hb.
- Methaemalbuminaemia.
- Haemoglobinuria.
- Haemosiderinuria.

HAEMOLYSIS

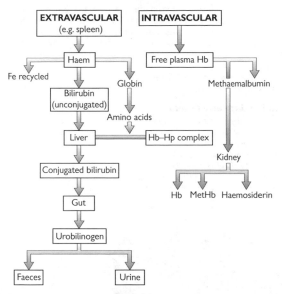

Fig. 3.8 Increased red cell breakdown may be extravascular (outside the circulation, predominantly spleen, liver and marrow) or intravascular (within the vessels).

What is the cause?

Genetic
- RBC morphology (e.g. spherocytes, elliptocytes).
- Hb analysis.
- RBC enzyme assays.

Acquired
- Immune—check DAT.
- Non-immune: check RBC morphology (e.g. TTP/HUS).
- Is there some other underlying disease?
- Consider PNH (rare).

🖰http://www.umm.edu/blood/anehemol.htm
🖰http://www.emedicine.com/med/topic979.htm

Modified from Lewis SM, Bain BJ & Bates I, eds. (2001) Dacie & Lewis *Practical Haematology*, 9th edition, Churchill Livingstone, Edinburgh.

Reticulocytes

These are immature RBCs formed in the marrow and found in small numbers in normal peripheral blood. They represent an intermediate maturation stage in marrow between the nucleated RBC and the mature RBC (the reticulocyte lacks a nucleus but retains some nucleic acid). Measuring the number of reticulocytes in the blood may help determine whether the anaemia is due to ↓ RBC production. The reticulocyte count is also a useful measure of response to haematinic (iron, B_{12} or folate) replacement therapy.

Detection and measurement
- Demonstrated by staining with supravital dye for the nucleic acid.
- Appear on blood film as larger than mature RBCs with fine lacy blue staining strands or dots.
- Some modern automated blood counters using laser technology can measure levels of retics directly.
- Usually expressed as a % of total red cells, e.g. 5%, though absolute numbers can be derived from this and total red cell count.

Spherocytes

Fig. 3.9 Blood film of numerous spherocytes (small darker red cells) and reticulocytes (larger red cells) in autoimmune haemolytic anaemia.

Sample: EDTA.

Normal range: 0.5–2.5% (50–100 × 10^9/L).

Causes of ↑ reticulocyte counts
Marrow stimulation due to
- Bleeding.
- Haemolysis.
- Response to oral Fe therapy.
- Infection.
- Inflammation.

- Polycythaemia (any cause).
- Myeloproliferative disorders.
- Marrow recovery following chemotherapy or radiotherapy.
- Erythropoietin administration.

Causes of ↓ reticulocyte counts
Marrow infiltration due to

- Leukaemia.
- Myeloma.
- Lymphoma.
- Other malignancy.

Marrow underactivity (hypoplasia) due to

- Fe, folate or B_{12} deficiency. *Note*: return of retics is earliest sign of response to replacement therapy.
- Immediately post-chemotherapy or radiotherapy.
- Autoimmune disease especially RA.
- Malnutrition.
- Uraemia.
- Drugs.
- Aplastic anaemia.
- Red cell aplasia.

Howells MR et al. (1986) Erythropoiesis in pregnancy. *Br J Haematol* **64**, 595–599.

Serum haptoglobins

Haptoglobins (Hp) are plasma proteins synthesised by the liver, whose function is the removal of free plasma haemoglobin. Hp molecules bind free Hb and are taken up by the reticuloendothelial system for degradation. Hp–Hb complexes do not appear in the urine because their large size prevents them passing through the renal tubules.

The Hp–Hb complex is cleared by the reticuloendothelial system at a rate of 15mg/100mL/h which means that even very mild haemolysis will cause the disappearance of Hp from the circulation. The serum haptoglobin should be measured in patients with suspected intravascular haemolysis. However, the Hp level is frequently reduced in patients with extravascular haemolysis, and the Hp level cannot be used to determine whether the basic haemolytic process is intra- or extravascular. It should generally be accompanied by estimation of the serum methaemalbumin, free plasma haemoglobin and urinary haemosiderin.

Sample: clotted blood.

Normal range: (expressed as Hb binding capacity in mg/dL): 30–250mg/dL.

Conditions with ↓ haptoglobins
Haemolysis including

- Incompatible blood transfusion.

- Autoimmune haemolytic anaemia.
- Sickle cell disease.
- Thalassaemia major.
- PNH.

Others
- 1% population have genetic lack of haptoglobin.
- Lower levels in infancy.

Note: it takes about 1 week after haemolysis has stopped for haptoglobin levels to return to normal.

Conditions with ↑ haptoglobins (acute phase protein, like ferritin)
- Any disorder with ↑ ESR.
- Carcinoma especially if bony secondaries.
- Any inflammatory disorder.
- Trauma.
- Surgery.
- Steroid therapy.
- Androgen therapy.
- Diabetes mellitus.

Rougemont A *et al.* (1988) Hypohaptoglobinaemia as an epidemiological and clinical indicator for malaria. Results of two studies in a hyperendemic region in West Africa. *Lancet* **2**, 709–712.

Serum bilirubin

Two forms are found: prehepatic bilirubin (unconjugated) and bilirubin conjugated to glucuronic acid (conjugated). Generally serum bilirubin levels are 17–50µmol/L in haemolysis (mainly unconjugated). *Beware*: serum bilirubin levels may be normal even if haemolysis is present; a level >85µmol/L suggests liver disease.

The serum bilirubin may be modestly ↑ (e.g. 20–30µmol/L) in dyserythropoietic disorders such as vitamin B_{12} or folate deficiency or myelodysplasia, due to ineffective erythropoiesis where the RBCs are destroyed in the marrow before ever being released into the circulation.

Urobilin & urobilinogen

Urobilinogen is the reduced form of urobilin, formed by bacterial action on bile pigments in the GI tract. Faecal and urinary urobilinogen ↑ in haemolytic anaemias.

Urinary haemosiderin

Usage
The most widely used and reliable test for detection of chronic intravascular haemolysis. Results from the presence of Hb in the glomerular filtrate.

Principle

Free Hb is released into the plasma during intravascular haemolysis. The haemoglobin binding proteins become saturated resulting in passage of haem-containing compounds into the urinary tract of which haemosiderin is the most readily detectable.

Method

1. A clean catch sample of urine is obtained from the patient.
2. Sample is spun down in a cytocentrifuge to obtain a cytospin preparation of urothelial cells.
3. Staining and rinsing with Perl's reagent (Prussian blue) is performed on the glass slides.
4. Examine under oil-immersion lens of microscope.
5. Haemosiderin stains as blue dots within urothelial cells.
6. Ignore all excess stain, staining outside cells or in debris, all of which are common.
7. True +ve only when clear detection within urothelial squames is seen.

Cautions

An iron-staining +ve control sample should be run alongside test case to ensure stain has worked satisfactorily. Haemosiderinuria may not be detected for up to 72h after the initial onset of intravascular haemolysis so the test may miss haemolysis of very recent onset—repeat test in 3–7 days if –ve. Conversely, haemosiderinuria may persist for some time after a haemolytic process has stopped. Repeat in 7 days should confirm.

Causes of haemosiderinuria

Table 3.6

Common causes	Red cell enzymopathies, e.g. G6PD and PK deficiency, but only during haemolytic episodes
	Mycoplasma pneumonia with anti-I cold haemagglutinin
	Sepsis
	Malaria
	Cold haemagglutinin disease
	TTP/HUS
	Severe extravascular haemolysis (may cause intravascular haemolysis)
Rarer causes	PNH
	Prosthetic heart valves
	Red cell incompatible transfusion reactions
	Unstable haemoglobins
	March haemoglobinuria

Plasma haemoglobin

In health, haemoglobin is contained within RBCs but during intravascular haemolysis excessive quantities of Hb may be released from ruptured RBCs. Normally haptoglobins mop up free Hb. If there are insufficient haptoglobins to cope with the free Hb, the kidneys clear the Hb leading to haemoglobinuria. Some Hb may be broken down in the circulation to haem and globin; haem can bind to albumin producing methaemalbumin (→ methaemalbuminaemia).

▶The finding of free Hb in plasma is *highly suggestive* of intravascular haemolysis.

Sample: sodium citrate (but discuss with haematology laboratory before sending sample).

Causes of ↑ plasma haemoglobin

Table 3.7

Mild ↑ (50–100mg/L)	Moderate↑ (100–250mg/L)	Severe↑ (>250mg/L)
Sickle/thalassaemia	AIHA	Incompatible blood transfusion
HbC disease	Sickle cell disease Thalassaemia major HbSC Prosthetic heart valve March haemoglobinuria	PNH PCH Blackwater fever

Normal range: 10–40mg/L (up to 6mg/L).

Pitfalls: any RBC damage occurring during blood sampling may result in an erroneously high reading. Great care must be taken during venepuncture.

Crosby WH, Dameshek W. (1951) The significance of hemoglobinemia and associated hemosiderinuria, with particular reference to various types of hemolytic anemia. *J Clin Lab Med* **38**, 829.

Schumm's test

Use: detection of methaemalbumin (seen after all haptoglobins used up in a haemolytic process, usually implies the haemolysis is predominantly intravascular).

This spectrophotometric test for methaemalbumin (which has a distinctive absorption band at 558nm) should be requested in patients with suspected intravascular haemolysis and may be abnormal in patients with significant extravascular (generally splenic) haemolysis. It should be accompanied by estimation of the serum haptoglobin level, free plasma haemoglobin and urinary haemosiderin.

Sample: heparinised or clotted blood.

Positive result in

- Intravascular haemolysis.
- Mismatched blood transfusion.
- RBC fragmentation syndromes.
- G6PD deficiency with oxidative haemolysis.
- PNH.
- March haemoglobinuria.
- Unstable Hbs.

Winstone NE. (1965) Methemalbumin in acute pancreatitis. *Br J Surg* **52**, 804–808; Hoffbrand AV, Lewis SM, Tuddenham EGD, eds. (2000) *Postgraduate Haematology*, 4th edition, Butterworth-Heinemann, Oxford.

Hereditary haemolytic anaemias

There are many inherited causes for haemolytic anaemia which fall into 3 major groups shown in Table 3.8.

Table 3.8

Mechanism	Example
Red cell membrane disorders	Hereditary spherocytosis Hereditary elliptocytosis
Red cell enzyme disorders	G6PD deficiency Pyruvate kinase deficiency
Haemoglobin disorders	Sickle cell anaemia Thalassaemia

Red cell membrane disorders

Hereditary spherocytosis

This is the best known inherited membrane abnormality leading to a reduced red cell lifespan and sometimes severe anaemia. Inheritance is usually autosomal dominant, and there is often a positive family history.

Osmotic fragility test

Principle of the test

The test measures the ability of red cells to take up water before rupturing (lysing). This is determined by the volume:surface area ratio. Normal red cells can ↑ their volume by up to 70% before lysing (because they are disc shaped, and have the capacity to take in extra water easily). Spherocytic red cells have an ↑ volume: surface area ratio and are able to take up less water than normal red cells before lysing (they are spheres and as such they are 'full' already).

Sample: EDTA (need normal control sample sent at the same time).

Method
- RBCs are incubated in saline at various concentrations. This results in cell expansion and eventually rupture.
- Normal RBCs can withstand greater volume increases than spherocytic RBCs.
- A positive result (confirming HS) seen when RBCs lyse in saline at near to isotonic concentration, i.e. 0.6–0.8g/dL (normal RBCs will simply show swelling with little lysis).
- Osmotic fragility is more marked in patients who have not undergone splenectomy, and if the RBCs are incubated at 37°C for 24h before performing the test.

Other supportive tests
- There will be a positive family history of HS in many cases.
- The blood film shows ↑↑ spherocytic RBCs.
- Anaemia, ↑ reticulocytes, ↑ LDH, unconjugated bilirubin, urinary urobilinogen with ↓ haptoglobins.
- DAT –ve.

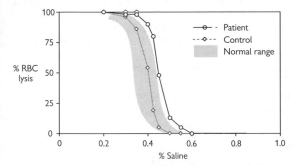

Fig. 3.10 Test and control samples subjected to varying concentrations of saline The broad grey band represents the normal range. The red cells in the test sample (from a patient with hereditary spherocytosis) lyse at higher concentrations of saline than that seen in the normal control which suggests that HS is a likely diagnosis.

Beware: this test is not diagnostic of HS, but will be +ve in any condition in which there are increased numbers of spherocytic red cells. Use this test in conjunction with a history, blood film and family studies (HS is inherited as an autosomal dominant, so one of the parents and some siblings should be affected).

🖰http://www.uq.edu.au/vdu/HDUAnaemiaHeridSphere.htm
🖰http://www.bcshguidelines.com/pdf/hereditaryspherocytosis.pdf

Parpart AK et al. (1947) The osmotic resistance (fragility) of human red cells. *J Clin Invest* **26**, 636; Weatherall DJ, Provan AB. (2000) Red cells I: inherited anaemias. *Lancet* **355**, 1169–1175.

Red cell enzyme assays

Numerous red cell enzymes are responsible for maintaining the integrity of the RBC in order to allow it to function efficiently in O_2 delivery and CO_2 removal. RBC enzyme defects lead to shortened RBC survival (i.e. haemolysis) and anaemia. Although there are numerous enzymopathies that may cause haemolysis, the most useful starting assays are for G6PD and pyruvate kinase.

Of course, one should start by taking a detailed history from the patient, asking about previous haemolytic episodes, family history, ethnic origin and possible drug toxicities.

Sample: fresh EDTA or heparin. The enzymes are stable for 6 days at $4°C$ and 24h at $25°C$.

Methods: these are too numerous and complex to list here.

Essentially there are 3 methods for analysis of G6PD
- Brilliant cresyl blue decolorisation test.
- Methaemoglobin reduction test.
- UV spot test.

Normal range: varies between laboratories (check with your local lab).

Pitfalls: during a haemolytic episode in patients with G6PD deficiency the oldest RBCs are destroyed first. Younger RBCs (and especially reticulocytes) have higher levels of the enzyme than older cells. It follows therefore that if the enzyme level is assayed during an acute episode the G6PD level obtained may be falsely normal. This will rise further as reticulocytes pour into the peripheral blood, as happens during recovery from the acute attack. It is better to wait until the acute attack is over and the patient is in steady-state.

http://www.rcpa.edu.au/pathman/haemolys.htm

Arya R et al. (1995) Hereditary red cell enzymopathies. *Blood Rev* **9**, 165–175; Beutler E. (1992) The molecular biology of G6PD variants and other red cell enzyme defects. *Annu Rev Med* **43**, 47–59; World Health Organization Scientific Group. (1967) Standardization of procedures for the study of glucose-6-phosphate dehydrogenase. *Technical Report Series*, **No. 366**, WHO, Geneva.

Haemoglobin abnormalities

There are 2 main classes of haemoglobin abnormalities.

Table 3.9

Abnormality	Example
Structural Hb variants	Sickle haemoglobin, HbD, HbE
Imbalanced globin production	Thalassaemias (α, β, etc.)

Structural haemoglobin variants

If the amino acid change results in an electrical charge difference, this may be detected by protein electrophoresis (separates proteins on the basis of charge). Investigation requires full clinical history, FBC, blood film and Hb electrophoresis.

Thalassaemias

β thalassaemia is diagnosed from the blood indices, blood film, HbA_2 and HbF levels. For a thalassaemia the investigation is more complex requiring DNA analysis to detect α globin deletions. Globin chain synthesis, which examines the ratio of α:β globin production, is performed less with the advent of DNA-based methods.

Weatherall DJ, Provan AB. (2000) Red cells I: inherited anaemias. *Lancet* **355**, 1169–1175.

Haemoglobin analysis

Haemoglobin electrophoresis

Electrophoresis is an electrical method for separating molecules on the basis of size (for DNA fragments) or overall electrical charge (for proteins). Hb electrophoresis allows the separation of different Hbs *providing* they have differing charges (Hb molecules with the same charge will move together on the gel and cannot be distinguished). The methods used take advantage of the fact that amino acid side chains on the globin molecules can be ionised. The net overall charge of a protein depends on the pH of the solution it is in and the pKs of the amino acids (the pK is the pH at which half the side chains are ionised).

Normal adult haemoglobins:
HbA   97% total
HbA_2 2.0–3.2%
HbF   0.5%

Electrophoretic methods used
• Cellulose acetate (at pH 8.6).
• Citrate agar (at pH 6.0).

- Isoelectric focusing (IEF).
- High-performance liquid chromatography (HPLC).

Due to space limitations each of these methods will be discussed only briefly. Other texts deal with this topic in considerable detail.

Sample: peripheral blood EDTA.

Cellulose acetate

This test is commonly performed in the diagnosis of abnormal haemoglobin production (haemoglobinopathies or thalassaemia). Because some Hbs have the same net charge they will run together, e.g. HbS will run in the same band as HbD and HbG, and HbC will run with HbE. To resolve these bands electrophoresis is next carried out at acid pH.

Citrate agar

This is similar to cellulose acetate where Hbs are separated at an acid pH (pH 6.0) to separate out Hbs that run together at alkaline pH.

Isoelectric focusing

This is a high resolution method for separating different Hb molecules. The basic principle of the test relies on the fact that all proteins and amino acids have a pH at which their net charge is zero. This is termed the isoelectric point. At this pH there is no net movement in the presence of an externally applied electric field. The Hb molecules are subjected to a pH gradient. This method has the advantage of high resolution but is more expensive than standard electrophoresis.

Fig. 3.11 Isoelectric focusing of haemoglobin.

High-performance liquid chromatography

This chromatographic technique has been around for 20 years or more, and is being increasingly used for analysis of haemoglobin molecules. Haemoglobins are passed through a matrix column and eluted from the column at varying times, during which their absorbance is measured. Detection of standard haemoglobin variants is simple; the advantage of HPLC is that novel haemoglobin variants can also be detected, and HPLC can separate proteins that cannot be resolved using other means. HPLC is more expensive than all the techniques mentioned above.

Fig. 3.12 HPLC analysis showing sickle trait (HbA + HbS).

Fig. 3.13 HPLC analysis showing β thalassaemia trait (elevated HbA_2).

When should you request these tests?
Haemoglobin analysis is usually carried out
- When the MCV is ↓↓ but Hb normal or slightly ↓.
- In patients from ethnic groups known to be associated with high levels of haemoglobin disorder, e.g. sickle or thalassaemia.

Investigation of possible thalassaemia

1. Check FBC and look at MCV.
2. Is the MCV normal (>76fL)? If so, thalassaemia is unlikely.
3. Does the FBC show anything else? ↑ RCC with ↓ MCV and MCH are likely in thalassaemia.
4. Measure the HbA$_2$: this is generally ↑ in β thalassaemia trait (carrier).
5. Carry out HPLC.
6. Measure HbF level.
7. Look at distribution of HbF in RBCs (HbF is present in *all* RBCs in African HPFH (hereditary persistence of fetal haemoglobin), but not present in all cells in carrier for δβ thalassaemia.
8. Assess iron status (common cause of ↓ MCV—don't miss this!).
9. Look for RBC inclusions (e.g. H bodies in α thalassaemia or Heinz bodies in unstable haemoglobin disorders).
10. Carry out DNA analysis, examining both α and β globin genes.

♐http://sickle.bwh.harvard.edu/menu_thal.html

Investigation of sickle haemoglobin

Sickle Hb is the result of a point mutation in the β globin gene resulting in a glu → val switch at position 6 of the β globin protein. Sickle haemoglobin (HbS) forms long filaments (tactoids) reducing its solubility when O$_2$ tension is reduced. This forms the basis of the sickle solubility test.

Sample: any anticoagulant.

Sickled red cells

Fig. 3.14 Blood film of homozygous sickle cell anaemia (HbSS). Note the sickle-shaped (crescent) red cells.

The patient's blood is mixed with sodium dithionite solution and left to stand. A positive sickle sample should be used as a control. When the tubes are examined a clear solution implies that there is no sickle Hb; a turbid solution confirms the presence of sickle Hb in the patient's sample.

▶A positive result will be obtained for sickle carriers (HbAS) and sickle cell homozygotes (HbSS). If a positive result is obtained Hb electrophoresis must be carried out to determine whether the patient is a carrier or has homozygous sickle cell anaemia.

🕭http://sickle.bwh.harvard.edu/menu_sickle.html

Steinberg MH et al., eds. (2001) *Disorders of Hemoglobin. Genetics, Pathophysiology, and Clinical Management*, Cambridge University Press, Cambridge.

Molecular diagnosis of sickle cell disease

This is useful for prenatal diagnosis. The β globin genes of the fetus are amplified using PCR (cells are obtained by amniocentesis or CVS) and digested with a bacterial restriction enzyme, e.g. Mst II. If the sickle mutation is present no digestion will occur (the mutation removes the restriction site).

Neonatal haemoglobin screening

• Obtain blood from neonate (e.g. heel prick) in babies at risk of sickle or β thalassaemia major (e.g. mother has gene for HbS, C, D^{Punjab}, E, O^{Arab}, β or δβ thalassaemia).
• Universal neonatal screening is generally used in areas where there is a high incidence of haemoglobinopathy.

📖OHCM p640.

Estimation of haemoglobin A_2 $(\alpha_2\beta_2)$

Normal adults have 3 types of haemoglobin: HbA, HbA_2 and HbF. HbA $(\alpha_2\beta_2)$ is the major Hb and HbA_2 is a minor adult haemoglobin, which is very useful for the diagnosis of β thalassaemia trait. HbA_2 levels are ↑ in the heterozygote (carrier state) and this is a specific test for this genotype. The test is carried out using a column chromatography method.

Sample: EDTA.

Normal range: 2.0–3.2%.

Causes of ↑ HbA_2

• β thalassaemia trait (HbA_2 level is ~3.9–6.5%).

Causes of ↓ HbA_2

• Iron deficiency.
• δ thalassaemia.

Estimation of fetal haemoglobin (HbF)

HbF makes up >50% of the total Hb at birth but decreases to ~5% by 5 months of age (as γ chain production is replaced by β chains). HbF levels may be raised in some haemoglobinopathies.

Sample: EDTA.

↑ *HbF found in*

- β thalassaemia trait.
- β thalassaemia major.
- Hereditary persistence of fetal haemoglobin.
- Homozygous sickle cell disease (HbSS).
- Sickle/β^+ thalassaemia (some cases).
- Sickle/β^0 thalassaemia (some cases).
- Juvenile chronic myeloid leukaemia.
- Multiple myeloma (uncommon and never measured).
- Acquired aplastic anaemia.

Haemoglobin H bodies (β_4)

HbH, consisting of a tetramer of β globins (β_4), is found in α thalassaemia. The β chains form tetramers due to the relative lack of α globins with which to pair. The demonstration of HbH allows the detection of α thalassaemia trait (either $-\alpha/-\alpha$ or $--/\alpha\alpha$) and HbH disease ($--/-\alpha$).

Method

The HbH body test involves staining RBCs with brilliant cresyl blue; HbH bodies are seen as large dark inclusions in the red cells.

Sample: fresh EDTA.

►*Note*: the presence of HbH confirms α thalassaemia but the *absence* of HbH bodies does not exclude the diagnosis.

Heinz bodies

These are red cell inclusions made up of insoluble denatured globin protein. Heinz bodies are seen when the RBCs are stained with methyl violet stain.

Sample: fresh EDTA.

Interpretation: Heinz bodies are seen close to the RBC membrane. These are normally removed by the spleen and are therefore more frequent following splenectomy.

Causes of Heinz bodies

- Oxidative haemolysis:
  - Chlorates, phenacetin, other drugs.

- G6PD, PK deficiencies and other enzymopathies.
- Unstable haemoglobins.

Sevitt S *et al.* (1973) Acute Heinz-body anaemia in burned patients. *Lancet* **2**, 471–475.

Testing for unstable haemoglobins

Globin gene mutations may lead to amino acid substitutions that render the haemoglobin molecule unstable, leading to haemolysis. Most mutations causing unstable Hb are autosomal dominant and >80% affect the β chain. Affected individuals are heterozygotes. Heinz bodies in RBCs are intracellular Hb precipitates. Unstable Hbs can be detected electrophoretically or using the heat precipitation test, in which lysed RBCs are heated to 50°C for 1h.

Sample: fresh EDTA.

Interpretation: normal fresh haemolysates should be stable for 1h at 50°C. If there is an unstable Hb a precipitate will be seen in the tube.

Examples
- Hb Köln.
- Hb Gun Hill.

Molecular tests for diagnosis of thalassaemia

Although most haematology labs can diagnose β thalassaemia trait and β thalassaemia major, there are occasions when molecular tests are required, e.g. antenatal diagnosis where a couple are at risk of having a child with β thalassaemia major or hydrops fetalis (absence of α globin, usually lethal). In addition, the diagnosis of α thalassaemia is difficult and requires DNA analysis either using Southern blotting or PCR amplification of globin genes.

β thalassaemia

There are >100 β globin mutations now known but fortunately each population tends to have its own group of mutations (this avoids having to test for all known mutations). It is important that you include the ethnic group on the request form since this will assist the lab who will then screen for mutations commonly found in the ethnic group of the patient. Details of these mutations can be found in the beta and delta thalassemia repository.

Methods used for molecular diagnosis of β thalassaemia

The methods used are complex and outwith the scope of this small book (see references below).

How the ARMS PCR technique works

- This is amplification refractory mutation system PCR.
- Specific point mutations are known for the β globin mutations.
- PCR primers are designed to bind with the mutated sequence.
- If the patient has the mutation there will be PCR amplification.
- If the patient lacks the mutation there is no binding of the primers to the patient's DNA, and no amplification.
- So, a band on the gel means the mutation is present (and the reverse is true—if the band is absent then that particular mutation is absent).

Other techniques including reverse dot blots and DNA sequencing are sometimes needed if ARMS PCR fails.

Methods used for molecular diagnosis of α thalassaemia

Whereas β thalassaemia is usually the result of point mutations (single base changes), the α thalassaemias are usually the result of deletions of chunks of DNA in the region of the α globin genes. Southern blotting is useful in detecting deletions since the DNA band sizes after digestion with restriction enzymes will differ to the wild type (i.e. normal).

UK Haemoglobinopathy Reference Laboratory

This is based at the John Radcliffe Hospital in Oxford (UK). Difficult cases (e.g. α thalassaemia) can be sent to this lab (after discussing the case first); they will perform α globin gene analysis and send a detailed report containing the genotype of the patient. See end of chapter for contact details (📖 p284).

Bowden DK *et al.* (1992) A PCR-based strategy to detect the common severe determinants of a thalassaemia. *Br J Haem* **81**, 104–108; Lewis SM, Bain BJ, Bates I, eds. (2001) *Dacie & Lewis Practical Haematology*, 9th edition, Churchill Livingstone, Edinburgh.; Huisman TH, Carver MF. (1988) The beta- and delta-thalassemia repository (9th edition, Part 1). *Hemoglobin* **22**, 169–195.

Acquired haemolytic anaemias

Determining the cause of haemolytic anaemia can be a complex process. Having excluded inherited disorders of haemoglobin, RBC membrane or enzymes we are left with a diverse group of disorders with a common phenotype of increased RBC destruction (and ↓ RBC lifespan).

Immune

- Autoimmune (primary, or 2° to SLE or CLL).
- Alloimmune (e.g. transfusion reactions, haemolytic disease of the newborn).
- Antibody can be warm (IgG) or cold (IgM usually).

RBC damage

- Drugs.
- Poisons.
- Burns.

RBC fragmentation syndromes

- DIC.
- TTP/HUS.
- March haemoglobinuria.

Investigations

There is little point investigating the cause of haemolytic anaemia until you have shown that haemolysis is *actually* occurring.

Look for the acquired cause

- FBC and peripheral film:
  - Spherocytes (suggests warm antibody; also present in HS).
  - ↑ WBC, e.g. might suggest underlying lymphoproliferative disorder such as CLL.
  - RBC fragments (suggests physical damage to the RBC, e.g. MAHA, TTP/HUS, burns, March haemoglobinuria, mechanical heart valves).
  - Parasites, e.g. malaria.
  - Infections, e.g. *Clostridium*, *Bartonella*, *Babesia*.
- Antiglobulin test (DAT):
  - IgG or IgG + complement (C3d) on RBC.
  - DAT is usually +ve in immune-mediated haemolysis.
- Renal function (abnormal in TTP/HUS).
- Coagulation screen (DIC with RBC fragmentation).
- LFTs (abnormal in Zieve's syndrome).
- USS for splenomegaly.
- Cold agglutinins:
  - IgM, usually against I or i proteins, RBC membrane proteins.
- Ham's test or immunophenotype if suspect PNH.

Table 3.10

Mechanism	Examples
Autoimmune	***Warm antibody (IgG mainly)*** Idiopathic haemolytic anaemia
	Secondary to other autoimmune diseases (e.g. SLE), lymphoid malignancies (e.g. CLL), infections, drugs (e.g. penicillins, methyldopa)
	Cold antibodies (IgM mainly) Cold agglutinin syndromes, cold haemagglutinin disease (CHAD), 2° to infection
Alloimmune	Haemolytic transfusion reactions, haemolytic disease of the newborn (HDN)
Infections	Many, including malaria, meningococcal, pneumococcal, viral
Chemical or physical	Drugs, burns, drowning
RBC fragmentation syndromes	Mechanical heart valves, microangiopathic haemolytic anaemia (MAHA, seen in DIC, HUS, TTP, pre-eclampsia, SLE, carcinoma)
Membrane disorders	Examples are Liver disease, PNH

Ham's acid lysis test

This is a test for the rare acquired red cell membrane disorder called paroxysmal nocturnal haemoglobinuria (PNH). Its pathophysiology is complex and involves an abnormality of the red cell membrane in PNH making it prone to complement-mediated lysis and episodes of marked intravascular haemolysis leading to free haemoglobin in the urine (haemoglobinuria).

Principle
- Abnormal sensitivity of RBCs from patients with PNH to the haemolytic action of complement.
- Complement is activated by acidification of the patient's serum to pH of 6.2 which induces lysis of PNH red cells but not normal controls.

Sample: EDTA, heparin, citrate, oxalate.

Result: +ve result indicates PNH.

Specificity: high—similar reaction is produced only in the rare syndrome HEMPAS (a form of congenital dyserythropoietic anaemia type II) which should be easily distinguished morphologically.

Sensitivity: low—as the reaction is crucially dependent on the concentration of magnesium in the serum.

Bleeding time

This is a test of primary haemostasis, and mainly of platelet function *in vivo*, rather than a laboratory test. You will generally need to arrange this test through the haematology department who will carry out the test for you.

Procedure

A disposable spring-loaded blade is used to make 2 incisions of fixed depth into the skin of the forearm whilst a sphygmomanometer is inflated to 40mmHg. Blood from the incisions is mopped up using circular filter paper (care needs to be taken to avoid disturbing the clot which forms on the cut surface).

Normal range: up to 7min (varies depending on method used; >9min is abnormal). Longer in ♀.

Uses: previously felt to be the best screen for acquired or congenital functional or structural platelet disorders. If bleeding time normal and history is negative (i.e. no major bleeding problems in past) this excludes an underlying platelet disorder.

Precautions

▶Don't carry out bleeding time if platelet count is <100 × 10^9/L (will be prolonged). Aspirin will interfere with test—ask patients to stop aspirin 7 days before test carried out.

Causes of prolonged bleeding time

- Low platelet count.
- Platelet function defect (acquired, e.g. aspirin, paraprotein, MDS).
- von Willebrand's disease.
- Vascular abnormalities, e.g. Ehlers–Danlos.
- Occasionally low factor V or XI.
- Afibrinogenaemia.

Pitfalls

Highly operator-dependent, with low reproducibility. Because of this, the test is seldom used now.

📖OHCM p644.

Mielke CH Jr. (1982) Aspirin prolongation of the template bleeding time: influence of venostasis and direction of incision. *Blood* **60**, 1139–1142; Parkin JD, Smith IL. (1985) Sex and bleeding time. *Thromb Haemost* **54**, 731.

Prothrombin time (PT)

This tests the extrinsic coagulation pathway and is useful for detecting coagulation deficiencies, liver disease and DIC. The PT is also the main monitor for coumarin therapy (e.g. warfarin), expressed as a ratio—the *international normalized ratio* (INR). The test measures the clotting time of plasma in the presence of a tissue extract, e.g. brain (thromboplastin). The test measures prothrombin but also factors V, VII and X.

Sample: citrate.

↑ PT

- Oral anticoagulation therapy (vitamin K antagonists).
- Fibrinogen deficiency (factor I).
- Prothrombin deficiency (factor II).
- Deficiency of factors V, VII or X (in V or X deficiency the APTT will be ↑).
- Liver disease especially obstructive.
- Vitamin K deficiency.
- DIC.

Fig. 3.15 Coagulation cascade showing the factors assayed using the various clotting tests. Modified from Provan D et al. (2004) *Oxford Handbook of Clinical Haematology*, 2nd edition OUP, Oxford.

Activated partial thromboplastin time (APTT)

Other terms: somewhat confusingly the APTT may be called kaolin cephalin clotting time (KCCT), partial thromboplastin time with kaolin (PTTK).

What is the APTT testing?

This is a test of the intrinsic coagulation system, and depends on contact factors + factors VIII, IX and reactions with factors X, V, II and I. The APTT is sensitive to circulating anticoagulants (e.g. lupus anticoagulant) and heparin.

Sample: citrate.

Uses

- Heparin monitoring.
- Screening for haemophilia A and B (VIII and IX deficiency, respectively).
- Screening for coagulation inhibitors.

Normal range: 26.0–33.5s (often expressed as ratio, APTR).

↑ APTT

- DIC.
- Liver disease.
- Massive blood transfusion.
- Heparin treatment.
- Circulating anticoagulant.
- Modest ↑ in patients taking oral anticoagulants.
- Haemophilia.

Is there an inhibitor present?

The APTT will be long if there is an inhibitor such as the lupus anticoagulant present. This can be determined by mixing the patient's plasma with an equal volume of normal control plasma and repeating the APTT. If the APTT is long because of an inhibitor it will not fully correct when normal plasma is added. However, if the APTT is long because of a deficiency it will correct with the normal plasma.

⤷http://www.labtestsonline.org/understanding/analytes/coag_cascade/coagulation_cascade.html

Denson KW. (1988) Thromboplastin—sensitivity, precision and other characteristics. *Clin Lab Haematol* **10**, 315–328; Turi DC, Peerschke EI. (1986) Sensitivity of three activated partial thromboplastin time reagents to coagulation factor deficiencies. *Am J Clin Pathol* **85**, 43–49; van den Besselaar AM *et al.* (1987) Monitoring heparin therapy by the activated partial thromboplastin time—the effect of pre-analytical conditions. *Thromb Haemost* **57**, 226–231.

Thrombin clotting time (TCT)

This is affected by the concentration of factor I (fibrinogen) and the presence of fibrin or fibrinogen degradation products and heparin.

Sample: citrate

↑ TCT
- Low fibrinogen, e.g. DIC.
- ↑ FDPs/XDPs/D-dimers.
- Heparin*.
- Dysfibrinogenaemia (inherited, mutation in fibrinogen gene leads to amino acid change and non-functional fibrinogen).

*If suspected, check reptilase time, similar to TCT but not affected by heparin.

D-dimers

D-dimers are produced during polymerisation of fibrinogen as it forms fibrin. Measurement of D-dimer levels is more specific for this process than the older FDP (fibrinogen/fibrin degradation products) test and is now being used to detect the presence of DIC and other coagulation disorders. The test measures fibrin lysis by plasmin and is a sensitive indicator of coagulation activation (e.g. such as that seen in DIC). The assay uses a monoclonal antibody specific for D-dimers; it will not cross-react with fibrinogen or fibrin.

Sample: citrate (clotting screen bottle).

↑ D-dimers seen in
- DIC.
- DVT.
- PE.

Summary of clotting tests in a variety of disorders

Table 3.11

PT	APTT	TCT	Platelets	Diagnosis
N	N	N	N	Platelet function defect., XII deficiency, normal
↑	N	N	N	VII deficiency, early oral anticoagulation
N	↑	N	N	VIIIC/IX/XI/XII deficiency, vWD, circulating anticoagulant, e.g. lupus
↑	↑	N	N	Vitamin K deficiency, oral anticoagulant V/VII/X/II deficiency
↑	↑	↑	N	Heparin, liver disease, fibrinogen deficiency
N	N	N	↓	Thrombocytopenia (any cause)
↑	↑	N	low	Massive transfusion, liver disease
↑	↑	↑	low	DIC, acute liver disease

Modified from Dacie JV, Lewis SM. (1995) *Practical Haematology*, 8th edition, Churchill Livingstone, Edinburgh.

▶▶Disseminated intravascular coagulation (DIC)

DIC is a medical and haematological emergency. DIC may be seen in a variety of situations and is characterised by generalised bruising and bleeding, usually from venepuncture sites, post-operatively and spontaneously.

Diagnosis requires FBC, clotting screen and evidence of rapid consumption of fibrinogen. Classic (acute) DIC, where the test results fit the bill, is easy to spot. The situation may be more subtle and you are strongly advised to discuss the case with a haematology registrar or consultant if you are in any doubt about the diagnosis of DIC.

▶▶Laboratory diagnosis

FBC	↓ platelets ± red cell fragments seen on the blood film
PT	↑ in moderately severe DIC
APTT	usually ↑
Fibrinogen	↓ (falling levels significant—but remember this is an acute phase protein so level may be *normal* even in florid DIC)
D-dimers	↑

⌖http://www.emedicine.com/emerg/topic150.htm

Conditions associated with DIC

Table 3.12

Disorder	Example
Infectious disease	Septicaemia Viraemia
Obstetric emergency	Placental abruption Eclampsia Amniotic fluid embolism Placenta praevia Septic abortion
Surgical	Cardiac bypass
Malignant disease	Metastatic cancer Acute leukaemia (esp. AML M3, i.e. acute promyelocytic leukaemia)
Shock	Trauma Severe burns
Transfusion	ABO mismatched transfusion
Miscellaneous	Snake bites (some) Liver cirrhosis

Platelet function tests

These are specialised tests carried out by the coagulation laboratory for the investigation of patients with suspected platelet dysfunction. Because of their complexity, the platelet function tests will not be described in detail here.

Patients generally present with bleeding or bruising problems and have had normal coagulation results. Because of the labour-intensive nature and cost of these assays you will need to arrange these tests after discussion with your local haematology medical staff.

Sample: blood collection needs to be optimal with non-traumatic venepuncture, rapid transport to the lab with storage at room temperature and testing within a maximum of 2–3h.

Current tests
- Platelet count.
- Morphology.
- Adhesion.
- Aggregation.
- Platelet release.
- Bleeding time.

Platelet count
Normal range 150–400 $\times$ 10^9/L. Adequate function is maintained even when the count is <0.5 normal level, but progressively deteriorates as it drops. With platelet counts <20 $\times$ 10^9/L there is usually easy bruising and petechial haemorrhages (although more serious bleeding can occur).

Morphology
Large platelets are biochemically more active; ↑ mean platelet volume (MPV >6.5) is associated with less bleeding in patients with severe thrombocytopenia. Altered platelet size is seen in inherited platelet disorders.

Platelet adhesion
Adhesion to glass beads now rarely performed in routine lab practice, but potentially useful in vWD diagnosis.

Platelet aggregation
Most useful of the special tests is performed on fresh sample using aggregometer.

Aggregants used
- Adenosine 5-diphosphate (ADP) at low and high concentrations. Induces 2 aggregation waves: primary wave may disaggregate at low concentrations of ADP; the second is irreversible.
- Collagen has a short lag phase followed by a single wave and is particularly affected by aspirin.
- Ristocetin-induced platelet aggregation (RIPA) is carried out at a high (1.2mg/mL) and lower concentrations and is mainly used to diagnose vWD.

- Arachidonic acid.
- Adrenaline (epinephrine), not uncommonly reduced in normal people.

Platelet release

ELISA or RIA are used to measure the granule proteins β-thromboglobulin (β-TG) and heparin neutralising activity (HNA). These are sensitive markers of platelet hyper-reactivity and beyond the scope of the routine laboratory.

Practical application of tests

Their main role is in diagnosis of inherited platelet functional defects. In acquired platelet dysfunction secondary to causes such as renal and hepatic disease, DIC and macroglobulinaemia, platelet function is rarely tested.

Yardumian A et al. (1986) Laboratory investigation of platelet function: a review of methodology. J Clin Pathol **39**, 701–712.

Thrombophilia screening

Thrombophilia describes acquired or inherited disorders that predispose to arterial or venous thromboembolism (VTE). Thrombophilia should be suspected when the blood clot affects an unusual site, the patient is young, has recurrent thrombotic episodes, or has a strong family history of VTE.

Causes: ▢*Symptoms & Signs*, (p82).

Which patients should be screened for possible thrombophilia?

- Arterial thrombosis, e.g. patients <30 years, without obvious arterial disease.
- Venous thrombosis:
  - Patients <40 years with no obvious risk factors.
  - Unexplained recurrent thrombosis.
  - VTE and family history of thrombosis in first degree relatives.
  - Unusual site, e.g. mesenteric, portal vein thrombosis.
  - Unexplained neonatal thrombosis.
  - Recurrent miscarriage (≥3).
  - VTE in pregnancy and the OCP.

Screen

- Exclude medical causes (check ESR, LFTs, AIP, fasting lipids).
- FBC (exclude thrombocytosis).
- Clotting screen for acquired defects (PT, APTT, LA/ACL, ↑ fibrinogen).
- Screen for inherited thrombophilia:
  - First line PC, PS, AT, APCR.
  - Check for presence of the factor V Leiden mutation in APCR +ve
  - patients (DNA analysis).
  - Consider testing plasminogen, factor XII, homocysteine levels, prothrombin variant.
- DNA analysis for prothrombin gene mutation.

Thrombophilia investigations are time-consuming and expensive and you should discuss with the local haematology medical or lab staff before sending samples. *Note:* some thrombophilia tests cannot be carried out in the 'acute' phase of a VTE event or while the patient is taking warfarin.

↗http://peir.path.uab.edu/coag/article_208.shtml
↗http://www.bcshguidelines.com/pdf/BJH512.pdf

Cattaneo M et al. (1998) Interrelation of hyperhomocyst(e)inemia, factor V Leiden, and risk of future venous thromboembolism. *Circulation* **97**, 295–296; Dahlback B. (1997) Resistance to activated protein C as risk factor for thrombosis: molecular mechanisms, laboratory investigation, and clinical management. *Semin Hematol* **34**, 217–234; Lane DA et al. (1996) Inherited thrombophilia: Part 1. *Thromb Haemost* **76**, 651–662; Lane DA et al. (1996) Inherited thrombophilia: Part 2. *Thromb Haemost* **76**, 824–834.

Antithrombin, proteins C&S

These proteins are the body's *natural anticoagulants*; hence deficiencies may lead to thromboembolic disease.

Antithrombin (AT)

Used to be called ATIII but there was never an ATI or ATII so now abbreviated to AT. A useful measure in thrombophilia screening since low levels of AT are found in 4.5% patients with unexplained VTE.

↓ AT levels

- Hereditary (40–60% normal level), autosomal dominant.
- Chronic liver disease.
- Protein wasting disorders.
- Heparin therapy.
- 3rd trimester of pregnancy.
- Acute leukaemia.
- Burns.
- Renal disease.
- Gram –ve sepsis.

Protein S

- Reduced levels predispose to VTE. Individuals with 30–60% normal level may suffer recurrent thrombosis.

↓ *Protein S*

- Inherited (autosomal dominant).
- Pregnancy.
- Oral anticoagulants, e.g. warfarin.
- Nephrotic syndrome.
- Liver disease.

Protein C

- Similar to protein S; autosomal dominant inheritance in genetic cases.

↓ *Protein C*

- Hereditary.
- Liver disease.
- Malignancy.
- Warfarin therapy.
- Pregnancy.

Bone marrow examination

This is a key investigation in haematology. It may be diagnostic in the follow-up of abnormal peripheral blood findings, and is an important staging procedure in defining the extent of disease, e.g. lymphomas. It is a helpful investigative procedure in unexplained anaemia, splenomegaly or selected cases of pyrexia of unknown origin (PUO).

Preferred sites: posterior iliac crest is the usual site (allows aspirate and biopsy to be obtained). The sternum is suitable only for marrow aspiration, and is not a test for the squeamish.

The marrow aspirate provides
- Cytology of nucleated cells.
- Qualitative and semiqualitative analysis of haematopoiesis.
- Assessment of iron stores (if Perls' iron stain used).
- Smears for cytochemistry (helps in the diagnosis of leukaemias).

Marrow cells can also be used for
- Chromosomal (cytogenetic) analysis.
- Immunophenotype studies using monoclonal antibodies.

Marrow trephine biopsy provides information about
- Marrow cellularity.
- Identification and classification of abnormal cells.
- Immunohistochemistry on infiltrates.

Contraindications
None, other than physical limitations, e.g. pain or restricted mobility. Avoid sites of previous radiotherapy (inevitably grossly hypocellular and not representative).

Procedure
1. BM aspiration may be performed under LA alone, but short acting IV sedative (e.g. midazolam) is preferred when trephine biopsy is performed. General anaesthetic used in children.
2. Place patient in (L) lateral position, or use right if s/he cannot lie on left side.
3. Infiltrate skin and periosteum over the posterior iliac spine with local anaesthetic.
4. Make a small cutaneous incision before introducing the aspirating needle, which should penetrate the marrow cortex 3–10mm before removal of the trocar.
5. Aspirate no more than 0.5–1mL marrow initially (to avoid dilution of sample with blood).
6. Make smears promptly (▶the sample clots rapidly!).
7. If further samples are needed, e.g. for immunophenotyping, cytogenetics, etc., these can be aspirated after making initial slides.
8. For trephine biopsy use Islam or Jamshidi needle.
9. Advance the needle through the same puncture site to penetrate the cortex.

10. Remove the trocar and, using firm hand pressure, rotate the needle clockwise and advance as far as possible.
11. Remove the needle by gentle anticlockwise rotation.
12. Following the procedure apply simple pressure dressings.
13. Minor discomfort at the location may be dealt with by simple analgesia such as paracetamol.

Table 3.13

Tests carried out on bone marrow

Chromosomes	Standard cytogenetic analysis, looking for rearrangements suggestive of acute or chronic leukaemias and myelodysplasia
	Fluorescence *in situ* hybridisation (FISH) looking for additions or losses of chromosomes, as well as more subtle changes seen in leukaemias and lymphomas
DNA or RNA analysis	Using PCR to look for mutations or translocations which help classify leukaemias and lymphomas; also useful for monitoring disease levels in some disorders
Immunophenotype	Cell surface marker profile helps in the diagnosis of most leukaemias and lymphomas; may also be used to monitor disease levels post-treatment
Microbiology	E.g. TB culture (not routine, but occasionally useful in cases of PUO)
Cytochemical stains	To help define type of leukaemia

Cytochemistry tests (leukaemia diagnosis)

These staining methods have been around for many years (for decades they were all that was available), but remain extremely useful in the diagnosis and classification of leukaemias. Modern technologies such as flow cytometry and nucleic acid analysis have refined leukaemia and lymphoma diagnosis but the examination of well-stained cytochemistry bone marrow smears remains the cornerstone of good haematology practice.

After performing a bone marrow aspirate and spreading the material onto glass slides, the air-dried unfixed microscope slides are passed to the cytochemistry lab who will fix and stain the slides according to the likely diagnosis (stains for AML differ to those for ALL, for example). Positive results with particular stains will point to a specific diagnosis. This will then be augmented by flow cytometric or molecular assays.

Auer rods ≡ AML

Fig. 3.16 AML marrow showing myeloblasts (leukaemic cells) and an Auer rod in one cell. Auer rods are pathognomonic of AML since they do not occur in any other disorder.

Table 3.14

Cytochemical stain	Substrate/cell
Myeloperoxidase (MPO)	Lysosomal enzyme found in neutrophils and monocytes
Sudan black (SB)	Phospholipids in neutrophil granules
Chloroacetate esterase	Stain specific esterase in granulocytes and mast cells. Makes it easier to diagnose AML M4 subtype
α-naphtholacetate esterase (ANAE)	Esterase stain, useful for diagnosis of AML subtypes
Acid phosphatase	Enzyme found in many different WBCs. Useful for T cell malignancies
Periodic acid-Schiff (PAS)	Detects glycogen in cells. Granulocytes have diffuse staining whereas lymphocytes staining is much coarser

Table 3.15

	Acute lymphoblastic leukaemia		Acute myeloid leukaemia		
	B lineage	T lineage	M1–3	M4–5	M6–7
Myeloperoxidase	–	–	+/++	+	–
Sudan black	–	–	+/++	+	–
Chloroacetate esterase	–	–	–/++	–	–
α-naphthol acetate esterase	–	–	–	++	–
Acid phosphatase	–	+ (focal)	–	+ (diffuse)	+ (focal)
Periodic acid–Schiff	+ (blocks)	–	–	+ (fine granular)	+

+, Positive; ++, strongly positive; –, negative.

From Hoffbrand AV, Lewis SM, Tuddenham EGD. (2000) *Postgraduate Haematology*, 4th edition, Butterworth-Heinemann, Oxford.

http://www.rcpa.edu.au/pathman/cytochem.htm

Neutrophil alkaline phosphatase

Uses

This is a cytochemical stain used to demonstrate the presence and quantity of the neutrophil enzyme alkaline phosphatase. Historically the NAP score was of value in differentiating 'reactive' states from myeloproliferative disorders, such as CML, polycythaemia rubra vera, etc.—now more often features in examination MCQs! (*Note*: sometimes termed leucocyte alkaline phosphatase, LAP.)

Procedure

Best performed on fresh blood films, made without the use of anticoagulant. EDTA samples may be used but are less satisfactory. The film should be made, air dried, fixed and then stained—all within 30min. Positive NAP activity is indicated by the presence of bright blue granules in the neutrophil cytoplasm (the nucleus is stained red).

Scoring: films are scored from 0 to 4 on the basis of stain intensity:

0 negative, no granules seen
1 weak positive, few granules
2 positive, few–moderate numbers of granules
3 strongly positive
4 very strong

Red cell

NAP stain
in cytoplasm

Fig. 3.17 NAP stained blood film: shows positively stained neutrophils. Red cells do not take up the stain.

Interpretation & significance

Table 3.16

High NAP score	Low NAP score
Polycythaemia rubra vera (PRV)	Chronic myeloid leukaemia
Leukaemoid reaction	Paroxysmal nocturnal haemoglobinuria
Neutrophilia—any cause	Acute myeloid leukaemia
Myelofibrosis	
Essential thrombocythaemia	
Hepatic cirrhosis	
Hodgkin's disease	
Aplastic anaemia	
Down's syndrome	
Cushing's disease	

The NAP score is affected by corticosteroids, oestrogens and pregnancy ($\uparrow$ NAP). In Hodgkin's disease the NAP score offers no advantage over simpler tests such as ESR for assessment of disease activity. Occasionally of value in a patient with aplastic anaemia who is developing PNH—the NAP score is seen to fall (both of these are very rare disorders). NAP score has been replaced in most hospitals by flow cytometry and other methods.

Lewis SM, Bain BJ, Bates I, eds. (2001) *Dacie & Lewis Practical Haematology*, 9th edition, Churchill Livingstone, Edinburgh.

Blood transfusion

Due to space limitations it is inappropriate to go into major details about the investigations used in transfusion medicine. However, we have provided the more important tests in current use which include:

- Blood group & antibody screen.
- Cross-match (compatibility test).
- Direct antiglobulin test (DAT).
- Antiplatelet and antineutrophil antibody testing.

Safe transfusion practice

Each year patients are transfused with the wrong blood. The commonest error is clerical and generally involves the cross-match sample being taken from the wrong patient and so the compatibility test is performed on the wrong sample. Occasionally the staff carrying out the transfusion connect the blood up to the wrong patient. In any event, the result varies from no symptoms to shock and possible death.

How to minimise errors

- First, ask yourself: *does this patient really need to be transfused* with blood or blood products (e.g. FFP, platelets, etc.)? For example, a post-operative patient who is asymptomatic with a Hb of 9g/dL probably does not require red cell transfusion. Use clinical judgement in helping decide whether or not to proceed with transfusion.
- Before taking the blood sample check that you are taking blood from the correct patient—ask for his/her name and check the identity bracelet.
- Label the patient's blood bottle at the bedside (i.e. no prelabelling of bottles:
  - Many transfusion labs insist on 1, 2, 5, 6 & 7 and either 3 or 4 from:

    1. Surname & forename (correctly spelt)
    2. dob
    3. Hospital/A&E/new NHS number
    4. First line of address
    5. Sex
    6. Time and date blood taken
    7. Signature of person taking blood

- Ensure details on form match those on the bottle.
- Complete the request form properly:
  - State what is required (e.g. 2 units of packed cells, etc.).
  - Detail any previous transfusions, reactions, antibodies (if known).
  - Let the lab know when you want the blood or blood product.

▶▶Adhesive patient labels are fine for forms but are not suitable for specimen bottles, and are usually not accepted by transfusion labs. Transfusion specimens should be labelled by hand—at the bedside.

> **If this sounds cumbersome and bureaucratic:**
>
> Remember many people die annually because they are transfused with the **wrong blood**. In most cases clerical error is to blame—people have filled out bottles in advance and failed to check patient identity.

~⊕http://www.blood.co.uk/
~⊕http://www.transfusionguidelines.org.uk/
~⊕http://www.scotblood.co.uk/
~⊕http://www.bcshguidelines.com/pdf/tme203.pdf

McClelland B. (2001) *Handbook of Transfusion Medicine*, 2nd edition, HMSO, London.

▶▶Transfusion reactions

Rapid temperature spike (>40°C) at start of transfusion indicates transfusion should be stopped (suggests acute intravascular haemolysis).

If slow rising temperature (<40°C), providing patient not acutely unwell, slow IVI. Fever often due to antibodies against WBCs (or to cytokines in platelet packs).

▶▶Immediate transfusion reaction

Intravascular haemolysis (→ haemoglobinaemia & haemoglobinuria). Usually due to anti-A or anti-B antibodies (in ABO mismatched transfusion). Symptoms occur in minutes/hours. *May be fatal.*

Table 3.17

Symptoms	Signs
Patient restless/agitated	Fever
Flushing	Hypotension
Anxiety	Oozing from wounds or venepuncture sites
Chills	Haemoglobinaemia
Nausea & vomiting	Haemoglobinuria
Pain at venepuncture site	
Abdominal, flank or chest pain	
Diarrhoea	

Immediate transfusion reaction or bacterial contamination of blood

If predominantly extravascular may only suffer chills/fever 1h after starting transfusion—commonly due to anti-D. Acute renal failure is not a feature.

Mechanism

Complement (C3a, C4a, C5a) release into recipient plasma → smooth muscle contraction. May develop DIC or oliguria (10% cases) due to profound hypotension.

Initial steps in management of acute transfusion reaction

- Stop blood transfusion immediately.
- Replace giving set, keep IV open with 0.9% saline.
- Check patient identity against donor unit.
- Insert urinary catheter and monitor urine output.
- Give fluids (IV colloids) to maintain urine output >1.5mL/kg/h.
- If urine output <1.5mL/kg/h insert CVP line and give fluid challenge.
- If urine output <1.5mL/kg/h and CVP adequate give frusemide 80–120mg.
- If urine output still <1.5mL/kg/h consult senior medical staff for advice.
- Contact blood transfusion lab before sending back blood pack and for advice on blood samples required for further investigation (see below).

Complications

Overall mortality ~10%.

꠵http://www.emedicine.com/emerg/topic603.htm

Urgent investigations

Your local blood transfusion department will have specific guidelines to help you with the management of an acute reaction. The following guide lists the samples commonly required to establish the cause and severity of a transfusion reaction. *If you are uncertain about the laboratory procedure or management of a patient who appears to have suffered a severe reaction you must notify your hospital's haematology medical staff* who will provide advice. ▶▶Delays may threaten the patient's life.

1. Check compatibility label of blood unit matches with patient's id band, forms and casenotes.
2. If mistake found *tell the blood bank urgently*—the unit of blood intended for your patient may be transfused to another patient.
3. Take blood for:

—haematology	FBC
	DAT
	plasma haemoglobin
	repeat cross-match sample
	coagulation screen
—chemistry	U&E
—microbiology	blood cultures

4. Check urinalysis and monitor urine output.
5. Do ECG and check for evidence of $\uparrow[K^+]$.
6. Arrange repeat coagulation screens & biochemistry 2–4 hourly.

Febrile transfusion reactions

Seen in 0.5–1.0% of blood transfusions. Mainly due to anti-HLA antibodies in recipient serum or granulocyte-specific antibodies (e.g. sensitisation during pregnancy or previous blood transfusion).

Delayed transfusion reaction

Occurs in patients immunised through previous pregnancies or transfusions. Antibody weak (so not detected at pre-transfusion stage). 2° immune response occurs—antibody titre $\uparrow$.

Symptoms and signs
- Occur 7–10 days after blood transfusion.
- Fever, anaemia and jaundice.
- ± Haemoglobinuria.

Management
- Discuss with transfusion lab staff.
- Check DAT and repeat compatibility tests.
- Transfuse patient with freshly cross-matched blood.

Bacterial contamination of blood products

Uncommon but *potentially fatal* adverse effect of blood transfusion (affects red cells and blood products, e.g. platelet concentrates). Implicated organisms include Gram –ve bacteria, including *Pseudomonas, Yersinia* and *Flavobacterium*.

Features

Include fever, skin flushing, rigors, abdominal pain, DIC, ARF, shock and possible cardiac arrest.

Management—as per *Immediate transfusion reaction*

- Stop transfusion.
- Urgent resuscitation.
- IV broad-spectrum antibiotics if bacterial contamination suspected.

Antiglobulin test

The old term is Coombs' test. Direct antiglobulin test (DAT) detects antibodies or complement or both on the RBC surface and the indirect antiglobulin test (IAT) detects presence of antibodies in serum. A useful investigation when investigating haemolytic anaemia.

Sample: EDTA.

Interpretation

- Positive DAT in most AIHA.
- Lymphoproliferative disorders, e.g. CLL.
- Drug-induced haemolysis (e.g. α-methyl dopa, L-dopa).
- Haemolytic disease of the newborn, e.g. Rhesus HDN.

Note: As with many tests in medicine, things are never entirely black or white—a +ve DAT does not necessarily imply that haemolysis is actively occurring and a –ve DAT does not exclude haemolysis.

Coombs RRA. (1945) A new test for the detection of weak and 'incomplete' Rh agglutinins. *Br J Exp Pathol* **26**, 255; Kelton JG. (1985) Impaired reticuloendothelial function in patients treated with methyldopa. *NEJM* **313**, 596–600.

Kleihauer test

Uses

To (1) determine whether fetal red cells have entered the maternal circulation, and if so (2) determine the volume of such fetal cells.

Background

If an Rh (D)-negative mother has a baby that is Rh (D) +ve she may develop antibodies (maternal anti-D) against fetal red cells. This may result in fetal red cell destruction termed *Rhesus haemolytic disease of the newborn*, a serious haemolytic disorder which is seen less today due to greater understanding of the underlying mechanism and our ability to prevent it. Sensitisation to the fetal red cells occurs when fetal RBCs enter the maternal circulation, e.g. at birth or through obstetric manipulations, e.g. amniocentesis, previous pregnancies, etc.

Fetal RBCs in the mother's circulation can be detected and quantified (in mL) using the Kleihauer test, which exploits the resistance of fetal red cells to acid elution (acid washes adult Hb out of the mother's red cells but the fetal RBCs contain HbF which is not washed out). The Kleihauer test should be performed on all Rh (D) –ve women who deliver a Rh (D) +ve infant.

Fetal cells appear as darkly staining cells against a background of ghosts (these are the maternal red cells). An estimate of the required dose of anti-D can be made from the number of fetal cells in a low power field.

Sample: maternal peripheral blood EDTA.

Calculating the volume of fetal RBCs in maternal circulation

Basically, a calculation is made by the laboratory staff based on the number of fetal RBCs seen in the Kleihauer film. The actual calculation is:

> 1800* x ratio of $^{fetal}/_{adult}$ RBCs x $^4/_3$ (correction factor)
> for example, if there are 1% fetal RBCs in maternal circulation
> 1800 x $^1/_{100}$ x $^4/_3$ = 24mL.
> *1800 is the maternal red cell volume

A 4mL bleed (i.e. 4mL fetal RBCs) requires 500IU anti-D given IM to the mother with a further 250IU anti-D for each additional mL of fetal RBCs.

Don't panic!

The lab carrying out the Kleihauer test will tell you the volume of fetal RBCs detected since they will count the cells and do the calculation for you. After this you will need to calculate the dose of anti-D to give the mother but *if you are unsure either discuss with the haematology medical staff* or contact your local transfusion centre.

Chanarin I, ed. (1989) *Laboratory Haematology: an Account of Laboratory Techniques*, Churchill Livingstone, Edinburgh.

Erythropoietin assay

Erythropoietin (Epo) is the hormone produced largely by the kidney that drives red cell production. The typical anaemia found in renal disease is a result of failure of Epo production. Epo assays are of value in renal medicine and haematology. For example, in the assessment of polycythaemic states an ↑ Epo level may be appropriate (e.g. in hypoxia where the body is attempting to increase O_2 availability to tissues) or inappropriate (e.g. some tumours). The Epo assay is carried out using a radioimmunoassay method and is not available in all haematology laboratories (may need to be sent to another hospital or lab).

Normal range: 35–25mU/mL, steady state level, no anaemia. May rise to 10,000mU/mL in hypoxia or anaemia.

Causes of ↑ Epo (appropriate)

- Anaemias.
- High altitude.
- Hypoxia:
  - Lung disease.
  - Sleep apnoea syndromes.
- Cyanotic heart disease (e.g. R → L shunts).
- High affinity haemoglobins.
- Cigarette smoking.
- Methaemoglobinaemia.

Causes of ↑ Epo (inappropriate)

- Renal disease:
  - Hypernephroma.
  - Nephroblastoma.
  - Post-renal transplant.
  - Renal cysts.
  - Renal artery stenosis.
- Hepatoma.
- Uterine fibroids.
- Cerebellar haemangioblastoma.
- Phaeochromocytoma.

Other causes of ↑ Epo

- Androgen therapy.
- Cushing's disease.
- Hypertransfusion.
- Neonatal polycythaemia.

Causes of ↓ Epo

- Renal failure.
- Polycythaemia vera.
- Rheumatoid arthritis, and other chronic inflammatory diseases.
- Myeloma and other cancers.

Cotes PM *et al.* (1986) The use of immunoreactive erythropoietin in the elucidation of polycythemia. *NEJM* **315**, 283–287.

Immunohaematology

Immunohaematology is the study of the effects of the immune system on the blood and its components. This includes red cells, white cells, platelets and coagulation proteins.

Tests for antiplatelet and antineutrophil antibodies

These tests are usually requested by the haematology department for patients with either thrombocytopenia or neutropenia, respectively. These assays are used to detect the presence of specific antibodies against platelet or neutrophil antigens on the cell surface.

Antibodies may be *alloantibodies* (e.g. antibody produced by the mother against fetal antigens) or *autoantibodies*, which are antibodies produced by the patient against his/her own antigens.

Antiplatelet antibody tests

Generally platelet immunofluorescence tests (PIFT) or monoclonal antibody immobilisation of platelet antigens (MAIPA) are used. These are useful for detecting even weak antibodies or where there are only a few antigenic sites per cell.

Table 3.18

Disorders with neutrophil-specific alloantibodies

- Neonatal alloimmune neutropenia.
- Febrile transfusion reactions (HLA antibodies).
- Transfusion-related acute lung injury (TRALI).

Disorders with neutrophil-specific autoantibodies

- Primary autoimmune neutropenia.
- Secondary:
  - SLE.
  - Evans' syndrome (AIHA + ↓ platelets).
  - Lymphoproliferative disorders (e.g. CLL).
  - Immune dysfunction (e.g. HIV, GvHD).

Elegant though these tests are, they are actually not useful in clinical practice for the diagnosis of neutropenia or thrombocytopenia where the cause is autoimmune since these are largely clinical diagnoses. (Platelet-associated IgG or IgM may be high in autoimmune thrombocytopenia. However, it may also be high in non-immune causes of thrombocytopenia.) Where these tests are of value is in the neonatal setting where the neonate has low platelets or neutrophils.

Roitt I. (2001) *Essential Immunology*, 10th edition, Blackwell Science, Oxford.

Immunophenotyping

This describes the identification and counting of cell types using powerful monoclonal antibodies specific for cell surface proteins.

Uses

- Diagnosis and classification of leukaemias and lymphomas.
- Assessment of cellular DNA content and synthetic activity.
- Determination of lymphocyte subsets, e.g. $CD4^+$ T cells in HIV infection.
- Assessment of clonality.
- Allows identification of prognostic groups.
- Monitoring of minimal residual disease (MRD, the lowest level of malignancy that can be detected using standard techniques).

Terminology and methodology

Cell surface proteins are denoted according to their cluster differentiation (CD) number. Most cells will express many different proteins and the pattern of expression allows cellular characterisation. Monoclonal antibodies recognise specific target antigens on cells. Using a panel of different antibodies an immunophenotypic *profile* of a sample is determined. Immunophenotyping is used in conjunction with standard morphological analysis of blood and marrow cells. The antibodies are labelled with fluorescent markers and binding to cell proteins is detected by laser. For each analysis thousands of cells are assessed individually and rapidly. Some antibodies can detect antigens inside cells.

Sample: heparin.

Monoclonal antibodies (MoAbs)

These are so-called because they are derived from single B lymphocyte cell lines and have identical antigen binding domains (idiotypes). It is easy to generate large quantities of MoAbs for diagnostic use.

- Cell populations from e.g. PB or BM samples are incubated with a panel of MoAbs, e.g. anti-CD4, anti-CD34, which are directly or indirectly bound to a fluorescent marker antibody.
- Sample is passed through a fluorescence-activated cell sorter (FACS) machine.
- FACS instruments assign cells to a graphical plot by virtue of cell size and granularity detected as forward and side light scatter by the laser.
- Allows subpopulations of cells, e.g. mononuclear cells, in blood sample to be selected.
- The reactivity of this cell subpopulation to the MoAb panel can then be determined by fluorescence for each MoAb.
- A typical result for a CD4 T lymphocyte population is shown:
  CD3, CD4 +ve; CD8, CD13, CD34, CD19 −ve.

Leukaemia diagnosis: common patterns (profiles)

AML   CD13+, CD33+, ± CD34, ± CD14 +ve.
cALL   CD10 and TdT +ve.
T-ALL   cCD3, CD7, TdT +ve.

B-ALL   CD10, CD19, surface Ig +ve.
CLL   CD5, CD19, CD23, weak surface Ig +ve.

Table 3.19

Surface immunophenotyping	Leukaemias
	Lymphomas
	CD4:CD8 ratios in HIV infection
DNA content of tumours	Ploidy
	S phase analysis
	Proliferation markers
TdT measurement	In leukaemias & lymphomas
BMT/stem cell transplantation	
Antiplatelet antibody detection	
Reticulocyte counts & maturation	
Apoptosis	
Detection of small numbers of cells	E.g. fetal cells in mother's circulation, microorganisms in blood

Clonality assessment

Particularly useful in determining whether there is a monoclonal B cell or plasma cell population.

▶ Monoclonal B cells from e.g. NHL will have surface expression of κ or λ light chains but not both.
▶ Polyclonal B cells from e.g. patient with infectious mononucleosis will have both κ *and* λ expression.

⤷http://pleiad.umdnj.edu/hemepath/immuno/immuno.html
⤷http://www.bcshguidelines.com/pdf/CLH135.PDF
⤷http://www.bcshguidelines.com/pdf/clh253.pdf
⤷http://www.bcshguidelines.com/pdf/clh190.pdf

Adapted from Provan D et al. (2004) *Oxford Handbook of Clinical Haematology*, 2nd edition, Oxford University Press, Oxford.

Cytogenetics

Uses

* The study of chromosomes.
* Looks at the number of chromosomes in each cell.
* Detects structural abnormalities between chromosome pairs.

Chromosome abnormalities may be constitutional (inherited) or acquired later in life. Cytogenetic analysis of chromosome structure and number has been used for many years for the study of disorders such as Down's syndrome. Acquired chromosomal abnormalities are found in malignancies, especially haematological tumours. The analysis and detection of cytogenetic abnormalities is known as *karyotyping*. Because of the complexity of this subject area we will concentrate on two main areas where chromosome analysis is of value.

- Prenatal diagnosis of inherited disorders:
  - Detection of common aneuploidies (gain or loss of chromosomes).
  - Detection/exclusion of known familial chromosome abnormalities.
- Detecting acquired chromosome abnormalities for:
  - Diagnosis of leukaemia subtypes, e.g. t(15;17) characteristic of AML M3 subtype.
  - Markers of prognostic information in a variety of diseases such as leukaemias, e.g. t(9;22) in acute leukaemias, N-myc amplification in neuroblastoma.
  - Monitoring response to treatment (in CML the Philadelphia chromosome, t(9;22), should disappear if the malignant cells are killed).

Principal indications for cytogenetic analysis are therefore

- Haematological malignancies at diagnosis (assuming the bone marrow is infiltrated).
- Infiltrated solid tumour tissue at diagnosis.
- Patients with equivocal morphology (e.g. type of leukaemia not clear using microscopy and other markers).
- FISH analysis when required in certain treatment protocols, e.g. MRC.
- Confirmation of disease relapse.
- Accelerated phase or blast crisis in CML.

Cytogenetic assays are expensive (around £250 for a leukaemia or lymphoma karyotype) and if there is any doubt as to whether the test is indicated we would suggest you discuss the case with one of your seniors or the cytogenetics staff. Arranging karyotyping before or during pregnancy is generally carried out by the obstetrician in charge of the woman's care.

Table 3.20 Cytogenetic terminology

Constitutional	Present at conception or arising during embryonic life
Acquired	Arise later in fetal life or after birth
Translocation	Exchange of material between chromosomes
Deletion	Loss of part of a chromosome
Duplication	Part of a chromosome is gained
Inversion	Part of a chromosome is rotated through 180°
Diploid	46 chromosomes (somatic cell)
Haploid	23 chromosomes (germinal cell, e.g. egg or sperm)
Trisomy	Extra copy of a chromosome
Monosomy	Loss of a chromosome
Aneuploidy	Loss or gain of certain chromosomes, e.g. monosomy or trisomy

Cytogenetics: prenatal diagnosis

This allows both the detection of genetic diseases associated with specific chromosomal abnormalities, thereby offering the possible prevention of an affected child. With the advent of chorionic villus sampling (CVS) in the first trimester, karyotyping can be done at an early stage of development. Pre-implantation genetic diagnosis allows abnormalities to be detected even before implantation has occurred.

Sample: amniotic fluid (15–16 weeks' gestation).

Tests available

- α-fetoprotein level.
- Chromosome analysis.
- Biochemical tests, e.g. acetylcholinesterase.

Sample: CVS (9–12 weeks' gestation).

Tests available

- DNA analysis.
- Chromosome analysis.
- Biochemistry tests.

Procedure (brief)

1. Cells are obtained using amniocentesis, CVS or fetal blood sampling.
2. Cells are cultured in medium.
3. Cell division is arrested at metaphase using e.g. colchicine.
4. Chromosomes are spread onto slides and stained.
5. Chromosomes are examined directly using light microscopy or with the aid of a computerised image analysis system.

Fig. 3.18 Diagram showing method of chorionic villus sampling.

Fig. 3.19 Normal karyotype showing metaphase chromosomes (22 autosomes, 1–22, and 2 sex chromosomes, XX or XY depending on sex of patient).

Chromosome anatomy

Note the banding pattern which helps identify individual chromosomes, along with position of the centromeres (mitotic spindle attaches to these during cell division), short (*p*) and long (*q*) arms, and telomeres (chromosome ends).

🖰http://www.pathology.washington.edu/galleries/Cytogallery/
🖰http://www.infobiogen.fr/services/chromcancer/Anomalies/Anomliste.html

Rooney DE. (2001) *Human Cytogenetics*, Vol 2, 2nd edition, Oxford University Press, Oxford.

p (short) arm

centromere

q (long) arm

telomere

Fig. 3.20 Chromosome anatomy: note short (*p*) arms and long (*q*) arms.

Cytogenetics: haematological malignancies

Uses
- Aids the diagnosis and classification of haematological malignancy.
- Assessment of clonality.
- Identification of prognostic groups.
- Monitoring response to therapy.
- Determining engraftment and chimerism post-allogeneic transplant.

Terminology
- Normal somatic cell has 46 chromosomes; 22 pairs and XX or XY.
- Numbered 1–22 in decreasing size order.
- 2 arms meet at centromere—short arm denoted p, long arm is q.
- Usually only visible during condensation at metaphase.
- Stimulants and cell culture used—colchicine disrupts the spindle apparatus thereby arresting cells in metaphase.
- Chromosomes are G-banded using Giemsa or Leishman's stain to create characteristic banding patterns along the chromosome. The regions and bands are numbered, e.g. p1, q3, etc.

Common abnormalities
- Whole chromosome gain, e.g. trisomy 8 (+8).
- Whole chromosome loss, e.g. monosomy 7 (–7).
- Partial gain, e.g. add9q+, or partial loss, e.g. del5q– .
- Translocation—material exchanged with another chromosome; usually reciprocal, e.g. t(9;22)—the Philadelphia translocation.
- Inversion—part of chromosome runs in opposite direction, e.g. inv(16) in M4Eo.
- Many translocations involve breakpoints around known oncogenes, e.g. bcr, ras, myc, bcl-2.

Molecular cytogenetics
- Molecular revolution is further refining the specific abnormalities in the genesis of haematological malignancies.
- Techniques such as FISH (fluorescence *in situ* hybridisation) and PCR (polymerase chain reaction) can detect cryptic abnormalities.
- Bcr-abl probes are now used in diagnosis and monitoring of treatment response in CML.
- IgH and T cell receptor (TCR) genes are useful in determining clonality of suspected B and T cell tumours, respectively.
- Specific probes may be used in diagnosis and monitoring of subtypes of acute leukaemia, e.g. AML, e.g. *PML-RARA* in AML M3, t(9;22), t(12;21), and 11q23 rearrangements in paediatric acute lymphoblastic leukaemias.

Table 3.21

Karyotypic abnormalities in leukaemia and lymphoma

CML

t(9;22)	Philadelphia chromosome translocation creates bcr-abl chimeric gene.

AML

t(8;21)	AML M2, involves AML-ETO gene—has better prognosis.
t(15;17)	AML M3 involves PML-RARA gene—has better prognosis.
inv(16)	AML M4Eo—has better prognosis.
−5, −7	Complex abnormalities have poor prognosis.

MDS

−7, +8, +11	Poor prognosis.
5q− syndrome	Associated with refractory anaemia and better prognosis.

Myeloproliferative disease

20q− and +8	Common associations.

ALL

t(9;22)	Philadelphia translocation, poor prognosis.
t(4;11)	Poor prognosis.
Hyperdiploidy	Increase in total chromosome number—good prognosis.
Hypodiploidy	Decrease in total chromosome number—bad prognosis.

T-ALL

t(1;14)	Involves tal-1 oncogene.

B-ALL and Burkitt's lymphoma

t(8;14)	Involves myc and IgH genes, poor prognosis.

CLL

+12, t(11;14)	

ATLL

14q11	

NHL

t(14;18)	Follicular lymphoma, involves bcl-2 oncogene.
t(11;14)	Small cell lymphocytic lymphoma, involves bcl-1 oncogene.
t(8;14)	Burkitt's lymphoma, involves myc and IgH genes.

Heim S, Mitelman F. (1995) *Cancer Cytogenetics*, 2nd edition, Wisley-Liss, New York; Kingston HM. (1994) *ABC of Clinical Genetics*, 2nd edition, BMJ Books, London; Sandberg AA. (1990) *The Chromosomes in Human Cancer and Leukemia*, 2nd edition, Elsevier Science, New York.

HLA (tissue) typing

The HLA (human leucocyte antigen) system or MHC (major histocompatibility complex) is the name given to the highly polymorphic gene cluster region on chromosome 6 which codes for cell surface proteins involved in immune recognition.

Uses

Tissue typing patients (to ensure compatibility between donor and recipient) who are undergoing transplantation to reduce the likelihood of rejection or graft-versus-host disease in the following types of transplant:
- Heart.
- Lung.
- Liver.
- Kidney.
- Bone marrow.
- Stem cells.

The gene complex is subdivided into 2 regions

Class 1   The A, B and C loci.
            These proteins are found on most nucleated cells and interact with CD8+ T lymphocytes.
Class 2   Comprised of DR, DP, DQ loci present only on B lymphocytes, monocytes, macrophages and activated T lymphocytes.
            Interact with CD4+ T lymphocytes.

- Class 1 and 2 genes are closely linked so one set of gene loci is usually inherited from each parent though there is a small amount of cross-over.
- There is ~25% chance of 2 siblings being HLA identical.
- There are other histocompatibility loci apart from the HLA system but these appear less important generally except during HLA matched stem cell transplantation when even differences in these minor systems may cause GvHD.

Typing methods

Class 1 and 2 antigens were originally defined by serological reactivity with maternal antisera containing pregnancy-induced HLA antibodies. There are many problems with the technique and it is too insensitive to detect many polymorphisms. Molecular techniques are increasingly employed such as SSP. Molecular characterisation is detecting enormous class 2 polymorphism.

Importance of HLA typing

- Matching donor/recipient pairs for renal, cardiac and marrow stem cell transplantation.
- Degree of matching more critical for stem cell than solid organ transplants.
- Sibling HLA-matched stem cell transplantation is now treatment of choice for many malignancies.

- Unrelated donor stem cell transplants are increasingly performed but outcome is poorer due to HLA disparity. As molecular matching advances, improved accuracy will enable closer matches to be found and results should improve.

Functional tests of donor/recipient compatibility

- MLC (mixed lymphocyte culture)—now rarely used.
- CTLp (cytotoxic T lymphocyte precursor assays)—determine the frequency of cytotoxic T lymphocytes in the donor directed against the recipient. Provides an assessment of GvHD occurring.

HLA-related transfusion issues

- HLA on WBC and platelets may cause immunisation in recipients of blood and platelet transfusions.
- May cause refractoriness and/or febrile reactions to platelet transfusions.
- Leucodepletion of products by filtration prevents this (the National Blood Service removes the WBCs at source routinely nowadays).
- Diagnosis of refractoriness confirmed by detection of HLA or platelet-specific antibodies in patient's serum.
- Platelet transfusions matched to recipient HLA type may improve increments.

⬠http://www.ebmt.org/4Registry/Registry_docs/HLA%20MANUAL%2003_2004.pdf
⬠http://content.nejm.org/cgi/content/full/343/10/702?ijkey=oOilwRsUqacag
⬠http://medind.nic.in/jaa/t03/i3/jaat03i3p79.pdf

Southern blotting

This technique has been around since the mid-1970s. It explained much about the physical structure of genes and was a major advance in the diagnosis of many single gene disorders. The method is simple and elegant, but time-consuming. Not used as much today with the advent of PCR technology. Southern blotting relies on the physical nature of DNA whereby single strands are able to recognise and bind to their complementary sequences (Fig. 3.21).

Sample: EDTA sample (heparin can be used but beware inhibitory effect on PCR amplification; if any chance PCR required, send EDTA).

Procedure

1. Genomic (i.e. total) DNA is extracted from WBC in EDTA blood sample.
2. DNA is digested with bacterial restriction endonucleases (enzymes cleave DNA at specific sequences—each enzyme recognises a different DNA sequence).
3. After digestion of the DNA, the fragments are separated on the basis of size using agarose gel electrophoresis (smallest fragments travel the farthest).
4. The fragments are transferred to a nylon membrane and fixed permanently to the membrane using UV light.
5. Membranes are 'probed' using specific (known) gene probes that are radioactively labelled using ^{32}P.
6. The location of specific binding is detected by placing the membrane next to radiographic film (standard x-ray film).
7. The film is developed using standard techniques and the autoradiograph generated will show bands corresponding to the position of binding of the labelled probe.
8. Fragment sizes are calculated and the presence or absence of mutations are worked out by determining whether enzyme cutting sites have been lost through mutation.

⊕http://www.accessexcellence.org/RC/VL/GG/southBlotg.html
⊕http://users.rcn.com/jkimball.ma.ultranet/BiologyPages/G/GelBlotting.html

Southern EM. (1975) Detection of specific sequences among DNA fragments separated by gel electrophoresis. *J Mol Biol* **98**, 503–517 (▶▶Southern's classic paper and probably *the* most cited molecular biology paper ever).

DNA from blood, marrow, fetal cells, etc.

Digestion by restriction enzyme, e.g. Mst II (chops the DNA up)

Digested products separated using agarose gel electrophoresis (small fragments move furthest)

Separated fragments exposed to radiolabelled probe, e.g. for β globin gene

Transferred to nylon filter which is then placed next to x-ray film. A black band is seen where the probe has bound to the patient's DNA fragment

Fig. 3.21 Southern blotting method.

Applications
- Historically many diseases caused by single base changes (loss of restriction enzyme cutting site) have been diagnosed using Southern blotting.
- Globin gene disorders:
  - Sickle cell anaemia (mutation in β globin gene).
  - Thalassaemia (mutations or deletions in α or β globin genes).
- Clotting disorders:
  - Haemophilia.
- Analysis of immunoglobulin or T cell receptor genes to detect clones of cells in suspected leukaemia or lymphoma.
- Detection of chromosomal translocations in leukaemia and lymphoma (e.g. t(9;22) in CML, t(14;18) in follicular lymphoma).

PCR amplification of DNA

The ability to use an enzyme to amplify specific DNA sequences has revolutionised modern diagnostic pathology. Whereas Southern blotting might take up to 1 week to produce a result, PCR can do the same thing in 2–3h! PCR is now in routine use in the analysis of oncogenes, haematological malignancies, general medicine, infectious disease and many other specialties. Because the system amplifies the starting DNA up to a million-fold there need only be one cell as starting material; in practice much more DNA is required but because of the extreme sensitivity of the technique PCR has been used in forensic medicine where there may be only a few cells available for analysis (e.g. blood or semen stain).

Advantages

- Requires very little DNA.
- DNA quality does not matter (can be highly degraded, e.g. with age and still be amplified—DNA from Egyptian mummies has been amplified).
- Rapid results.

Disadvantages

- Expensive, but less so than it used to be.
- DNA sequence of the gene of interest must be known in order to design the short PCR primers (oligos). With the near completion of the Human Genome Project this is less of a problem now.
- Highly sensitive, and contamination of samples may occur (DNA fragments float through the air constantly; if these drop into the reaction tube a false +ve result may be obtained).

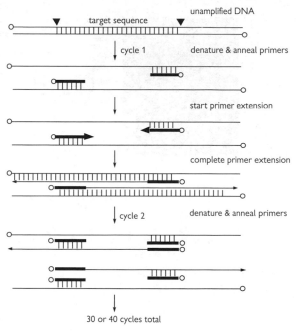

Fig. 3.22 PCR amplification method.

Procedure (in brief)
- Two short DNA primers on either side of the gene of interest bind to the fragment of interest.
- The region between the primers is filled in using a heat-stable DNA polymerase (Taq polymerase).
- After a single round of amplification has been performed the whole process is repeated.
- This takes place 30 times (i.e. through 30 cycles of amplification) leading to a million-fold increase in the amount of specific sequence.
- After the 30 cycles are complete a sample of the PCR reaction is run on agarose gel and bands are visualised.
- Information about the presence or absence of the region or mutation of interest is obtained by assessing the size and number of different PCR products obtained after 30 cycles of amplification.

Fig. 3.23 Detection of residual leukaemia using PCR. Patients 1 and 2 have undergone chemotherapy but as can be seen (arrow) there is still some leukaemia-specific DNA sequence present, i.e. they have minimal residual disease.

Applications

- PCR is currently used to amplify immunoglobulin genes, HIV loci, tuberculosis genes and many other targets that are of use in molecular medicine (cystic fibrosis, haemophilia, thalassaemia, sickle cell disease and many others).
- PCR can be used to quantitate mRNA species in blood samples and tissue samples. Allows gene 'activity' to be measured.

🖰http://nobelprize.org/chemistry/educational/pcr/
🖰http://allserv.rug.ac.be/~avierstr/principles/pcr.html

Saiki RK. (1988) Primer-directed enzymatic amplification of DNA with a thermostable DNA polymerase. *Science* **239**, 487–491 (classic PCR method paper).

In situ hybridisation & FISH

Like PCR and other techniques, *in situ* hybridisation and FISH are conceptually simple techniques that rely on the ability of a DNA probe to 'find' its counterpart on a chromosome, bind, and if a fluorescent tag is present it will light up the region of binding (this modification is termed fluorescence *in situ* hybridisation, or FISH). These techniques have evolved from standard cytogenetic analysis of metaphase chromosomes in which meta phase chromosomes were prepared on glass slides to which specific labelled probes were applied.

Sample: discuss with your local cytogenetics or haematology lab (they will have specialised medium for maintaining cells from blood or marrow so that they will divide and be suitable for hybridisation studies).

In situ hybridisation

The location of binding of the probe is detected by visualising the signal produced after coating microscope slides with photographic emulsion, which generate a black area around the probe which is labelled with ^{32}P.

FISH

A further modification based on the original principles, whereby specific gene probes are hybridised to chromosomes without the need for metaphase preparations (interphase cells can be used). Instead of ^{32}P the probes are labelled with fluorescent dye and hybridisation may be detected as red, blue or other coloured dots over the cells.

Slide containing cells

Fig. 3.24 FISH analysis. Metaphase chromosomes are placed on microscope slide, and the probe (e.g. for the gene of interest) is applied. The chromosome region to which the probe binds will fluoresce—highlighting its exact location in the genome.

Applications of FISH

- Used in the analysis of trisomies (chromosome gains) and monosomies (chromosome losses) associated with leukaemias and lymphomas. The presence of trisomy is detected as three fluorescent dots within the cell whilst monosomy is seen as a single fluorescent dot within the cell.
- FISH has been used widely within paediatric leukaemias, such as ALL, where abnormalities of chromosome number are common.

⌐Ɪhttp://www.slh.wisc.edu/cytogenetics/procedures/fish/fish-method.php

Sinclair PB *et al.* (1997) Improved sensitivity of BCR-ABL detection: a triple-probe three-color fluorescence in situ hybridization system. *Blood* **90**, 1395–1402; Vaandrager JW. (1996) Direct visualization of dispersed 11q13 chromosomal translocations in mantle cell lymphoma by multi-color DNA fiber fluorescence *in situ* hybridization. *Blood* **88**, 1177–1182; Mathew P *et al.* (1997) Detection of the t(2;5)(p23;q35) and NPM-ALK fusion in non-Hodgkin's lymphoma by two-color fluorescence in situ hybridization. *Blood* **89**, 1678–1685.

Specialised haematology assays

The following laboratories provide specialised molecular, biochemical and cellular investigations for rare haematological disorders. Please contact the laboratory before tests are requested to confirm the specimen(s) required.

Thalassaemia disorders

Dr John Old
National Haemoglobinopathy Reference Laboratory, Institute of Molecular Medicine, John Radcliffe Hospital, Headington, Oxford OX3 8DU
Tel: 01865-222449; Fax: 01865-222500
E-mail: *jold@hammer.imm.ox.ac.uk*

Professor Swee Lay Thein
Haematological Medicine, King's College Hospital, Denmark Hill, London SE5 9RS
Tel: 020-7346-1682; Fax: 020-7346-6168
E-mail: *sl.thein@kcl.ac.uk*

Dr Mary Petrou
Perinatal Centre, University College Hospital, 84–86 Chenies Mews, London WC1E 6HX
Tel: 020-7388-9246; Fax: 020-7380-9864
E-mail: *m.petrou@ucl.ac.uk*

Dr Tom Vulliamy
Haematology, ICSTM, Hammersmith Hospital, London W12 0HS
Tel: 020-8383-1136; Fax: 020-8742-9335
E-mail: *t.vulliamy@ic.ac.uk*

Haemoglobin variants, unstable and altered affinity haemoglobins

Dr John Old
National Haemoglobinopathy Reference Laboratory, Institute of Molecular Medicine, John Radcliffe Hospital, Headington, Oxford OX3 8DU
Tel: 01865-222449; Fax: 01865-222500
E-mail: *jold@hammer.imm.ox.ac.uk*

Professor Sally Davies[1] & Joan Henthorn[2]
Department of Haematology, Central Middlesex Hospital, Acton Lane, London NW10 7NS
1 Tel: 020-8453-2112; Fax: 020-8965-1115
E-mail: *sally.davies@dol.gso.gov.uk*
2 Tel: 020-8453-2323

Dr Barbara Wild
Haematological Medicine, King's College Hospital, Denmark Hill, London SE5 9RS
Tel: 020-7737-4000 Ext 2283; Fax: 020-7346-3514
E-mail: *barbara.wild@kcl.ac.uk*

Glycolytic defects, G6PD deficiency other erythroenzymopathies

Dr Mark Layton

Haematology, ICSTM, Hammersmith Hospital, London W12 0HS
Tel: 020-8383-2173; Fax: 020-8742-9335
E-mail: m.layton@ic.ac.uk

Dr Barbara Wild

Haematological Medicine, King's College Hospital, Denmark Hill, London SE5 9RS
Tel: 020-7737-4000 Extn 2283; Fax: 020-7346-3514
E-mail: barbara.wild@kcl.ac.uk

Porphyrias

Dr Allan Deacon

Clinical Biochemistry, King's College Hospital, Denmark Hill, London SE5 9RS
Tel: 020-7346-3856; Fax: 020-737-7434

Dr Michael Badminton[1] & Ms J Woolf/Dr S Whatley[2]

Porphyria Service, Medical Biochemistry, University Hospital of Wales, Cardiff CF14 4XW
1 Tel: 02920-748349; Fax: 02920-748383
E-mail: badminton.mn@cardiff.ac.uk
2 Tel: 02920-743565

Red cell membrane defects

Dr May-Jean King

International Blood Group Reference Laboratory, Southmead Road, Bristol BS10 5ND
Tel: 0117-991-2111; Fax: 0117-959-1660
E-mail: may-jean.king@nbs.nhs.uk

Immunology & allergy

Serum immunoglobulins *288*
IgG subclasses *290*
IgD *292*
Serum free light chains *294*
Cryoglobulins *294*
β_2-microglobulin *295*
Acute phase proteins (CRP, ESR, SAA) *296*
Amyloidosis *298*
Serum complement components *300*
C1 esterase inhibitor *300*
Haemolytic complement (lytic complement function tests) *302*
Immune complexes *302*
Autoimmunity *304*
Rheumatoid factor (RF) *304*
'Autoantibody screen' *305*
Double-stranded DNA antibodies (ds-DNA) *307*
Antibodies to extractable nuclear antigens (ENA) *307*
Antiphospholipid antibodies *309*
Other patterns of autoantibodies identified on
  'autoantibody screen' *309*
Autoantibodies in autoimmune hepatitis *310*
Gastric parietal cell and intrinsic factor antibodies *311*
Thyroid disease *312*
Islet cell antibodies (ICA), anti-GAD antibodies,
  insulin-receptor and insulin antibodies *313*
Adrenal antibodies & other endocrine autoantibodies *314*
Classification of autoimmune polyglandular syndromes *314*
Endomysial (EMA) & tissue transglutaminase (tTG)
  antibodies *315*
Autoimmune skin diseases *316*
Autoantibodies & neurological disease *317*
Vasculitic syndromes *318*
Allergic disease *319*
Skin prick tests *320*
Specific IgE: 'RAST tests' *321*
Mast cell tryptase *322*
Drug allergy testing *322*
Cellular function assays *323*
Lymphocyte function tests *324*
Neutrophil & macrophage function *324*
NK cell function *325*
Immunology websites *325*

Serum immunoglobulins

Units: g/L.

Normal range (adults):

	IgG	5.8–15.4g/L
	IgA	0.64–2.97g/L
	IgM (♂)	0.24–1.90g/L
	IgM (♀)	0.75–2.30g/L

Principles of assay

The 3 main classes of immunoglobulins (Igs) are measured by either rate nephelometry or turbidimetry on automated analysers. Principles are similar, dependent on immune complex formation, using antisera specific for the class of antibody. Rarely radial immunodiffusion may be used—this is slow and less accurate. For automated analysers, coefficients of variation should be in the 5–10% range. Results are standardised against international standards. In the UK, an EQA scheme operates. Laboratories should provide normal ranges, which vary according to age and sex. Unfortunately many laboratories do not adjust ranges for age and sex, which may lead to confusion.

Indications for testing

Measurement of serum immunoglobulin is indicated in the following:

- Suspected immunodeficiency (1° or 2°); diagnosis and monitoring.
- Suspected myeloma, plasmacytoma; diagnosis and monitoring.
- Lymphoma.
- Liver disease (primary biliary cirrhosis, hepatitis, cirrhosis).
- Sarcoidosis (diagnosis).
- Post-bone marrow/stem cell transplantation; monitoring.

Interpretation

Measurement of serum immunoglobulins does not provide categorical diagnosis in any disease. Normal serum immunoglobulins do *not* exclude immunodeficiency. In all cases, measurement of immunoglobulins *must* be accompanied by serum electrophoresis, and immunofixation to look for paraproteins (*see below*).

Causes of hypogammaglobulinaemia

- X-linked agammaglobulinaemia (absent B cells; all immunoglobulins low/absent).
- Common variable immunodeficiency (reduced T/B cells; low immunoglobulins).
- Hyper-IgM syndrome (normal/raised IgM, low/absent IgG, IgA).
- Selective IgA deficiency (absent IgA, normal IgG, IgM).
- Severe combined Immunodeficiency (mainly children; all immunoglobulins low; absent T cells).
- Lymphoma (reduced IgM, IgA normal, IgG normal or low; disease, chemotherapy or radiotherapy).
- SLE (rare).

- Infections:
  - HIV (rare).
  - Herpes viruses (rare, Epstein–Barr virus in X-linked lympho-proliferative disease).
  - Acute bacterial infections.
  - Measles/rubella.
- Drugs (immunosuppressives, e.g. cyclophosphamide, azathioprine, chemotherapy).
- Plasmapheresis.
- Renal loss (IgM normal IgG and IgA reduced).
- Gastrointestinal loss (IgM normal, IgG and IgA reduced).

Causes of hypergammaglobulinaemia

- Chronic infection—all immunoglobulins ↑.
- Osteomyelitis.
- Bacterial endocarditis.
- Tuberculosis.
- Chronic inflammation.
- SLE, rheumatoid arthritis—all immunoglobulins ↑.
- Sjögren's syndrome—↑ IgG (all IgG$_1$).
- Sarcoidosis—↑ IgG and IgA, IgM usually ↔.
- Liver disease:
  - Primary biliary cirrhosis (IgM, may be very high e.g. >30g/L with small monoclonal bands on a polyclonally raised background.
  - Alcohol-related (↑ IgA, polyclonal, β–γ bridging on electrophoresis).
  - Autoimmune hepatitis (↑ IgG, IgA; IgM ↔).
- Hodgkin's disease—IgE ↑ (also eosinophilia).
- Viral infections:
  - Acute common viral infections: ↑ IgM, ↔ IgG and IgA.
  - HIV—all immunoglobulins ↑ (IgG very high but *polyclonal*).
  - EBV—all ↑.

Critical action

All patients with recurrent infections* should be reviewed by an immunologist or paediatric immunologist. Any patient with recurrent infections and ↓ serum immunoglobulins has an immunological problem until proven otherwise.

Patients with unusual infections, or with illness caused by opportunist or normally non-pathogenic organisms infections, and patients with infections in unusual sites (without good reason) should all be referred for further investigation.

---

*Recurrent infections can be pragmatically defined as 2 or more major microbiologically/virologically proven infections, requiring hospitalisation, within one year. One major, and recurrent minor infections should also be referred, where minor are documented infections requiring treatment in the community.

IgG subclasses

Units: g/L.

Normal range (adults):

IgG$_1$	2.2–10.8g/L
IgG$_2$	0.5–8.0g/L
IgG$_3$	0.05–0.9g/L
IgG$_4$	0.0–2.4g/L

Principles of test

As for serum immunoglobulins, IgG subclasses are normally measured by nephelometry or turbidimetry. Radial immunodiffusion is still occasionally used.

Indications for testing

There are no absolute indications for testing, as significant immunodeficiency can occur in the presence of normal subclasses, and conversely, complete genetic absence of a subclass may be completely asymptomatic. Measurement usually performed as part of the work up of patients with recurrent infections.

Interpretation

Low levels may be significant in the context of presentation with recurrent infections. Deficiency of IgG$_3$, which is involved in immunity against viruses, associated with asthma, and intractable epilepsy. IgG$_2$ deficiency may be seen in patients with IgA deficiency and may be associated with poor responses to polysaccharide antigens, such as the capsular polysaccharides of bacteria.

Raised IgG$_1$ with normal or reduced IgG$_2$, IgG$_3$ and IgG$_4$ is seen in Sjögren's syndrome and is a specific pattern, which may occasionally be helpful in diagnosis.

Evaluation of specific antibody production (anti-bacterial and anti-viral antibodies)

Units: variable: u/L, IU/mL, µg/mL.

Ranges: variable, check with reporting laboratory.

Pneumococcal antibodies	>20u/L (asplenics >35)
Tetanus antibodies	>0.1IU/mL (minimum protective level)
Haemophilus influenzae type B	>1.0µg/mL (full protection; asplenics >1.5)

Principles of test

Measurement of antibody production against defined pathogens or antigens purified from pathogens plays an important role in the investigation of suspected immunodeficiency. Most assays carried out by enzyme-linked immunoassay, but some viral antibodies are still measured by haemagglutination or complement fixation. Pre- and post-immunisation samples should be run on the same run for direct comparison as the coefficients of variation for the assays tend to be high: 15–25%! An EQA scheme exists. Assays have tended to focus on agents for which there are safe and effective vaccines. Live vaccines should *never* be given to any patient in whom immunodeficiency is suspected.

Antibodies normally assayed in immunology laboratories include: pneumococcal polysaccharides (which may be further differentiated as IgG_1 and IgG_2) *Haemophilus influenzae* type B (Hib) and tetanus. Diphtheria antibodies are not run by many laboratories as the assays' performance has been so poor. Meningococcal C polysaccharide antibodies are run by a few specialised laboratories, but correlation with known clinical status has been poor. ASOT may be helpful.

Viral antibodies may be valuable, to natural exposure and immunisation antigens such as polio, measles, mumps, rubella, chickenpox, EBV and hepatitis B (if immunised).

Indications for testing

These assays should be used in the work-up of patients with suspected immunodeficiency, or in monitoring change in such patients. Responsiveness to immunisation is a helpful marker of immunological recovery post-bone marrow transplant. Annual monitoring of levels may be valuable in asplenic patients, as such patients lose immunity more rapidly than a eusplenic population.

Interpretation

The interpretation is entirely dependent on the context. Assays for pneumococcal polysaccharides measure a composite of responses to the 23-strains in the Pneumovax vaccine. This can be misleading as not all strains represented in the vaccine are equipotent as immunostimulators. This means that a 'normal' response, may actually mean a good response to the immunogenic strains masking failure of response to the less immunogenic strains. For this reason evaluation of such patients should be carried out by an immunologist with an interest in immunodeficiency. More weight should be placed on changes in response to immunisation than on actual values.

A 'normal' response to immunisation has never been standardised, publications frequently using different criteria, rendering comparison impossible. The following is a useful working definition:

A 4-fold rise in titre, which rises to well within the normal range.

Antibody deficiency in adults

This usually presents with upper and lower respiratory tract infections (*Streptococcus pneumoniae*, *Haemophilus*, *Staphylococcus*, *Klebsiella*), leading to chronic bronchiectasis and sinusitis. Gastrointestinal infections (*Salmonella, Giardia, Campylobacter*). Skin infections (recurrent boils); autoimmune features (ITP, haemolytic anaemia, diabetes, thyroid disease) only in CVID not XLA. Increased incidence of lymphoma.

Normal serum immunoglobulins *do not exclude* antibody deficiency (IgG subclass deficiency, specific failure of antibody production against polysaccharides). Use test immunisation with killed or purified component vaccines to test humoral responses.

Asplenia

Patients are at increased risk of overwhelming sepsis: *Streptococcus pneumoniae, Haemophilus influenzae, Staphylococcus aureus, Meningococcus, Klebsiella* species, *Capnocytophaga canimorsus* (from dog-bites), fulminant malaria and babesiosis. Risk is lifelong. Asplenia may result from trauma, involvement in malignancy, removal for diagnosis (rarely performed for this indication today), coeliac disease and sickle disease, and rarely due to congenital absence. Serum immunoglobulins and IgG subclasses are normal, but responses to polysaccharide antigens are often poor, especially in patients with lymphoma. Blood film will show Howell–Jolly bodies. Absence of the spleen (if not known from records) will be shown by ultrasound.

IgD

IgD is rarely measured in clinical practice, as its main function is as a membrane receptor. Elevated levels may be seen in the periodic fever syndrome, hyper-IgD syndrome, due to deficiency of mevalonate kinase, and in IgD-secreting myeloma (very rare). Measurement is usually by radial immunodiffusion.

Electrophoresis & immunofixation

Units: not applicable to electrophoresis (qualitative). Paraprotein quantitated by scanning densitometry reported in g/L.

Normal range: N/A.

Principles of testing

In serum or urinary electrophoresis, the relevant body fluid is applied to an electrolyte-containing agarose gel. A current is applied across the gel and causes the proteins to migrate through the gel on the basis of their charge, and to a lesser extent size, until they reach a neutral point in the electric field. The proteins are then visualised with a protein binding stain. If the total protein is known, then the electrophoretic strip can be scanned and the absorption by the stain measured, which will be proportional to the amount of protein in the particular region in the gel. Thus any monoclonal bands can be measured directly. This is useful for patients with myeloma, as immunochemical methods for measurement of immunoglobulins may be inaccurate in patients with myeloma.

Immunofixation is the technique by which monoclonal immunoglobulins are identified by overlaying the electrophoresed strips with anti-sera against heavy and light chains. These precipitate with the monoclonal proteins in the gel and unbound anti-sera can be washed free prior to staining.

The same techniques can be carried out with urine, although this may require concentration to provide the clearest results.

Indications for testing

Electrophoresis and, if necessary, immunofixation of serum is an integral part of measurement of serum immunoglobulins. *All* requests for serum immunoglobulins must have electrophoresis carried out—failure to do so will lead to important abnormalities being missed. There is no place for carrying out electrophoresis as a stand-alone test.

Interpretation

Serum electrophoresis gives valuable information, not only of immunological status but also of other organ systems. Reports are poorly understood by clinicians and not explained by laboratories. The following reports may be seen:

Table 4.1

Report	Interpretation
Reduced albumin	Chronic inflammation, nephritic syndrome
Absent α1 band	Absent/reduced alpha-1-antitrypsin
Increased α2 band	Chronic inflammation/infection; also seen in nephrotic syndrome, due to selective retention of alpha-2-macroglobulin
Increased β	Seen in pregnancy (raised β-lipoprotein) and iron deficiency (transferrin)
β–γ bridging	Caused by raised polyclonal IgA, e.g. cirrhosis
Increased γ	Caused by polyclonal increase in IgG: infection/inflammation
Faint band(s) on polyclonal background	Caused by monoclonal escape during polyclonal response to infection/inflammation (does NOT indicate myeloma)
Monoclonal band in γ	Due to myeloma, lymphoma, and MGUS*
Absent/reduced γ	Due to inherited or acquired immunoglobulin deficiency (further investigation essential)

*MGUS = monoclonal gammopathy of uncertain significance—most evolve to myeloma given time (years).

Monoclonal proteins may polymerise to give more than one band. Some patients will have more than one clone present producing different immunoglobulins.

Densitometry cannot be used where the monoclonal protein overlies the beta-region, as the figures include non-immunoglobulin proteins.

Serum free light chains

Modifications in the techniques for measurement of free, as opposed to bound, light chains have been proposed as a valuable adjunct to monitoring light-chain only myelomas, which had previously been monitored by measurement of 24-hour urinary light chain excretion. The urinary measurement can be problematic where there is renal impairment, and as light chains are nephrotoxic, as the disease advances, urinary measurements become less accurate.

'Bence Jones proteins'; urine electrophoresis and immunofixation

Bence Jones proteins are urinary free light chains, i.e. unbound to heavy chains. During normal antibody synthesis a small excess of light chains are produced which are excreted. Hypergammaglobulinaemic states, such as rheumatoid arthritis, chronic infection, may therefore be accompanied by excretion of polyclonal free light chains. Monoclonal free light chains are seen in myeloma, and may be the only marker in light-chain only myelomas, which do not produce any heavy chains at all. Testing is carried out as for serum.

Cryoglobulins

Units: usually reported qualitatively but a 'cryocrit' can be measured in a similar way to a manual haematocrit using capillary tubes.

Normal range: tiny amounts of cryoglobulins may be found in normal individuals.

Principle of test

Cryoglobulins are immunoglobulins that precipitate when serum is cooled. The temperature at which this occurs determines whether disease will result. If the blood circulates through a part of the body where the temperature is below the critical temperature, then the protein will precipitate in the capillaries causing obstruction, vascular damage and eventually necrosis. The temperature of the hand is approximately 28°C at ambient room temperature. To check for the presence of cryoglobulins, take blood using a warmed syringe into warmed bottle and transport to laboratory at 37°C, using a thermos flask with either pre-warmed sand or water at 37°C. The laboratory will allow the blood to clot at 37°C and then cool the serum. Cryoglobulins will form a precipitate as the temperature drops. The precipitate is then washed and redissolved for analysis by electrophoresis and immunofixation.

Cryoglobulins are not the same as cold agglutinins (a feature of *Mycoplasma pneumoniae* infection)—see Chapter 3.

Indications for testing

All patients with Raynaud's phenomenon of new onset, or with winter onset of purpuric or vasculitic lesions on the extremities should be tested.

Chronic hepatitis C infection is often accompanied by type II cryoglobulinaemia and a characteristic syndrome: 'mixed essential cryoglobulinaemia' = autoimmune phenomena, arthritis, ulceration, glomerulonephritis, neuropathy. C3 normal, C4 ↓. Patients with myeloma, SLE. Sjögren's syndrome and rheumatoid arthritis also at risk.

Interpretation

Table 4.2

Type	Nature of cryoprecipitate
Type I	All monoclonal immunoglobulin; myeloma, lymphoma
Type II	Monoclonal immunoglobulin with rheumatoid factor activity; myeloma, lymphoma, connective tissue diseases,infections (esp. HCV, SBE)
Type III	Polyclonal rheumatoid factor: connective tissue diseases, infections

Cryofibrinogen

This is found less commonly than cryoglobulins. It will not be detected unless both EDTA and heparinised blood samples are sent warm to the laboratory. The main association is with occult malignancy (and thrombophlebitis migrans). Also associated with: connective tissue disease, pregnancy, OCP use, diabetes mellitus and cold urticaria.

β₂-microglobulin

Units: mg/L.

Normal range: 1–3mg/L.

Principles of test

The test measures free β_2-microglobulin, which normally forms the light chain of HLA class I molecules but is shed when there is increased lymphocyte turnover. It is usually rapidly cleared by the kidneys. Measurement is usually by automated analyser, nephelometry or turbidimetry. RID is still used.

Indications for testing

The main indication is as part of the routine monitoring of patients with myeloma and HIV.

Interpretation

Levels ↑ in:

- HIV infection (surrogate marker of progression).
- Myeloma (marker of tumour mass).
- Lymphoma.
- Common variable immunodeficiency (correlation with severity).
- Renal dialysis (depending on type of membrane).

Acute phase proteins (CRP, ESR, SAA)

Units: CRP mg/L
                            ESR mm/hour
                            SAA mg/L

Normal ranges: CRP 0–6mg/L
                            ESR—see Chapter 3
                            SAA—not measured routinely

Principles of test

As serum proteins C-reactive protein (CRP) and serum amyloid A (SAA) are amendable to measurement by nephelometry or turbidimetry. Measurement of the ESR is covered in Chapter 3.

Indications for testing

Acute and chronic infections, vasculitis, connective tissue disease, arthritis.

Interpretation

Clinicians are usually confused by ESR and CRP—they do not give the same information and should be used together. CRP is like blood glucose while ESR is like HbA_{1c}. CRP rises within hours of onset of inflammation/infection and falls quickly once treatment is instituted. It is therefore useful for rapid diagnosis and for monitoring response. The ESR rises slowly, being dependent in part on fibrinogen, a long-lived protein, and falls equally slowly (see Fig. 4.1). In active SLE, the ESR is high, but the CRP is not elevated. CRP is driven by IL-6 and may be ↑ in myeloma.

Fig. 4.1 Time course of acute phase response proteins. ESR in acute phase response parallels fibrinogen level.

Table 4.3

Level of CRP	Common associations
Little or no change: (<4–100mg/L)	Most viral infections Active SLE Systemic sclerosis & CREST Inactive RA Myeloma Most tumours
Moderate elevation: (100–200mg/L)	EBV/CMV infection Bacterial infection Active rheumatoid arthritis Polymyalgia rheumatica Temporal arteritis Lymphoma Hypernephroma
Large elevation: (>200mg/L)	Severe bacterial sepsis Legionella Active vasculitis (Wegener's, rheumatoid)
Huge elevation (>400mg/L)	Overwhelming sepsis (deep tissue abscess) Fulminant Legionella At this level, death usually ensues!

Levels in very young children may be much lower for a given stimulus. A very small number of patients do not make inflammatory responses that exceed the normal range, but seem to run on a lower 'normal' range (10-fold less): ultra-sensitive assays for low level CRP are available.

Amyloidosis

Amyloid refers to the deposition of altered proteins in tissues in an insoluble form. The precursor protein varies according to the cause, and can often be measured specifically. Amyloid is usually confirmed by special stains on histological examination of biopsies. Measurement of serum immunoglobulins and electrophoresis, β_2-microglobulin and CRP is essential if amyloid is suspected.

Table 4.4

Amyloid protein	Protein precursor	Clinical syndrome
AL, AH	Light or heavy chain of immunoglobulin	Idiopathic, multiple myeloma, gamma-heavy chain disease
AA	Serum amyloid A	Secondary, reactive: inflammatory arthritis, familial Mediterranean fever, hyper-IgD syndrome, TRAPS (periodic fever), Behçet's, Crohn's disease
Aβ_2M	β_2-microglobulin	Dialysis amyloid
ACys	Cystatin C	Hereditary cerebral angiopathy with bleeding (Iceland)
ALys, AFibA	Lysozyme, fibrinogen Aa	Non-neuropathic hereditary amyloid with renal disease
AIAPP	Islet amyloid polypeptide	Diabetes mellitus type II; insulinoma
AANF	Atrial natriuretic peptide	Senile cardiac amyloid
ACal	Procalcitonin	Medullary carcinoma of the thyroid
AIns	Porcine insulin	Iatrogenic
ATTR	Transthyretin	Familial amyloid polyneuropathy, senile cardiac amyloid
Aβ	Aβ-protein precursor	Alzheimer's disease
AprP	Prion protein	Spongiform encephalopathies

Serum complement components

Units: g/L.

Normal ranges:

Complement C3	0.68–1.80g/L
Complement C4	0.18–0.60g/L

Factor B (rarely measured routinely)
Other components usually reported as percentage of normal human plasma

Principles of test

C3, C4 and factor B are usually measured by rate nephelometry or turbidimetry. Other components are measured by radial immunodiffusion (RID) or simply by double diffusion, where presence or absence is the only result of interest. Complement breakdown products are measured by RID or enzyme-linked assay (EIA).

Indications

Valuable in suspected

- SLE (C3, C4, C3d).
- Complement deficiency (C3, C4, haemolytic complement).
- Anaphylaxis (anaphylatoxins C4a, C5a).
- Hereditary angioedema (C3, C4, C1q, C1 esterase inhibitor, immuno-chemical *and* functional).

Complement deficiency is common (esp. C4 and C2 deficiency); predisposes to recurrent neisserial disease, bacterial infections (C3 deficiency) and immune complex disease (lupus-like). Anyone with more than one episode of systemic neisserial disease has a complement deficiency until proven otherwise.

C1 esterase inhibitor

Units:
Immunochemical: g/L
Functional: reported as percentage activity compared to normal fresh plasma

Normal range:
Immunochemical: 0.18–0.54g/L
(paediatric ranges not well defined, but lower than adults)
Functional: 80–120% normal plasma

Principles of tests

Immunochemical measurement carried out by RID; functional assay is usually a colorimetric assay.

Indications for testing

Key indication is angioedema occurring *without* urticaria at any age. If urticaria is present, diagnosis is *never* C1-esterase inhibitor deficiency. C4 is a useful screen: normal C4 during an attack excludes C1-esterase inhibitor deficiency.

Interpretation

C1-esterase inhibitor deficiency causes hereditary angioedema.

Two types

Type I (common, 80%)
Absence of immunochemical C1-esterase inhibitor (C1-inh).

Type II (rare 20%)
Presence of non-functional C1-inh; immunochemical levels normal or high.

Both are inherited as autosomal dominants. Presents with angioedema, NO urticaria; may involve larynx and gut, usual onset at puberty. C4 absent during acute attacks. Treat with purified C1-inh (FFP may be a substitute but can make attacks worse); maintenance therapy with danazol, stanozolol or tranexamic acid to decrease frequency of attacks. Pregnancy/oral contraceptive exacerbate.

Rare acquired form due to autoantibody to C1-inh (SLE, lymphoma); C1q levels are reduced and a paraproteins may be present.

Haemolytic complement (lytic complement function tests)

Units: can be reported in arbitrary units, or percentage of normal plasma but better reported as normal, reduced or absent.

Normal range: present (80–120% of reference plasma).

Principles of test

Haemolytic complement assays screen for the integrity of the classical, alternate pathways and the terminal lytic sequence, and use either antibody coated sheep cells (CH100, classical pathway) or guinea-pig red cells (CAPCH100, alternate pathway). Either a gel or liquid assay can be used, but the gel is easier! Both tests must be performed in parallel.

Indications for testing

Any patient in whom deficiency of a complement component is suspected.

Interpretation

Reduced levels of haemolytic activity will be seen during infections and during immune complex diseases such as serum sickness and SLE. Testing for absence of a component needs to be undertaken a minimum of 4–6 weeks after recovery from infection. Absence of both CH100 and APCH100 indicates a deficiency in the terminal lytic sequence C5–C9 (C9 deficiency will give slow lysis). Absence of CH100 indicates a missing component in the classical pathway C1–C4. Absence of APCH100 indicates deficiency in alternate pathway (factor D, factor B, C3).

Follow-up testing to identify missing component will be performed by laboratory automatically (if they are doing their job!).

Critical action

Anyone who has a single episode of neisserial meningitis with an unusual strain or a second episode *must* be assumed to have a complement deficiency until proven otherwise. *Refer* after recovery to immunologist for investigation.

Immune complexes

Used in the past to monitor connective tissue disease activity, but the many different assays have given different results and have proven impossible to standardise: therefore no longer recommended for routine clinical use.

Complement breakdown products

Measurement of specific complement breakdown products such as C3bi and C3d are more valuable as markers of complement turnover. A number of different assays are available—your laboratory will advise. Special samples are usually required.

Factor H and factor I

Deficiency of either of these factors may lead to haemolytic-uraemic syndrome (HUS). Measurement is possible in specialised centres, with follow-up genetic testing.

Autoimmunity

Autoantibodies are usually divided into organ specific and organ non-specific, but clinical testing rarely follows this pattern. They are therefore covered in convenient groups, associated with types of testing.

Rheumatoid factor (RF)

Units: titre (particle agglutination assay)
IU/mL (nephelometry, EIA)

Normal range: titre <1/20 <16 yrs
titre <1/40 16–65 yrs
titre <1/80 >65 yrs
<30IU/mL

Principles of test
Tests detect autoantibodies binding to human immunoglobulin: these can be of any class but assays commonly recognise IgG and IgM autoantibodies. Suggestions that IgA RF may be helpful have not been widely accepted. Assays use either agglutination of immunoglobulin coated particles (visual assay) or latex particle enhanced nephelometry.

Indications for testing
Difficult to think of any indications where this test is essential. Widely abused by clinicians.

Interpretation
Not a diagnostic test for rheumatoid arthritis! Only positive in 70–80%. High titre in patient with known rheumatoid arthritis is risk factor for extra-articular manifestations.

RF also found in:
- Healthy elderly (asymptomatic).
- Chronic bacterial (SBE) & viral infections (HIV, HCV).
- Acute viral infections (transient, esp. Adenovirus).
- Myeloma (often type II cryoglobulins).
- Lymphoma.
- Connective tissue diseases (SLE, Sjögren's, systemic sclerosis, polymyositis, UCTD).

Antibodies to cyclic citrullinated peptide (anti-CCP) may be more valuable in identifying and monitoring RA.

'Autoantibody screen'

Another abused test! Usually used as an immunological fishing expedition. Multiple tissues (rodent), often with human Hep-2 cell line; gives rapid and semi-quantitative results for the following autoantibodies:

- Anti-nuclear antibodies (*see below for patterns*).
- Anti-ribosomal antibodies.
- Anti-mitochondrial antibodies.
- Anti-smooth muscle antibodies.
- Anti-liver-kidney microsomal antibodies.
- Anti-gastric parietal cell antibody.

Where Hep-2 cells are used other patterns of nuclear and cytoplasmic fluorescence may be seen. See Fig. 4.2 for examples.

Principles of test

The traditional method is to overlay suitably diluted serum into frozen sections of rodent liver kidney and stomach, and human Hep-2 cells. Bound antibody in the serum is then identified using a fluoresceinated anti-human IgG (or IgM, IgA) as second stage. Slides are then read manually. Enzyme-based immunoassays are being introduced for screening, including multiplex bead-laser array systems. These can be very specific when purified or recombinant antigens are used, but lose out because of their inability to pick up unexpected patterns.

Enzyme-linked assays are used for confirming antigens such histone antibodies and ds-DNA antibodies.

Indications

The correct use of testing is to identify which specific autoantibody is being sought as part of the differential diagnosis.

Interpretation

Because of the multiple patterns detected in this system, the interpretation for each is covered separately.

Table 4.5 Patterns of anti-nuclear antibodies (ANA)

Homogeneous	SLE, drug-induced SLE (ds-DNA or histones)
Coarse speckled	UCTD*, SLE (U1-RNP)
Fine speckled	SLE, Sjögren's (Ro and La)
Nucleolar	Systemic sclerosis, polymyositis, SLE
Centriole	Commonest in mycoplasma pneumonia; also scleroderma
PCNA (proliferating cell nuclear antigen)	SLE—highly specific but rare
Centromere	'CREST' syndrome, limited scleroderma, Raynaud's, never diffuse scleroderma; may be confused with multi-nuclear dot pattern, which is seen in mitochondrial antibody negative primary biliary cirrhosis
Nuclear matrix Nuclear mitotic spindle	SLE and UCTD Non-specific: SLE, RhA, CREST, UCTD and Sjögren's syndrome
Histones	SLE, drug-induced SLE (>90% of patients); other connective tissue diseases (low frequency)

* UCTD = undifferentiated connective tissue disease (previously mixed connective tissue disease). *Note*: ribosomal antibodies associated with SLE especially neuro-lupus (cytoplasmic pattern not nuclear).

Titre of antibodies does NOT correlate with disease activity.

Anti-nuclear antibodies may be seen transiently after viral infections, especially in children. Therefore observe low titre antibodies occurring in the absence of clinical symptoms compatible with a juvenile arthritis.

Fig. 4.2 ANA on Hep-2 cells with a speckled pattern (L) and homogeneous pattern (R).

Double-stranded DNA antibodies (ds-DNA)

Units: IU/mL.

Normal range: varies according to assay

<30IU/mL	Negative
30–50IU/mL	borderline
>50IU/mL	Positive

Principles of assay

Original and still best assay is Farr assay: a radioisotope based assay. EIA tends to be widely used, but is less specific, due to frequent contamination with single-stranded DNA. Crithidia assay used only rarely as quick fluorescent screen (kinetoplast is pure ds-DNA).

Indications

Suspected SLE or autoimmune hepatitis; used to monitor SLE, in conjunction with complement studies.

Interpretation

Sensitive and specific for SLE and AIH: positive result is significant (in correct clinical context).

Antibodies to extractable nuclear antigens (ENA)

Units: reported qualitatively.

Normal range: dependent on antibody, normally negative.

Principles of test

Usually carried out by enzyme-linked immunoassay. However, counter-current immunoelectrophoresis and Western blotting are still widely used, especially for rare antibodies. EIA is much more sensitive than other methods, and has led to clinical confusion.

Indications

Should always be carried out in patients with suspected connective tissue disease. Monitoring at yearly intervals should be carried out in diagnosed patients as the antibody pattern may change with time and this may correlate with changes in the clinical profile.

Interpretation

Reported qualitatively; normally laboratories will carry out a six-antigen screen: Ro, La, RNP, Sm, Jo-1 and Scl-70.

Table 4.6 Antibodies to ENA

Ro/SS-A	SLE, Sjögren's, neonatal lupus, neonatal congenital complete heart block (cause of ANA-negative lupus, as not picked up by standard ANA screen, which does not include Hep-2 cells)
La/SS-B	SLE, Sjögren's, neonatal lupus, neonatal congenital complete heart block (rare)
(U1)-RNP	Mixed (undifferentiated) connective tissue disease (if present alone); SLE (if present with ds-DNA)
Sm	Highly specific marker for SLE (mainly West Indians; rare in Caucasians)
Jo-1	Polymyositis, dermatomyositis; transferase syndrome (fibrosing lung disease; 65% positive); many other specificities are known (all recognising tRNA-transferases)
Scl-70	Systemic sclerosis (diffuse scleroderma); only 30% of patients are positive
Pm-Scl (PM1)	Scleroderma–myositis overlap
Ku, Ki	Rare: SLE, UCTD, Sjögren's syndrome, polymyositis
Mi-2	Rare: steroid-responsive polymyositis

Table 4.7 Diagnosis and monitoring of SLE

Antinuclear antibodies double-stranded DNA antibodies	Both +ve
C3 & C4	Both ↓
Complement breakdown products	↑ in active disease (C3d)
CRP	Normal
Anti-Ro	Often +ve in ANA-negative lupus
Anti-Sm	+ve in West Indian lupus
Cardiolipin antibodies & lupus anticoagulant (dRVVT)	These should usually be checked (see below)
Ribosomal P antibodies	May be a marker for neuropsychiatric lupus

Monitor with CRP (differential between infection and flare of disease), C3, C4, C3d and ds-DNA antibodies (no value from serial ANA); rising titre DNA antibodies often heralds relapse (actual titre not related to disease activity).

Antiphospholipid antibodies

Principles of testing

Many types of antibodies to phospholipids are recognised. However routinely available tests are IgG and IgM anti-cardiolipin antibodies, detected by EIA, and the presence of a 'lupus anti-coagulant', detected using the dilute Russell viper venom test (dRVVT). *Both* tests must be carried out together as either may be positive without the other but the clinical significance is the same. Antibodies to β_2-glycoprotein I are also important as the protein is key co-factor for pathogenic antibodies. Other specificities are available only as research tools.

Indications

Patients with unexplained venous or arterial thrombosis; recurrent miscarriage (>3), connective tissue disease, early TIAs or stroke (<60 years). Livedo reticularis is a cutaneous marker.

Interpretation

Prolonged APTT and reduced platelet count (80–120 $\times$ 10^9/L) are typical features. May get false +ve VDRL.

Persistent positive IgM anti-cardiolipin antibodies as only marker of syndrome unusual but clinically significant.

Hughes' syndrome = anti-phospholipid antibodies without evidence of other connective tissue disease or vasculitis. Presents with recurrent miscarriage, thrombosis or strokes. Fulminant disease causes multi-organ failure.

Antibodies also found in SLE, but NOT cerebral lupus, Behçet's and Sneddon's syndrome. Also seen after EBV infection (asymptomatic and disappear).

Treatment is lifelong warfarinisation if symptomatic (heparin in pregnancy) if symptomatic; aspirin may be acceptable if asymptomatic (but no controlled studies). No indication for intensive immunosuppression.

Other patterns of autoantibodies identified on 'autoantibody screen'

Anti-mitochondrial antibodies (AMA) and anti-M2 antibodies

Units: reported as titre (AMA). Anti-M2 reported as positive or negative.

Normal range: not usually detectable in health.

Principles of testing

AMA are identified on fluorescent screen and previously unknown positives should be followed up with EIA or blot-based test for anti-M2 antibodies.

Indications

Suspected liver disease, especially with ↑ alkaline phosphatase (and in females); investigation of unexplained pruritus (early feature of primary biliary cirrhosis).

Interpretation

95% of PBC patients positive for anti-mitochondrial antibodies (anti-M2, against dihydrolipoamide acyltransferase, E2). Remainder may have antibodies against S100 antigen of nuclear membrane (Nsp-II pattern; multi-nuclear dots) or gp210, another nuclear antigen. Type of antibody present has no influence on prognosis or response to therapy. Marked elevation in IgM.

Autoantibodies in autoimmune hepatitis

Units: reported as titres (anti-smooth muscle antibodies (ASMA), anti-liver–kidney microsomal (LKM) antibodies). Anti-liver cytosol (LC-1) and soluble liver antigen (SLA) reported as positive or negative.

Normal range: not usually detectable in health.

Principles of testing

ASMA and LKM are identified on fluorescent screen and previously unknown positives should be followed up with EIA or blot-based test for anti-LC and anti-SLA antibodies. Also do ANCA (*see below*).

Indications

Suspected autoimmune liver disease (abnormal LFTs, alcohol and viral infections excluded).

Interpretation

Antibodies to HCV or HCV PCR +ve = exclusion criteria for auto-immune hepatitis.

Autoimmune hepatitis

- Type 1 (AIH-1) is ANA+, smooth muscle Ab (SMA)+, P-ANCA+, and soluble liver antigen (SLA) Ab+. Typically occurs in adults and has a better prognosis and responds well to therapy.
- Type 2 (AIH-2) is typically liver–kidney microsomal (LKM-1, LKM-3) Ab+ and liver cytosol (LC-1) Ab+. AIH-2 is seen in children and has a worse prognosis with poor response to therapy.
- In serological studies AIH-1 50% are ANA+/SMA+, 15% are ANA+ only and 35% are SMA+ only; however there are biopsy proven serologically negative hepatitis. 8% of AIH-1 are SLA+ only. 43% of AIH-2 are LC-1+ only. Therefore necessary to do SLA and LC-1 tests. Prognosis is dependent on type and early diagnosis.
- Liver–kidney microsomal antibodies are also associated with drug-induced hepatitis (esp. halothane) and chronic hepatitis C or D.

- Non-actin smooth muscle antibodies may be seen in SLE and after viral infections (especially adenovirus).
- Sclerosing cholangitis may be associated with atypical P-ANCA (see below).

Gastric parietal cell and intrinsic factor antibodies

Units: GPC may be reported as titre or simply positive/negative (as titre of no clinical value); IF antibodies reported positive/negative.

Normal range: GPC antibodies found in healthy normals without evidence of B_{12} deficiency or gastritis—may be at risk of later pernicious anaemia. IF antibodies only found in PA.

Principles of testing
GPC antibodies are detected as part of the 'autoantibody screen'; IF antibodies usually detected by either radioimmunoassay or EIA, but assays are inconsistent. There is a robust EQA scheme for GPC antibodies but none currently for IF antibodies.

Indications for testing
GPC antibodies should be checked in all patients with thyroid disease, as there is a close association ('thyrogastric disease'). Also check in patients with unexplained macrocytosis ± low B_{12}. Positive antibodies identified incidentally should be followed up with a blood count and if the MCV is high, a B_{12} level. Intrinsic factor antibodies may help in patients with high MCV and low B_{12} to confirm pernicious anaemia (but Schilling test is gold standard).

Interpretation
Gastric parietal cell antibodies found in 90% of patient with pernicious anaemia and in 40% of patients with other organ-specific autoimmune diseases; antigen is b-subunit of gastric H^+/K^+ ATPase. Anti-intrinsic factor antibodies are of two types: those that block B_{12} binding to IF (70% of patients with PA) and those that block uptake of the B_{12}–IF complex (35% of patients with PA).

Thyroid disease

Thyroid microsomal antibodies; thyroid peroxidase antibodies

Units: variable—check with laboratory.

Normal range: low levels of antibodies may be found in asymptomatic individuals, although higher levels may indicate predisposition to later development of thyroid disease.

Principles of testing

Previously, particle agglutination assays for thyroid microsomal antibodies were the mainstay; now being replaced by thyroid peroxidase (EIA). Thyroglobulin antibodies not monitored now except as part of monitoring for thyroid carcinoma (interfere with assays for thyroglobulin, which is used as a tumour marker). Antibodies to TSH-receptor may be stimulating or blocking, but these can only be identified by bioassay or radio-immunoassay in specialised laboratories.

Indications for testing

Suspected thyroid disease and as reflex testing when thyroid function is abnormal; often now combined with thyroid testing on same analyser. Also check in patients with pernicious anaemia. Use thyroid peroxidase (or microsomal) antibodies. Other antibodies are for specialist use only.

Interpretation

Table 4.8

Thyroid peroxidase (thyroid microsomal)	95–100% Hashimoto's thyroiditis 70% Graves' disease Highest titres seen in Hashimoto's
Thyroglobulin antibodies	Add little to diagnosis (also found in other endocrinopathies and thyroid carcinoma).
Antibodies to TSH-R (stimulating or blocking)	95% Graves' patients

Islet cell antibodies (ICA), anti-GAD antibodies, insulin-receptor and insulin antibodies

Units: qualitative (previously measured in JDF units).

Normal range: 0.4% of normal population positive for ICA.

Principles of testing

Islet cell antibodies can be detected by immunofluorescence on pancreatic sections; other antibodies detected by EIA.

Indications for testing

All newly diagnosed early onset diabetics should be tested; they should also be tested for coeliac disease using endomysial or tissue transglutaminase antibodies. May be used to screen normoglycaemic first degree relatives for likelihood of developing diabetes.

Interpretation

Islet cell antibodies found in 75–86% of type I diabetics but only 10% type II diabetics and 2–5% first-degree relatives. Levels decline with time and may disappear completely in longstanding type I patients. Antigen is glutamic acid decarboxylase, GAD (similar antibodies cause stiff man (person!) syndrome although a different epitope on the molecule is recognised). Other target antigens for autoantibodies, with high specificity for diabetes, are:

- Insulin/proinsulin (seen at diagnosis in 40% type I diabetics).
- Insulin receptor (associated with acanthosis nigricans and insulin resistance).
- Pancreatic decarboxylase.
- β-cell granule protein.

Monitoring is of no value.

Note: IgE antibodies to porcine or bovine insulin may occur in insulin allergy, due to exogenous 'foreign' insulin.

Adrenal antibodies & other endocrine autoantibodies

Units: qualitative.

Normal range: not detectable.

Principles of testing
Usually detected by immunofluorescence on appropriate tissue (adrenal, ovary, testis, parathyroid, pituitary). EIA for 21-hydroxylase, 17-hydroxylase and P450 side-chain cleavage enzymes (targets of adrenal antibodies) in research centres.

Indications for testing
Suspected autoimmune endocrinopathy (adrenal insufficiency, premature ovarian failure, hypoparathyroidism).

Interpretation
Positives indicate autoimmune disease of relevant organ.

Classification of autoimmune polyglandular syndromes

Table 4.9

Syndrome	Major criteria	Minor criteria
Type I	Candidiasis Adrenal failure Hypoparathyroidism	Gonadal failure Alopecia Malabsorption Chronic hepatitis
Type II (Schmidt's syndrome)	Adrenal failure Thyroid disease IDDM	Gonadal failure Vitiligo Non-endocrine autoimmunity (myasthenia)
Type III	Thyroid disease	*either* IDDM *or* Pernicious anaemia *or* Non-endocrine autoimmunity (myasthenia)

Endomysial (EMA) & tissue transglutaminase (tTG) antibodies

Units: qualitative.

Normal range: not usually detected in healthy individuals. Positive IgA EMA or tTG with normal biopsy probably indicates risk of later development of coeliac disease.

Principles of testing

Originally identified as anti-reticulin R1 antibodies on 'autoimmune screen'. Later identified as anti-gliadin antibodies by modified immunofluorescence or by EIA. EMA detected by immunofluorescence on monkey oesophagus (also umbilical vein, but this is difficult to read); purified recombination human tissue transglutaminase used for EIA (assays with guinea pig tTG are less sensitive).

Indications for testing

Patients with malabsorption, wheat intolerance, 'irritable bowel'; children with type I diabetes (and suggested that they should be monitored every year!). Suspected dermatitis herpetiformis. Unexplained hyposplenism, small bowel lymphoma.

Interpretation

IgA endomysial antibody has nearly 100% sensitivity & specificity for coeliac disease. Antigen is tissue transglutaminase. In IgA deficiency (commoner in coeliac), IgG endomysial antibody is as good a diagnostic test. Gliadin antibodies (IgG or IgA) are not sensitive and specific and should no longer be used: they are found in a range of bowel diseases and in healthy individuals. Reticulin R1 antibodies may be picked up on routine autoantibody screen; these may also be found in inflammatory bowel disease, especially with liver involvement, and non-specific bowel disease (post-infectious, allergic, etc.). Also found in dermatitis herpetiformis (typical rash). Strong association with juvenile type I diabetes mellitus.

Antibodies disappear with strict gluten-free diet, over 6–12 months. Persistent positivity of IgA endomysial antibodies in a patient on a GFD is an indication of incomplete/non-compliance with diet.

Gliadin antibodies & neurological disease

Gluten sensitivity enteropathy is also associated with neurological disease, typically a cerebellar ataxia. Reports have suggested that gliadin antibodies are a marker for this syndrome; the lack of specificity of gliadin antibodies means that it is unlikely that these antibodies can be used as an accurate diagnostic test and specific tests (EMA and tTG) should be used instead.

Autoimmune skin diseases

Units: normally reported qualitatively.

Normal range: antibodies when detected are highly disease-specific.

Principles of testing
Autoantibodies to components of the skin can be detected either by direct immunofluorescence on a skin biopsy of affected tissue, or indirectly in the patients serum, using monkey oesophagus as a substrate. Saline splitting of the skin may be used to identify the precise location of the antigenic target to differentiate between epidermolysis bullosa acquisita (antigen on the dermal side) and pemphigoid (antigen on the epidermal side).

Indications for testing
Bullous (blistering) skin diseases.

Interpretation
Bullous pemphigoid
Antibodies bind to dermal–epidermal junction and recognise hemidesmosome antigens (BP 230 (BPAG1) and BP 180 (BPAG2)); detect by direct immunofluorescence on skin biopsies or in serum (only 70% of patients have detectable circulating antibodies in serum). Linear basement membrane deposition of IgG and C3 on direct immunofluorescence.

Herpes gestationis
Antibodies to BP 180 (BPAG2) binding to dermal–epidermal junction on direct immunofluorescence of biopsies, often negative for serum antibodies. Linear basement membrane deposition of IgG and C3 on direct immunofluorescence.

Pemphigus
Antibody binds to cell surface of stratified squamous epithelium, recognises desmosomal proteins desmoglein I & III. 80–90% of patients have detectable antibody in serum. Chicken-wire pattern of immunofluorescence in epidermis. May occur as a paraneoplastic phenomenon in patients with lymphoma, but antigenic specificity is for desmoplakin I & II.

Dermatitis herpetiformis
Granular deposits of IgA at dermal–epidermal junction in dermal papillae on direct immunofluorescence; EMA and tTG antibodies will be positive.

Autoantibodies & neurological disease

Principles of testing

Most neurological autoantibodies of interest are rare and are available from the Neuroimmunology Research Laboratory in Oxford. A variety of methods are used; some assays are reported with numeric values.

Indications for testing

These are restricted to very specific neurological syndromes.

Interpretation

Acetylcholine receptor antibodies (ACRAb) associated with myasthenia gravis (90%); reported numerically as high and low positives distinguish different clinical phenotypes. May also be found in asymptomatic relatives. Striated muscle antibodies (immunofluorescence on striated muscle section) strongly associated with underlying thymoma.

Lambert–Eaton myasthenic syndrome occurring with small cell carcinoma of the lung, associated with autoantibodies to voltage gated calcium channels, alpha & beta subunits. Same tumour also associated with retinal autoantibodies. Antibodies to voltage-gated potassium channels are associated with neuromyotonia.

Anti-ganglioside antibodies associated with Guillain–Barré syndrome (GM-1, GD1a) and variants (Miller–Fischer—GQ1b, GT1a), chronic variants (chronic inflammatory demyelinating polyneuropathy) and neuropathy associated with paraproteins.

Myelin associated glycoprotein associated antibodies (MAG) associated with paraproteinaemic neuropathy especially with Waldenström's macroglobulinaemia.

Antibodies to myelin basic protein found in multiple sclerosis but not useful diagnostically.

Anti-Yo (Purkinje cell antibodies) found in paraneoplastic cerebellar degeneration (gynaecological or breast tumours associated); anti-Hu (anti-neuronal nuclear antibodies, ANNA) associated with paraneoplastic neuropathies and myelopathies (small cell carcinoma). Anti-Ri (anti-neuronal nuclei) associated with cerebellar ataxia and opsiclonus (small cell carcinoma, gynaecological or breast tumours associated).

Anti-neuronal antibodies in CSF of 74% of patients with cerebral lupus; also associated with anti-ribosomal P antibodies.

Anti-GAD antibodies found in stiff-person syndrome; same antigen to that found in pancreatic islets; diabetes usually occurs in stiff person syndrome. Antibodies appear to inhibit the production of γ-aminobutyric acid (GABA), an inhibitory neurotransmitter. Rasmussen's encephalitis associated with autoantibodies to GluR3 receptor, which cause hyperexcitability of neurones.

Vasculitic syndromes

ANCA

Units: usually expressed as titre (qualitative EIAs are used in some centres).

Normal range: in adults, normally undetectable.

Principles of testing
Screening is usually carried out by immunofluorescence on ethanol-fixed human neutrophils; rapid EIA screening tests exist for positive–negative testing in emergencies. EIA to specific antigens is an essential follow-up. Distinction between anti-nuclear and perinuclear staining may require the use of Hep-2 cells.

Indications for testing
Suspected vasculitis; acute glomerulonephritis.

Interpretation
Two main patterns recognised: C-ANCA (mostly Wegener's; 90% of Wegener's ANCA +ve) and P-ANCA (some Wegener's, microscopic polyarteritis, Churg–Strauss syndrome, glomerulonephritis, sclerosing cholangitis, autoimmune hepatitis ulcerative colitis).

C-ANCA pattern due to antibodies against proteinase-3; P-ANCA pattern due to antibodies against myeloperoxidase, lactoferrin, cathepsin, elastase. Follow-up EIA required to identify antigenic specificity: minimum PR3 and MPO ELISA; other antigens available through supra-regional referral laboratories.

In Wegener's, monitoring titre of ANCA is useful: rising titre in a patient in clinical remission heralds relapse.

ANCA may be seen as epiphenomenon in states of chronic neutrophil activation and turnover, e.g. cystic fibrosis.

Anti-GBM disease (Goodpasture's syndrome)

Units: qualitative (quantitation available through reference centres— used only to follow patients post-plasmapheresis or transplant).

Normal range: not detectable in health.

Principles of testing
Usually carried out by EIA; screening by immunofluorescence is not sensitive. Biopsies will show linear IgG deposition in glomeruli (and alve-oli). Antibodies recognise the NC1 region in the α3 chain of type IV collagen.

Indications for testing
Acute glomerulonephritis, particularly if associated with pulmonary haemorrhage.

Interpretation

Positive antibodies confirm Goodpasture's syndrome. Urgent plasmapheresis is required and monitoring reduction of antibody with treatment is advisable. Disease may recur in transplanted kidneys, so monitoring of antibody is advised. Some patients may be both ANCA and anti-GBM antibody +ve.

Allergic disease

Total IgE

Units: kU/L.

Normal range: <100kU/L (>14 years old).

Principles of testing

Previously carried out by radioimmunoassay, now by enzyme immunoassay.

Indications for testing

There are FEW indications for testing. Screening for atopic disease; investigation of suspected hyper-IgE syndrome (Job's syndrome, a rare immunodeficiency), Churg–Strauss vasculitis. Gating requests for RAST tests on the basis of IgE is scientifically unsound (*see below*).

Interpretation

Significant allergic disease is possible with low levels of total IgE (including anaphylaxis). Only patients with undetectable IgE (<7kU/L) are unlikely to have allergic disease. Conversely, levels above the normal range are compatible with no clinical allergic disease. IgE >1,000kU/L associated with atopic eczema; IgE >50,000kU/L confirms hyper-IgE syndrome (although patients may have lower levels—diagnosis is clinical). Raised levels are also seen in parasitic infections of the bowel, filariasis, lymphoma (especially Hodgkin's disease) and Churg–Strauss vasculitis.

⁀ http://www.worldallergy.org
⁀ http://www.aaaai.org/professionals.stm
⁀ http://www.medscape.com/allergy-immunologyhome

Skin prick tests

Units: mm wheal size, compared to histamine and saline controls.

Normal range: no wheal.

Principles of testing

This remains the gold standard for allergy diagnosis. It identifies IgE-mediated reactions (type I), such as inhalant allergy, anaphylaxis, food allergy. It is dependent on triggering release of histamine from cutaneous mast cells. Solution of allergen or controls (histamine or saline) placed on skin, and priced through by lancet. After 15 minutes wheal will be visible. Positive is at least 2 mm greater than negative control. Histamine control must be positive. Not interpretable if patient is dermographic (negative = positive). Can use factory prepared allergens; also use double-prick technique with fresh foods (prick food then patient)—useful where allergens are labile, e.g. fruits.

Indications for testing

Mainstay for diagnosis of all types of allergic disease. Contraindicated when there is significant skin disease, previous severe allergic reactions (use RASTs first), patients on anti-histamines (need to be off drug for a week). Other drugs will interfere, e.g. calcium channel blockers, tricyclic anti-depressants.

Interpretation

Results can only be interpreted in the context of the clinical history. Testing should be tailored to individual patients to answer specific questions. May need to be followed up by open or blinded challenges, where negative results are obtained in patients with good histories.

Good specificity for inhalant allergens and some foods (nuts, fish); results comparable with RAST testing.

Many known families of cross-reactivity between biological families:
- Latex allergy associated with food reactions: banana, avocado, kiwi fruit, chestnut, potato, tomato, cannabis, lettuce. Also birch pollen allergy commoner.
- Birch pollen allergy (asthma, rhinitis) with food-related reactions to nuts, apples, plums, cherries, carrots and potatoes ('oral allergy' syndrome).
- Mugwort pollen and celery.
- Ragweed pollen with melon and banana.

Specific IgE: 'RAST tests'

Units: reported as Grades 1–6. Also as continuous numeric scale in IU/mL.

Normal range: Grades 0 & 1 indicate insignificant specific IgE.

Table 4.10

Grade	IU/mL
0	<0.35
1	0.35–0.70
2	0.70–3.50
3	3.50–17.50
4	17.5–50.0
5	50–100
6	>100

Principles of testing

Previously tested by radioimmunoassay (hence acronym RAST = radio-allergosorbent test); now identified by enzyme-linked or fluorimetric assays.

Indications for testing

'RAST' tests are expensive and should be reserved for cases where skin prick testing is not possible: extensive skin disease, patient on anti-histamines, severe reactions, small children, dermographic patients. Testing *must* be guided by history—do not request 'allergen screen'.

Interpretation

Presence of specific IgE does *not* equate to allergic disease—indicates sensitisation only. Must be interpreted in the context of the clinical history. Numerical value does *not* correlate with severity of clinical reactions.

RAST tests of little value for identifying allergy to fruits and vegetables as the allergens are labile and drugs (unreliable). False positives possible when total IgE is very high due to non-specific binding (less of a problem with newer assays).

Mast cell tryptase

Units: mg/L.

Normal range: 2–24mg/L.

Principles of testing
Measured by EIA. Analyte is stable in clotted blood.

Indications for testing
Valuable test for the investigation of acute ?allergic reactions. Released when mast cells degranulate and stable in serum for up to 24 hours. Also useful for monitoring patients with mastocytosis.

Interpretation
Raised levels indicate mast cell degranulation and will help distinguish anaphylactic and anaphylactoid reactions from other causes of reactions (vasovagal, hyperventilation, carcinoid, phaeochromocytoma, etc.).

Drug allergy testing

Investigation of severe drug allergy is a specialised field and all patients should be referred to an appropriate expert for an opinion, usually a consultant in allergy or clinical immunology in a regional centre. Testing will usually involve skin prick testing followed by intradermal testing and patch testing and if necessary blind challenge.

Patch tests

Units: scored qualitatively.

Normal range: negative.

Principles of testing
This test identifies cell-mediated reactions = delayed type hypersensitivity (type IV reactions). It should not be confused with skin prick testing. Allergens in petrolatum jelly are placed in contact with the skin for 48 hours under occlusion with aluminium cups. Test result is read at 96 hours, looking for eczematous change and blistering. Usually carried out by dermatology departments.

Indications for testing
Investigation of contact reactions, e.g. eczema.

Interpretation
Positive results are invariably significant. Common allergens include metals such as nickel and chromium, dyes and chemical in leather, rubber chemicals (accelerators), cosmetic chemicals. Panels of allergens used depending on clinical history.

Cellular function assays

Investigation of cellular function of lymphocytes, neutrophils, macrophages and NK cells are restricted to specialised regional immunology laboratories. The tests are labour-intensive and difficult to standardise, with the exception of basic lymphocyte markers. EQA schemes are available only for basic lymphocyte markers.

All tests, other than basic lymphocyte markers, should only be requested after discussion with a consultant immunologist. Their role is in the investigation of suspected cellular immunodeficiency, particularly severe combined immunodeficiency (SCID) and primary disorders of neutrophils. In such cases urgent referral of the patient to an appropriate paediatric or adult immunologist is more appropriate than fiddling around trying to get tests done, as the immunologist will have direct and immediate access to the appropriate tests. Lives have been lost due to delay in transfer while inexperienced clinicians have tried to make diagnoses.

Lymphocyte surface markers

Units: cells/mL.

Normal range

Table 4.11

CD3+ (total T cells)	690–2540
CD19+ (total B cells; CD20 is equivalent)	90–660
CD3+CD4+ (T helper cells)	410–1590
CD3+CD8+ (cytotoxic T cells)	190–1140
CD16+CD56+ (NK cells)	90–590

Principles of testing

Lymphocyte surface markers should be carried out on a single platform flow cytometer, which will give a direct absolute count, not requiring a total lymphocyte count from a haematology analyser. Absolute counts are the preferred value; percentages are not useful. Fresh samples are required for optimum results. Many other surface markers are available to answer more specific immunological questions, but these will usually be of interest only to clinical immunologists. An EQA scheme operates.

Indications for testing

There are no absolute indications. Investigation of lymphocyte subsets is an important part of the work-up of any patients with suspected primary or secondary immunodeficiency and of patients with unexpected lymphopenia. Serial measurements are valuable in patients undergoing bone marrow or stem cell transplantation, with primary immunodeficiencies, in patients on any immunosuppressive therapy and with HIV on therapy with HAART.

Interpretation

Results can only be interpreted in the context of the clinical question. Lymphocyte surface marker analysis *cannot* be used as a surrogate for HIV testing, as many acute viral and bacterial infections, as well as other medical problems, will give rise to a reduction in CD4+ T cells.

Critical action

Baby <6 months with lymphocyte count <2 × 10^9/L = SCID until proven otherwise: *immediate* referral to SCID BMT Unit (In UK, Newcastle General Hospital, Newcastle upon Tyne and Great Ormond Street Hospital for Sick Children, London). Look at the differential white count not just the total white count!

Lymphocyte function tests

These are highly specialised and should only be carried out on the recommendation of a clinical immunologist.

Indications for testing

There are no absolute indications for testing but it is usually carried out as part of the specialised work-up of patients with known or suspected severe combined immunodeficiency and in the monitoring of immunological reconstitution post bone marrow transplant.

Interpretation

Is complex and dependent on the precise clinical circumstances.

Neutrophil & macrophage function

This is a specialised test. Samples do not transport well and results are often abnormal if the patient has active infection or is on antibiotics. It is preferable to refer patients to a clinical immunologist who will organise testing if appropriate.

Indications for testing

Patients with deep-seated abscesses, recurrent major abscesses (exclude diabetes, staphylococcal carriage and hidradenitis suppurativa first), major oral ulceration, unusual fungal or bacterial infections (pseudomonas, serratia, staphylococci, aspergillus). Atypical granulomatous disease, including atypical Crohn's disease. Genetic defects of neutrophil function may present at any age.

Interpretation

Interpretation is complex; defects of oxidative metabolism may indicate chronic granulomatous disease; defects of phagocytosis are recognised. Also myeloperoxidase deficiency. Neutropenia may be chronic or cyclical. Genetic testing to follow-up may be required.

NK cell function

Is rarely required. Main indication is in recurrent severe infection with herpes viruses. Assays are complex and need specialist interpretation. Always discuss cases with a clinical immunologist.

Immunology websites

Immunology and general medicine

⤷ http://www.specialtylabs.com/books/default.asp
⤷ http://www.emedicine.com/

European Federation of Immunological Societies

⤷ http://www.efis.org/

American Academy of Allergy, Asthma & Immunology

⤷ http://www.aaaai.org/professionals.stm

Infectious & tropical diseases

Introduction to infectious diseases 328
Investigating the infectious diseases/tropical
  medicine case 334
Culture techniques 335
Serology 340
Antigen tests 344
Collection of specimens 346
Molecular diagnostics 350
Haematology 352
Radiology 354
Gastrointestinal tract investigations 356
Immunology 358
Biochemical tests 358
Tissue biopsy & deep aspiration specimens 360
Other tests 364
Clinical investigation in action: PUO
  (pyrexia of uncertain origin) 366
Further reading 376

Introduction to infectious diseases

'Everything about microscopic life is terribly upsetting... how can things so small be so important?' (Isaac Asimov—1920–92).

An old enemy

Infectious diseases have had a huge impact on the human species. Throughout history mighty armies have been humbled by microbiology. After the introduction of effective antibiotics during the Second World War, there was great optimism that the fight against infectious diseases had been won. In recent years this hope has been dramatically dashed. Almost all new diseases are infections, and some of the 21st century's most pressing problems are pathogens which have only appeared in the 30 years prior to this book being written. Globally the most important of the newer organisms are HIV and hepatitis C, though old enemies such as TB, pneumococcus and malaria are still killing millions throughout the world.

New challenges

As we enter the 21st century several factors are serving to increase the relative importance of infection over other areas of medicine. New infections such as SARS and avian influenza are continually emerging. Anti-microbial resistance is increasing, methicillin-resistant *Staphylococcus aureus* (MRSA) being the most infamous example. There are more immunosuppressed patients as a result of increased use of chemotherapy agents and organ transplantation. Tourists and other travellers are making their way to ever more remote parts of the world. Migration of populations has always spread disease and this continues to do so. Most alarmingly, there are concerns of bioterrorism. All of these factors mean that the infectious differential diagnosis—even in the developed world—grows ever longer.

It is always worth bearing in mind that the infectious diseases in a differential diagnosis are often treatable; accordingly it is always better to consider treatable options over incurable ones. Furthermore, some infectious diseases like MDR-TB and avian influenza have major public health consequences.

A challenge to the clinician

The same infectious disease is often capable of causing a wide variety of clinical pictures. HIV, for example, is a great mimicker. This is not so surprising given the genetic variety of mankind, hence individually tailored responses to a bewildering variety of infecting agents. Some clinical syndromes can be caused by many quite different pathogens. Good examples include pneumonia, hepatitis and endocarditis.

Furthermore, some infectious diseases can resemble non-infectious diseases. For example, amoebic colitis can resemble ulcerative colitis, syphilis can present with serious psychiatric symptomatology, a brain abscess or a tuberculoma can resemble a brain tumour, and tuberculosis of the vertebral column can resemble metastatic malignancy. Getting it wrong can be catastrophic for the patient.

Other diseases can mimic infections

Non-infectious diseases can resemble infection. Examples include gout of the first metatarso-phalangeal joint rather than cellulitis, cervical lymphadenopathy due to lymphoma rather than tuberculosis, familial Mediterranean fever as a cause of PUO, SLE leading to Libman–Sachs endocarditis, adult Still's disease as a cause of fever and neutrophilia, and an inflammatory carcinoma of the female breast resembling a pyogenic breast abscess.

The importance of epidemiological factors

Epidemiology is fundamental to determining which, if any, infecting agents and, therefore, investigations are relevant in a given patient.

Geography: this is very important.

Some infections are common the world over and include
- *Salmonella* infections.
- Pneumococcal pneumonia.
- Gonorrhoea.
- Thrush (candidiasis).
- Tuberculosis.
- Influenza.
- Epstein–Barr virus.
- HIV (although sub-Saharan Africa is the worst affected area).
- Hepatitis C.
- Herpes simplex.
- Threadworm (*Enterobius*).

Some infectious diseases are only common in the developing world, e.g.
- Malaria.
- Syphilis.
- Diphtheria (although still common in Eastern Europe).
- Rheumatic fever.
- Enteric fever (typhoid and paratyphoid).
- Hepatitis E.
- Poliomyelitis.
- Rabies (although Eastern Europe has significant disease).
- Viral haemorrhagic fever.
- Onchocerciasis (river blindness).
- Schistosomiasis.
- Leishmaniasis (although commonly found around the Mediterranean sea).
- Ascariasis.
- Cutaneous myiasis (e.g. tumbu fly).

Some infectious diseases are common in some parts of the developed world but not in others. These include
- Lyme disease.
- Babesiosis.
- Ehrlichiosis.
- Histoplasmosis.
- Hydatid disease.
- Anisakiasis.

Indeed, in the USA, only certain areas are endemic for

- Lyme disease.
- Coccidioidomycosis.
- Babesiosis.
- Histoplasmosis.

Travel history: this is important for many reasons. Travel exposes patients to new infectious agents to which they have no immunity. The clinician must therefore be aware of the distribution of common infections. Great variation in antibiotic resistance patterns can be observed in different parts of the world; this clearly has in impact on choice of empirical treatment. Finally, travel often has an impact on patterns of sexual and risk-taking behaviour.

Fig. 5.1 The importance of taking a geographic history. Malaria, which can be life-threatening, is a very common disease in many parts of the world (see *map*), but is not indigenous to most parts of the developed world. Making a diagnosis depends heavily upon the clinician eliciting the clues in the patient's history. Even if s/he has been taking antimalarial drugs, a patient who has been on holiday to Kenya, Thailand or Brazil may die if the disease is not diagnosed. Clinical suspicion should lead to blood films (on 3 consecutive days) and a platelet count. Bear in mind that the patient may not have been taking adequate prophylaxis, may have been missing tablets, or may not have been absorbing them.

Sexual and drug-taking activity: searching and personal questions may need to be asked. This is always difficult to do, even with great experience. Patients will rarely admit to high risk sexual activity or the use of illegal substances and may need to be pressed. The clinician must maintain a high clinical suspicion at all times, even and especially when the patient does not fit a social stereotype. Bear in mind that any patient may have a 'double life' that even his/her spouses is unaware of. It is dangerous for the clinician to assume that being married equates to sexual fidelity or even heterosexuality.

It may not be immediately obvious that the fever, rash and hypotension in a woman may be related to her tampon usage (toxic shock syndrome), yet menstruation can be a difficult subject to discuss in some cultural settings. TB of the female genital tract may present as infertility or menorrhagia. 'Lumpy semen' may be indicative of *Schistosoma haematobium* infection, and a 'urinary tract infection' in a 19 year old man may be gonorrhoea.

Social and professional: pets, hobbies and jobs may well be important. The patient with pneumonia and a budgerigar could have psittacosis. The tropical fish salesman with a chronic rash on his hand could have *Mycobacterium marinum* infection (aka 'fish tank granuloma'). The jaundiced volunteer cleaning out canals at weekends could have leptospirosis related to contact with rats. The cat owned by the middle-aged lady with recurrent axillary lymphadenopathy may be the key to her problem.

Sexual history
e.g. HIV, syphilis, PID, herpes simplex, etc.

Contact with animals (job, hobbies, pets, etc.)
e.g. tuberculosis, brucella, psittacosis, leptospirosis, etc.

Travel history
(holidays, business, military, etc.)
e.g. malaria, VHF, Legionnaire's disease, gastroenteritis, etc.

Drug-injecting history
e.g. HIV, HCV, HBV, endocarditis, deep sepsis

Menstrual history
Toxic shock syndrome

Fig. 5.2 Infection and history taking.

Assessing the patient

The recognition of an infectious disease in a patient (or the absence of one) goes far beyond the petri dish, the microbiology bench and PCR testing technology. The *Andromeda Strain* phenomenon (with all due credit to Michael Crichton MD) should be borne in mind. The disease in front of you might be the first ever presentation! Almost the only significant new human diseases that will appear in the future will be infectious diseases, and they will keep appearing till the end of the human species.

Assessment should include
- A detailed history.
- Full physical examination (including temperature).
- The generation of a differential diagnosis.
- Laboratory tests.
- Non-invasive procedures (including radiological tests where appropriate).
- Invasive procedures.
- The making of a definitive diagnosis (wherever possible).

When considering the possibility of an infective process, one should always consider the basic infection groups
- Bacteria (including primitive forms).
- Mycobacteria.
- Fungi.
- Viruses.
- Protozoa.
- Helminths.
- Prions.
- Myiasis.

Investigations available to the ID or general physician

Many tests will be performed with a view to making a diagnosis. Investigation of a patient should be rational and evidence-based wherever possible. Although the interrogative armamentarium of the infectious diseases and tropical medicine physician is enormous—as with any other branch of medicine, the history and examination will point the way. Results will emerge which, while not producing a diagnosis as such, will nevertheless require following up. For example, low C5 levels in recurrent meningococcal septicaemia may need immunological assessment. IgG deficiency leading to recurrent pneumonia may require regular infusions of gamma globulins. A low CD4+ cell count, which is not due to HIV infection, could be a feature of sarcoidosis.

Making a diagnosis alone is not the only issue at stake. Some tests must be done if a patient is going to be treated safely. Examples might include: G6PD levels before administering primaquine for hypnozoite eradication in malaria; TB cultures for antibiotic sensitivity prior to starting empirical therapy; exclusion of pregnancy before using certain antibiotics such as doxycycline and ciprofloxacin. Other tests relate to the fact that some infectious diseases are dangerous to others: prime examples of this would be multi-drug-resistant tuberculosis and SARS, both of which are potentially dangerous for the population at large and need to be identified (or at least suspected wherever appropriate) and treated in an isolation unit.

Investigating the infectious diseases/tropical medicine case

Available diagnostic techniques include

Direct detection

- Microscopy:
  - Direct: e.g. faecal parasites (± iodine) or malarial and trypanosomal blood films.
  - Special stains: these include Gram and Ziehl–Nieelsen stains.
  - Electron microscopy: for viruses and other pathogens.
- Presence of toxin (e.g. *Clostridium difficile*).
- Antigen detection (◫*Serology*, p340).
- Molecular assays (◫*Molecular diagnostics*, p350): these include gene probes, amplification assays (e.g. polymerase chain reaction, PCR).

Culture

- Almost all body fluid and tissues can be cultured. As a general principle, the larger the sample sent, the greater the yield. It is good practice to forewarn the laboratory before sending any unusual samples. Laboratory preparation and specialist containers may be required. Adequate clinical details should be written on any request forms. The choice of culture technique can vary dramatically depending on the organism that is being sought. There may be only one chance to culture the correct bacteria so it should not be wasted.
- Identification through special growth media, culture temperature or atmosphere. ⌁http://textbookofbacteriology.net
- Identification of individual colonies by biochemical reactions (e.g. catalase or coagulase).
- Identification with specific antisera (i.e. latex agglutination.)
- Identification using molecular-based methods (e.g. specific probes, restriction enzyme patterns, DNA sequencing).
- Antimicrobial susceptibility testing, if indicated.

Serology (◫*Serology*, p340).

Other tests as appropriate (see appropriate sections)

- Biochemistry.
- Haematology.
- Immunology.
- Molecular tests.
- Radiology.
- Stool & bowel contents.
- Tissue biopsy and deep aspiration specimens.
- Other tests.

Culture techniques

Microorganisms exist in nature as mixed populations. Diagnosis of an infection means identifying the relevant pathogen in the face of this plethora of 'pretenders to the crown'. Furthermore, different organisms can cause the same disease (e.g. pneumonia) and require very different treatment and management and have different prognoses. While some specimens (e.g. stool, sputum) contain extremely large numbers of a varied organisms, some specimens (e.g. blood, CSF, urine) should be sterile unless infected or contaminated during their collection.

Microbiological culture assists with the aetiological diagnosis of bacterial, fungal, protozoal or viral illness by enabling identification and susceptibility testing of the isolated organism(s). Bacterial culture was the first to evolve, but useful data on other pathogenic groups can also be obtained through the use of culture-based methodologies (although options for treatment are currently more limited for viruses and fungi than for bacteria). Furthermore, culture of viruses and fungi usually takes longer than most bacterial culture; therefore the data obtained is most valuable for the late confirmation of the diagnosis or for epidemiological purposes (e.g. for predicting the appropriate constituents for a polyvalent influenza vaccine).

Bacteria

3 major steps are involved in extracting pure cultures from a diverse population of microorganisms and identifying a pathogen.

1. An isolation plate is created—to do this, the mixture must be diluted until the various individual microorganisms have been dispersed far enough apart on an agar surface so that, after incubation, they will form visible colonies isolated from the colonies of their neighbours. Specialised culture media (such as selective media, differential media, enrichment media, and combination selective and differential media—a great many exist) may be used to supplement mechanical techniques of isolation. Culture can be aerobic or anaerobic. (*Note*: specimens for the isolation of anaerobic pathogens require special care as anaerobic bacteria die in the presence of oxygen. Such specimens should therefore be transported in a reduced container.) Lastly temperature can be used to further select for pathogenic organisms, for example *Campylobacter jejuni* is unusual as it will grow at 41°C.

2. A pure culture is created—to achieve this, an isolated colony will be selected out and carefully 'picked off' the isolation plate for transferring to a new sterile medium. Following incubation all the organisms in the new culture will be descendants of the same organism.

3. The organism can then be identified through various manoeuvres
- The colony appearance and susceptibility to specific antibiotic disks.
- The microscopic appearance.
- The staining responses (e.g. Gram +ve vs. Gram –ve).

- The use of a range of biochemical tests designed to uncover characteristics typical of a particular organism, e.g. catalase reaction, sugar fermentation. The presence of the enzyme coagulase is useful for distinguishing *Staphylococcus aureus* from less pathogenic coagulase-negative staphylocci (normal skin commensals).
- The use of antisera (direct serology) for culture confirmation:
  - Agglutination and latex agglutination tests are used on colonies to identify *Escherichia coli* 0157, *Streptococcus pneumoniae*, serogroups of *Neisseria meningitidis*, *Shigella* and *Salmonella*, Lancefield groups of β-haemolytic streptococci and serotypes of *Haemophilus influenzae*.
  - Detection of specific antigens by DFA (direct fluorescent antibody) staining can be used to identify colonies of *Streptococcus pyogenes*, *Bordetella pertussis* and the species and serotypes of *Legionella*.
  - The Quellung reaction, which employs specific antisera to interact with capsular polysaccharides of *Streptococcus pneumoniae*, can be used to confirm the identification of the pneumococcus as well as to determine the serotype of the cultured organism.

Ideally, specimens for bacterial culture should be taken *before* antibiotics are administered. This may not always be feasible but the information yielded may well be less than ideal.

Bacteriological diagnosis at the bench

http://www.medmicro.mds.qmw.ac.uk/underground/diagnose/diagnose.html

Fig. 5.3 Bacteriological diagnosis at the bench.

Antibiotic sensitivity

Once a bacterium is isolated, it can be cultured in the presence of antibiotic(s) to assess if it is susceptible to that agent or not (i.e. resistant). The minimum inhibitory concentration (MIC) is the lowest antibiotic concentration at which the microorganism under assessment shows no visible growth *in vitro*. The MIC can provide the clinician with precise information about the infecting bacterium's degree of antibiotic susceptibility and enable him/her to avoid antibiotics to which the organism shows resistance.

For organisms exhibiting unusual resistance patterns, susceptibility panels using methodologies such as broth microdilution, gradient diffusion, and/or disc diffusion have been created to assist clinicians.

On occasions, these data will need to be linked to testing of blood levels for some antibiotics (e.g. gentamicin, vancomycin, cycloserine). Serum bactericidal test (sbt) can be used to determine whether concentrations of the antibiotic in a patient's serum are capable of killing the infecting microorganism.

Viruses

Viral culture differs from bacterial culture, i.e. viruses require a very different type of medium to grow in. They grow in cell cultures, and are detected through the cytopathic effects that appear in cell culture. New techniques appear regularly. Indeed, viral culture is being used less commonly as molecular techniques such as PCR become more effective.

The appropriate type of specimen to collect, the best means of transport and the most appropriate cell culture to use will vary with the particular virus suspected, the specimen site and the time of the year.

- The choice of specimen is very important: numerous viruses enter via the mucosa of the upper respiratory tract, yet that virus may compromise multiple or distant tissues and organs.
- Swabs can be used to collect a variety of specimens from the body surfaces for viral detection, e.g. nose, throat, eye, skin and rectum. A nasopharyngeal aspirate may be the more appropriate specimen if influenza is suspected. Deeper specimens, such as blood and CSF, will be appropriate for some viruses. Different viruses will need different collection approaches—for example, heparin, citrate and EDTA are all acceptable for the detection of CMV by culture or by antigenaemia testing, but for some other viruses only citrate should be used if they are to be cultured.
- Unlike many bacterial or fungal pathogens, the time of year is important to keep in mind when making a diagnosis of certain viral diseases. For example, enteroviruses (e.g. poliomyelitis) circulate almost exclusively in the summer months and influenza likewise circulates during the winter months.
- Timing is important when collecting specimens for viral detection. They should be collected as early as possible after the onset of symptoms as once viral shedding ceases, culture will be impossible and serological and molecular techniques may be the only way of diagnosing the viral pathogen.
- Some viruses cannot be cultured—e.g. viral agents of diarrhoea (caliciviruses, astroviruses and coronaviruses), hepatitis (HCV, HBV).

(a)

(b)

Fig. 5.4 Diagnosing viral infections using cell culture: (a) enterovirus cytopathogenic effect from a sample of stool in monkey kidney tissue culture, and (b) normal monkey kidney tissue culture. From Grist NR et al. (1987) *Diseases of Infection—an Illustrated Textbook*, Oxford University Press, Oxford.

Cell culture techniques enable detection of a wide range of viral pathogens and can allow for dual or mixed viral infections to be diagnosed. Once specimens arrive at the laboratory, they are processed and inoculated into a variety of cell cultures that support the growth of common viral isolates. The inoculated cell cultures are then examined daily for the development of a viral cytopathic effect. Viruses vary in their cell culture requirements, and laboratories must use more than one cell line for culture. For example, the respiratory viral pathogens, influenza and parainfluenza viruses favour replication in primary cell lines such as primary Rhesus monkey kidney (RhMK) cells. However, respiratory syncytial virus (RSV) and adenoviruses prefer heteroploid cell lines such as human epidermoid larynx carcinoma (Hep-2) cells.

Among the newer viral culture techniques are shell vial spin amplification cultures. These offer a more rapid turnaround time than traditional viral cultures for detection of the more common respiratory viruses and some other agents. Rather than having to examine for a cytopathic effect, fluorescein-labelled monoclonal antibodies are employed to detect antigens of replicating viruses. This system can be utilised for detecting CMV, HSV, influenza A and B, parainfluenza 1, 2 and 3, adenovirus and RSV, and can detect, for example, HSV in as little as 1 or 2 days.

Laboratory assays for antiviral susceptibility testing include phenotypic and genotypic assays. Phenotypic assays require growth of the virus *in vitro*, and are useful for HSV and CMV for aciclovir and ganciclovir, respectively. These assays cannot be used in the viruses for which *in vitro* culture systems are not available such as HBV. In these circumstances genotypic assays (□*Molecular diagnostics*, p350) may be available and useful.

Fungi

Unlike bacterial and viral diseases, direct microscopy can often be used to diagnose fungal infections (based on distinctive morphological characteristics of the invading fungi (e.g. tinea) and/or the judicious use of special stains such as methylene blue). However, histopathological diagnoses should be confirmed by culture wherever possible. Conversely, although diagnoses are usually made by isolating the causative fungus from bodily samples, the presence of a fungus in a culture from a non-sterile site does not mean that it is pathological (e.g. *Candida* isolation from sputum). Fungal infection can only be definitively established with evidence of tissue invasion. There are also a range of serological tests available for systemic mycoses (□*Serology*, p340), but few provide definitive diagnoses by themselves. A recent innovation which is proving useful is galacotomannon. This is an antigen released in blood by invasive aspergillosis, and when taken serially it can be used for both diagnosis and treatment response.

Fungal culture techniques are similar to the bacterial scenario. They are most useful for detecting the dimorphic fungi, which manifest both mycelial and yeast forms. This group includes *Candida* spp., *Cryptococcus neoformans*, *Blastomyces dermatidis*, *Histoplasma capsulatum* and *Coccidioides immitis*.

Protozoa

Protozoa of the genera *Acanthamoeba* and *Naegleria* may cause fatal CNS disease. *Acanthamoeba* spp. are free-living amoebae associated with keratitis; they may also cause a granulomatous encephalitis. Another free-living amoeba, *Naegleria fowleri*, is able to cause an acute fulminant meningoencephalitis, and is usually associated with a history of swimming in freshwater lakes or brackish water. In suspected cases, CSF and other suspicious clinical material may be cultured on a non-nutrient agar plate seeded with a 'lawn' of a Gram-negative bacteria (such as *E. coli*). Pathogenic amoebae can be identified microscopically.

Worldwide the most important protozoan infection is malaria. This can be cultured but this is rarely of use clinically. The mainstay of malarial identification is direct microscopy.

Serology

Immunological methods are in wide usage to detect pathogens present in clinical samples. Serology refers to the laboratory usage of antigen–antibody reactions for such diagnostic purposes. Diagnosis is made by detecting antibody or antigen in blood and/or other bodily fluids, or by the identification of pathogens in culture.

Both *direct* and *indirect* serological tests exist

Indirect serological techniques employ antigen–antibody reactions to detect specific antibodies manufactured in response to an antigen or antigens on an infecting pathogen's surface. These antibodies are found circulating in the patient's blood or present in other body fluids.

Direct serological techniques employ antibodies to detect specific antigens. Because this technique can be used to identify and type cultured organisms (☐*Culture techniques*, p335), it not only has individual clinical value but also has important epidemiological applications.

Hepatitis B (HBV) is a good example of an infection where both antigen and antibody profiles are diagnostically, therapeutically, prognostically and epidemiologically important:

- Antibody detection of specific antibody, e.g. antihepatitis Be antigen (anti-Hbe antibody), anti-Hepatitis B surface antigen (anti-Hbs antibody).
- Antigen detection, e.g. hepatitis B 'e' antigen (HbeAg), hepatitis B surface antigen (HBsAg).

HBsAg (hepatitis B surface antigen)
Tests:
1) HBsAg can be measured in plasma
2) Generates anti-HBs antibodies, which can be measured in plasma (useful in assessing response to vaccination)

(a)

HBcAg (hepatitis B core antigen, Dane particle)
Contains viral DNA.
HBeAg (e antigen) arises out of HBcAg
Tests:
1) HBeAg can be measured in plasma
2) Generates anti-HBc antibodies and anti-Hbe antibodies
3) Plasma hepatitis B DNA levels

(b)

Hepatitis D (HDV, delta agent)
Can only infect when patient is HBV-infected
Tests:
1) Antibodies to delta agent (anti-HDV)
2) Delta antigen

(c)

Fig. 5.5

Antibody tests

A wide variety of methodologies for assessing antibody response are available, such as immunofluorescence, agglutination, ELISA and complement fixation. This is complex and beyond the range of this book.

⍆ www.eawag.ch/publications_e/proceedings/oecd/proceedings/Torrance.pdf

Sub-classification of organisms, through serogrouping, is very valuable epidemiologically, e.g. while investigating an outbreak of meningococcal (*Neisseria meningitides*) disease; if the culprit is determined to be type C, vaccination can be utilised to control the outbreak.

In the 'direct fluorescent antibody' (DFA) technique, a fluorescent monoclonal antibody is used to react with an antigen specific for a given organism (e.g. herpes simplex virus) and a positive result will be detected microscopically. If the fluorescent antibody does not react with the antigen, the antibodies will be washed off the slide and the antigen will not fluoresce.

General principles

1. ↑ specific IgM levels indicates a 'new' infection.
2. ↑ specific IgG levels indicates a 'new' or a 'previous' infection, or, in some cases, immunity generated by vaccination.
3. Increasing IgG ('rising titre') when two samples ('paired sera') are taken with an appropriate intervening interval between them indicates a 'new' infection or re-infection. Diagnosis (as indicated by seroconversion)

necessitates a diagnostic antibody titre or a four-fold increase in antibody titre.

4. *Seroconversion* is said to have occurred in situations 1 and 3.

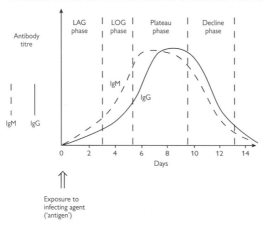

Fig. 5.6 Relative rate of appearance and disappearance of IgM and IgG.

Viral antibody tests

These can be very useful because, once viral shedding has ceased, viral culture is of no further value. They include tests for HIV-1, HIV-2, HTLV-1, HTLV-2, hepatitis A, hepatitis B, hepatitis C, delta agent (hepatitis D), hepatitis E, EBV, CMV, dengue, Ebola fever, Lassa fever, RSV, mumps, measles, rubella, influenza, parainfluenza, St Louis encephalitis, West Nile virus, yellow fever, SARS and many more.

🔗 http://www.mic.ki.se/Diseases

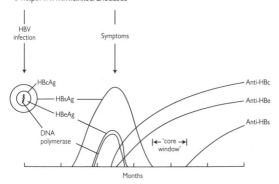

Fig. 5.7 Hepatitis B antigens and antibodies.

Bacterial antibody tests

These include ASO (for streptococcal infection), anti-DNAse B (for streptococcal infection) and anti-staphylococcal (for *Staphylococcus aureus infections*) tests.

Can also test for: cat scratch fever (*Bartonella henselae*), *Bordetella pertussis*, Lyme disease (*Borrelia burgdorferii*), *Brucella abortus*, *Burkholderia pseudomallei* (melioidosis), *Campylobacter jejuni*, *Chlamydia* spp., Q fever (*Coxiella burnetti*), *E. coli 0157*, *Francisella tularensis*, *Helicobacter pylori*, *Legionella pneumophila*, *Leptospira interrogans*, *Listeria monocytogenes*, *Mycoplasma pneumoniae*, *Neisseria meningitidis*, *Neisseria gonorrhoeae*, *Rickettsia prowazekii*, *Salmonella* spp., *Treponema pallidum* (including TPHA, VDRL, FTA-ABS, IgM-FTA, IgM-ELISA), *Yersinia enterocolitica/ Y. pseudotuberculosis*, (Widal test).

⌖http://www.mic.ki.se/Diseases

Protozoal antibody tests

Include tests for malaria (*Plasmodium* spp.), amoebiasis, toxoplasmosis, leishmaniasis (kala azar), African trypanosomiasis (sleeping sickness), American trypanosomiasis (Chagas' disease), babesiosis, *Toxoplasma gondii*.

⌖http://www.mic.ki.se/Diseases

Helminthic antibody tests

Include tests for *Echinococcus granulosus* (hydatid disease), *Echinococcus multilocularis* (alveolar echinococcosis), *Microsporidium* spp., *Pneumocystis jiroveci* (formerly *Pneumocystis carinii*), schistosomiasis (bilharzia), strongyloidiasis, filariasis, onchocerciasis, *Trichinella spiralis*, *Toxocara* canis, *Taenia solium* (cysticercosis, or pork tapeworm), paragonimiasis (Chinese lung fluke), gnathostomiasis.

⌖http://www.mic.ki.se/Diseases

Fungal antibody tests

Include tests for *Aspergillus fumigatus*, *Aspergillus niger*, *Aspergillus nidulans*, *Aspergillus versicolor*, *Blastomyces dermatitidis*, *Candida albicans*, *Coccidioides immitis*, *Cryptococcus neoformans*, *Histoplasma capsulatum*, *Mukorazeen*.

⌖http://www.clinical-mycology.com/

Note: in the case of complement fixation (CF) antibody assays for antibodies to coccidiomycosis, these are specific and do not require proof of rising levels. They can provide indispensable confirmatory evidence for a diagnosis of coccidiomycosis as well as an indication of the relative risk of extrapulmonary dissemination. In a case of chronic meningitis, a positive CF for anti-coccidioidal antibodies in the CSF often provides the only definite diagnostic indication of the need for aggressive antifungal therapy.

Antigen tests

Antigen measurement is achieved through techniques such as complement fixation and immunodiffusion. A variety of bodily fluids can yield diagnostically-useful antigens, including serum, urine, CSF and fresh stool—the choice depends upon the clinical context.

Viral antigen tests

Include mumps, cytomegalovirus, influenza, HIV, hepatitis B, respiratory syncytial virus, parainfluenza viruses, adenovirus, rota virus and varicella-zoster virus.

Bacterial antigen tests

Include *Legionella pneumophila* (serotype 1) and *Borrelia burgdorferii* (in urine), β-haemolytic streptococci, pneumococcus, *Clostridium difficile*, *Haemophilus influenzae*, *Neisseria meningitidis*, *Helicobacter pylori*, *Campylobacter jejuni*.

Helminthic antigen tests

Filariasis.
⬦http://www.who.int/mediacentre/facs102/en/

Protozoal antigen tests

Include giardiasis, *Trypanosoma cruzi* (Chagas' disease).

Fungal antigen tests

Include *Cryptococcus neoformans*, *Histoplasma capsulatum*, mannoprotein antigen in *Candida albicans*.[1]
⬦http://www.clinical-mycology.com/

1 Sendid B et al. (1999) New enzyme immunoassays for sensitive detection of circulating *Candida albicans* mannan and antimannan antibodies: useful combined test for diagnosis of systemic candidiasis. *J Clin Microbiol* **37**, 1510–1517.

Collection of specimens

Principles of good specimen collection

- Good-quality specimen and clinical information produce the most valuable data.
- Optimal time of collection: e.g. take bacterial specimens before administering antibiotics.
- Collect the optimal type of specimen wherever possible: e.g. pus is preferable to a 'pus swab'.
- Acquire expertise in specimen collection: ensure minimal contamination by normal flora (e.g. mid-stream specimen of urine (MSU), use of a tongue depressor for throat swab collection).
- Freshness of specimens: rapid transport to the laboratory is essential (especially for anaerobic organisms, and for 'hot stools' for parasite diagnosis).
- Collect the appropriate number of specimens at the appropriate intervals: e.g. paired antisera should be taken at least 1–6 weeks apart if a diagnostic rising titre is to be demonstrated.
- Be aware of biological hazards: category 3 organisms (e.g. tuberculosis, *Burkholderia pseudomallei*, hepatitis C, HIV) and category 4 organisms (e.g. viral haemorrhagic fever, possible bioterrorism cases such as smallpox).

Surface specimens include

Anal/anorectal: e.g. gonococcus (*Neisseria gonorrhoeae*).

Cervical swab: e.g. HSV, gonococcus, HPV.

Ear swab: e.g. otitis externa, otitis media, bacterial and fungal infections.

Foreign bodies: almost always infected if causing trouble! (includes iatrogenic foreign bodies, such as arthroplasties, cardiac valves, pacemakers, ventriculo-peritoneal shunts, etc.). Foreign bodies in the ear, nose or vagina can lead to prolonged (and often unpleasant) discharges.

Genital ulcers: dark ground microscopy for syphilis organisms. Also chancroid, *Entamoeba histolytica*.

Indwelling catheters: include urinary catheters, IV cannulae, Portacaths, etc. If a catheter is thought to be the source of an infection, cultures should performed, and if the catheter or cannula is removed, this should be sent for culture. Urinary catheters are always colonised by bacteria. Intravascular foreign bodies such as central venous catheters and prosthetic heart valves are often colonised by bacteria which are normally non-virulent such as coagulase –ve staphylococci.

Laryngeal swab: can be useful for tuberculosis.

Nasal, pharyngeal, gingival and throat: e.g. meningococcus, *Staphylococcus aureus* carriage, streptococcal infections, pertussis, adenovirus. Nasopharyngeal aspirates are useful diagnosing for influenza and RSV through direct immunofluorescence (DIF) tests and culture. In lepromatous leprosy, a swab from the anterior nares may reveal acid-fast bacilli indicative of this infection.

Ophthalmic: e.g. bacterial conjunctivitis, adenovirus, rabies (from corneal impressions.[1] For trachoma, direct fluorescein-labelled monoclonal antibody (DFa) and enzyme immunoassay (eia) of conjunctival smears is useful.

⇱http://www.emedicine.com/OPH/topic118.htm

Skin: • abscess—culture for bacteria and other, unusual, organisms; • dermal scrapings, nail clippings: fungal infections (tinea—includes pedis, capitis, cruris, versicolor forms); • petechial rash scrapings: meningococcus (occasionally gonococcus).

Throat: e.g. *Candida albicans*, diphtheria, gonococcus, croup organisms.

Urethral: e.g. *Chlamydia*, gonococcus.

Vagina (high vaginal swab): e.g. *Staphylococcus aureus* in toxic shock syndrome (including toxin testing), *Gardnerella*, gonococcus.

Normally sterile fluids include

Amniotic fluid: bacterial infection can cause premature delivery, and rDNA was detected by PCR (☐*Molecular diagnostics*, p350) in samples from 15 (94%) of 16 patients with positive amniotic fluid cultures.[2] Hydrops fetalis can be caused by congenital infections (e.g. CMV, parvovirus B19, toxoplasmosis, syphilis and Chagas' disease), and making a diagnosis may involve analysis of amniotic fluid with cultures, PCR, etc.

Ascites: consider TB (consider laparoscopy for biopsying peritoneal lesions for culture as well as histology, ☐*Gastrointestinal tract investigations*, p356).

Blood: multiple samplings at separate times from separate body sites may need to be taken, e.g. in endocarditis. For some organisms and pathologies, an extended period of culture may be needed.

Cerebrospinal fluid (CSF): possibilities include e.g. meningococcus, pneumococcus, *Listeria monocytogenes*, TB, fungi (e.g. *Cryptococcus neoformans*), viruses (☐*Tissue biopsy & deep aspiration specimens*, p360).

Ejaculate (semen): if the semen contains a high number of leucocytes, this may be an indication of either infection or inflammation. WBCs are considered significant if >1 million found in each mL of ejaculate. STDs, e.g. gonorrhoea or *Ureaplasma*, and prostate infections come into the differential diagnosis. *Schistosoma haematobium* (bilharzia) may cause haemospermia, and be found in ejaculate.[3] Acute mumps orchitis can be associated with loss of spermatozoa.

Ocular fluids (intra-): include aqueous humor, vitreous humor. Bacterial, fungal and parasitic problems can affect the interior of the eye.

Pericardial fluid: the most common organisms will include staphylococci, streptococci, pneumococci, *Haemophilus influenzae*, meningococci and tuberculosis.

Pleural fluid: numerous pathologies, including underlying bacterial pneumonia, tuberculous pleurisy, parasitic infections (such as strongyloidiasis) and fungal diseases (such as histoplasmosis).

Synovial fluid (joint aspirate): bacterial infections can be very destructive and the options are legion. TB must always be borne in mind. Viral arthritides are usually self-limiting and treatment is supportive.

Urine: standard culture and sensitivity, e.g. midstream specimen (MSU), catheter specimen (CSU)—useful for diagnosing cystitis, pyelonephritis, prostatitis, etc. (prostatic massage may be helpful for improving diagnosis of prostatic infections); EMU ('early morning urines') for tuberculosis and a terminal specimen for *Schistosoma haematobium* (bilharzia) best collected around midday.

Normally infected fluids include

Pus: e.g. abscess contents, wound swab/aspirates, drainage swabs. Usually bacterial (consider both aerobic and anaerobic), but amoebic and hydatid options need to be considered when the lesion is in the liver.

Saliva: normally contains a wide range of commensal flora. Cannulation of a parotid gland duct may yield a specific pathogen that is causing a problem in that gland.

Sputum: includes tracheal aspirate, induced sputum (obtained with physiotherapy assistance) and bronchoalveolar lavage (BAL), which may be needed in sicker patients unable to produce sputum or in conditions where copious sputum production may not be a feature (such as *Pneumocystis carinii* pneumonia in HIV infection). Culture and sensitivity assists with identifying a vast range of organisms, including and especially tuberculosis (always ally sputum culture to direct microscopy).

Stool: vast range of uses (📖*Gastrointestinal tract investigations*, p356). Includes direct microscopy for parasites, ova and cysts, i.e. giardia and Ascariasis, culture for *Salmonella*, *Campylobacter*, *Shigella*, *E. coli* 0157, typhoid and paratyphoid, *Plesiomonas shigelloides*, enteroviruses and antigen detection of rotavirus. 'Hot stools' (from patient to the microbiology bench in less than 1h) may be helpful for amoebae, strongyloides larvae, etc.

1 Zaidman GW, Billingsley A. (1998) Corneal impression test for the diagnosis of acute rabies encephalitis. *Ophthalmology* **105**, 249–251; **2** Hitti J et al. (1997) Broad-spectrum bacterial rDNA polymerase chain reaction assay for detecting amniotic fluid infection among women in premature labor. *CID* **24**, 1228; **3** Torresi J, Yung A. (1997) Usefulness of semen microscopy in the diagnosis of a difficult case of Schistosoma haematobium infection in a returned traveler. *J Travel Med* **4**, 46–47.

Molecular diagnostics

These tests are expensive and are often only available in larger or specialist laboratories, but their potential power is considerable. While a full understanding of these complex technologies can present some conceptual difficulties to the average clinician, they are destined to become an increasingly important part of mainstream clinical practice. HIV viral load and anti-retroviral drug resistance are considered mainstream tests, while examination of the CSF for JC virus DNA by PCR is the method of choice for the diagnosis of progressive multifocal leucoencephalopathy.

The areas of greatest value include

- Detection and quantification of viruses to monitor therapy, e.g. HCV, HIV, HBV, CMV.
- Detection of slow-growing organisms, e.g. TB, atypical mycobacteria.
- Diagnosis of pathogens which are potentially too dangerous for the laboratory staff to handle, e.g. viral haemorrhagic fever, smallpox.
- Detection of organisms killed by antibiotics prior to culture samples being taken, e.g. meningococcal sepsis.
- Detection of organisms that cannot be cultured, e.g. hepatitis C virus (HCV).
- Detection of unusual diseases, e.g. helminthic diseases, fungi.
- Detection of toxins elaborated in small quantities by bacteria, e.g. toxic shock syndrome toxins.
- To quantify the level of an infection (e.g. viral load in HIV disease).
- Detection of mutations manifesting resistance to antimicrobial agents (genotypic resistance testing), e.g. HIV, CMV, TB.
- Elucidation of pathogens that are as yet 'undiscovered'.

Available molecular techniques include

PCR (polymerase chain reaction): this test uses probes to look for the presence of the genes of infecting organisms (📖*PCR*, p280).

There are numerous PCR tests available, and it is particularly valuable for hepatitis C (including for genotyping), HIV and TB. A universal eubacterial PCR (for genus and species identification of prokaryotes) and universal fungal PCR (genus and species identification of fungi) are available. HBV DNA quantification is accomplished through PCR.

Choosing the appropriate sample for the application of PCR testing is important (e.g. biopsy of possible Kaposi's sarcoma lesion and KSHV (HHV-8); BAL fluid and PCP; small bowel biopsy and Whipple's disease; CSF and meningococcal disease, herpes simplex virus or *Mycobacterium tuberculosis*). Note: fluid samples for PCR usually have a higher yield when not spun in a centrifuge.

LCR (ligase chain reaction): works through specific probe amplification through the use of DNA-ligase. Greatest value in *Chlamydia* infection.

TMA (transcription-mediated amplification): uses an isothermal amplification system. Amplified telomerase products are rna, detected using a non-isotopic hybridisation protection (HPA) system. Identification of HCV, tuberculosis, gonococcus and *Chlamydia* are among its potential uses.

Branched chain DNA (bDNA): a signal amplification methodology able to quantify HIV RNA levels.

NASBA (nucleic acid sequence-based amplification): a quantitative test for HIV RNA, also of value with CMV.

Hybridisation with nucleic acid probes: detects specific ribosomal RNA, and is most widely used for culture confirmation of an organism (e.g. fungi, mycobacteria).

Sequencing: organisms are identified by direct sequencing of amplified gene fragments. Has been applied to tuberculosis, *H. pylori*, enteroviruses and HIV (for assessing drug resistance).

Restriction fragment length polymorphisms (RFLP): restriction enzymes are used to cut up DNA into pieces, and the fragments are then subjected to gel electrophoresis (such as Southern blotting, 📖*Southern blotting*, p278). The patterns produced can be used to identify organisms.

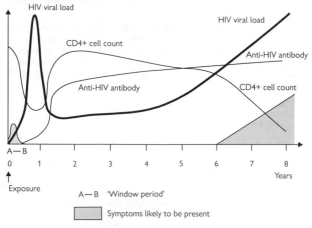

Fig. 5.8 The immunological profile of HIV disease.

Shanson DC. (1999) *Microbiology and Clinical Practice*, 3rd edition, Butterworth-Heinemann, Oxford.

Haematology

Many infectious diseases manifest haematological changes that are diagnostically valuable.

Blood film: the blood smear examination provides general data on the size and appearance of cells as well as data on particular cell segments, while pathogens may be seen, e.g. malaria, African trypanosomiasis, Chagas' disease, babesiosis, borreliosis, bartonellosis, ehrlichiosis, filaria (time of day the blood is taken may be significant in this condition), haemolysis and evidence of hyposplenism. Thick and thin blood films should be considered, especially where malaria is concerned; at least 3 blood films each taken 24h apart should be performed. Blood films are also useful in assessing if a patient has DIC—*below*.

Bone marrow examination: culture (for e.g. TB, brucellosis, *Mycobacterium avium intracellulare*, typhoid/paratyphoid, CMV), microscopy (for e.g. leishmaniasis), and establishing cell line integrity (e.g. WBC abnormalities). An aspirate is generally useful for culture purposes and for establishing what cells are present in the marrow, but a trephine is needed if structural information is needed (e.g. to establish if granulomata suggestive of tuberculosis are present).

Coagulation studies, fibrin degradation products, D-dimers: useful where DIC is suspected. DIC is a common association of severe sepsis (especially meningococcal disease). Coagulation abnormalities are also present in conditions such as viral haemorrhagic fevers, *Plasmodium falciparum* malaria, rickettsial diseases, etc. D-dimers may assist with the diagnosis of deep venous thrombosis, although this is not universally accepted.

Cold agglutinins: a haemagglutination-based test. Can be caused by *Mycoplasma pneumoniae* (most commonly), influenza A, influenza B, parainfluenza and adenoviruses.

Differential white cell count in peripheral blood: useful associations include (1) eosinophilia and parasitoses, (2) neutrophilia and bacterial sepsis, (3) neutropenia and atypical pneumonias, (4) atypical lymphocytes and Epstein–Barr virus (EBV), (5) neutropenia and pyrexia.

ESR—together with the CRP (□*Biochemical tests*, p358), the rate of erythrocyte sedimentation is sensitive to the extent of a body's response to a lesion or disease. The ESR is important for pointing to the possible existence of an organic disease, but a normal result does not exclude the presence of disease. An ↑ ESR points to the need for additional investigations and, if ↓, is very useful in monitoring the course of a disease. Procalcitonin (PCT) may eventually prove to have even greater value in a similar role.
⌖http://www.pubmedcentral.nih.gov/articlerender.fcgi?artid=29013)

Ferritin levels: ↓ in iron deficiency, e.g. associated with hookworm infestation of the bowel (*Ancyclostoma duodenale*, *Necator americanus*) or *Helicobacter pylori*-associated gastritis. Ferritin levels are often extremely high in Still's disease, an important non-infective cause of pyrexia and neutrophilia. Serum iron and TIBC may be helpful in a fuller evaluation (Biochemical tests, p358).

Glucose 6-phosphate dehydrogenase: useful in therapy of benign malarias, e.g. *Plasmodium vivax* and *P. ovale* (a deficiency will cause therapeutic problems with primaquine usage to kill the hypnozoite phase and prevent relapse).

Hb concentration and red cell parameters (especially MCV): useful in e.g. anaemia of chronic infection, haemolysis, iron deficiency (microcytosis) associated with hookworm infestation of the bowel or *H. pylori*-associated gastritis, macrocytosis due to vitamin B_{12} deficiency with Diphyllobothrium *latum* (fish tapeworm) infestation.

Hb electrophoresis: can detect haematological conditions such as thalassaemia, sickle cell disease (see *below*), etc.

Haemolysis screen (including reticulocyte count): may be abnormal in e.g. DIC, EBV, viral haemorrhagic fever, *E. coli* 0157 gastroenteritis due to haemolytic uraemic syndrome, rickettsial infections, dengue, gas gangrene. Haptoglobin levels can be useful (Biochemical tests, p358) since they are generally ↓/absent in haemolysis.

Monospot test (Paul Bunnell test): diagnostic of EBV infection.

Sickling test: uncovers sickle cell disease, known to be associated with *Salmonella* osteomyelitis, chronic leg ulcers, etc.

Thrombocytopenia: characteristic in some conditions, e.g. HIV disease, *Plasmodium falciparum* malaria and dengue.

Vitamin B_{12} levels: ↓ in *Diphyllobothrium latum* infestation, tuberculosis of the terminal ileum, etc.

Radiology

Plain x-rays
- *Chest*: the potential diagnoses are legion, including pneumonia, TB, pleural effusion/empyema, bronchiectasis, *Pneumocystis carinii* pneumonia (PCP), tropical eosinophilia and other parasite-related diseases (e.g. paragonimiasis), occupational risks for infections (e.g. silicosis and TB), post-varicella calcification.
- *Plain abdominal x-ray*: e.g. bowel dilatation, perforation, calcification of adrenal glands and lymph nodes (e.g. TB, histoplasmosis), 'babies head' sign of schistosomal bladder calcification.
- *Dental radiography (orthopantomogram)*: occult dental sepsis.
- *Elsewhere*: e.g. limbs for osteomyelitis, skeletal muscles for calcified cysticercosis lesions, joints for Charcot changes (such as in syphilis).

More sophisticated imaging

ERCP: using contrast medium and radiographs to define the anatomy of the biliary tree and pancreatic duct. Useful for HIV-associated biliary tree disease (including porta hepatis nodal lymphoma), parasites (e.g. *Clonorchis sinensis*, *Ascaris lumbricoides*) and pancreatic disease such as tuberculosis.

IVP (IVU): defines renal anatomy. Renal infection such as pyelonephritis, renal calculi, malignancy or anatomical abnormalities (including congenital) leading to recurrent infections. CT-IVP is generally considered superior now (see *below*).

MRI, including with contrast enhancement
- *Cranial*: variant CJD or vCJD (exhibits bilateral pulvinar high signal), encephalitis, rabies, sagittal sinus thrombosis. MRI is also more sensitive than CT when looking for infective space occupying lesions such as tuberculoma, especially in and around the cerebellum.
- *Elsewhere in the body*: defining solid lesions, fluid-filled lesions, etc.
- *MRCP* (MRI used with ERCP): further defines the hepatopancreatic-biliary tree anatomy.
- New techniques such as cardiac MRI imaging show great promise in the diagnosis of valvular disease.

Computed tomography (CT), including with contrast enhancement
- *Cranial*: e.g. brain abscess, paranasal sinus disease, middle ear disease, orbital sepsis, cysticercosis, mastoid air cells.
- *Chest*: e.g. cardiac lesions (possibly with associated endocarditis risk), mediastinum (e.g. lymphadenopathy, including retrosternal), lung lesions such as bronchiectasis, lung abscess, other non-infectious pathologies.
- *Abdomen*: delineates intra-abdominal abscesses and abnormalities in retroperitoneal and mesenteric lymph nodes, defects in the spleen, liver, kidneys, adrenals, pancreas and pelvis.
- *CT-IVP* (CT-IV pyelography): powerful tool for defining the anatomy of the urinary tract.

- *Spiral CT scan*: e.g. for defining pulmonary emboli as a cause of PUO.
- New techniques such as 'virtual colonoscopy' and cardiac CT scanning are in advanced stages of development. May have value in diagnosing colonic and cardiac disease (including valvular disease) respectively.

Ultrasound
- Abdomen: evidence of pancreatic, liver, renal and biliary tree/ gallbladder abnormalities (e.g. abscess, hepatic cyst, presence or absence of spleen, ascites, gallstones, etc.).
- *Thoracic*: pleural effusion, empyema (can assist with drainage).
- *Echocardiography*: to help exclude the cardiac vegetations of endocarditis, TB pericarditis (with effusion), myocarditis. *Note*: both transthoracic and transoesophageal (TOE) approaches are available, each yielding data of differing value in different situations.
- *Doppler* studies of blood vessels: to exclude deep vein thrombosis (DVT), such as in the legs.
- *Biopsy*: to specifically pick out an area for sampling, e.g. liver lesion, lymph node, mediastinal mass.
- *Drainage*: to specifically pick out an area for draining, e.g. liver abscess, pleural effusion.

Radionuclide scanning
- *Indium (^{111}In)-labelled granulocyte scan*: helps localise many infectious or inflammatory processes (i.e. deep sepsis). This test is particularly valuable in PUO investigation.
- ^{99m}*Technetium bone scan*: bone and joint sepsis.
- *V/Q scan*: to exclude pulmonary embolus as cause of PUO, to delineate consolidation, abscess, bronchiectasis, etc.

PET (positron emission tomography)
- Has enormous potential for locating localised infective processes, especially in the brain. Limited availability at time of writing.

📖These techniques are all described in detail in *Radiology*.

Gastrointestinal tract investigations

Biopsy-based

Duodenal biopsy (Crosby capsule and endoscopic methods, ± electron microscopy): e.g. Whipple's disease, giardiasis, cryptosporidium, strongyloidiasis.

Gastric biopsy: H. pylori.

Laparoscopy: useful to exclude TB and other infections in the presence of ascites (biopsies should be sent for histology, culture and sensitivity).

Liver biopsy: 🕮 *Tissue biopsy and deep aspiration specimens*, p360.

Oesophageal biopsy: e.g. candidiasis, cytomegalovirus (e.g. in advanced HIV disease).

Sigmoidoscopy and bowel biopsy: e.g. amoebiasis, pseudomembranous colitis (*Clostridium difficile infections*), exclusion of idiopathic colitis and Crohn's disease.

GI contents-based

Baermann concentration technique: the method of choice for the detection of *Strongyloides stercoralis*.

Capsule endoscopy: involving the swallowing of a pill-sized capsule containing digital video recording equipment which broadcasts to a receiver outside of the body. Enormous potential for diagnosing pathology within the gastrointestinal tract, including small bowel infective processes such as tuberculosis (see ⏀http://www.nzma.org.nz/journal/116-1183/633/).

Duodenal aspirate: e.g. giardiasis, cryptosporidium, strongyloidiasis.

Enterotest (string test): e.g. giardiasis, cryptosporidium, strongyloidiasis.

Hot stools: 🕮 *Culture techniques*, p335.

Salivary amylase: mumps.

Stool culture and sensitivity: 🕮 *Culture techniques*, p335.

Stool microscopy: for ova, cysts, parasites (e.g. amoebae, helminths such as *Ascaris lumbricoides*).

Stool electron microscopy: good for viruses, e.g. rotavirus and norovirus.

Stool chromatography: *Clostridium difficile* toxin, though microscopy of cell cultures in the presence and absence of a specific *Clostridium difficile* antibody is used more commonly.

Sellotape® (adhesive) strip test: for the threadworm, *Enterobius verminformis*. To perform this test, roll some clear adhesive tape around 4 fingers of a hand, sticky side out, while an assistant spreads the buttocks. In good lighting, identify the involved perianal area, and apply the tape 1–2 times to the affected perianal area. Place the tape on a slide with the clean side downwards, trim the tape, label the slide and send to the laboratory.

Toxin tests the definite diagnosis of botulism food poisoning is the examination of faeces for *Clostridium botulinus* and toxin (EMG is also helpful). In wound botulism (common in drug injectors), the organism may grow in material taken directly from the wound(s): also useful with *Clostridium difficile, E. coli* 0157.

GI tract function

D-xylose absorption test for malabsorption syndromes, such as Whipple's disease and tropical sprue.

^{13}C breath test for detection of H. pylori:
⌐ᗺhttp://www.infai.de/scripten/iquery.cgi?res=ae1

Immunology

Cutaneous hypersensitivity tests are discussed elsewhere (&Other tests, p364).

Complement (especially 'terminal' complements C5 to C9): deficiencies can lead to recurrent meningococcal sepsis, pneumococcal disease, etc.

Cytokine studies: currently experimental.

Differential white cell count (&Haematology, p352): neutropenia is associated with bacterial sepsis.

Immune globulins: deficiencies lead to recurrent infections (some cases may be hereditary, and family history is important). Levels may also be higher—IgM tends to be ↑ in brucellosis, malaria, trypanosomiasis and toxoplasmosis.

Splenic dysfunction: indicated by a history of surgical removal (not always clear!) or a condition associated with hyposplenism (e.g. coeliac disease/ dermatitis herpetiformis), an abnormal blood film, and absent spleen on abdominal imaging. This state may be associated with recurrent meningo-coccal infection and life-threatening pneumococcal sepsis. Once diag-nosed, the patient will need appropriate vaccinations and advised to always carry a warning card and/or wear a MedicAlert® bracelet or similar.

T cell subsets: the absolute CD4+ (T4) cell count and the CD4+/CD8+ (T4/T8) cell ratio is of value. HIV disease, tuberculosis and sarcoidosis are associated with reduced CD4+ cell levels, HIV with a reversed CD4+/CD8+ cell ratio.

Biochemical tests

A number of biochemical tests are useful in the diagnosis and assessment of a range of infectious illnesses.

α-fetoprotein (AFP): ↑ in hepatocellular carcinoma (associated with HCV and HBV). Note: much higher AFP than in other causes of hepatocellular damage.

Arterial blood gases: assessment of sepsis, assessment of pneumonia.

CA-125: ↑ in peritoneal tuberculosis.

C-reactive protein (CRP): together with the ESR, a valuable method for monitoring infections. CRP is an acute phase reactant, ↑ in bacterial infections and ↓ in viral infections. PCT (procalcitonin) may be of value.

Creatinine phosphokinase (CPK) level: ↑ in Legionella pneumophila infec-tion[1]. Also ↑ with zidovudine (AZT) usage in HIV disease.

Glucose metabolism: diabetes mellitus is a common association of infec-tion, particularly TB. Consider performing a fasting glucose level, an oral glucose tolerance test (OGTT) or checking haemoglobin A_{1c} levels.

Haptoglobin levels part of haemolysis screen (📖*Haematology*, p352). Iron levels (serum iron), total iron binding capacity (TIBC): iron ↓ (TIBC↑) in iron deficiency, e.g. associated with hookworm infestation of the bowel (*Ancyclostoma duodenale*, *Necator americanus*) or *H. pylori*-associated gastritis. Serum ferritin may be helpful.

Lactate levels may be ↑ in HIV-associated mitochondrial toxicity syndrome. Also high in severe sepsis syndrome.

Lipid abnormalities (cholesterol, triglycerides): HIV drug toxicity.

Liver function tests abnormalities are present in many conditions, e.g. hepatitis, leptospirosis, yellow fever, antimicrobial drug toxicity (e.g. in TB).

- *Alkaline phosphatase (AP)*: in the serum of healthy adults, AP mostly originates from the liver. Biliary obstruction, often associated with sepsis, leads to an ↑ in serum concentration of AP.
- *Bilirubin*: determination of the bilirubin levels (conjugated and unconjugated) is important in the differential diagnosis of jaundice.
- *γGT*: ↑ in serum concentration of γGT is most sensitive indicator of liver damage.

Pancreatic amylase level ↑ with pancreatitis in, e.g. mumps (consider also salivary amylase), toxicity with antiretroviral drugs (e.g. dideoxyinosine or DDI).

Pleural fluid analysis: analysis for LDH levels is useful (as well as albumin, total protein and amylase). An exudate, which implies infection in the differential diagnosis, is defined by at least one of the following criteria: pleural fluid/serum total protein ratio >0.5, pleural fluid/serum LDH ratio >0.6, or pleural fluid LDH >$^2/_3$ upper limits of normal of serum LDH.

Pregnancy test: some infections, e.g. varicella, genital herpes (simplex) and TB, are often more serious in pregnancy. The use of some antibiotics, e.g. ciprofloxacin and tetracyclines, is relatively contra-indicated in pregnancy. There is the potential to prevent vertical transmission of HIV if diagnosed prior to delivery.

Procalcitonin (PCT): shows considerable promise for detecting and following 'inflammation induced by microbial infections' (⏴http://www.pubmedcentral.nih.gov/articlerender.fcgi?artid=29013).
Serum Na^+ levels: hyponatraemia strongly associated with Legionnaire's disease[1].

Synacthen test: TB and histoplasmosis can damage the adrenal glands, leading to an Addisonian state.

Vitamin D levels: if deficient, may lead to difficulties with resolving TB infections (consider checking levels in patients with darkly pigmented skins, especially those with a culture of wearing clothing over most of their body surface).

1 Kociuba KR et al. (1994) Legionnaires' disease outbreak in south western Sydney, 1992. Clinical aspects. Med J Aust **160**, 274–277.

Tissue biopsy & deep aspiration specimens

Whatever part of the anatomy they are taken from, biopsy specimens should be evaluated both histopathologically (with specialised stains used wherever appropriate) and by culture for bacteria, mycobacteria, fungi, viruses and prions (using specialised culture techniques where appropriate).

Bone marrow biopsy: 🕮*Haematology*, p352. Important for TB, brucellosis, MAI, typhoid/paratyphoid, leishmaniasis.

Cerebrospinal fluid (CSF): while the main objective of a lumbar puncture is usually to obtain fluid for microscopy, culture and sensitivity, there are other useful tests that can be performed. The opening pressure should be between 10–20cm H_2O—infective and other processes may alter this. While the usual approach to obtaining CSF is through a lumbar puncture, if the pressure is high a cisternal puncture can be performed instead (normally the advice and help of a neurosurgeon would need to be sought). In neonates, foramenal puncture is a possibility.

Along with the Gram-staining process and microscopy, other tests to consider include a complete blood cell count and differential, measurement of glucose and protein levels, Ziehl–Neelsen staining for tuberculosis, and bacterial, mycobacterial, viral and fungal cultures. On occasions, other tests that might be considered include:

- Wet mount (for amoebae such as *Acathamoeba*; 🕮*Culture techniques*, p335).
- PCR for herpes simplex virus, herpes varicella-zoster, enteroviruses tuberculosis, JC virus, cryptococcosis (🕮*Molecular diagnostics*, p280, 350).
- Antibodies to specific pathogens (e.g. arboviruses; 🕮*Serology*, p340).
- India ink capsule stain (for cryptococcosis).
- Cryptococcal antigen (🕮*Serology*, p340).
- VDRL etc. for syphilis (🕮*Serology*, p340).
- 14-3-3 protein—specific protein marker present in CSF of patients with vCJD.
- Xanthochromia to help exclude subarachnoid haemorrhage.
- Bilirubin presence: seen in leptospirosis.
- Cytology to help exclude carcinomatous meningitis.
- Assessing comparative CSF protein-cellular levels if Guillain–Barré syndrome (recognised association of infections such as *Campylobacter* gastroenteritis) is being considered.

Liver biopsy

Indications are numerous and include assessment of viral hepatitis (especially HBV and HCV, including possible cirrhosis and/or hepatocellular carcinoma), assessment of PUO (including TB) and determining if a patient has a medication-induced liver disease. On <1% of occasions does the liver biopsy overestimate the amount of hepatic damage.

The biopsy is commonly preceded by an USS examination of the liver to determine the best and safest biopsy site. Sometimes the biopsy is conducted under ultrasonic guidance. Coagulation status should be optimal at the time of biopsying.

The risks of the traditional liver biopsy (not performed under ultrasound guidance) include

- Pain (1 in 5 patients).
- Haemorrhage (1 in 500 patients).
- Bleeding requiring transfusion or surgery (1 in 1000 patients).
- Pneumothorax and/or puncture of the gallbladder, kidney or bowel (1 in 1000 patients).
- Death (1 in 5000 patients).

⁀ᵂhttp://pages.prodigy.com/hepc/hepc6.htm.

Equivalent figures are not available for USS-guided liver biopsy, but the technique is well established. Liver biopsy material should be subjected to microbiological culture as well as to histological assessment.

Assessing hepatitis C
(HCV)

1. Counsel and test for antibodies to HCV.

2. If antibody-positive, test blood for HCV RNA (the 'hepatitis C PCR test')

3. If PCR-positive, organise liver ultrasound and biopsy, and check hepatic enzymes and coagulation profile. Histology looks at inflammation, focal necrosis, bridging necrosis and fibrosis, and the histological appearance is scored, e.g. Knodell score (X/22).

4. If score is high (e.g. Knodell score ≥6/22), consider treatment for HCV. Vaccinate against HBV & HAV.

5. If score is low (e.g. Knodell score <6/22), observe patient regularly, watch HCV RNA levels, re-biopsy liver at ~2–3 years. Vaccinate against HBV & HAV. Watch α-fetoprotein levels.

Fig. 5.9 Assessing hepatitis C.

Lymph node sampling

The likely pathologies depend upon whether or not the lymphadenopathy is regional or generalised, and upon the site.

Biopsy: for histology and culture, especially for TB, for tropical infections such as chancroid, and for other relevant infections such as the cat scratch fever (*Bartonella henselae*). If regional, the differential diagnosis varies with the site; if intra-abdominal, for example, TB, *Yersinia enterocolitica* and adenovirus should be considered.

Fine needle aspirate (FNA): useful as full biopsy for culture purposes, but no structural information available (similar to the aspirate *vs.* trephine issue in bone marrow sampling; ▢*Haematology*, p352).

Respiratory samples

Sputum tests

Microscopy: can perform direct microscopy (e.g. for *Aspergillus* spp., eggs of paragonimiasis), Gram stain, ZN, PCP (silver staining needed).

Induced sputum: e.g. for TB, PCP, *Aspergillus*.

Tracheal aspirate: used in ill individuals. May produce similar material.

Bronchoscopy

Bronchoalveolar lavage (BAL): useful for TB and other mycobacteria, PCP, fungi, melioidosis, resistant bacteria (e.g. *Pseudomonas*), RSV, paragonimiasis.

Lung biopsy: useful for TB and other mycobacteria, PCP (needs silver staining), IFT or PCR), fungi, melioidosis, resistant bacteria (e.g. *Pseudomonas*), RSV, paragonimiasis.

Open lung biopsy

When not feasible to obtain intrathoracic tissue by less invasive means.

Pleural disease: effusion, empyema, biopsy

Consider e.g. TB, pneumococcal sepsis, underlying neoplasm (and rarer conditions, like strongyloidiasis). Biochemical analysis of pleural fluid can help (📖*Biochemistry*, p359). An empyema will have ↑ white cell count, ↑ protein, ↓ pH, LDH changes compatible with an exudate, and, possibly, organisms visible and/or culturable within the fluid. A pleural biopsy can be obtained with an Abraham's needle, but in recent times pleuroscopy may have developed into a better option.

⬐http://blue.temple.edu/~pathphys/pulmonary/pleural_disease.html

Skin biopsy

Biopsy and hair sampling

- Useful for e.g. TB, Kaposi's sarcoma (caused by HHV-8 and associated with HIV), onchocerciasis (see below), the aetiology of warts (common viral warts versus molluscum contagiosum—the distinction can be important in view of the therapeutic options and the potential for malignant change in some sites, such as the female cervix).
- The identification of pathogenic arthropod parasites, e.g. myiasis (the invasion and feeding on living tissues of humans or animals by dipterous larvae, such as that of the tumbu fly), scabies, lice, ticks and chigger fleas, depends on the offending agent being seen and correctly recognised or the appropriate specimen (e.g. excision biopsy) being taken and examined histologically.

Skin snips

- Filarial infestations: examination of skin snips will identify microfilariae of *Onchocerca volvulus* and *Mansonella streptocerca*. Skin snips can be obtained using a corneal-scleral punch, or more simply a scalpel and needle. The sample must be allowed to incubate for 30min to 2h in saline or culture medium, and then examined microscopically for microfilariae that would have migrated from the tissue to the liquid

phase of the specimen. In onchocerciasis, nodulectomy is also of value, as is examination of the eye with a slit lamp.
- Leprosy: acid-fast bacilli are present in the skin.
- Ebola virus: these have diagnostic value.
〜http://www.uct.ac.za/microbiology/promed21.htm

Other tissues and collections are numerous and include
- Bone infection/abscess/osteomyelitis: consider e.g. pyogenic sepsis, TB, atypical mycobacteria, sickle cell disease, ectopic ova of schistosomi-asis. History is important, e.g. with a history of fight trauma to a hand, anaerobic bony infection may be more likely.
  〜http://www.worldortho.com/database/etext/infection2.html
- Brain lesions and abscesses: biopsy and drainage useful for e.g. TB, herpes simplex, rabies, cysticercosis, encephalitis, vCJD, JC virus and toxoplasmosis (in HIV infection).
- Cervix: HPV, HSV, *Neisseria gonorrhoeae*.
- Joint infections: aspirate synovial fluid and consider e.g. pyogenic sepsis, TB. An acute attack of gout (diagnosed through identifying the birefrin-gent crystals of sodium urate) can mimic an acute infective arthritis and should be excluded.
  〜http://www.rheumatology.org/publications/primarycare/number6/hrh0033698.html
- Liver abscess: consider *Streptococcus milleri*, hydatid disease, amoebic dysentery, necrotic hepatocellular carcinoma in hepatitis C or hepatitis B, obstruction of biliary tree by *Ascaris lumbricoides* or liver flukes such as *Clonorchis sinensis*.
- Muscle biopsy:
  - Cardiac: may point towards a myocarditis or Chagas' disease.
  - Skeletal: may be used to identify parasites, including e.g. trichinosis, cysticercosis.
- Nerve biopsy: peripheral nerve biopsy (e.g. posterior auricular nerve) may reveal tuberculoid leprosy.
- Ocular:
  - Vitreous humor: e.g. intraocular infections, including fungal, HSV, HVZ, pyogenic bacterial.
  - Cornea: e.g. rabies, CJD.
  - Retina: e.g. herpes varicella-zoster, toxocariasis, CMV.
- Paranasal sinus aspirates: e.g. bacteria, fungal (such as mucomycosis).
- Pericardial biopsy: particularly important for establishing a diagnosis in a chronic pericarditis, e.g. tuberculosis, fungal.
- Peritoneal infection: via laparoscopic tissue sampling and ascites sam-pling (📖*Gastrointestinal tract investigations*, p356).
- Splenic aspiration: useful in the diagnosis of visceral leishmaniasis (kala-azar) by microscopic examination and culture and demonstration of the organism.
  〜http://www.who.sci.eg/Publications/RegionalPublications/Specimen_Collection/
- Tonsillar biopsy: of particular value for diagnosing vCJD: also consider MRI scanning (📖*Radiology*, p354), EEG and 14-3-3 protein in CSF.
  〜http://www.mad-cow.org/~tonsil_human.html

Other tests

Antibiotic plasma concentration monitoring

- Some drugs are toxic if the plasma levels rise too high and their use is futile if the levels are too low. Monitoring serum drug levels ensures that plasma drug levels remain within the therapeutic range. Antimicrobial drugs that may require this approach include gentamicin, netilmicin, vancomycin, kanamycin, amikacin, tobramycin, chloramphenicol, streptomycin, cycloserine, amphotericin B, 5-fluorocytosine, ketoconazole, fluconazole and itraconazole.

Cardiac

- ECG: serial ECGs can be of value in rheumatic fever, pericarditis, myocarditis and toxic shock syndrome. Also of value in conditions where cardiac conduction mechanism has been damaged, e.g. Chagas' disease (American trypanosomiasis) and with a valve root abscess in severe infective endocarditis. In cholera and enteric fever (typhoid and paratyphoid), the cardiac rate will often be slower than one might anticipate for the degree of fever.
- Echocardiography.

Dermatological tests

- Tuberculosis skin tests: measure delayed hypersensitivity. The Mantoux test usually involves the intradermal injection of 10 tuberculin units of purified protein derivative (ppd), and the response is quantified. The reaction is read at 48–72h. Most useful epidemiologically, their individual clinical value being relatively limited. Multiple puncture techniques (the Heaf and Tine tests) are likely to be more convenient for large group study. Interpretation of these tests is more difficult in patients inoculated with the BCG vaccine.
- Casoni test: immediate hypersensitivity skin test employed to detect sensitisation to hydatid antigen (*Echinococcus granulosus*). No longer used.
- Histoplasmin test: a +ve intradermal skin reaction to histoplasmin (the histoplasmin test) may be only sign of past infection with *Histoplasma capsulatum*. Main value is epidemiological. A similar skin test exists for *Coccidioides immitis*.
- Mazzotti (DEC) test: for filariasis. This test relied on the intense pruritic response induced by microfilariae after treatment with the antifilarial agent diethylcarbamazine (DEC). Used in a minute quantity, it can nevertheless be associated with side effects, ranging from mild discomfort, fever, headaches and intolerable pruritus to tachypnoea, tachycardia, and even pulmonary oedema.
- Schick test: for assessing susceptibility to diphtheria. A small amount of diphtheria toxin is injected into the skin; in individuals with low levels of specific antibody the injection will produce an area of redness and

swelling, indicating that vaccination is needed. When the patient is immune to diphtheria, serum antibody to diphtheria toxin will neutralise the injected toxin, and no skin reaction will develop. Seldom used.
- Skin testing for antibiotic allergy: this can be performed in the same way as for other allergens.

Narcotics and anabolic steroids screen
- If positive, these may point towards occult drug use and a concomitant risk of blood-borne viruses (e.g. HIV, hepatitis C, hepatitis B). vCJD has been transmitted through anabolic steroid injecting.

Neurological
- EEG: may help with making a diagnosis of encephalitis (e.g. in patients with HSV encephalitis, the EEG may exhibit focal unilateral or bilateral periodic discharges localised in the temporal lobes), of brain abscess or of cerebral cysticercosis. It may also be of value in vCJD.
- Lumbar puncture: material for culture and sensitivity can be obtained, but much additional information is also gathered, for example, the opening pressure is usually elevated in infections (📖 *Tissue biopsy & deep aspiration specimens*, p360).
- EMG: offers rapid bedside confirmation of the clinical diagnosis of botulism. It shows a pattern of brief, small, abundant motor unit potentials. In Guillain–Barré syndrome (associated with *Campylobacter* gastroenteritis) EMG may be helpful in excluding 1° muscle disease.
- Nerve conduction studies: helpful with diagnosing neuropathies (e.g. HIV, leprosy, Guillain–Barré syndrome).

Ophthalmology
- Slit lamp examination: can help with the diagnosis of infective and parasitic ocular problems, e.g. uveitis (syphilis, Reiter's syndrome), *Onchocerca volvulus* larvae, toxocariasis, toxoplasmosis, candidiasis.

Pulmonary
- Pulmonary function tests: bronchial hyperreactivity can be assessed for (often provoked by infection) and interstitial lung disease checked for (which can include, for example, tuberculosis, fungal infections, etc.).

Clinical investigation in action: PUO (pyrexia of uncertain origin)

Common problem in hospital medicine, with huge potential differential diagnosis.

PUO is best defined as a body temperature ≥38.3°C centrally (rectally) for 3 weeks or longer without the cause being discovered, despite extensive investigation for at least 1 week.

Assessment should include

Observation of the fever pattern
▶Some conditions, such as typhoid and malaria, may exhibit characteristic fever patterns.

Complete and repeated detailed history, with emphasis on the recognised differential diagnosis including
- Travel history.
- Antimalarial usage.
- Vaccination history.
- Past use of medical services in foreign parts may be especially important (e.g. blood transfusions, splenectomy post-trauma, needlestick assaults).
- Drug-using history (including illicit drugs and especially injecting).
- Exposure to certain agents and/or animals (e.g. pet ownership, occupational risk of animal contact, such as veterinary medicine, nursing, farming, meat packing).
- Hobbies (e.g. caving is linked to histoplasmosis and canal fishing to leptospirosis).
- Sexual history (and risk taking).
- Menstrual history.

Complete and repeated physical examination, including re-evaluation of previous findings, e.g.
- Check the skin, eyes, nail beds, lymph nodes, heart and abdomen.
- A new sign, e.g. cardiac murmur, may have developed over time.

The judicious use of repeated tests also critical, depending upon context
- Laboratory and radiological tests, taking into account new data, e.g. blood cultures, blood films, autoantibody screen, radiological findings.
- Non-invasive procedures, taking into account new data, e.g. genito-urinary assessment, such as high vaginal swab.
- Invasive procedures, e.g. liver biopsy, bone marrow biopsy, laparoscopy, Waldeyer's ring assessment by otolaryngologist.

Common groups of causes of a PUO in an adult are
- Infections.
- Connective tissue diseases.
- Occult neoplasms (esp. leukaemia, lymphoma and renal carcinoma).

A list of relevant pathologies might include

HIV, tuberculosis, endocarditis, osteomyelitis, malaria, syphilis, zoonoses (e.g. brucellosis, Lyme disease, tularaemia), viral hepatitis (especially hepatitis C and B), typhoid/paratyphoid, pelvic inflammatory disease, chronic meningococcaemia, dental sepsis, tumours such as lymphoma, renal carcinoma, liver metastases, familial Mediterranean fever, multiple pulmonary emboli, drugs, rheumatological (Still's disease, temporal arteritis, SLE, vasculitis), atrial myxoma, factitious fever, Munchausen's syndrome, Munchausen's syndrome by proxy.

With improved non-invasive and microbiological techniques, most cases of PUO are found not to be caused by infections but rather by other systemic diseases, such as sarcoidosis, SLE and temporal arteritis. However, there are also infectious diseases capable of causing prolonged fever that should always be considered and factored into the assessment because they are often treatable and/or transmissible to others and will have serious consequences if missed.

Endocarditis

Endocarditis is a deep-seated infection that behaves like a deep-seated abscess—indeed, an abscess can form adjacent to an infected cardiac valve or shunt. The diagnosis involves thoughtful clinical assessment, including whether or not there is a history of injecting drug use, and requires multiple blood cultures and cardiac assessment. Assess clinically for likelihood, e.g. background of injecting drug use, congenital heart disease, prosthetic valves, rheumatic fever, scarlet fever. Endocarditis may manifest changing cardiac murmurs over a period of time, as well as a number of additional signs.

- Establish diagnosis: echocardiography (especially TOE)—to look at valves, cardiac chambers, shunts, etc.
- Establish aetiology:
  1. Blood cultures (multiple)—consider culturing for unusual organisms such as fungi, HACEK organisms (*Haemophilus species* e.g. *H. parainfluenzae*, *H. aphrophilus*, and *H. paraphrophilus*, *Actinobacillus actinomycetemcomitans*, *Cardiobacterium hominis*, *Eikenella corrodens*, and *Kingella* spp.), *Listeria monocytogenes*, etc.
  2. Serology—Q fever (*Coxiella burnetti*) phase I and II, *Candida albicans*.
- Assess clinical status:
  1. ECG—tachycardia, conduction abnormalities.
  2. CXR—cardiac size, pulmonary emboli with right-sided endocarditis.
  3. U&E—to assess renal compromise, if any.
  4. Haematology—WBC.
  5. Inflammatory markers—ESR, CRP.
  6. Proteinuria—to assess renal compromise, if any.
  7. Blood-borne virus status—HIV, hepatitis C, hepatitis B if there is a history of drug injecting.
- Assistance with therapy:
  1. Antibiotic sensitivity testing,
  2. Serum antibiotic levels (e.g. gentamicin, vancomycin).
- Prevention: dental assessment—for prevention in the future. Endocarditis warning card. MedicAlert® bracelet.

Tuberculosis

Consider pulmonary vs. extrapulmonary disease and other epidemiological parameters.

- Establish diagnosis/aetiology:
  1. Radiological evidence.
  2. Bodily fluids (e.g. sputum, early morning urines, gastric washings, CSF) and biopsies (*see below*)—always consider performing induced sputum even with a normal CXR; histology may show caseating granulomata.
  3. PCR testing.
  4. Mantoux test.
  4. CA-125 levels—abdominal TB in women.
- Assess clinical status:
  1. Inflammatory markers—ESR, CRP.
  2. T cell subsets—low CD4+ cell count characteristic.
  3. Body weight.
  4. HIV testing—may be an association, especially in people from sub-Saharan Africa.
  5. Glucose metabolism—may be an association (fasting glucose, OGTT, HbA$_{1c}$).
- Assistance with therapy:
  1. Antibiotic sensitivity testing.
  2. Serum antibiotic levels (e.g. cycloserine).
  3. Liver function tests.
  4. Skin testing.
  5. Vitamin D levels.
  6. Gene probes (for rifampicin resistance).
- Prevention: notify cases to public health authorities. Contact tracing.

CASEOUS GRANULOMA

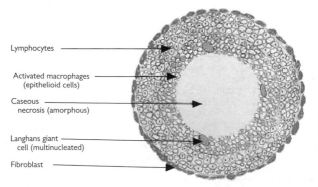

Lymphocytes

Activated macrophages (epithelioid cells)

Caseous necrosis (amorphous)

Langhans giant cell (multinucleated)

Fibroblast

Fig. 5.10 Caseating granulomata are the principal histological feature of tuberculosis together with acid-fast bacilli (detected using the Ziehl–Neelsen stain). In any tissue affected by tuberculosis, caseating granulomata may be present and are accordingly of immense assistance diagnostically.

Tuberculosis and biopsies: when a biopsy is being obtained of any organ or tissue, the possibility of extrapulmonary TB should be borne in mind. If histology is performed, caseating granulomata may be seen, and appropriate staining for acid-fast bacilli (such as the Ziehl–Neelsen stain) may reveal the presence of TB organisms. However, wherever possible material should always be sent to the microbiology laboratory and appropriate cultures for TB should be set up, both for diagnostic and for drug sensitivity purposes. Molecular techniques, including gene probes and PCR, will increasingly augment the diagnostic armoury for TB in the future. In many instances, having a biopsy taken is an unpleasant experience for a patient and remembering to perform a TB culture at the outset may prevent the patient from having to undergo an unpleasant procedure more than once.

Malaria (fever in the returning traveller)
Always consider malaria in the febrile individual returning from overseas. A detailed geographical history and malaria prophylaxis history is essential. Always consider the possibility of a coexistent second diagnosis (especially in *P. falciparum* infestation), such as *Salmonella* septicaemia (so-called 'algid malaria').
● Establish diagnosis/aetiology:
   1. Thick and thin blood films: perform 3 (each 24h apart).
   2. Molecular tests.
   3. Platelet count—thrombocytopenia suggestive of *P. falciparum*.
   4. Haematology—WBC.
   5. Inflammatory markers—ESR, CRP.
   6. Malaria antibodies—not useful in acute situation, but useful epidemiologically.
● Assess clinical status:
   1. Blood cultures—to exclude algid malaria.
   2. Haemoglobinopathy—assess for sickle cell disease.
   3. Assess the very ill patient thoroughly for possible cerebral malaria (includes LFTs, blood film for haemolysis, coagulation status, CXR, ECG, arterial blood gases, glucose levels, lactate levels, etc.). Note that severe *Plasmodium falciparum* malaria can present as a diarrhoeal illness.
● Assistance with therapy:
   1. G6PD levels.
   2. Tests of hearing—deafness can occur with quinine.
● Prevention: avoid blood donation.

Jaundice (acute)
Jaundice can be pre-hepatic, post-hepatic or a combination of both. Epidemiological factors are important (drug injecting, travel, unsafe food, unsafe sex, job, hobbies, vaccination history, alcohol, prescribed medications, herbal remedies, etc.). The patient may have an acute exacerbation of a chronic disease e.g. hepatitis C. Always remember Courvoisier's law (distended gall bladder in a patient with obstructive jaundice means cancer) and Charcot's triad (the characteristic presentation of acute cholangitis, with biliary colic, jaundice and spiking fevers with rigors). Haemolysis may lead to jaundice without liver disease being present.

- Establish diagnosis:
  1. LFTs—conjugated and unconjugated bilirubin levels.
  2. Urinalysis.
  3. Stool examination—colour, flushability.
  4. Haemolysis screen—blood film, coagulation studies, antiglobulin test, etc.
  5. Hepatobiliary ultrasound—serial scans can assess hepatobiliary status sequentially.
  6. α-fetoprotein levels—may suggest hepatocellular carcinoma associated with hepatitis C and hepatitis B infection.
- Establish aetiology:
  1. Serology—e.g. hepatitis A through to E, EBV, CMV, toxoplasmosis, leptospirosis, hantavirus, yellow fever.
  2. Blood culture.
  3. Stools for ova, cysts and parasites (e.g. *Clonorchis sinensis*, ascariasis).
  4. Monospot for EBV.
  5. Hepatobiliary ultrasound—obstruction by malignancy or parasites, liver parenchyma status, gallstones.
  6. ERCP/MRCP—may diagnose parasitic invasion of biliary tree, CMV/cryptosporidial disease, porta hepatis lymphadenopathy associated with HIV, etc.
  7. Paracetamol levels.
- Assistance with therapy:
  1. HIV testing—if appropriate: co-infection with HIV, HCV and HBV an increasing problem world-wide.
  2. Ethanol assessment—γGT levels, ↑ MCV.
  3. Molecular tests: PCR testing for HCV, circulating DNA levels in HBV.
  4. Antigens—hepatitis B.
- Prevention:
  1. Notify cases to public health authorities; safe sex education; safe drug-injecting education possible once viral diagnosis of HCV, HBV and/or HIV established.
  2. Assess family, sexual partners, etc. for possible infection (HIV, HBV, HCV) and/or need to vaccinate (HBV).
  3. Vaccination strategies: HBV, HAV as appropriate.

Diarrhoea

Diarrhoea can be acute *vs.* chronic, or acute on chronic. For example, a gastroenteritis illness may uncover pre-existing inflammatory bowel disease, such as Crohn's disease, or malabsorption (such as coeliac disease or pancreatic insufficiency). Drugs such as opiates can lead to 'overflow' diarrhoea. Also bear in mind that where there is one bowel pathogen, another one might be present. Antibiotic resistance is common among some bowel pathogens. Diarrhoea can appear infective, but, for example, might be endocrine in origin (e.g. carcinoid syndrome, Zollinger–Ellison syndrome, medullary carcinoma of thyroid), while the possibility of bowel cancer must always be borne in mind. Note that the presence of *Streptococcus bovis* in blood cultures is *always* highly indicative of the presence of a bowel cancer until proven otherwise. Irritable bowel disease is being increasingly diagnosed. Malaria can present as diarrhoea (*see earlier*).

- Establish diagnosis:
  1. Examine stools.
  2. Keep stool chart on ward.
- Establish aetiology:
  1. Stool culture and sensitivity.
  2. Stool microscopy for ova, cysts and parasites.

Pneumonic illness

Pneumonia is multi-aetiological. If recurrent, this throws up certain diagnostic possibilities that must be considered. Many epidemiological considerations are important, such as travel history, occupation, pet keeping, hobbies, sexual activity, etc. Osler's triad of rigors, pleuritis and rust-coloured sputum is said to be characteristic of pneumococcal pneumonia.

- Establish diagnosis/aetiology:
  1. CXR (or CT chest).
  2. Serology: atypical pneumonia organisms (*Legionella pneumophila, Mycoplasma pneumoniae, Coxiella burnetti, Chlamydia psittaci*), hantavirus, RSV, influenza.
  3. Sputum including induced sputum, bronchoscopy and BAL: microscopy and culture.
  4. Blood cultures.
  5. Serum Na^+ level—↓ in *Legionella*.
  6. Antigen—pneumococcal (blood), *Legionella* (urine).
  7. Nasopharyngeal aspirate (NPA) for viral culture—RSV, influenza.
  8. Cryoglobulins, e.g. *Mycoplasma pneumoniae*.
  9. Molecular—various PCR tests.
  10. HIV test—if appropriate.
- Assess clinical status:
  1. Arterial blood gases.
  2. Ultrasound of chest—if effusion developing (drain if necessary).
  3. Pulmonary function tests if appropriate.
- Assistance with therapy:
  1. Antibiotic sensitivity testing.
  2. If recurrent: consider tuberculosis testing (see *earlier*), HIV testing, immunoglobulin levels (to check for deficiency), assessing for hyposplenism, checking terminal complement levels (C5–C9).
- Prevention:
  1. Notify appropriate cases to public health authorities (e.g. *Legionella*, tuberculosis); isolate as necessary.
  2. Vaccination strategies: influenza, *Pneumococcus*, *Haemophilus influenzae* B (Hib).
  3. Stop smoking, if relevant.

Meningitic illness (headache and photophobia)

Meningitis can be extremely serious, particularly bacterial, mycobacterial, fungal and protozoal forms, but viral meningitis is generally less serious. Meningitic infection is often mimicked by much less serious infections, such as urinary tract infection (especially in women), throat infections (ASO, monospot), atypical pneumonias and sinusitis (especially ethmoidal, sphenoidal). A similar picture can also be generated by a subarachnoid haemorrhage. Meningococcal infection can be life-threatening without ever causing meningitis. If a bacterial meningitis is recurrent, certain diagnostic possibilities must be considered. Brain abscess (consider injecting drug use, congenital heart disease, immunodeficiency, etc.) and, under certain circumstances, encephalitis can present in a similar fashion to meningitic illnesses. Where the patient has a marked petechial rash and a history of travel to Africa, Ukraine or South America, even viral haemorrhagic fever (particularly the Congo-Crimean variety) comes into the picture.

- Establish diagnosis/aetiology:
  1. LP/cisternal puncture/foramenal puncture (in neonates): for CSF pressure, microscopy, bacterial and mycobacterial culture (including special cultures, e.g. for *Listeria*), viral culture, biochemistry (e.g. protein, glucose), differential cell count, viral PCR, xanthochromia, India ink stain, cryptococcal antigen testing.
  2. CT scan of head: sometimes necessary to exclude a space-occupying lesion prior to performing LP, CT is little better than a clinical assessment in the exclusion of raised intracranial pressure. When ↑ ICP is found, cisternal puncture and foramenal puncture is possible in skilled hands.
  3. CXR and assessment for atypical pneumonia if appropriate (*see earlier*).
  4. NPA (*see earlier*).
  5. Petechial rash sampling: aspirate material from a fresh purpuric lesion using a small-needle insulin syringe, Gram stain and culture.
  6. Molecular: meningococcal PCR (blood and CSF), pneumococcal PCR (blood and CSF).
  7. Serology: urine and blood for cryptococcal antigen; blood for pneumococcal antigen; urine and saliva for mumps antigen; ASO, antibodies to mumps, EBV, *Cryptococcus, Neisseria meningitidis*.
  8. Nasopharyngeal swab for meningococcus.
  9. Stool for enteroviral culture.
  10. Monospot test for EBV.
- Assess clinical status:
  1. CT scan/MRI scan of head: assess for raised intracranial pressure, exclude SAH (xanthochromia), sagittal vein thrombosis; exclude skull fracture, especially of cribriform plate or middle ear (this can lead to recurrent pneumococcal meningitis—if there is a nasal drip, test fluid for glucose to exclude presence of CSF as CSF contains glucose).
  2. Differential WBC in blood.
  3. Inflammatory markers: ESR, CRP.
  4. Coagulation screen and platelet count: for meningococcal sepsis.
  5. Arterial blood gases: to assess acid-base balance in severe cases.
  6. Synacthen test (☐*Short synacthen test*, p193): adrenal failure in severe meningococcal sepsis (Waterhouse–Friederichsen syndrome).
  7. HIV test—suggested by some pathologies, and may be the overall underlying problem.
  8. TB assessment—may be the underlying pathology.

- Assistance with therapy:
  1. Antibiotic sensitivity testing,
  2. Serum antimicrobial levels, e.g. amphotericin, flucytosine.
- Prevention:
  1. Notify relevant cases to public health authorities; isolate as necessary.
  2. Vaccination strategies: meningococcus A and C, pneumococcus, influenza, Hib.
  3. History of skull fracture: may need neurosurgery, etc.

1. A detailed travel history and a high index of suspicion are essential in making the diagnosis of VHF. A recent travel history to an area where one of these viruses are known to be particularly prevalent is suggestive, particularly Africa (e.g. Uganda and Ebola, Nigeria and Lassa) and South America — the incubation period ranges from 3 to 21 days, depending upon the variety. Many VHF cases presenting together may suggest a bioterrorism attack.

Biohazard

5. Almost always, the true diagnosis will not be a VHF, but they must be considered where appropriate. Strict adherence to isolation and infection control precautions has prevented secondary transmission in almost all cases.

2. VHFs are severe febrile illnesses that can be complicated by a haemorrhagic tendency, petechiae, hypotension (and even shock), flushing of the face and chest, and oedema. Constitutional symptoms such as headaches, myalgia, vomiting and diarrhoea may occur. Some VHFs manifest particular features not shared by the others.

3. Once suspected, VHFs are category 4 pathogens, so precautions for healthcare workers must be instituted and the case notified to the proper authorities. Isolation measures and barrier nursing procedures are indicated (Marburg, Ebola, Lassa and Congo-Crimean HF viruses may be particularly prone to aerosol nosocomial spread), usually in a special infectious diseases/tropical medicine unit staffed with clinicians with expertise in the field. Intensive supportive care may be required.

4. Diagnosis requires clinical expertise in infectious diseases/tropical medicine. The differential diagnosis includes malaria, yellow fever, dengue, typhoid/ paratyphoid fever, non-typhoidal salmonellae, typhus and other rickettsial diseases, leptospirosis, shigella dysentery, relapsing fever (borreliosis), fulminant hepatitis and meningo coccal disease. Antigen tests, antibody detection and viral culture are all available for most of the VHFs. The patient should be fully investigated and treated accordingly.

Fig. 5.11 Investigating a possible case of viral haemorrhagic fever (VHF) case.

Urethritis (with or without haematuria)

Pain on micturition can simply represent a urinary tract infection, or there may be—a sexually transmitted disease such as gonorrhoea present. The patient's sexual and travel history is important. Renal calculi can produce clinical pictures resembling infection, as can dermatological condition such as Stevens–Johnson syndrome. Urinary tract infections are more common during pregnancy. Prostatitis can be a problem in older men.

- Establish diagnosis/aetiology:
  1. Urine collection (MSU): culture (bacterial infections), microscopy (parasites, etc. such as schistosomiasis—use terminal specimen), molecular techniques (LCR for *Chlamydia*).
  2. Sexually transmitted diseases and pelvic inflammatory disease: perform HVS and urethral swabs, screen for gonococcus (includes throat and anal swabs).
  3. Calcular disease: exclude with urine microscopy, radiology, etc.
  4. Prostatitis: prostatic massage, cryptococcal antigen.
  5. Tuberculosis—can present like any other UTI.
  6. Reiter's syndrome: slit lamp examination of the eye, urine and stool culture/LCR for *Chlamydia*.
- Assess clinical status:
  1. Biochemistry: exclude renal failure (urea, creatinine, etc.).
  2. Markers of inflammation: CRP, ESR.
  3. White cell count.
  4. Check all other mucosal surfaces of the body (mouth, conjunctivae, nose, etc.) to help exclude Stevens–Johnson syndrome.
- Assistance with therapy:
  1. Pregnancy test.
  2. PSA to exclude prostatic carcinoma (recurrent UTIs in older men).
  3. Radiology of renal tract: ultrasound, IVP (to exclude underlying renal tract anatomical problems, TB involvement, calculi, etc.).
- Prevention:
  1. History of unsafe sex, recent new sexual partner, drug injecting: consider VDRL, HIV, viral hepatitis testing.
  2. Tuberculosis: notify, contact trace, etc.
  3. Calculi: exclude hypercalcaemia, hyperuricaemia, etc.

Red painful swollen lower leg

One of the most difficult things in medicine is to distinguish effectively between a distal deep venous thrombosis, and cellulitis—and a combination of both! Less commonly a ruptured Baker's cyst of the knee can present in almost the same way, the key is in the history. Sometimes the problem is in the tissues, and sometimes in the joints (even gout and pseudogout can look like cellulitis) or the bone (osteomyelitis). Ulceration may be present on the legs. Venous and arterial insufficiency may complicate the picture—infected legs in older people can be very difficult to treat with antibiotics alone. Recent long-haul air travel may point more towards thrombosis, but swollen legs with compromised veins can easily get infected. Although rare syphilis, yaws and *Mycobacterium ulcerans* can cause leg ulcers that are potentially amenable to treatment. Pyoderma gangrenosum can resemble infection of the leg, but is associated with non-infectious systemic diseases.

- Establish diagnosis/aetiology:
  1. Exclude DVT (and possible embolic disease on occasions).
  2. Swabs: from ulcers, between the toes.
  3. Blood cultures.
  4. ASO titre, antistaphylococcal titres (on occasions), VDRL.
  5. Joint assessment: urate levels for gout, assess (if relevant) for pseu-dogout, rheumatological screen, synovial fluid analysis (if relevant), Lyme disease titres (depends on the travel history, etc.).
  6. Leg ulcers in the young: consider sickle cell disease, hereditary spherocytosis.
- Assess clinical status:
  1. White cell count.
  2. Inflammatory markers: ESR, CRP.
  3. Assess blood vessel integrity: e.g. compression ultrasound for venous problems, lower limb arteriography.
- Assistance with therapy:
  1. Exclude diabetes.
  2. X-ray, bone scanning—is osteomyelitis present?
- Prevention:
  1. Treat diabetes if present.
  2. Treat other underlying conditions if present.
  3. Patient advised to take care in future (e.g. DVT avoidance while travelling).

Vesicular rash

Many vesicular rashes are infective, many are not. In particular, the distribution of the rash should be carefully assessed and joint assessment and management with a dermatologist is often valuable. If atopic, eczema herpeticum comes into the picture. Staphylococcal impetigo can cause vesiculation. If there is a relevant travel history, rickettsial pox and monkey pox, come into the picture. Erythema multiforme, which often has an infective basis but can also be produced by medications, can produce a vesiculating rash (so check the mouth, eyes and genitalia, and determine the medication history). Non-infective blistering conditions include dermatitis herpetiformis (coeliac disease), pompholyx and pemphigus.

- Establish diagnosis/aetiology:
  1. Vesicular fluid—EM, IFT, culture, etc.
  2. Serology—HSV, HVZ, rickettsial pox, coxsackievirus, ASO titre.
- Assess clinical status:
  1. CXR—chickenpox (if compromised, ABGs will be needed).
  2. EEG if cerebral symptoms present (e.g. cerebellar encephalitis can occur with HVZ).
  3. Monkey pox, small-pox, rickettsial pox: the patient will be ill and will require full assessment, even possibly intensive care.
- Assistance with therapy: pregnancy test—HVZ a bigger problem in pregnancy.
- Prevention:
  1. Avoid precipitants with erythema multiforme.
  2. Manage atopy optimally.

Further reading

Chin J ed. (2000) *Control of Communicable Diseases Manual*, 17th edition, American Public Health Association, Washington DC, USA.

Cohen J, Powderly WG eds. (2003) Infectious Diseases, 2nd edition, Mosby, St Louis, USA.

Cook GC, Zumla AI eds. (2002) *Manson's Tropical Diseases*, 21st edition, WB Saunders, Philadelphia, USA.

Mandell GL, Douglas JE, Dolin R, Bennett RE, eds. (2004) Principles and Practice of Infectious Diseases, 6th edition, Churchill Livingstone, London, UK.

Peters W, Pasvol G. (2001) Color Atlas of Tropical Medicine and Parasitology, 5th edition, Mosby-Year Book, St Louis, USA.

Shanson DC. (1999) Microbiology and Clinical Practice, 3rd edition, Butterworth-Heinemann, Oxford, UK.

Steffen R, Dupont HL, Wilder-Smith A. (2003) Manual of Travel Medicine and Health, 2nd edition, BC Decker, Ontario, Canada.

Cardiology

Cardiac catheterisation *380*
Cardiac markers of myocardial necrosis *384*
Cardiac volumetric imaging: magnetic resonance &
    computerised tomography *386*
Echocardiography *394*
Electrocardiogram (ECG) *416*
Electrocardiographic monitoring *420*
Exercise testing *423*
Myocardial perfusion imaging *428*
Radionuclide ventriculography *432*
Swan–Ganz catheterisation *434*
Tilt table testing *436*

Cardiac catheterisation

Principle
Cardiac catheterisation is an invasive procedure during which catheters are placed within the cardiac chambers, coronary arteries and great vessels to provide information on cardiac anatomy, pressures, disease states, function and oxygen saturations.

Indications
- Diagnosis of suspected coronary artery disease (after appropriate non-invasive assessment, or if results are equivocal).
- Assessment of coronary artery disease burden and suitability for intervention, e.g. percutaneous angioplasty, coronary artery bypass surgery or cardiac transplantation.
- Measurement of intra-cardiac pressures in patients with valvular heart disease (largely superseded by TOE).
- Detailed measurement of left and right ventricular cardiac output and pulmonary hypertension in patients considered for cardiac transplantation or with suspected congenital heart disease.
- Evaluation of O_2 saturations in cardiac chambers to identify cardiac shunting.
- Myocardial biopsy in patients with cardiomyopathy of unknown cause.
- Monitoring of cardiac transplantation success/rejection.

Contraindications
- Pregnancy is an absolute contraindication to coronary angiography.
- Relative contraindications include:
  - Severe peripheral vascular disease.
  - Aortic aneurysm.
  - Renal failure.
  - Unstable cardiac failure or arrhythmias.
  - Haemodynamic instability.
  - Sensitivity to contrast agents.

Patient preparation
The patient is fasted for 4 hours prior to the procedure. Intravenous access is required, together with haemodynamic and electrocardiographic monitoring. Sedation may be used according to patient request or operator direction. It is important that the patient understands the risks of the procedure and gives informed, written consent. The contrast agents used can provoke renal failure in susceptible patients. Metformin should be withdrawn for 48 hours prior to the procedure. In patients with renal impairment, pre-treatment with acetyl-cysteine is advised, or a less nephrotoxic contrast agent may be considered. Contrast agent volume should be minimised.

Procedure
1. The patient lies flat on a couch and appropriate monitoring is applied.
2. Local anaesthetic is used and an aseptic technique employed. For a left heart procedure, arterial access is required. The proximal femoral

artery is the most commonly employed, but the radial or brachial arteries provide alternative routes, especially if peripheral vascular disease is present.
3. The chosen artery is cannulated using the Seldinger technique and an access sheath inserted.
4. Fluoroscopic screening is used to monitor the passage of a guidewire and catheter to the cardiac structures.
5. Catheters are pre-shaped according to the structure being examined. Typically, a Judkin's left 4 catheter is used for the left coronary artery, Judkin's right 4 catheter for the right coronary artery, and an angled pigtail catheter is placed in the left ventricle and/or aorta for examination of these structures.
6. A contrast agent is injected for image acquisition. Images of the coronary arteries are acquired in multiple planes in order to optimally identify coronary artery stenoses. Continuous pressure transducers can be used for dynamic left heart pressure monitoring, e.g. left atrium, left ventricle and aorta.
7. Evaluation of the right heart necessitates venous access. The most common access point is the femoral vein, but the central veins, e.g. subclavian or internal jugular vein, can also be used.
8. A right heart or Swan–Ganz catheter is passed towards the right heart. Right-sided pressures, e.g. vena cavae, right atrium, right ventricle, pulmonary artery and pulmonary wedge pressure (indirect left atrial pressure), can be measured.
9. Blood samples obtained from these sites can be analysed for oxygen saturation and used to identify the presence and site of cardiac shunts, e.g. atrial or ventricular septal defects. Cardiac output studies can also be performed.

Risks

Cardiac catheterisation is an invasive technique and so there are inherent risks to the procedure (1:200 patients). Full cardiopulmonary resuscitation facilities should be immediately available.

These risks include
- Trauma to arterial/venous access site, including haematoma, occlusion, aneurysm, pseudoaneurysm, nerve damage.
- Aortic/coronary artery dissection.
- Cerebrovascular accident (embolus).
- Myocardial infarction (embolus/dissection).
- Arrhythmias.
- Pulmonary oedema (left main stem stenosis).
- Renal failure (see patient preparation).
- Vasovagal response to arterial access/sheath removal.

Additionally the patient is exposed to ionising radiation and so screening/image acquisition times should be reduced as much as possible. Serial studies should be avoided.

Possible results

Results from a left heart study can provide information on
- Left ventricular size and function.
- Aortic and mitral valve integrity.
- Aortic size and disease.
- Coronary artery anatomy and distribution of disease, to aid decisions regarding prognosis and need for further intervention.
- Left heart pressures.
- Myocardial microscopic content, where biopsy is taken.
- Congenital abnormalities.

A right-sided study can provide information on
- Right ventricular size and function.
- Tricuspid and pulmonary valve integrity.
- Pulmonary artery anatomy, function.
- Right heart pressures.
- Presence of congenital abnormalities, e.g. shunts.

Advantages over other tests

Invasive coronary angiography has high spatial and temporal resolution for the evaluation of coronary artery disease and is the current gold standard imaging technique for this application. However cardiac CT is rapidly becoming an accurate alternative means of depicting coronary artery atheroma. Advances in echocardiography and cardiac magnetic resonance have reduced the need for right heart catheterisation but the latter is still the only means with which to obtain direct histopathological information from myocardial structures.

Pitfalls

The procedure is invasive and the risks involved are not insignificant. Whilst coronary angiography is the gold standard for the demonstration of anatomical coronary arterial lesions, it provides little information regarding their physiological significance on the myocardium. The information should therefore be used in conjunction with haemodynamic imaging techniques, e.g. stress nuclear imaging, echocardiography or cardiac magnetic resonance. The soft tissues *per se* are not directly imaged and so their size and integrity can only be estimated.

Scanlon PJ et al. (1999) ACC/AHA Guidelines for Coronary Angiography: Executive Summary and Recommendations. *Circulation* **99**, 2345–2357.

Cardiac markers of myocardial necrosis

Principle

When cardiac muscle is damaged, certain substances, e.g. myoglobin, creatine kinase, troponins I and T, are released into the bloodstream and may be measured by biochemical assays. Such assays can be helpful in making the diagnosis of acute coronary syndromes or myocardial contusion. Myoglobin and creatine kinase (CK and CK-MB) are relatively non-specific cardiac markers of myocardial necrosis (CK is also released by skeletal muscle) that are elevated within 2–4 hours of myocyte damage. Troponins (cTnT and cTnI) are cardiac muscle proteins that are released into the peripheral circulation more slowly. They may be undetectable within the initial 12 hours after myocardial infarction (Fig. 6.1) but they are highly specific for cardiac injury.

Fig. 6.1 Changes in levels of cardiac markers following acute myocardial infarction.

Acute coronary syndromes are categorised into unstable angina, ST-segment elevation myocardial infarction (STEMI) and non-ST-segment elevation myocardial infarction (NSTEMI) on the basis of the clinical history, ECG changes and cardiac markers of myocardial necrosis. Ischaemic chest pain and/or ischaemic ECG changes, in the absence of cardiac damage, are classified as unstable angina. In the presence of cardiac damage (as evidenced by a typical rise and fall in cardiac markers, ideally a troponin) a myocardial infarction is diagnosed. The categorisation into STEMI or NSTEMI is determined by the nature of any accompanying ECG changes.

Indications

Cardiac markers of myocardial necrosis are useful

- In conjunction with the clinical history and 12-lead ECG to diagnose and to categorise suspected acute coronary syndromes.
- To stratify risk in acute coronary syndromes.
- To ascertain the extent of any myocardial injury following coronary revascularisation procedures.
- To identify myocardial contusion following thoracic trauma.

Procedure

A 10mL venous blood sample is sufficient, ideally taken 12 hours after the patient's most severe symptoms. Repeat sampling may be necessary, especially if a sample has been taken too soon after symptom onset.

Risks

In patients who have had thrombolysis for acute myocardial infarction, bleeding or haematoma formation may occur spontaneously at venepuncture sites.

Possible results

In the appropriate clinical setting of chest pain typical of acute myocardial infarction ± ECG changes:

- An elevated troponin is diagnostic of STEMI or NSTEMI.
- Acute myocardial infarction (STEMI and NSTEMI) can be confidently excluded if troponin is within normal limits 18 hours after the onset of symptoms.

Pitfalls

Creatine kinase may be elevated in skeletal muscle injury as well as with myocardial infarction. Direct estimation of CK-MB, the isoenzyme that is more specific for cardiac muscle, may be helpful. Troponins are much more specific for cardiac injury, but may also be elevated in cardiac failure, arrhythmias, renal failure or pulmonary embolus and so the clinical context should always be taken into account. Timing of blood samples is critical since values may be normal if blood is taken too soon after symptom onset. Troponins may remain elevated for 7–10 days following a cardiac event and so the diagnosis of re-infarction using troponins alone may be unreliable. Troponin assays vary between hospitals so always check local laboratory normal ranges.

Ammann P. *et al.* (2004) Raised cardiac troponins. *BMJ* **328**, 1028–1029; ESC/ACC. (2000) Myocardial infarction redefined. *J Am Coll Cardiol* **36**, 959–969; Timmis A. (2000) Acute coronary syndromes: risk stratification. *Heart* **83**, 241–246.

Cardiac volumetric imaging: magnetic resonance & computerised tomography

Principle

Cardiac volumetric imaging is now established as a powerful tool to visualise anatomy, size and function of cardiac structures, i.e. valves, chambers, myocardium, pericardium and great vessels. Advanced technology magnetic resonance imagers and multislice computerised tomography scanners are increasingly available to clinicians. These techniques provide information regarding aetiology and severity of most congenital and acquired cardiac abnormalities.

Indications

The indications for cardiac magnetic resonance (CMR) and computerised tomography (CT) are shown in Table 6.1. CMR is especially useful in patients with ischaemic heart disease, where a comprehensive assessment of left ventricular function, reversible myocardial ischaemia and myocardial viability can be made. Cardiac CT is of particular value in screening for coronary artery disease and for assessment of the great vessels and coronary arteries.

Indications for CMR and CT

Table 6.1

Condition	MRI	CT
Congenital heart disease	+++	++
Anatomy, size or mass of the cardiac chambers (left atrium, left ventricle, right atrium, right ventricle)	++++	+++
Global and regional left ventricular function	++++	+++
Screening (cardiomyopathy, including arrhythmogenic right heart)	++++	+
Valvular heart disease (aortic, mitral, tricuspid and pulmonary)	+++	+
Prosthetic heart valves	+++	+
Cardiac masses	+++	++
Pericardial disease	+++	++
Aortic disease	+++	++++
Coronary artery anatomy and patency	++	++++
Screening for coronary artery disease	+	++++
Myocardial perfusion	+++	−
Stress study in ischaemic heart disease	++++	−
Myocardial viability	++++	+

Contraindications
- Presence of any ferrous metal, e.g. intracranial clips, intraocular foreign bodies, shrapnel (MRI).
- Temporary or permanent pacing systems (MRI).
- Internal cardioverter–defibrillator (ICD) systems (MRI).
- Clinically dehiscing Starr–Edwards valve prostheses manufactured between 1960 and 1964 (MRI).
- Severe claustrophobia (more of an issue with MRI).
- Allergy to non-ionic contrast agents (CT).
- Haemodynamic instability.
- Pregnancy is a relative contraindication to MRI but an *absolute* contraindication to CT.

Patient preparation

A patient questionnaire is performed to exclude contraindications. Patients should be relaxed and have the procedure explained so that they are able to cooperate effectively. Breath-holding techniques should be practised prior to the scan to achieve optimal image quality. Height and weight are required for indexing cardiac measurements. Where stressors are to be used, a 12-lead ECG should be obtained. Intravenous access is required for contrast agent administration.

Procedure

The patient is positioned on the imaging couch. Electrodes are attached to allow image acquisition to be gated to the electrocardiogram. For CMR a cardiac coil is selected and earplugs supplied. Images are then acquired in order to evaluate the clinical problem.

The following MRI sequences are commonly performed

T1 weighted images

These are used for anatomical assessment and contribute, with optional contrast agent enhancement, towards tissue characterisation.

Cine sequences

Cine sequences are used for anatomical assessment and particularly for cardiac function. Repetitive short axis slices from cardiac base to apex are summated to calculate left ventricular function. This is an extremely accurate method since it avoids geometrical assumptions created by regional wall abnormalities. It is therefore a gold standard method for the calculation of left ventricular ejection fraction, mass and other cardiac volumes. The technique can be used in conjunction with pharmaceutical stress (e.g. dobutamine) in a manner analogous to stress echocardiography to identify regional reversible myocardial ischaemia.

First pass contrast agent imaging

Myocardial perfusion is assessed by imaging the first pass of a T1 shortening contrast agent, e.g. gadodiamide. The contrast agent passes through the right heart and lungs to the left heart. It is carried into the myocardium by the coronary circulation, giving rise to a rapid increase in myocardial signal intensity. Myocardial areas with reduced blood flow have slower and reduced signal change. The effect is enhanced by use of pharmaceutical stressors, e.g. adenosine, and can be used for the identification of myocardial infarction and reversible ischaemia. In contrast to nuclear perfusion imaging, high spatial resolution allows detection of subendo-cardial as well as transmural ischaemia.

Delayed contrast agent imaging
Gadodiamide is an interstitial contrast agent and it accumulates in tissue where extracellular membranes are damaged within 10–15 minutes after administration. This is a powerful tool to delineate between myocardial scar tissue (increased signal intensity) and viable or hibernating myocar-dium (no change in signal intensity on delayed imaging).

Velocity encoded imaging
Velocities can be encoded into grey scale to measure motion of cardiac structures and flow within great vessels. This has similar applications to echocardiographic Doppler imaging and can be used to quantify valvular disease, e.g. stenosis or regurgitant volumes, and congenital heart disease, e.g. cardiac shunts.

Magnetic resonance angiography
A volume (3-dimensional) image acquisition is performed after a bolus of gadodiamide reaches an area of interest within the great vessels. This technique is useful for evaluating aortic disease, congenital heart disease and the presence of renal artery stenosis.

Cardiac CT

An infusion of iodinated contrast agent is given and a volumed image acquisition is attained during a 15–20 second breath-hold. Where coronary arteries are the area of interest, a coronary artery calcification score is performed initially, and this data can then be used to guide further imaging. A β-blocker may be required to lower heart rate to optimise image resolution. Images are then post-processed to reconstruct them to attain clinical information according to scan indication.

Risks

If appropriate screening is carried out to exclude patients with contra-indications then MRI carries minimal risk. Patients who are haemodynamically unstable, e.g. acute aortic dissection, should undergo an alternative form of imaging. CT exposes the patient to ionising radiation and so this should limit its application.

Possible results

Figure 6.2 shows the types of images that can be acquired by CMR imaging.

Advantages over other tests

Volumetric imaging is non-invasive and facilitates excellent temporal and spatial definition of soft tissues. It overcomes difficulties of echocardiography where acoustic window availability limits the scan. CMR uses no ionising radiation, and so is ideal for serial imaging. A very comprehensive examination can be performed and allows dynamic assessment of the heart and great vessels at a single visit. Multislice CT provides very accurate information regarding coronary artery disease and is a non-invasive alternative to traditional coronary angiography.

Pitfalls

CMR image quality may be impaired by artefact in some patients, especially if metal is present, e.g. non-ferrous surgical clips, spinal rods or prosthetic valves. Rapid heart rates degrade image quality in multi-slice CT.

Higgins CB, De Roos A. (2003) *Cardiovascular MRI and MRA*. Lippincott, Williams and Wilkins.

Fig. 6.2A Examples of volumetric imaging techniques: (A) MRI Black blood sequence illustrating aortic coarctation bypass.

Fig. 6.2B MRI cine sequence of aortic stenosis.

Fig. 6.2C MRI cine sequence demonstrating huge inferoposterior left ventricular aneurysm containing thrombus.

Fig. 6.2D MRI delayed enhancement study delineating subendocardial scar tissue in the anteroseptal wall following myocardial infarction.

Fig. 6.2E MRI first pass perfusion: (i) prior to contrast injection, (ii) contrast agent appears in the right ventricle, (iii) left ventricle, (iv, arrow) opacifies normally-perfused myocardium, (v, arrow) but identifies an inferoseptal subendocardial perfusion deficit.

Fig. 6.2F MRA of a severe ascending aortic aneurysm.

Fig. 6.2G CT of type II aortic dissection and associated thrombus.

Echocardiography

Principle

Echocardiography is the use of ultrasound to visualise anatomy, size and function of cardiac structures, i.e. valves, chambers, myocardium, pericardium and great vessels. The technique provides information regarding aetiology and severity of most congenital and acquired cardiac abnormalities.

Imaging modalities

Several imaging modalities are available including 2-dimensional (2-D), motion-mode (M-mode), Doppler and contrast agent enhancement (Fig. 6.3).

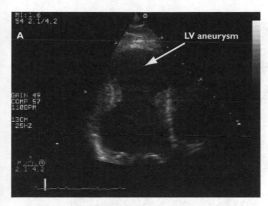

Fig. 6.3A 2-D TTE image of left ventricle demonstrating an apical aneurysm.

Fig. 6.3B 2-D TOE image of rheumatic heart disease (mitral and aortic stenosis).

Fig. 6.3C Colour Doppler of eccentric jet of severe mitral regurgitation secondary to mitral valve prolapse. (**Colour plate 1**.)

Fig. 6.3D Normal M-mode through mitral valve leaflets.

Fig. 6.3E Laminar pulse wave Doppler flow in a patient with mitral stenosis.
(**Colour plate 2.**)

Fig. 6.3F Continuous wave Doppler of tricuspid regurgitation, with pulmonary
artery systolic pressure calculated as 54mmHg (plus right atrial pressure).
(**Colour plate 3.**)

2-D imaging

2-D echocardiography allows real time visualisation of cardiac anatomy, abnormalities of cardiac structures and their motion. Image quality is enhanced by use of harmonic imaging and contrast opacification. With some systems, 3-dimensional imaging is also possible.

M-mode imaging

M-mode imaging samples movement of cardiac structures along a single scan line, creating a graph of the motion of sampled structures against time. It is useful for accurate timing of cardiac events and measurement of cardiac dimensions.

Doppler

Doppler is the comparison of transmitted ultrasound beam frequency with received ultrasound frequency reflected from moving structures, e.g. soft tissues (Doppler tissue imaging) or blood cells. The direction of motion and its velocity can be assessed. When blood cells reflect ultrasound as they move towards the transducer, they compress ultrasound wavelength, whereas if they are moving away, ultrasound wavelength lengthens. The change in frequency between the transmitted and reflected wavelengths is the Doppler shift frequency.

Continuous wave (CW) Doppler

CW Doppler acquires velocity data along the ultrasound beam's entire path. Blood flow of varying strengths and velocities is demonstrated in blood vessels and through the cardiac valves. The signal is represented graphically on a spectral display. Flow away from the transducer is reflected below the zero line, flow towards the transducer is positive in deflection. Signal density and shape give an indication of severity of any abnormalities.

CW Doppler velocity data can be used to measure the pressure gradients between the cardiac chambers according to the Bernoulli equation. The data thus obtained can be used to calculate the severity of valvular stenosis, expressed in terms of mean and peak pressure gradients and effective orifice area. The pressure half-time can be used to estimate severity of diastolic valvular lesions, i.e. mitral stenosis and aortic regurgitation. It is defined as the time taken for the peak gradient to fall to half its original value. It is inversely related to effective orifice area.

Pulse wave (PW) Doppler

The velocity of blood is sampled within a small area. Since this involves only a small sample volume, it localises blood flow. It is particularly useful for evaluating low velocity flow such as cardiac inflow and outflow tract velocities. At higher velocities it is limited by the problem of aliasing.

Colour Doppler

Colour Doppler colour codes direction and velocity of blood flow through cardiac structures. Blood flow in the direction away from the ultrasound probe is depicted as blue whereas blood flowing towards the probe is red. Increased blood flow velocity is reflected by colour mixing, or turbulence. This is a useful screening tool for abnormal jets of blood and can be used to estimate the severity of some abnormalities.

Contrast echocardiography
Microbubbles, consisting of a gas core encapsulated by a protein shell, can be used as contrast agents to improve image quality. Typically they are used in conjunction with harmonic imaging to allow opacification of left ventricular volume and thereby assess wall motion. Research is continuing into their use to assess myocardial perfusion.

Transthoracic and transoesophageal echocardiography

Transthoracic echocardiography (TTE), where the ultrasound beam is directed to the heart from outside the chest wall, is the most commonly performed examination. In certain clinical situations, more information is obtained by directing the ultrasound beam towards the heart from the oesophagus, and this is termed transoesophageal echocardiography (TOE). TOE allows image acquisition without interference of the chest wall, i.e. ribs, soft tissues and lungs. Ultrasound beam attenuation is small and a high frequency transducer can be used, giving rise to higher spatial resolution than with TTE. This facilitates improved definition of the posterior cardiac structures, i.e. valves, atria and aorta. Relatively small structures such as cardiac vegetations may be visualised with greater accuracy.

Indications
Indications for TTE and TOE are shown in Table 6.2.

Indications for TTE and TOE

Table 6.2

Condition	TTE	TOE
Congenital heart disease	++	+++
Suitability for percutaneous closure of atrial septal defect	−	++++
Anatomy, size and function of the cardiac chambers (left atrium, left ventricle, right atrium, right ventricle)	+++	++++
Global and regional left ventricular function	+++	+++
Valvular heart disease (aortic, mitral, tricuspid and pulmonary)	+++	++++
Assessment for mitral valvuloplasty	+	++++
Prosthetic heart valves	++	++++
Infective endocarditis (and its complications)	++	++++
Guide to safe cardioversion (atrial fibrillation)	−	+++
Intra-operative assessment of valve disease/repair/replacement	−	+++
Pulmonary hypertension	++	+++
Unexplained pulmonary hypertension/right sided dilatation	+	++++
Cardiac source of embolus in TIA/CVA/peripheral embolism	+	+++
Cardiac masses	++	+++
Pericardial disease	+++	++
Aortic disease	+	+++
Screening (cardiomyopathy)	+++	++

Contraindications

Transthoracic echocardiography is a very safe imaging technique with no known side effects. Contraindications to transoesophageal echocardiography include:

- Cervical spine instability, e.g. rheumatoid arthritis, ankylosing spondylitis.
- Oesophageal disease e.g. stricture, carcinoma, oesophageal varices.
- Haemodynamically unstable patients, including significant hypoxia.

Patient preparation

For both procedures, the patient is made comfortable on an imaging couch in the left lateral position with the head end raised to at least 60°. Cardiac electrodes should be applied to obtain an electrocardiographic trace. Aqueous gel is used on the probe to aid ultrasound beam conduction. For TOE, the patient should be nil by mouth for at least 4 hours prior to the procedure and intravenous access sited. Any loose teeth or dentures should be removed. The throat should be sprayed with a local anaesthetic, e.g. xylocaine, and a bite guard inserted prior to intubation. The patient may be sedated according to the clinical situation, patient wishes or operator recommendation. Antibiotic prophylaxis is not required.

Procedure

For TTE, the probe is applied to the chest in standard imaging positions (parasternal, apical, subcostal and suprasternal) and the following imaging planes (Fig. 6.4) are acquired with use of all available modalities:

- Parasternal (long axis and short axis).
- Apical (2, 3, 4, 5 chamber).
- Subcostal and suprasternal.

For TOE, the probe is passed gently over the tongue towards the cricopharyngeal muscles. Gentle continuous pressure is applied and the patient is encouraged to swallow until the probe lies within the oesophagus. Views of the cardiac structures are acquired from varying levels within the oesophagus, gastro-oesophageal junction and stomach.

Risks

TTE is extremely safe. TOE is a semi-invasive procedure and so informed written consent should be obtained. Intubation of the oesophagus carries a risk of approximately 1 per 2000 of oesophageal trauma. There is a small risk of laryngospasm and cardiac arrhythmia (usually supraventricular). This usually resolves spontaneously on probe withdrawal. Neither technique should be performed on a haemodynamically compromised patient where an interventional procedure is delayed by inappropriate image acquisition, e.g. aortic dissection, cardiac tamponade.

Advantages over other tests

TTE is cheap, non-invasive and requires no ionising radiation ensuring that serial examinations are without risk. It is portable and can easily be used at the bedside. The technique provides a comprehensive assessment of cardiac anatomy, function and blood flow. In the future, additional information on myocardial perfusion may be available. TOE has similar advantages to transthoracic echocardiography, with the difference that it is a semi-invasive technique. Its superior imaging abilities compared with TTE are discussed above. It is a powerful tool for intra-operative use and in patients with limited transthoracic windows.

Pitfalls

Transthoracic image quality may be limited by inadequate acoustic windows in patients with obesity, lung disease, chest wall deformities and those undergoing artificial ventilation. Structures at the posterior aspect of the heart are not well visualised. Optimal transoesophageal image quality is obtained at the posterior aspect of the heart and so the apex of the heart is less well seen. Image quality may be compromised in patients with hiatus hernia. Not all patients tolerate the procedure and so images relating to the suspected pathology should be acquired first in case the procedure has to be abandoned prematurely.

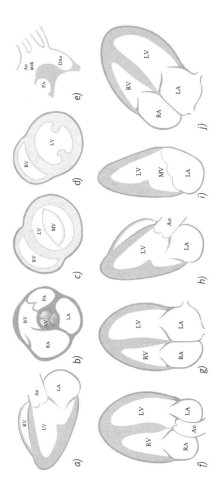

Fig 6.4 Transthoracic imaging planes: (a) parasternal long axis, (b) parasternal short axis at level of aortic valve, (c) mitral valve, (d) papillary muscles, (e) suprasternal notch, (f–i) apical 5,4,3, and 2 chamber views, (j) subcostal plane.
LA = left atrium; LV = left ventricle; RA = right atrium; RV = right ventricle; Ao = aorta; PA = pulmonary artery;
AV = aortic valve; MV = mitral valve; DAo = descending aorta.

Possible results

Anatomy and size of the cardiac chambers
Normal anatomy is demonstrated to exclude congenital heart disease. Each cardiac chamber and its connections are systematically identified and the presence of any shunts excluded. The size of the cardiac chambers and walls are assessed. Normal values are shown in Table 6.3.

Normal values for cardiac dimensions (M-mode)

Table 6.3

Parameter	Normal range
Left atrium	31–45mm
Aortic root	25–38mm
LV diastolic diameter	35–57mm
LV systolic diameter	24–35mm
Septum diastolic diameter	7–12mm
Posterior wall diastolic diameter	9–12mm

Causes of chamber abnormalities include

- *Left atrial dilatation*: mitral valve disease, aortic valve disease, systemic hypertension, coronary artery disease, dilated cardiomyopathy, restrictive cardiomyopathy, hypertrophic cardiomyopathy, constrictive pericarditis.
- *Left ventricular dilatation*: mitral regurgitation, aortic regurgitation, severe aortic stenosis, systemic hypertension, ischaemic heart disease, dilated cardiomyopathy.
- *Left ventricular hypertrophy*: systemic hypertension, left ventricular outflow obstruction (aortic stenosis, supra-aortic membrane, sub-aortic membrane), hypertrophic cardiomyopathy (asymmetric), aortic coarctation, infiltrative cardiomyopathy (amyloidosis), restrictive cardiomyopathy.
- *Aortic root dilatation*: systemic hypertension, collagen disorders, e.g. Marfan syndrome, syphilitic aortitis, aortic coarctation, aortic valve disease, aortic aneurysm, aortic dissection.
- *Right atrial dilatation*: tricuspid valve disease, pulmonary valve disease, pulmonary hypertension, dilated cardiomyopathy, restrictive cardiomyopathy, constrictive pericarditis.
- *Right ventricular dilatation*: primary pulmonary hypertension, secondary pulmonary hypertension, e.g. mitral stenosis, pulmonary emboli, lung disease, left to right shunts, tricuspid regurgitation, pulmonary regurgitation, right ventricular cardiomyopathy (including arrhythmogenic), right ventricular infarction.
- *Right ventricular hypertrophy*: primary pulmonary hypertension, secondary pulmonary hypertension, e.g. mitral stenosis, pulmonary emboli, lung disease, left to right shunts, pulmonary stenosis, right ventricular outflow tract obstruction.

- *Pulmonary trunk dilatation*: pulmonary hypertension, collagen disorders, e.g. Marfan syndrome, pulmonary atresia, pulmonary valve disease, idiopathic pulmonary artery dilatation.

Global and regional left ventricular systolic function

The size, shape and function of the left ventricle (LV) are evaluated with 2-dimensional imaging ± contrast opacification. Commonly measured echocardiographic parameters of LV function include ejection fraction, fractional shortening, stroke volume and cardiac output. It should be remembered that, when calculated from the M-mode image, only the function of the base of the heart is assessed. This should not be extrapolated to global LV function unless the entire ventricle is normal. Ejection fraction can also be calculated from apical diastolic and systolic views (using the modified Simpson's rule). This is more reflective of global LV function but is still limited since it is a 2-D measurement and requires geometric assumptions. A more subjective assessment can be made by visually estimating LV function as normal or as having mild, moderate or severe impairment. Causes of impaired left ventricular systolic function are:

- Ischaemic cardiomyopathy.
- Hypertensive cardiomyopathy.
- Dilated cardiomyopathy.
- Valvular heart disease.

Regional wall motion abnormalities are confined to specific walls or segments of the left ventricle. Systolic wall thickening is defined in Table 6.4.

Categorisation of regional wall motion

Table 6.4

Severity	Description
Normal	>50% increase in systolic wall thickness compared with diastole
Hypokinetic	<50% increase in systolic wall thickness compared with diastole
Akinetic	Absent systolic wall thickening
Dyskinetic	Outward systolic wall motion

Causes of regional wall motion abnormalities are almost exclusively related to coronary artery disease

- Myocardial infarction.
- Left ventricular aneurysm.
- Myocardial hibernation.
- Myocardial ischaemia.
- Post cardiac surgery.
- Cardiac tumour.

Stress echocardiography

Dobutamine stress may be used in conjunction with left ventricular global and regional wall functional assessment. As well as allowing distinction between normal, ischaemic and infarcted myocardium, it also permits the assessment of myocardial viability (regional dysfunction that will improve with revascularisation) versus scar tissue (no effect on function from revascularisation). It should be noted that cardiac magnetic resonance is now proven to be a superior technique for identification of myocardial scar/viability. Resulting interpretation with respect to regional wall motion responses to low dose and peak dose dobutamine stress is shown in Table 6.5.

Interpretation of contractile responses to dobutamine stress

Table 6.5

Interpretation	Rest	Low dose	Peak dose
Normal	Normal	Increased	Hyperdynamic
Inducible ischaemia	Normal or reduced	No change or reduced from baseline	Reduced from baseline
Scar tissue	Absent	Absent	Absent
Viability	Absent	Improved	Improved or reduced compared with low dose (biphasic response)

Left ventricular diastolic function
Left ventricular filling during diastole is an important component of left ventricular functional assessment. Normal left atrial filling is passive throughout systole (S wave) and diastole (D wave) and is assessed from pulse wave Doppler sampling of pulmonary venous flow. Left ventricular filling is assessed from diastolic mitral valve flow. It is predominantly passive and early in diastole (E wave), with a small, later contribution from atrial systole (A wave). Diastolic dysfunction results in elevated left ventricular end diastolic pressure (LVEDP) and ultimately left atrial pressure (LAP) and so alters measured flow characteristics. There are three types of diastolic dysfunction (Table 6.6), depending on the degree of raised left atrial pressure that occurs in order to drive flow across the mitral valve.

Right heart function
Right heart failure is depicted by a dilated, poorly functioning right ventricle. Raised right-sided pressures are indicated by a dilated right atrium and inferior vena cava (seen on subcostal view).

Pulmonary hypertension
Systolic pulmonary artery pressure, assuming there is no pulmonary valve stenosis, can be estimated from the pressure gradient between right atrium and ventricle. This is measured from any tricuspid regurgitant jet (Bernoulli equation) summated with estimated right atrial pressure. Diastolic pulmonary artery pressure is measured by substituting end-diastolic velocity of pulmonary regurgitation into the Bernoulli equation, again summated with estimated right atrial pressure. If systolic pulmonary

Table 6.6

Characteristics	Abnormal relaxation	Pseudonormalisation	Restrictive
Haemodynamics	↑LVEDP Normal LAP Loss of passive gradient LA:LV LV filling from atrial systole	↑LVEDP ↑LAP LA:LV passive filling gradient restored Pulmonary vein: LA gradient lost	↑LVEDP ↑↑LAP LA:LV passive filling gradient ↑↑ Pulmonary vein: LA gradient lost
Mitral valve	(E:A reversal E↓ A↑)	Normal	(E↑↑, sharp descent, A↓)
Pulmonary venous flow	Normal	Diminished S wave Deeper broader A wave	Diminished S wave Deeper broader A wave
Doppler pattern (*mitral valve above pulmonary vein below*)			
LV impairment	Mild	Moderate	Severe
Significance	Slow early LV relaxation	Slow early relaxation, reduced compliance	Slow early LV relaxation Severely reduced compliance
Symptoms	Well at rest but SOB if heart rate increases	SOB on exercise and limited exercise tolerance	SOB on minimal exertion

artery pressure is raised but diastolic pressure is normal, this represents increased flow volume rather than pulmonary hypertension. Right atrial pressure is assessed by inferior vena cava diameter evaluation and its calibre reduction with inspiration (Table 6.7).

Estimation of right atrial pressure

Table 6.7

IVC size (cm)	IVC change with inspiration	Estimated RA pressure (mmHg)
<1.5	Collapse	0–5
1.5–2.5	Decreased >50%	5–10
1.5–2.5	Decreased <50%	10–15
>2.5	Decreased <50%	15–20
>2.5	No change	>20

Valvular heart disease
Echocardiography can identify and quantify valve abnormalities to decide whether long-term follow-up or referral for valve surgery is necessary.

Valves may be
- Stenosed (narrowed).
- Regurgitant (leaky).
- Infected (endocarditis).
- Affected by other cardiac pathological processes, e.g. cardiomyopathy, carcinoid.

Aortic stenosis
Aortic stenosis leads to left ventricular hypertrophy, increased left ventricular pressures and, if untreated, left ventricular failure and risk of sudden death.
- *Aetiology*: congenital abnormality (bicuspid, unicuspid or quadricuspid valve), calcific degenerative disease, rheumatic heart disease.
- *Differential diagnosis*: hypertrophic obstructive cardiomyopathy, sub-aortic membrane, supra-aortic membrane.
- *2-D findings*: thickened, calcified and/or fused aortic cusps with reduced excursion, left ventricular outflow tract dimension (to calculate aortic valve area), effects on left ventricle (hypertrophy/impaired systolic/diastolic function), post-stenotic dilatation of the ascending aorta/aortic coarctation.
- *Colour Doppler findings*: turbulent bright colour is seen through the valve.
- *CW/PW Doppler findings*: peak and mean valvular gradients; aortic valve area; dimensionless severity index (DSI) is a useful parameter particularly where left ventricular function is impaired.

Parameters of aortic stenosis severity

Table 6.8

	Mild	Moderate	Severe
Mean gradient (mmHg)	<25	25–50	>50
Peak gradient (mmHg)	<35	35–65	>65
Effective orifice area (cm²)	>1.5	1.0–1.5	<0.1
DSI	>0.5–1.0	0.2–0.5	<0.2

Aortic regurgitation

Aortic regurgitation leads to mild left ventricular hypertrophy, left ventricular dilatation and failure.

- *Aetiology*: congenital abnormality (bicuspid, unicuspid or quadricuspid valve), rheumatic heart disease, aortic leaflet prolapse, calcific or idiopathic degeneration, sub-aortic ventricular septal defect (VSD), infective endocarditis (presence of vegetations), aortic dissection (aortic root dissection flap), ascending aortic dilatation (hypertension, aortic stenosis, age), aortitis (syphilis, ankylosing spondylitis, giant cell arteritis, rheumatoid arthritis, Reiter's syndrome), degenerative disease, including collagen disease, e.g. Marfan syndrome.
- *2-D findings*: aortic valve anatomy (including calcification, prolapse, vegetations, presence of sub-aortic VSD), size of aortic root/aortic dissection flap/aortic coarctation, effects on left ventricle (hypertrophy/impaired systolic/diastolic function).
- *Colour Doppler findings*: a diastolic regurgitant jet is seen. The width of the jet (colour M-mode) comparative to left ventricular outflow tract diameter and its extent into the left ventricular cavity is measured.
- *CW/PW Doppler findings*: The density of the diastolic signal is assessed together with the pressure half time. Diastolic flow reversal in the aortic arch or descending aorta is indicative of significant aortic regurgitation, unless left ventricular diastolic pressure is high from a separate aetiology, e.g. myocardial infarction. It can be difficult to differentiate between mild and moderate aortic regurgitation, especially with transthoracic imaging (Table 6.9).

Parameters of aortic regurgitation severity

Table 6.9

	Mild	Moderate	Severe
Jet width (as % of left ventricular outflow tract)	<25	25–60	>60
Pressure half-time (ms)	>500	400–600	<400
Diastolic flow reversal	None	Aortic arch	Descending aorta

Mitral stenosis

Mitral stenosis causes left atrial dilatation, increased pulmonary venous pressures, pulmonary oedema, pulmonary hypertension, right heart failure and functional tricuspid regurgitation. TOE should be used to assess the suitability of the patient for percutaneous mitral valvuloplasty.

- *Aetiology*: rheumatic heart disease/calcification (valve leaflets, chordae or papillary apparatus), congenital abnormality (very rare), systemic lupus erythematosus (rare).
- *Differential diagnosis*: left atrial myxoma, obstruction of the valve by thrombus or vegetations.
- *2-D findings*: anatomy and degree of any calcification/fusion of the mitral valve leaflets and apparatus for suitability for valvuloplasty, effective orifice area (evaluated with planimetry), left atrial size (dilated), presence of left atrial thrombus, right heart size (hypertrophy) and function.
- *Colour Doppler findings*: turbulent flow is seen through the valve.
- *CW/PW Doppler findings*: peak and mean valvular gradients are calculated, pressure half time is measured and effective orifice area calculated. Pulmonary hypertension is estimated.

Parameters of mitral stenosis severity

Table 6.10

	Mild	Moderate	Severe
Mean gradient (mmHg)	<5	5–10	>10
Pressure half-time (ms)	<150	150–200	>200
Mitral orifice area (cm^2)	>1.5	1.0–1.5	<1.0
Tricuspid regurgitation peak velocity (m/s)	>2.7	Variable	>3.0

Mitral regurgitation

Mitral regurgitation causes left atrial dilatation, increased pulmonary venous pressures, pulmonary oedema, left ventricular failure, pulmonary hypertension, right heart failure and functional tricuspid regurgitation. TOE gives an optimal assessment of severity.

- *Aetiology*: rheumatic heart disease, mitral valve prolapse/redundant tissue, ischaemic heart disease (papillary muscle rupture/infarction/restriction of posterior leaflet), dilated/ischaemic cardiomyopathy (annular dilatation), hypertrophic obstructive cardiomyopathy (systolic anterior motion), infective endocarditis (presence of vegetations), congenital abnormality (very rare: note association of cleft mitral valve and primum atrial septal defect), systemic lupus erythematosus (rare).

- *2-D findings*: mitral valve anatomy (calcification, prolapse, redundant tissue, leaflet excursion, vegetations, annular size, apparatus integrity), left ventricular size and function (hypertrophy, dilatation), left atrial size (dilatation), right heart function (hypertrophy, dilatation) and pulmonary artery pressures.
- *Colour Doppler findings*: an abnormal systolic jet is seen through mitral valve into left atrium. The size of this is assessed. This can be deceptive with very eccentric jets associated with mitral valve prolapse.
- *CW/PW Doppler findings*: signal density and shape are characterised. Analysis of pulmonary venous flow with PW Doppler can be helpful.

Parameters of mitral regurgitation severity

Table 6.11

	Mild	Moderate	Severe
Jet length into left atrium (LA)	Proximal 1/3 of LA	Mid-third of LA	Extends to back of LA
Signal density on CW Doppler	+	++	+++
Pulmonary venous flow	Normal	Absent systolic component	Reversed systolic component
Tricuspid regurgitation peak velocity (m/s)	>2.7	Variable	>3.0

Tricuspid stenosis

Tricuspid stenosis causes right atrial dilatation and increased systemic venous pressures.

- *Aetiology*: rheumatic heart disease (occurs in 10% patients with mitral stenosis), carcinoid disease, endomyocardial fibrosis, systemic lupus erythematosus.
- *2-D findings*: tricuspid valve anatomy and degree of any doming, calcification, fusion of tricuspid valve leaflets and apparatus, size of right atrium and inferior vena cava (dilated).
- *Colour Doppler findings*: turbulent flow is seen through the valve.
- *CW/PW Doppler findings*: peak and mean valvular gradients are calculated, pressure half time is estimated and effective orifice area calculated. Pulmonary hypertension is calculated from the velocity of any tricuspid regurgitant jet. Peak E wave velocity is elevated (normal peak is <0.7ms^{-1}) and there is a slow deceleration time. A mean gradient of 2–3mmHg may be clinically significant.

Tricuspid regurgitation
- Tricuspid regurgitation leads to right atrial dilatation, right ventricular hypertrophy, and failure.
- *Aetiology*: rheumatic heart disease, infective endocarditis (intravenous drug abuse), functional (secondary to right ventricular dilatation, e.g. cardiac left to right shunts, right ventricular cardiomyopathy, pulmonary hypertension, permanent pacing system), carcinoid disease, Ebstein's anomaly, systemic lupus erythematosus, myxomatous degeneration, cardiac amyloidosis.
- *2-D findings*: tricuspid valve anatomy (site, calcification, prolapse, redundant tissue, leaflet excursion, vegetations, annular size, apparatus integrity), right ventricular size (dilated) and function, size of right atrium, inferior vena cava (dilated), presence of pacing wires.
- *Colour Doppler findings*: abnormal systolic jet is seen through tricuspid valve into right atrium. The size of this is assessed compared with the right atrium.
- *CW/PW Doppler findings*: The density of the signal and shape is assessed. Analysis of hepatic flow with PW Doppler can be helpful. Pulmonary arterial pressure can be measured but may be underestimated if there is severe tricuspid regurgitation.

Parameters of tricuspid regurgitation severity

Table 6.12

	Mild	Moderate	Severe
Jet area as a % of right atrium	<20%	20–34%	>34%
Signal density on CW Doppler	+	++	+++
Shape of CW Doppler signal	Pansystolic	Pansystolic	Triangular
Hepatic venous flow reversal	None	Absent systolic component	Pansystolic flow reversal

Pulmonary stenosis
Pulmonary stenosis causes right ventricular hypertrophy, and if left untreated, right heart failure.
- *Aetiology*: congenital, rheumatic heart disease, carcinoid.
- *Differential diagnosis*: right ventricular outflow obstruction (infundibular stenosis).
- *2-D findings*: pulmonary valve anatomy (calcification, leaflet thickening, doming), size of pulmonary trunk (post-stenotic dilatation), effects on right ventricle (hypertrophy/impaired function).
- *Colour Doppler findings*: turbulent systolic flow through pulmonary valve.
- *CW/PW Doppler findings*: The maximum gradient and pulmonary valve area are calculated.

Parameters of pulmonary stenosis severity

Table 6.13

	Mild	Moderate	Severe
Peak gradient (mmHg)	<25	25–50	>50
Effective orifice area (cm^2)	1.0–2.0	0.5–1.0	<0.5

Pulmonary regurgitation
- *Aetiology*: congenital, infective endocarditis (intravenous drug abuse), pulmonary hypertension, pulmonary artery dilatation, carcinoid disease, post pulmonary valvotomy.
- *2-D findings*: pulmonary valve anatomy (calcification, prolapse, vegetations), size of pulmonary trunk, effects on right ventricle (hypertrophy/impaired function).
- *Colour Doppler findings*: A diastolic regurgitant jet is seen. The width of the jet and its extent into the right ventricular outflow tract and cavity is measured.
- *CW/PW Doppler findings*: The density of the diastolic signal and its duration are estimated. Pulmonary regurgitation is haemodynamically significant if the jet is broad relative to the width of the pulmonary artery, extends >2cm into the right ventricular outflow tract and persists throughout diastole.

Prosthetic heart valves
Echocardiography is used for follow-up of prosthetic heart valves and potential dysfunction. It is important to consult tables of normal flow pattern values for each valve type according to its make and size. TOE is superior to TTE. The following parameters are assessed:
- Direct 2-dimensional imaging of the valve ring and leaflets.
- Presence of any rocking motion suggestive of valvular dehiscence.
- Forward blood flow through the valve.
- Valvular regurgitation (typical regurgitation on valve closure is normal).
- Infective endocarditis.
- Thrombus/pannus.

Infective endocarditis
The following features are characteristic of infective endocarditis
- Predisposing abnormal structure (valve lesion/congenital abnormality).
- Regurgitant lesion.
- Mobile echogenic masses (vegetations, usually in the path of regurgitant jets).
- Spread of infection to other valves (usually along the path of a regurgitant jet).
- Abscess (particularly around aortic root, prosthetic valves).
- Embolic potential (large, mobile vegetations, especially aortic valve). Valve destruction (degree of regurgitation and effect on cardiac chamber size and function).
- Chamber perforation and shunting.
- Prosthetic valve dehiscence.

Pericardial disease

The normal pericardium is poorly visualised with echocardiography since it is a very thin structure. Pericardial abnormalities that may be identified are:
- Pericardial effusion (fluid between the pericardial layers).
- Pericardial thickening or calcification (constrictive pericarditis).
- Pericardial masses, e.g. cysts or tumour.

Pericardial effusion

A pericardial effusion gives rise to echo-free space around the heart. The anatomical relationship of pericardial fluid with the descending aorta distinguishes pericardial (anterior) and pleural (posterior) effusions. If the effusion is organising or contains thrombus or tumour, then echodense structures may be identified within it. The width of this space is measured to give a rough guide as to the size of the effusion:
- Small   <1cm
- Moderate   1–2cm
- Large   >2cm

The most important assessment is whether fluid is causing any haemodynamic compromise, i.e. cardiac tamponade. This may occur regardless of the size of the effusion, particularly if it has accumulated rapidly. Features suggestive of tamponade include:
- Dilatation of inferior vena cava (>2.5cm), poor collapse with inspiration (<50%).
- Exaggerated reduction in transmitral velocities on inspiration (>40%).
- Right ventricular diastolic collapse.
- Low volume, poorly filled left ventricle.

Constrictive pericarditis

This is typically caused by tuberculosis and constrains left and right ventricular filling. On 2-D imaging the pericardium is thickened and appears bright when calcification is present. The period of left ventricular diastolic function is shortened. Systolic function is normal. Doppler shows:
- Exaggerated reduction of transmitral E wave velocity with inspiration.
- Shortened transmitral E wave deceleration time.
- Exaggerated flow reversal in the superior vena cava on expiration.

Cardiac masses

The most common intra-cardiac masses are thrombi and vegetations (infective endocarditis). Thrombus formation is increased in conditions causing slow blood flow such as mitral or tricuspid valve stenosis, or cardiomyopathy. The most common cardiac tumours are atrial myxomas and metastatic deposits. An atrial myxoma is typically a pedunculated, frond-like mass that arises from the interatrial septum. Metastatic deposits can be found anywhere within the heart, including the pericardium. Extrinsic masses may cause compression of cardiac structures. Atrial pectinate muscles, Eustachian valve, Chiari network, papillary muscles, fibrin strands, sutures on prosthetic valves, large vascular structures such as the aorta, coronary sinus or left ventricular aneurysms may be incorrectly interpreted as cardiac masses.

- *Atrial masses*: thrombus, myxoma, lipomatous hypertrophy of the interatrial septum, ruptured mitral valve apparatus, primary benign tumour, primary malignant tumour, secondary tumour.
- *Ventricular masses*: thrombus, ruptured mitral valve apparatus, primary benign tumour (fibroma, lipoma, rhabdomyoma, haemangioma), primary malignant tumour (rhabdomyosarcoma, fibrosarcoma, angiosarcoma), secondary tumour.
- *Valvular masses*: vegetations, thrombus/pannus, fibroelastoma.

Aortic disease

The aorta is a predominantly posterior structure and so the arch and descending aorta is best visualised by TOE.

- *2-D findings*: integrity of the walls is assessed for atheroma (irregular wall thickening), intramural haematoma or dissection flap. The latter may be indirectly suspected from the presence of pericardial effusion or aortic regurgitation. Its anatomy and extent is noted to allow classification. Presence of regional left ventricular wall motion abnormalities may indicate coronary artery involvement. The size of the aorta is measured at several sites to assess dilatation or coarctation (Table 6.14). The normal aortic wall thickness is ≤4mm.

Normal aortic dimensions

Table 6.14

Site	Normal range (mm)
Annulus	17–25
Sinus of Valsalva	22–36
Sinotubular junction	18–26
Arch	14–29
Descending	11–23
Abdominal	10–22

- *Doppler findings*: colour, CW and PW Doppler can all be used to distinguish between true (normal systolic velocity flow) and false (low or absent systolic flow) lumens in aortic dissection, to identify and determine severity of aortic regurgitation and aortic coarctation.

Congenital heart disease

It is important to recognise situs and connections of cardiac chambers and great vessels.

The right ventricle is recognized by the following features
- It is associated with the tricuspid valve.
- The tricuspid valve is sited more towards the apex than the mitral valve.
- The tricuspid and pulmonary valves are not continuous (compare aortic and mitral valves).
- It is trabeculated and contains a moderator band.

The ventricles should be connected to the correct outflow tract

- The aorta is a single vessel.
- The pulmonary artery bifurcates soon after its origin unless hypoplasia/atresia is present.

The atria should be connected to the correct inflow

- The pulmonary veins normally drain into the left atrium. Drainage into alternative structures, e.g. superior or inferior vena cavae, hepatic veins, is referred to as anomalous pulmonary venous drainage and is associated with a left to right shunt.

There should be no shunts between systemic and pulmonary systems; such shunts include atrial septal defect (abnormal connection between left and right atria—Table 6.15), ventricular septal defect (abnormal connection between left and right ventricles—Table 6.16) or patent ductus arteriosus (abnormal connection between aorta and pulmonary artery).

Types of atrial septal defect

Table 6.15

Atrial septal defects	Site	Associations
Ostium secundum	Fossa ovalis	Mitral valve prolapse
Ostium primum	Low septum	Atrioventricular valve abnormalities
Sinus venosus	Upper septum	Anomalous pulmonary venous drainage

Types of ventricular septal defect

Table 6.16

Ventricular septal defects	Site	Associations
Membranous	Infundibular septum	
Sub-aortic	Below aortic valve	Aortic regurgitation Fallot's tetralogy
Muscular	Muscular septum	
Atrioventricular	Posterior septum near atrioventricular valves	Atrioventricular valve abnormalities

If shunts are identified, they are quantified. Pulmonary artery pressure is assessed together with evidence of shunt reversal (right to left) indicating Eisenmenger's syndrome. Fallot's tetralogy is a relatively common congenital condition, composed of a subaortic ventricular septal defect, overriding aorta, right ventricular outflow tract or pulmonary valve stenosis and right ventricular hypertrophy.

Valves and outflow tracts should be morphologically normal
- *Aortic valve:* may be unicuspid, bicuspid, quadricuspid, or associated with a sub-aortic or supra-aortic membrane.
- *Pulmonary valve/right ventricular outflow tract* may be obstructed.
- *Mitral valve:* cleft leaflet associated with primum atrial septal defect, mitral stenosis, parachute valve.
- *Tricuspid valve:* ventricularization of site = Ebstein's anomaly.

Aortic and pulmonary arteries should be normal situs, size, anatomy and unobstructed:
- Left sided aortic arch, aortic coarctation.
- Pulmonary hypoplasia, atresia, affecting either of the pulmonary arteries after trunk bifurcation.

ACC/AHA/ASE 2003 Guidelines for the Clinical Application of Echocardiography
⬧ http://www.acc.org/clinical/guidelines/echo/index_clean.pdf

Chambers JB. (1995) *Clinical Echocardiography*, BMJ Books, London.

Electrocardiogram (ECG)

Principle
The electrocardiogram (ECG) records the heart's electrical activity. It can provide valuable information about not just arrhythmias but also a host of other disorders that affect the electrical activity of the myocardium such as ischaemia, cardiomyopathy and electrolyte disturbances.

Indications
- Investigation of suspected arrhythmias, both to 'capture' the cardiac rhythm whilst the patient is experiencing symptoms and also to look for predisposing abnormalities, e.g. short PR interval, pre-excitation (delta waves), conduction abnormalities, long QT interval.
- Investigation of chest pain, e.g. myocardial ischaemia or infarction, pericarditis, pulmonary embolism.
- Assessment of suspected cardiomyopathy and/or left ventricular failure (a normal ECG is unusual in the presence of left ventricular systolic dysfunction).
- Assessment of electrolyte disturbances, particular where these might have pro-arrhythmic potential, e.g. hyperkalaemia.
- Assessment of drug effects on the heart, e.g. digoxin, tricyclic antidepressants.

Contraindications
- None. However, always check if the patient has a known allergy to the self-adhesive pads used to attach the electrodes to the skin.

Patient preparation
- Explain what the procedure involves.
- Ask the patient to lie supine on a bed or examination couch.

- Prepare the skin by shaving, where necessary, and cleaning with alcohol wipes.
- Ask the patient to relax and lie still whilst the recording is in progress.

Procedure

- Having prepared the patient for the test, attach the chest and limb electrodes in the appropriate positions.
- Before recording the ECG, check that the calibration settings of the ECG machine are appropriate. Standard settings are an amplitude of 10mm/1mV and a paper speed of 25mm/s. Ensure that these settings are noted on the ECG.
- After recording the ECG, ensure that the patient's identification details and the time and date of the recording are noted on it.
- It is good practice to make a record on the ECG of any symptoms, e.g. chest pain, palpitations, that the patient was experiencing at the time of the recording, or to write 'asymptomatic' where appropriate.
- Ensure that the ECG is seen and reported by an appropriate staff member as soon as practicable.

Reporting the findings

Always use a systematic approach to ECG reporting to ensure nothing is overlooked.

Report the ECG in the following order

- *Heart rate*—bradycardia *vs.* tachycardia.
- *Rhythm*—regular *vs.* irregular, supraventricular *vs.* ventricular, broad complex *vs.* narrow complex.
- *QRS axis*—left or right axis deviation.
- *P wave*—presence or absence, inverted, tall (peaked) or wide (bifid).
- *PR interval*—long, short or variable.
- *Q waves*—are pathological Q waves present?
- *QRS complex*—large, small, broad or abnormally shaped.
- *ST segment*—elevated or depressed.
- *T wave*—tall, small or inverted.
- *QT interval*—short or long.
- *U wave*—are prominent U waves present?
- *Additional waves*—are delta or J waves present?

Possible results

The range of possible ECG results is almost endless. Some of the more significant findings, and their possible significance, are listed below:

Heart rate

Heart rate can be calculated in one of two ways

- By counting the number of large squares between two successive QRS complexes and dividing this number into 300, e.g. 4 large squares = 300/4 = 75 beats per minute. This method is preferred when the heart rhythm is regular.
- By counting the number of QRS complexes along a 15cm rhythm strip (30 large squares), and multiplying this number by 10, e.g. 8 complexes in 15cm = 8 × 10 = 80 beats per minute. This method is preferred when the heart rhythm is irregular.

Bradycardia is arbitrarily defined as a heart rate <60 beats per minute, **tachycardia** as a heart rate >100 beats per minute.

If the patient is bradycardic, consider
- Sinus bradycardia.
- Sick sinus syndrome.
- Second-degree and third-degree AV block.
- Escape rhythms, e.g. AV junctional escape rhythms, ventricular escape rhythms, asystole and drug-induced conditions.

If the patient is tachycardic, consider
- Narrow complex tachycardia, e.g. sinus tachycardia, atrial tachycardia, atrial flutter, atrial fibrillation, AV re-entry tachycardias.
- Broad complex tachycardia, e.g. narrow complex tachycardia with aberrant conduction, ventricular tachycardia, accelerated idioventricular rhythm, torsades de pointes.

Cardiac rhythm
To identify the cardiac rhythm ask the following questions
- How is the patient?
- Is ventricular activity (QRS complexes) present?
- What is the ventricular rate?
- Is the ventricular rhythm regular or irregular?
- Are the QRS complexes narrow or broad?
- Are there P waves (atrial activity)?
- What is the correlation between P waves and QRS complexes?

Being able to describe the cardiac rhythm in these terms will narrow down the range of possible diagnoses in most cases and you will, at least, be able to describe the key features of the rhythm clearly over the telephone to an expert.

Rhythms to consider include
- Sinoatrial nodal rhythms.
  - Sinus rhythm.
  - Sinus bradycardia.
  - Sinus tachycardia.
  - Sinus arrhythmia.
  - Sick sinus syndrome.
- Atrial rhythms.
  - Atrial tachycardia.
  - Atrial flutter.
  - Atrial fibrillation.
  - AV junctional rhythms.
  - AV re-entry tachycardias.
- Ventricular rhythms.
  - Ventricular tachycardia.
  - Accelerated idioventricular rhythm.
  - Torsades de pointes.
  - Ventricular fibrillation.

- Conduction disturbances.
- Escape rhythms.
- Ectopic beats.

QRS axis

- *Left axis deviation*: left anterior hemiblock, Wolff–Parkinson–White syndrome, inferior myocardial infarction, ventricular tachycardia (with left ventricular apical focus).
- *Right axis deviation*: left posterior hemiblock, right ventricular hypertrophy, Wolff–Parkinson–White syndrome, anterolateral myocardial infarction, dextrocardia.

P wave

- *P waves absent*: atrial fibrillation, sinus arrest or sinoatrial block (persistent or intermittent), hyperkalaemia.
- *P waves inverted*: dextrocardia, retrograde atrial depolarisation, electrode misplacement.
- *Tall or peaked P waves*: right atrial enlargement.
- *Wide, often bifid P waves*: left atrial enlargement.

PR interval

- *Short PR interval (<0.12s)*: AV junctional rhythm, Wolff–Parkinson–White syndrome, Lown–Ganong–Levine syndrome.
- *Long PR interval (>0.2s)*: first degree AV block, e.g. ischaemic heart disease, hypokalaemia, acute rheumatic myocarditis, Lyme disease, digoxin, beta-blockers, certain calcium channel blockers.
- *Variable PR interval*: second degree AV block (Mobitz type I, Mobitz type II, 2:1 AV block), third degree AV block.

Q waves

- *Pathological Q waves*: myocardial infarction, left ventricular hypertrophy, bundle branch block.

QRS complex

- *Large R or S waves*: incorrect ECG calibration, left ventricular hypertrophy, right ventricular hypertrophy, posterior myocardial infarction, Wolff–Parkinson–White syndrome (left-sided accessory pathway), dextrocardia, bundle branch block.
- *Small QRS complexes*: incorrect ECG calibration, obesity, emphysema, pericardial effusion.
- *Broad QRS complexes (>0.12s)*: bundle branch block, ventricular rhythms, hyperkalaemia.
- *Abnormally-shaped QRS complexes*: incomplete bundle branch block, fascicular block, Wolff–Parkinson–White syndrome.

ST segment

- *Elevated ST segments*: acute myocardial infarction, left ventricular aneurysm, Prinzmetal's (vasospastic) angina, pericarditis (concave appearance), high take-off.
- *Depressed ST segments*: myocardial ischaemia, acute posterior myocardial infarction, drugs e.g. digoxin (reverse tick), ventricular hypertrophy with 'strain'.

T wave
- *Tall T waves*: hyperkalaemia, acute myocardial infarction.
- *Small T waves*: hypokalaemia, pericardial effusion, hypothyroidism.
- *Inverted T waves*: normal (aVR, V1, sometimes V2–V3 and III), myocardial ischaemia, myocardial infarction, ventricular hypertrophy with 'strain', digoxin toxicity.

QT interval
- *Short QT interval*: hypercalcaemia, digoxin effect, hyperthermia.
- *Long QT interval*: hypocalcaemia, drug effects, acute myocarditis, hereditary syndromes (Jervell and Lange–Nielsen syndrome, Romano–Ward syndrome).

U wave
- *Prominent U waves*: hypokalaemia, hypercalcaemia, hyperthyroidism.

J wave
- *Present*: hypothermia.

Pitfalls
- A common error is to interpret an ECG in isolation. To avoid this error, always consider the clinical context in which it was recorded. Begin your assessment of the ECG by asking, 'How is the patient?' before rushing to conclusions about the clinical relevance of any abnormalities that may be present.
- A normal ECG does not necessarily exclude a significant cardiac problem, particularly when recorded whilst the patient is asymptomatic. This is particularly the case when investigating palpitations and chest pain.
- Technical artefacts are often mistaken for significant abnormalities. Follow the advice given above regarding patient preparation and how to perform the procedure to minimise the risk of artefact.

Houghton AR, Gray D. (2003) *Making Sense of the ECG*, 2nd edition, Arnold, London.

Electrocardiographic monitoring

Principle
Electrocardiographic monitoring allows continuous observation of a patient's electrocardiogram (ECG) in an ambulatory setting over an extended period of time. This is typically from 24 hours up to 14 months depending upon the technique used. There are three types of device available for ambulatory ECG monitoring:
- 24-hour ambulatory ECG (Holter) monitor.
- External loop recorder.
- Implantable loop recorder (Reveal™).

The choice of device is largely determined by how frequently the patient experiences symptoms, as the key to successful ECG monitoring is to maximise the chances of capturing a typical symptomatic event during the monitoring period. A Holter monitor is typically worn for 24–48 hours, but becomes somewhat impractical over longer periods. It is therefore ideally suited to patients with frequent (daily) symptoms. An external loop recorder (often called an event monitor) is carried for around 7 days and is therefore used for patients with less frequent symptoms. Instead of recording a continuous ECG they capture brief periods of the ECG, usually when activated by the patient. Transtelephonic monitors allow captured loops to be relayed to a cardiac centre by telephone, allowing an immediate analysis of the recorded ECG.

An implantable loop recorder (ILR) is used to detect infrequent events. It is used to monitor a patient's cardiac rhythm over an extended period (up to 14 months or its battery life). An ILR is implanted subcutaneously and contains a battery, a digital memory and diagnostic software to analyse the ECG recording. It records the ECG on a digital 'loop', continuously overwriting older ECG data with the most current data. It can store up to 42 minutes of ECG recording in its memory, either as one single 42-minute block or a number of shorter blocks, e.g. 3 blocks of 14 minutes each. Should a symptomatic event occur, the patient can 'freeze' the loop using an external handheld device that is held over the ILR ('patient activated mode'). Alternatively or additionally, the device can be programmed to detect and store abnormal cardiac rhythms automatically ('auto activated mode'). The device will usually store the ECG leading up to an event and also a short segment of ECG following the event. Stored ECG loops can subsequently be downloaded for further analysis via a telemetry device at the hospital clinic.

Indications

Where patients have symptoms suggestive of a paroxysmal arrhythmia (palpitation and/or dizziness/syncope), ECG monitoring can provide a diagnosis by capturing the cardiac rhythm during a typical event. This allows the underlying arrhythmia to be identified or, where the rhythm proves to be normal, an arrhythmic aetiology to be ruled out. The choice of method depends upon the frequency of the symptoms (see above).

Contraindications

None. However, always check if the patient has a known allergy to the self-adhesive pads used to attach the electrodes to the skin.

Patient preparation

For external monitoring no specific preparation is required apart from ensuring that the electrodes make good contact with the patient's skin, so that an ECG of diagnostic quality can be recorded. For the implantation of an ILR:
• Explain what the procedure involves.
• Obtain written informed consent.
• Check FBC (and clotting profile if bleeding risk).
• Local anaesthesia.
• Sedation if the patient is anxious.

The best site for the device is established by optimal ECG signal measurement prior to insertion.

Procedure

External monitors are attached to the patient's skin via electrodes, ensuring good contact is maintained. The recorder itself is carried on a belt or in a pouch. The patient should be given a diary with clear instructions on how to operate the monitor and how to note the timing and nature of any symptoms that occur. Some event monitors are carried by the patient and only applied to the skin during symptomatic episodes. The patient should be given clear instructions on how to operate such a monitor and a 'test run' should be conducted.

An ILR is implanted subcutaneously under aseptic technique and using local anaesthetic. The implantation takes around 15 minutes and can be done as a day case procedure. The device is self-contained since, unlike a pacemaker, there are no associated leads. The ILR is commonly implanted near the left deltopectoral groove or below the left breast. This requires an incision approximately 2cm in length. Once implanted, the device is interrogated using an external programmer to ensure that a high-quality ECG is being recorded. If not, the orientation of the device relative to the heart is adjusted until the ECG signal is optimised. The device is then secured in position using sutures and the incision is closed.

Risks

External monitoring carries no significant risks. Implantation of an ILR carries a risk of:
- Infection.
- Erosion through the skin (if patient is thin).

Possible results

Depending upon the underlying cause of the patient's symptoms, almost any cardiac rhythm disturbance (or indeed no rhythm disturbance whatsoever) may be revealed by ECG monitoring. The most important aspect of interpreting the results is to correlate recordings with symptoms. Patient activated recordings are, as one might expect, usually made in relation to a symptomatic episode. In this case, it's essential to find out precisely what symptoms were experienced at the time (including a witness account where appropriate). Auto activated recordings may be asymptomatic and made by the device without the patient being aware of a problem. The most useful outcome is to assess the ECG recorded during a typical symptomatic event. It is then usually straightforward to make a diagnosis and plan further treatment as appropriate.

Advantages over other tests

Ambulatory ECG monitoring allows the chance of capturing paroxysmal arrhythmias, an opportunity that is unlikely to arise with a 12-lead ECG recording unless the patient happens to be symptomatic at the time. Each of the methods of ECG monitoring has advantages over the others. External monitoring is non-invasive but can only be performed for relatively short periods. An ILR allows continuous ECG monitoring over a much longer period, making it extremely useful for investigating patients with infrequent but nonetheless troublesome symptoms. It does however involve an invasive procedure (with the attendant risks) and is more expensive than other forms of ambulatory monitoring. It can, however, prove very cost-effective if it avoids the need for multiple short-term ambulatory recordings.

Pitfalls

As with any other form of ambulatory monitoring, a failure to correlate symptoms with recorded events can lead to inappropriate diagnoses.

ACC/AHA 1999 Guidelines on Ambulatory Electrocardiography
✇ http://circ.ahajournals.org/cgi/reprint/100/8/886

ESC Task Force on Syncope. (2004) Guidelines on management (diagnosis and treatment) of syncope. *Eur Heart J* **25**, 2054–2072.

Exercise testing

Principle

Exercise testing permits the dynamic assessment of cardiac function. There are many different indications for exercise testing but the commonest is the investigation of suspected or known coronary heart disease.

Indications

- Assessment of likelihood of coronary heart disease (CHD) in patients with chest pain.
- Risk stratification of patients with known CHD and hypertrophic cardiomyopathy.
- Evaluation of response to treatment or revascularisation in CHD.
- Assessment of exercise-induced arrhythmias.
- Assessment of symptoms in valvular heart disease.
- Objective assessment of exercise capacity.

Contraindications

The absolute and relative contraindications to exercise testing are listed in Table 6.17.

Table 6.17

Absolute contraindications

Recent myocardial infarction (within 2 days)

Unstable angina (rest pain within previous 48 hours)

Uncontrolled cardiac arrhythmias (causing symptoms or haemodynamic compromise)

Symptomatic severe aortic stenosis

Uncontrolled symptomatic heart failure

Acute pulmonary embolus or pulmonary infarction

Acute myocarditis or pericarditis

Acute aortic dissection

Relative contraindications

Left main stem coronary stenosis

Moderate valvular stenosis

Electrolyte abnormalities

Uncontrolled hypertension (systolic >200mmHg, diastolic >110mmHg)

Tachyarrhythmias or bradyarrhythmias

Outflow obstruction, e.g. hypertrophic cardiomyopathy

Inability to exercise adequately

High-degree atrioventricular block

Patient preparation

Unless the exercise test is being performed to assess response to treatment, patients should be advised to discontinue anti-anginal drugs, e.g. β-blockers, calcium channel blockers, long acting nitrates, nicorandil and also digoxin 48 hours prior to the test. Patients should attend for the test wearing suitable clothing and footwear.

Procedure

The test should be carefully explained to the patient so that they are familiar with the exercise protocol being used. A resting ECG is recorded and the patient's blood pressure measured. An appropriately trained team comprising at least two personnel, trained in advanced life support, should supervise the test. Full resuscitation and defibrillation facilities must be readily available. Exercise can be performed using either an exercise treadmill or an exercise bicycle. A variety of protocols are available, of which the most common are the Bruce protocol and the Modified Bruce protocol (see Table 6.18). The workload during exercise normally increases at 3 minute intervals, with the blood pressure and ECG being recorded at each stage. The patient should be asked to report any symptoms during the test.

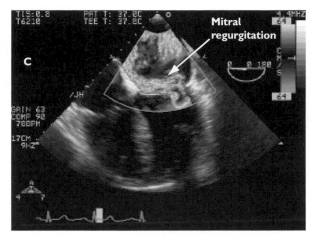

Plate 1 Colour Doppler of eccentric jet of severe mitral regurgitation secondary to mitral valve prolapse.

Plate 2 Laminar pulse wave Doppler flow in a patient with mitral stenosis.

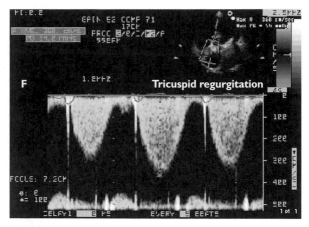

Plate 3 Continuous wave Doppler of tricuspid regurgitation, with pulmonary artery systolic pressure calculated as 54mmHg (plus right atrial pressure).

Plate 4 Endoscopic view of gastric antral vascular ectasia, one cause for blood transfusion-dependent iron deficiency anaemia, which may be treated using argon plasma coagulation.

Plate 5 Endoscopic image of a rectal carcinoid tumour.

Plate 6 Colour Doppler image of the patient in Fig. 13.27 shows abnormal vascularity in the wall of the gallbladder.

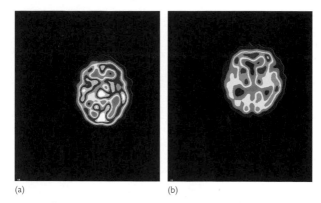

(a)　　　　　　　　　　　　　　　　(b)

Plate 7 ^{99m}Tc-HMPAO brain imaging. Transaxial tomographic slices: (a) normal and (b) dementia.

(a)　　　　　　　　　　　　　　　　(b)

Plate 8 ^{123}I-ioflupane brain receptor imaging: (a) normal dopamine receptors and (b) in Parkinson's disease.

Anterior

Posterior

(a)

Anterior   Posterior

(b)

Plate 9 ^{123}I-MIBG scan: (a) right intra-adrenal phaemochromocytoma; (b) whole body scan—right intra-adrenal phaeochromocytoma. Excludes multifocal, ectopic and malignant tumour.

Plate 10 Whole body ^{111}In-octreotide scan showing neuroectodermal tumour with hepatic metastases.

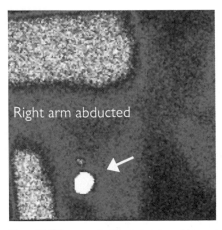

Right arm abducted

Plate 11 ^{99m}Tc-nanocolloid sentinel node study—anterior thorax, right arm abducted. Peri-tumoural, subcutaneous injection right breast and sentinel node (arrow).

Plate 12 ^{18}FDG PET scan—transaxial views showing CT (top left) correlation with PET (top right). The image fusion is shown bottom left.

Plate 13 Normal myocardial perfusion scan.

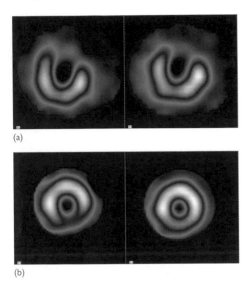

(a)

(b)

Plate 14 Myocardial perfusion scan: (a) in fixed perfusion loss (anterolateral infarction) and (b) in inferior stress-induced (reversible) ischaemia.

(a)

(b)

(c)

(d)

Plate 15 MUGA scan showing (a) LV regions of interest at end diastole and (b) end systole for ejection fraction calaculation; (c) amplitude image showing relative anteroseptal hypokinesis but (d) synchronous LV contraction.

Modified Bruce and Bruce protocols

Table 6.18

Protocol	Modified Bruce			Standard Bruce				
Stage	01	02	03	1	2	3	4	5
Speed (kph)	2.7	2.7	2.7	2.7	4.0	5.5	6.8	8.0
Slope (degrees)	0	1.3	2.6	4.3	5.4	6.3	7.2	8.1

Exercise should be stopped if there is
- A fall of >10mmHg in systolic blood pressure from baseline associated with ischaemia.
- Moderate–severe angina.
- Increasing ataxia, dizziness or near syncope.
- Evidence of poor perfusion.
- Difficulty in monitoring the ECG or blood pressure.
- Sustained ventricular tachycardia.
- 1.0mm or more ST elevation (in leads without Q waves, other than V_1 or aVR).

One should also consider stopping exercise if there is
- A fall of >10mmHg in systolic blood pressure from baseline even in the absence of ischaemia.
- >2mm of ST segment depression or marked axis shift.
- Arrhythmias (other than sustained ventricular tachycardia, see *above*).
- Fatigue, breathlessness or wheezing, leg cramps, claudication.
- Development of bundle branch block that cannot be distinguished from ventricular tachycardia.
- ↑ chest pain.
- Rise in blood pressure above 250/115.

At the end of exercise the patient may be permitted to sit. Monitoring of the ECG and blood pressure must continue until heart rate and blood pressure have returned to baseline and any ECG changes have resolved.

Risks

Exercise testing is generally well tolerated with a morbidity of 2.4 in 10,000 and a mortality of 1 in 10,000 (within 1 week of testing). Risks include arrhythmias and cardiac arrest, myocardial infarction and cardiac rupture and are more likely in those with a recent history of acute coronary syndrome. Facilities for resuscitation and defibrillation must be immediately available.

Possible results

Myocardial ischaemia is indicated by ≥1mm horizontal or downsloping ST segment depression 80msec after the J point. Some cardiologists use ≥2mm of ST segment depression as the diagnostic criterion—this increases the specificity of the test but reduces the sensitivity. Upsloping ST segment depression and T wave changes are not reliable indicators of ischaemia. A fall in blood pressure (or a failure of blood pressure to rise) during exercise can also indicate ischaemia, particularly if accompanied by ST segment depression and chest pain.

Generally speaking, the earlier and the more marked the ST segment changes, the more severe the underlying coronary artery disease. The prognostic value of exercise testing is well established. Patients can be risk stratified using the Duke Treadmill Score, calculated as follows:

Duke Treadmill Score =

Exercise time (Bruce protocol) − (5 × ST depression in millimetres) − (4 × exercise angina index)

where:
0 = no exercise angina
1 = exercise angina
2 = exercise angina that led to termination of test

The Duke Treadmill Score defines a high risk group with a score of equal to or greater than −11, with an annual cardiovascular mortality of ≥5%. Low risk patients have a score of equal to or greater than +5, with an annual cardiovascular mortality of 0.5%.

Almost any arrhythmia or conduction disturbance can occur during exercise testing. If the exercise test is being performed to investigate arrhythmias this can indicate a diagnostic result.

Advantages over other tests

Exercise testing is a relatively simple and inexpensive investigation with a strong evidence base that is useful in a large number of clinical situations. Alternative tests for myocardial ischaemia include stress echocardiography, cardiac magnetic resonance and myocardial perfusion imaging.

Pitfalls

Exercise test results are commonly reported as 'positive' or 'negative', giving the erroneous impression that the results are 'black or white'. The sensitivity and specificity of exercise testing varies widely between different patient populations, but in a 'typical' population has a modest sensitivity of 50% but a reasonably good specificity of 90%. False negative and false positive results are therefore not uncommon. If the pretest probability of CHD is low, e.g. an asymptomatic young woman, exercise testing is of little value as even a 'positive' result is unlikely to be true. Similarly if the pretest probability of CHD is high, e.g. a male in his 60s with typical anginal symptoms, a 'negative' result is also unlikely to be true. The test is therefore of most use in diagnostic decision-making when the pretest likelihood of CHD is intermediate.

ACC/AHA 2002 Guideline for Exercise Testing
⌁ http://www.acc.org/clinical/guidelines/exercise/exercise_clean.pdf

Myocardial perfusion imaging

Principle

Since myocardial perfusion abnormalities occur early following the onset of ischaemia, evaluation of regional myocardial perfusion heterogeneity is a sensitive marker for the presence of coronary artery disease. Myocardial perfusion imaging is most commonly performed with radionuclide imaging. Optional, but less readily available modalities include contrast echocardiography and contrast magnetic resonance imaging.

The radioisotopes thallium-201 or technetium-99m are taken up by the myocardium in proportion to blood flow. Images are then acquired by a gamma camera. The images are processed to provide colour mapping of myocardial perfusion. Information is obtained regarding the presence of reversible or fixed myocardial ischaemia. Late repetition of image acquisition allows redistribution of the isotope in areas of slow blood flow for assessment of myocardial viability.

As with all investigational methods for evaluation of ischaemia, perfusion imaging is enhanced by the addition of cardiac stress. This may be in the form of physical exercise, e.g. treadmill or bicycle, or with use of pharmacological stressors. The latter are particularly useful if the patient is physically unable to exercise sufficiently or has electrocardiographic abnormalities that prohibit accurate interpretation, e.g. left bundle branch block or ventricular pacing. The two most commonly used pharmacological stressors are the vasodilators, dipyridamole and adenosine. Adenosine is preferred as it has a very short half-life. Dobutamine can also be used in patients with contraindications to adenosine but it is a less effective vasodilator. Adenosine gives rise to a four- or five-fold hyperaemia, whereas dobutamine only has a two-fold vasodilatory effect. During adenosine stress, there is a four- to five-fold increase in blood flow to normal myocardial territories compared with the basal state. In the presence of coronary artery stenosis, there is impaired vasodilatation and a reduction in the stress:rest ratio, precipitating myocardial ischaemia.

Indications

- To assess the presence and degree of coronary artery stenoses in patients with suspected coronary artery disease.
- To assist in the management of patients with known coronary artery disease:
  - To determine likely prognosis and probability of future cardiac events, e.g. following myocardial infarction or during proposed non-cardiac surgery.
  - To guide proposed revascularisation procedures by determining the physiological significance of known coronary artery lesions, including the effects of anomalous coronary arteries, muscle bridging and coronary artery ectasia in Kawasaki's disease.
  - To assess the success of performed revascularisation strategies.
- To differentiate between areas of myocardial scar tissue and viable myocardium prior to proposed revascularisation.

Contraindications and risk

Pregnancy is a contraindication to nuclear imaging. Contraindications to physical exercise testing are listed in Table 6.17

Contraindications to adenosine are
- Known hypersensitivity to adenosine.
- Untreated 2nd or 3rd degree heart block, sick sinus syndrome, long QT syndrome.
- Asthma, chronic obstructive airways disease with known bronchospasm.
- Hypotension (systolic blood pressure <90mmHg).
- Acute coronary syndrome not successfully stabilised with medical therapy.
- Decompensated heart failure.
- Concomitant use of dipyridamole (within last 24 hours) or xanthines (within last 12 hours).

Contraindications to dobutamine include those for physical exercise testing and
- Known hypersensitivity to dobutamine.
- Glaucoma.
- Hypokalaemia.
- Concomitant use of β-blockade.

Patient preparation

β-blockers and rate-limiting calcium antagonists should be withdrawn for 48 hours prior to the test if physical exercise or dobutamine stress is planned. Xanthines and dipyridamole should be withdrawn for 24 hours prior to adenosine stress and any foods or drugs containing caffeine should be avoided. Peripheral intravenous access should be sited.

Procedure

The stress study is generally performed first, since if this is normal there may be no need to acquire resting images. The radioisotope is injected at peak stress so that myocardial uptake of the tracer reflects maximal blood flow and optimises visualisation of any perfusion deficit. The protocols for the varying forms of stress are given in Table 6.19.

Radionuclear exercise and imaging protocols

Table 6.19

Stress	Protocol	Injection time of radioisotope
Physical exercise	As directed by physician, e.g. Bruce, Sheffield, to ≥85% max predicted heart rate (MPHR)	1–2 min prior to cessation of peak exercise
Adenosine	140µg/kg/min for 6 min	3–4 min after start of infusion
Dipyridamole	140µg/kg/min for 4 min	4 min after infusion completion
Dobutamine	In 3 min stages: 5–10, 20, 30, 40µg/kg/min	When ≥85% MPHR and/or maximal dose dobutamine

Heart rate and blood pressure should be measured throughout physical or pharmaceutical stress. A 12-lead ECG should be observed continuously for evidence of ST segment or T wave changes suggestive of ischaemia and arrhythmias.

Redistribution imaging for assessment of myocardial viability can be performed 3–4 hours after stress imaging. To enhance redistribution imaging, particularly if any perfusion deficits seen with stress are severe, sublingual nitrate can be given, followed by a further resting injection of the radioisotope and image acquisition an hour later. This is known as a stress-redistribution-reinjection protocol.

A single or dual head gamma camera is used for image acquisition. This rotates 180° round the patient from 45° in the right anterior oblique position to 45° in the left posterior oblique position. The tomographic data are reconstructed into double oblique imaging planes. Stress and rest images are aligned carefully with accurate image registration for comparison. Image quality is assessed and then the long and short axis images are evaluated for myocardial perfusion deficits.

Risks

It should be remembered that the patient is exposed to ionising radiation, especially if sequential studies are planned. Physical or pharmaceutical stress may induce severe myocardial ischaemia, infarction and potentially life-threatening arrhythmias (0.01–0.05%).

The test should be stopped if the patient is physically unable to complete the test or if s/he develops

- Severe angina.
- ST segment elevation of >0.1mV in leads without Q waves.
- A fall in systolic blood pressure >10mmHg below baseline.
- A severe hypertensive response (blood pressure >250/115).
- Clinical loss of peripheral perfusion, i.e. pallor or cyanosis.
- Dizziness or near syncope.

Possible results

Perfusion deficits are identified as areas of reduced tracer uptake. These may be assessed qualitatively or semiquantitatively. Semi-quantitative classification expresses regional myocardial uptake as a percentage of the maximal uptake seen according to the following scale:

Absent	0–9%
Severely reduced	10–29%
Moderately reduced	30–49%
Mildly reduced	50–69%
Normal	70–100%

Perfusion deficits may be categorised as either reversible (present on stress imaging alone) or fixed (present on stress and rest imaging). When the redistribution protocol is followed, areas of reduced perfusion can be examined for the presence of viability (revascularisation will improve regional function) or scar tissue (revascularisation is futile). The size of the left and right ventricles can also be determined.

Possible results for myocardial perfusion imaging

Table 6.20

Myocardial perfusion	Stress	Rest	Clinical conclusion
	Normal/increased	Normal	Normal
	Reduced	Normal	Myocardial ischaemia (reversible defect)
	Reduced/absent	Reduced/absent	Myocardial infarction (fixed defect)
Late redistribution	**Rest**	**Delayed rest**	**Clinical conclusion**
	Reduced	↑ from baseline	Viable myocardium
	Reduced	Reduced	Myocardial infarction (scar)

Advantages over other tests

Radionuclide imaging is readily available and non-invasive. It is inexpensive compared with coronary angiography. In contrast to magnetic resonance imaging where the number of imaging planes that can be acquired may be limited, radionuclide imaging provides full myocardial coverage. There are many studies supporting the ability of the technique to give accurate diagnostic information and prognostic data.

Pitfalls

Qualitative or semiquantitative analytical techniques, whereby signal intensity is compared to the area of maximal myocardial uptake, may limit accuracy in the presence of triple vessel disease where there is globally reduced myocardial perfusion. Additionally, the study may be suboptimal if peak stress is not achieved. Radionuclide imaging has poor spatial resolution in comparison with other techniques. Perfusion defects limited to the subendocardium may not be visualised. Image quality can be degraded by patient movement and by artefacts. Such artefacts include attenuation from breast tissue in the anterior wall and inferior signal loss.

Anagnostopoulos C. *et al.* (2004) Procedure guidelines for radionuclide myocardial perfusion imaging. *Heart* **90**, Suppl 1.

Radionuclide ventriculography

Principle

Radionuclide ventriculography (RNV) is a technique to provide accurate assessment of cardiac chamber size, morphology and function. The patient's red blood cells are radiolabelled with ^{99m}Tc pertechnate *in vitro* or *in vivo*. The labelled blood pool within the cardiac chambers is then imaged with a gamma camera, gated to the electrocardiogram. Multiple image acquisitions are acquired throughout the cardiac cycle, typically over at least 16 systolic and 32 diastolic frames. These images can be assessed based on either the radioactive count or by geometric analysis.

Indications

- Prognostic estimation in patients with heart failure or coronary artery disease.
- Estimation of operative coronary risk for non-cardiac surgery.
- Diagnosis of coronary artery disease where conventional exercise testing is inadequately performed or result equivocal.
- Evaluation of the efficacy of revascularisation or medical management strategies in patients with coronary artery disease.
- Monitoring of cardiac function in patients undergoing chemotherapy.

Contraindications

The technique is contraindicated in pregnant or lactating women.

Patient preparation

No special preparation is required for a resting study. If an exercise study is to be performed, the patient should fast for 3–4 hours prior to the procedure. If pharmacological stress agents are used, the same preparation as for myocardial perfusion imaging should be followed. A resting ECG is helpful to exclude arrhythmias.

Procedure

For a resting study, the patient lies supine whilst anterior and left anterior oblique images are acquired. Stress studies may be performed with either physical exercise, e.g. bicycle ergometry, or with pharmacological stressors, e.g. dobutamine. Images are acquired at intervals once the heart rate has stabilised at each new level of exercise or stress. The patient should have haemodynamic and ECG monitoring throughout. Cardiopulmonary resuscitation facilities should be available. Images are then analysed to obtain the required morphological and functional parameters. High activity areas such as spleen or aorta may be filtered out for optimal assessment of cardiac parameters.

Risks

Technetium has a 6 hour half life. Although the heart receives the largest dose, 5% of the total radiation dose is sequestered by bone marrow, the most radio-sensitive body tissue. Radiation dose is up to 1100 MBq and so a typical examination carries a fatal cancer risk of 1 in 3300. Serial studies should be avoided where alternative forms of imaging suffice.

Possible results

- Dilatation or hypertrophy of the cardiac chambers and great vessels may be identified.
- Left and right ventricular ejection fractions can be measured. Normal left ventricular ejection fraction is 60–80% at rest and slightly more during exercise. Right ventricular ejection fraction is 46–70%. Both values decline with age. The extent of any global left ventricular dysfunction can therefore be identified.
- Regional wall dysfunction at rest, low and peak dose stress and during recovery may be described in a manner analogous to stress echocardiography in order to identify areas of reversible myocardial ischaemia, myocardial hibernation or scar.

Advantages over other tests

RNV is non-invasive and repeatable and provides serial measurements especially in patients who are difficult to scan echocardiographically or cannot tolerate magnetic resonance imaging. It can be used in critically-ill patients soon after acute myocardial infarction.

Pitfalls

Patients receive a significant radiation dose. Echocardiography is safer and cardiac magnetic resonance imaging is likely to replace this technique as the gold standard. Red cell labelling may be inefficient in chronic renal failure. Technical factors are important; in particular, radioactivity in the left atrium must be separated from that in the left ventricle to obtain an accurate ejection fraction. A poor ECG signal and inappropriate gating may render data uninterpretable, heart rate variability may compromise diastolic filling indices and inadequate frame counts decrease statistical reliability.

ACC/AHA/ASNC 2003 Guidelines for the Clinical Use of Cardiac Radionuclide Imaging
http://www.acc.org/clinical/guidelines/radio/index.pdf

Schwaiger M et al. (1999) Cardiological applications of nuclear medicine. *Lancet* **354**, 661–666.

Swan–Ganz catheterisation

Principle

A Swan–Ganz catheter is a multi-lumen catheter that is passed percutaneously from a central vein, e.g. femoral, subclavian or jugular to the right heart structures. It can be used to measure venous, right atrial, right ventricular, pulmonary artery and left atrial (indirect) pressures, to obtain blood samples for oxygen saturation estimation, to measure cardiac output and systemic vascular resistance and additionally to act as a central venous infusion port.

Indications

- Aid in the diagnosis of cardiovascular shock and pulmonary oedema.
- Management of complicated acute myocardial infarction, especially right ventricular infarction, cardiogenic shock.
- Management of patients with cardiac failure.
- Fluid therapy/inotropic delivery in severely ill patients, e.g. sepsis, burns, multi-organ failure, cardiac surgery, trauma.
- Diagnostic right heart catheterisation, including congenital heart disease, pulmonary hypertension, intracardiac shunts.

Contraindications

- Right-sided endocarditis.
- Prosthetic tricuspid or pulmonary valve.
- Right heart tumour or thrombus.
- Unstable ventricular arrhythmia.

Patient preparation

Local anaesthetic is injected into the skin at the site of venous access. The patient is positioned flat on a couch, generally with a head-down orientation if cephalad access is to be used. Pressure transducers are made ready and zeroed for accurate measurements. Fluoroscopic screening should be available if required.

Procedure

An access sheath is placed in the vein using a Seldinger technique. The Swan–Ganz triple lumen catheter is flushed with saline and the integrity of the flotation balloon assessed by inflation with air. Under fluoroscopic guidance or by observation of intra-cardiac pressure traces, the catheter is passed through the venous system towards the right heart and into a branch of the pulmonary artery. At each stage, pressure and oxygen samples can be measured. The balloon can be inflated to assist passage through the right heart. The balloon is wedged briefly into a pulmonary artery branch to obtain an assessment of indirect left atrial pressure (pulmonary artery wedge pressure). Cardiac output can be calculated using a thermodilution method. Iced saline at a known temperature is injected through the proximal lumen and a thermistor at the catheter tip measures the temperature rise in the blood-warmed saline as it passes through the tricuspid valve, right ventricle and pulmonary valve. Systemic peripheral resistance can also be estimated.

Risks

- Arterial puncture, pneumothorax, haemothorax.
- Sepsis.
- Pulmonary embolus or infarction (if right heart contains masses, or if balloon remains inflated in wedge pressure position).
- Pulmonary artery rupture (balloon over-inflation).
- Arrhythmia.

Possible results

Swan–Ganz catheterization can be used to assess pulmonary and systemic venous filling pressures and fluid status, right and left cardiac function, and also where indicated to provide information on valve dysfunction, intra-cardiac shunts, tamponade and pulmonary hypertension.

Advantages over other tests

This technique has traditionally been a useful adjunct to patient monitoring in the intensive care setting, in particularly for accurate pressure evaluation of the right heart and left atrium and for continuous cardiac output assessment. However, recently several less invasive devices have been designed for cardiac output monitoring, e.g. oesophageal Doppler.

Pitfalls

The procedure is generally well-tolerated but it is an invasive procedure not without risk. It is essential that the Swan–Ganz catheter is inserted only by suitably-trained individuals to assist diagnosis and to monitor treatment in carefully selected patients. If a non-invasive alternative is available then this should be preferentially employed. Care must be taken in data interpretation as misleading results may be obtained if the system is not systematically and accurately zeroed for serial measurements. Indirect left atrial pressure measurements may be inaccurate in patients with pulmonary disease.

Tilt table testing

Principle

On standing, gravity redistributes up to 800mL of blood to the legs. The normal compensatory response is increased sympathetic and decreased parasympathetic stimulation which maintains blood pressure with a small increase in heart rate. Head-up tilt table testing uses gravity-induced venous pooling to assess autonomic control and to attempt to reproduce symptoms of autonomic dysfunction of dizziness or collapse, i.e. neuro-cardiogenic (vasovagal) syncope.

Indications

Testing is appropriate in the investigation of sudden, unpredictable loss of consciousness thought to be neurally-mediated (vasovagal syncope, carotid sinus syncope or situational syncope) in the absence of structural heart disease.

Contraindications

Testing is not appropriate for frail patients who cannot weight-bear for up to an hour or those with a suspected psychogenic cause of syncope.

Patient preparation

The patient should be asked to omit all cardioactive drugs for 24 hours, if possible, and to fast overnight.

Procedure

The patient is laid supine and lightly strapped to a table with a weight-bearing footboard. Blood pressure, pulse and ECG are measured every 5 minutes for 15–20 minutes and then the table is mechanically tilted to about 70°. Recordings are made for a further 30 minutes. If responses are normal and symptoms not reproduced, an infusion of isoprenaline adjusted to achieve a heart rate 20% higher than resting for 20 minutes or carotid massage may provoke a response.

Risks

Syncopal symptoms (or in extreme cases loss of consciousness), hypotension and bradycardia may be induced, albeit transiently, so full cardiopulmonary resuscitation facilities should be available. Intravenous access is necessary.

Possible results

A normal response is a <20% decrease in blood pressure associated with a modest rise in pulse rate. The test is negative in the absence of a fall in blood pressure, fall in heart rate and lack of syncopal symptoms, and positive if syncopal symptoms are induced by hypotension and/or brady-cardia. A cardio-inhibitory response is characterised by a fall in heart rate (asystole in extreme cases), a vasodepressor response by a fall in blood pressure with no pulse change and a mixed response by a fall in both pulse and blood pressure.

Advantages over other tests

Monitoring of ECG and blood pressure during a 24 hour ambulatory period or during a Valsalva manoeuvre, measurement of plasma catecholamines, mineralocorticoids and glucose have a role in the investigation of autonomic dysfunction and syncope but only tilt table testing provides a dynamic objective, witnessed assessment.

Pitfalls

The test is time-consuming and requires technical and medical personnel trained in the conduct and interpretation of the procedure and in resuscitation.

ESC Task Force on Syncope. (2004) Guidelines on management (diagnosis and treatment) of syncope. *Eur Heart J* **25**, 2054–2072.

Gastroenterology

Endoscopy 440
Oesophagogastroduodenoscopy (OGD) 442
Enteroscopy 443
Flexible sigmoidoscopy & colonoscopy 444
Endoscopic retrogade cholangiopancreatography (ERCP) 445
Endoscopic ultrasound (EUS) 446
Wireless capsule endoscopy (WCE) 446
Tests for *Helicobacter pylori* 448
Faecal occult blood 449
Serological testing in inflammatory bowel disease 450
Tumour markers 450
Investigations for small bowel pathology 451
Tests of absorption 454
Tests for bacterial overgrowth 455
Tests for pancreatic exocrine function 456
Testing for neuroendocrine tumours 457
Gastrointestinal physiology 459
Non-invasive liver investigations 461
Specific biochemical tests 463
Liver biopsy 466
Investigations of ascitic fluid 468

Endoscopy

This allows direct visualisation of the gastrointestinal tract mucosa and offers further diagnostic investigations to obtain tissue for histology, cytology or microbiology, as well as therapeutic possibilities.

Consent (general)

Consent is a vital component of the endoscopy process. Patients should receive written information before attending for the procedure. This should describe pre-test preparation, the procedure itself, risks and possible complications, after-care advice (particularly for those patients requiring sedation) and contact details in the event of problems and include the consent form that the patient will be asked to sign.

Sedation

While the majority of oesophagogastroduodenoscopy (OGD) procedures can be performed using local anaesthetic spray to the oropharynx, sedation will be required for more complex or prolonged procedures. An IV combination of a sedative with amnesic effects such as midazolam or diazepam is usually combined with an analgesic such as pethidine or fentanyl. Finally, buscopan may act to reduce intestinal motility.

Antibiotic prophylaxis

This is recommended for patients with a high risk of endocarditis (prosthetic heart valve, previous endocarditis, surgically constructed systemic-pulmonary shunt or synthetic vascular graft less than 1 year old or severe neutropenia), when there is a high risk of bacteraemia during their procedure (oesophageal dilatation, laser or argon beam coagulation, or variceal sclerotherapy). All patients undergoing ERCP or PEG placement require antibiotic prophylaxis using ciprofloxacin or co-amoxiclav respectively.

Anticoagulation guidelines

For diagnostic OGD, colonoscopy, flexible sigmoidoscopy and enteroscopy, including simple biopsies and thermocoagulation techniques, it is possible to continue anticoagulation as long as the INR is within the therapeutic range. However, therapeutic procedures such as PEG placement, ERCP, polypectomy or dilatation require normal coagulation and specialist advice should be sought.

Risks and points for consent

Table 7.1 shows the common complications of endoscopic procedures with morbidity and mortality figures for each.

Table 7.1

Procedure	Risks	Morbidity	Mortality	Other issues
OGD	Perforation	0.0009%	0.0009%	Greatest risk for therapeutic procedures
	Haemorrhage	0.002%		
				Cardiorespiratory complications related to sedation—0.005%
Flexible sigmoidoscopy/ colonoscopy	Perforation	0.005%	0.001%	Cardiorespiratory complications related to sedation—0.01%
	Haemorrhage	0.001%		
Colonic polypectomy	Perforation	0.06%	0.007%	As *above*
	Haemorrhage	0.26%		
PEG placement	Perforation	Overall	1–2%	30 day mortality of approximately 10% (often resulting from underlying condition)
	Haemorrhage	risk		
	Infection	5–10%		
ERCP	Perforation	1.1%	1.0%	Greatest risk with dilated bile duct, placement of stent and high dose buscopan
	Haemorrhage	0.9%		
	Cholangitis	5%		
	Pancreatitis	3.8%		
				Risk of pancreatitis greatest with age <40 years, placement of stent and dilated bile duct
				Cardiorespiratory complications related to sedation—2.3%

Bramble MG. (2001) Antibiotic prophylaxis in gastrointestinal endoscopy (British Society of Gastroenterology guidelines). *Gut* **49**, 775–779; Christensen M, Matzen P, Schulze S, Rosenberg J. (2004) Complications of ERCP: A prospective study. *Gastrointest Endosc* **60**, 721–731; Eisen GM, Baron TH, Dominitz JA, et al. (2002) Guideline on the management of anticoagulation and antiplatelet therapy for endoscopic procedures. *Gastrointest Endosc* **55**, 775–779; Scapiro GD, Edmundowicz SA. (1996) Complications of percutaneous endoscopic gastrostomy. *Gastrointest Endosc Clin North Am* **6**, 409–422; Sieg A, Hachmoeller-Eisenbach U, Eisenbach T. (2001) Prospective evaluation of complications in outpatient GI endoscopy: a survey among German gastroenterologists. *Gastrointest Endosc* **53**, 620–627.

Oesophagogastroduodenoscopy (OGD)

- Endoluminal visualisation of oropharynx to second part of duodenum.
- Allows direct testing for *Helicobacter pylori*.
- In preparation for OGD, patients should be nil-by-mouth for 4–6h beforehand and for at least 30 minutes afterwards to allow local anaesthetic spray or sedation to wear off.
- Stop proton pump inhibitors 2 weeks before elective diagnostic OGD to prevent masking of appearances (risk of partial healing and thus misdiagnosing malignant oesophageal or gastric ulcers).

Alternative investigations

As an alternative procedure to OGD or enteroscopy, barium swallow, meal or follow through may be performed depending upon symptoms (for oesophageal, gastric or duodenal and jejunal pathology respectively). These investigations are limited by the inability to obtain tissue for histology or *H. pylori* testing and a lesser sensitivity for mucosal pathology.

Indications

Symptoms/signs

- Dysphagia.
- Haematemesis and melaena.
- Dyspepsia despite appropriate therapy.
- Iron deficiency anaemia.
- Weight loss.
- Vomiting or nausea.
- Investigation of suspected giardia or coeliac disease to obtain duodenal aspirates and biopsies.
- Investigation to obtain histology and cultures of *H. pylori*.
- Abnormal barium swallow, meal or early follow through.

Surveillance/screening

- Ensures healing of oesophageal and gastric ulceration.
- Barrett's oesophagus.
- Establishes response to a gluten-free diet in coeliac disease.
- Diagnosis of polyps in familial polyposis syndromes.

Therapeutic

- Treatment of bleeding lesions (peptic ulceration, angiodysplasia, varices, vascular malformations).
- Palliation of oesophageal cancers using stent placement, argon plasma coagulation or Nd:Yag laser therapy.
- Placement of percutaneous endoscopic gastrostomy or jejunostomy tubes.
- Direct placement of nasogastric or nasojejunal feeding tubes.
- Dilatation of strictures of the oesophagus or pylorus.
- Polypectomy.

Fig. 7.1 Endoscopy view of gastric antral vascular ectasia, one cause for blood transfusion-dependent iron deficiency anaemia, which may be treated using argon plasma coagulation. **(Colour plate 4.)**

Enteroscopy

- Similar to OGD but allows views of distal duodenum and jejunum using a 2.4m instrument.
- An overtube allows less looping but increases complications.
- Preparation is as for OGD but usually requires sedation, analgesia and buscopan.

Alternative investigations

Sonde enteroscopy uses a thinner endoscope with a balloon at its tip passing through the entire small bowel over 6-8h, with examination occurring on withdrawal of the instrument after deflation of the balloon. Intraoperative enteroscopy allows complete examination of the entire small bowel, often via an enterotomy. Barium investigations are limited by a lower sensitivity for mucosal pathology. Wireless capsule endoscopy may represent a future alternative.

Indications

Symptoms/signs
- Investigation of obscure gastrointestinal bleeding (following non-diagnostic OGD and colonoscopy).
- Investigation of lesions found on barium follow-through/CT scan abdomen.
- Investigation of severe iron deficiency anaemia (following non-diagnostic OGD and colonoscopy).

Therapeutic
- Treatment of bleeding lesions found at enteroscopy or by wireless capsule endoscopy.
- Polypectomy.

Flexible sigmoidoscopy & colonoscopy

- Allows examination from anus to splenic flexure (flexible sigmoidoscopy) or from anus to caecum/terminal ileum (colonoscopy).
- Flexible sigmoidoscopy may be performed without sedation.
- Colonoscopy usually requires a sedation and analgesia together with smooth muscle relaxant (buscopan).
- Preparation for flexible sigmoidoscopy—phosphate enema 30–60min prior to the procedure.
- Preparation for colonoscopy: oral preparation using 2 sachets of picolax on the day before the procedure with a low residue diet for the 3 days pre-procedure.

Alternative investigations
Alternative procedures are radiological: barium enema or CT colonography. Neither allows tissue to be taken, nor polypectomy, nor other therapeutic procedure to be performed.

Indications
Symptoms and signs
- Rectal bleeding (bright red ?flexible sigmoidoscopy and dark red ?colonoscopy).
- Positive faecal occult bloods (colonoscopy).
- Abnormal barium enema (depends upon site of pathology found).
- Iron deficiency anaemia (colonoscopy).
- Diarrhoea (colonoscopy with biopsies).

Surveillance/screening
- Ulcerative colitis or colonic Crohn's disease for more than 8 years.
- High risk of adenomatous colonic polyps or carcinoma or previous history of adenomatous polyps or carcinoma.
- Familial polyposis syndrome (FAP), hereditary non-polyposis colorectal carcinoma (HNPCC) or other family cancer syndromes.

Therapeutic
- Treatment of bleeding lesions (angiodysplasia, vascular abnormalities, haemorrhoids).
- Dilatation of benign strictures.
- Palliation of malignant strictures (placement of stents, argon plasma coagulation or Nd:Yag laser therapy).
- Decompression of sigmoid volvulus and non-malignant toxic megacolon.

Cairns S, Scholefield JH. (2002) Guidelines for colorectal cancer screening in high risk groups. *Gut* **51** (suppl V), V1–21.

Endoscopic retrograde cholangiopancreatography (ERCP)

- Side-viewing endoscope used to find the ampulla of Vater and enable cannulation of the biliary and pancreatic ducts for diagnosis and treatment using x-ray screening facilities.
- Using ERCP for diagnosis has been superseded by magnetic resonance cholangiopancreatography (MRCP) which yields the same information without the risks of ERCP.
- ERCP is first line only if therapies are required.
- ERCP requires sedation, an analgesic and buscopan.

Alternative investigations

MRCP allows imaging of the biliary and pancreatic systems but no therapeutic procedures are possible. A percutaneous transhepatic cholangiogram (PTC) allows imaging, stent placement and drainage of a dilated biliary tree using a trans-abdominal approach. PTC is indicated if therapeutic ERCP fails.

Indications

Symptoms and signs

- Endoscopic diagnosis of periampullary polyps and tumours.
- Obtaining bile/brushings for cytology in suspected cholangiocarcinoma.
- Investigation of dilated ducts found on ultrasound scan with contraindications to MRCP.
- Assessment of sphincter of Oddi pressures in suspected sphincter of Oddi dysfunction syndromes (SOD).

Therapeutic

- Biliary stenting.
    - Palliation of pancreatic, ampullary and cholangiocarcinomas.
    - Treatment of biliary leak following surgery.
    - Benign biliary stricture.
- Biliary sphincterotomy.
    - Gaining access to perform diagnostic or therapeutic procedures.
    - Choledocholithiasis.
    - Ampullary carcinoma.
    - Treatment of a biliary leak following surgery.
    - Treatment of sphincter of Oddi dysfunction.
    - Treatment of acute severe pancreatitis secondary to gallstones.
- Pancreatic stenting.
    - Drainage of pseudocysts (via stomach).
    - Following sphincterotomy for SOD.
- Pancreatic sphincterotomy.
    - Pancreatic stone disease.
    - Gaining access prior to stent placement.
    - Minor duct papillotomy in pancreatic divisum to prevent pancreatitis.

Endoscopic ultrasound (EUS)

- Combines endoscopy with ultrasound imaging to allow visualisation of organs such as the pancreas and accurate assessment of degree of invasion of luminal tumours.
- Higher frequency ultrasound probe allowed by proximity of probe to organ results in increased spatial resolution compared with transabdominal ultrasound, CT or MR scanning.
- Two different modes of imaging are possible: radial which allows a 360° view around the shaft of the instrument, or linear which is in line with the endoscope and allows 90° up to 270° views.
- Specialist technique provided in few centres at the present time.
- Pre-procedure preparation is as for OGD or ERCP.
- Consent procedures differ, depending upon indications and potential pathology likely to be found.

Alternative investigations

Transabdominal ultrasound, CT and MRI scanning allow views of the pancreas and liver, but do not allow such fine detail for diagnosis or therapy.

Indications

- Staging of oesophageal, gastric, pancreatic and distal biliary tumours.
- Diagnosis and staging for gastrointestinal stromal tumours.
- Fine needle aspiration of 'Trucut' biopsy of mediastinal or coeliac axis lymph nodes, pancreatic lesions or submucosal lesions.
- Defining mucosal abnormalities such as Barrett's oesophagus.
- Coeliac axis nerve block to treat pancreatic pain (chronic pancreatitis or pancreatic carcinoma).
- Evaluation and treatment of pancreatic pseudocysts.
- Detection of common bile duct stones.

Allum WH, Griffin SM, Watson A, et al. (2002) Guidelines for the management of oesophageal and gastric cancer. Gut **50** (suppl V), v1–23; Soriano A, Castells A, Ayuso C, et al. (2004) Preoperative staging and tumor resectability assessment of pancreatic cancer: prospective study comparing endoscopic ultrasonography, helical computed tomography, magnetic resonance imaging, and angiography. Am J Gastroenterol **99**, 492–501.

Wireless capsule endoscopy (WCE)

- Allows imaging of the entire small bowel by using an 11 × 27mm capsule ('M2A') with up to 7.5h of battery life.
- When swallowed, the capsule transmits images to aerials attached by adhesive pads to the abdominal wall and stored on a recorder attached round the waist.
- Propelled by the patient's own peristalsis so symptom-free.
- Views of the distal small bowel are improved by using one sachet of sodium picolax one day beforehand to remove residue.
- Specialist procedure but with a higher diagnostic yield than other small bowel investigations.
- Prior barium small bowel imaging may be advisable to rule out stricturing where WCE could precipitate obstruction.

Indications
- WCE has a role in visual diagnosis but is unable to obtain samples for subsequent analysis or allow therapeutic management.
- Occult gastrointestinal bleeding with non-diagnostic OGD and colonoscopy.
- Possible small bowel polyposis (e.g. Peutz–Jegher syndrome).
- Unexplained diarrhoea and malabsorption undiagnosed by other methods.

Points for consent
- 1–2% risk of obstruction reported especially if stricturing (e.g. small bowel Crohn's disease) or previous small bowel surgery.
- Contraindicated in patients with a pacemaker.

Table 7.2

Diagnostic yield of small bowel investigations for occult bleeding lesions

	Sensitivity	Specificity	Diagnostic yield
Enteroscopy	37%	97%	30–32%
Wireless capsule endoscopy	64%	92%	55–68%

Mylonaki M, Fritscher-Raven A, Swain CP. (2003) Wireless capsule endoscopy: a comparison with push enteroscopy in patients with gastroscopy and colonoscopy negative gastrointestinal bleeding. *Gut* **52**, 1122–1126; Swain P. (2003) Wireless capsule endoscopy. *Gut* **52**, 48–50.

Tests for *Helicobacter pylori*

Indications for testing

Dyspepsia: patients <55 years of age with a low probability of significant pathology do not require OGD. Non-invasive testing for *H. pylori* allows treatment of those found to be positive to assess effect on symptoms. However, all patients with alarm symptoms (weight loss, anaemia or dysphagia) should undergo urgent OGD. Ensure eradication in patients with confirmed peptic ulceration or MALT-lymphoma.

Non-invasive tests

Serology

Serum IgG antibodies to *H. pylori* may be detected by ELISA with sensitivity of 90% and a specificity up to 90%. IgG levels take up to 1 year to fall so are not useful to confirm response to eradication. Other organisms may cause cross-reactivity. False negatives occur in elderly or immunocompromised patients.

Urea breath test

Expired air is collected after ingestion of ^{13}C-labelled urea. If *H. pylori* present, bacterial urease breaks down urea → ammonium and bicarbonate then → carbon dioxide and ammonia. Expired $^{13}CO_2$ is collected into a tube 30min after ingestion and measured by mass spectrophotometer. This sample is compared with one collected prior to ingestion. This test is almost 100% sensitive and specific and remains the gold standard to confirm eradication.

Faecal antigen test

H. pylori antigens in faeces are measured using an immunochromatographic test. Sensitivity exceeds 91% and specificity exceeds 92%. Using commercial kits, this test may be performed in general practice or hospital out-patients for initial diagnosis or to confirm eradication.

Invasive tests (performed at OGD)

Investigations are based on biopsy samples. *H. pylori* density is usually greatest in the antrum, but during acid suppression the greatest concentration is found in the corpus. Colonisation may be patchy and biopsies are subject to sampling errors.

Histology

H. pylori can be detected on routine histology using the modified Giemsa stain. Sensitivity is 85% with a specificity of almost 100%.

Culture

This is useful in those few patients who have failed eradication to establish antibiotic sensitivities. Sensitivity is over 95% with specificity of almost 100%.

Rapid urease test

A biopsy is placed into a urea solution containing phenol red. *H. pylori* contains urease which releases ammonia from urea changing pH which is detected by the phenol red dye as a colour change from straw to pink/purple. Commercial kits such as the CLO test are available but many endoscopy units use 'homemade' versions. Specificity is 97% and sensitivity between 70–95%.

Calam J. (1996) *Clinicians guide to* Helicobacter pylori. Chapman and Hall Medical, London, UK; Gatta L, Perna F, Ricci C et al. (2004) A rapid immunochromatographic assay for *Helicobacter pylori* in stool before and after treatment. *Aliment Pharmacol Ther* **15**, 469–474.

Faecal occult blood

Indications

- Population screening for colorectal neoplasms—mortality can be decreased by 15 to 33% by population screening.
- Pre-menopausal women to establish whether iron-deficiency anaemia is related to gastrointestinal blood loss (in all other groups, the GI tract should be investigated in iron-deficiency anaemia using OGD and colonoscopy).

Investigation

- Simple and inexpensive, performed by the patient in their own home.
- Samples taken onto test card from 3 consecutive bowel motions and card sent to screening centre.
- Test card uses the 'guaiac' reaction with pseudoperoxidase in haemoglobin causing a colour change in an indicator dye.
- Dietary changes advised (avoid red meat, horseradish, broccoli and turnips as these have high perioxidase activity which may cause false positive results) and vitamin C tablets (high ascorbic acid activity).

Results

- Sensitivity of the non-hydrated test is 70%; this increases to 90% with rehydration but at the loss of specificity. Sensitivity improves with the number of samples taken.
- Individuals who are positive, require full colonoscopy.

Limitations

- Polyps and carcinomas may bleed intermittently but FOB are more likely to be positive with early-stage cancers than polyps.

False positives
- Rehydration of the sample, non-colorectal blood source (upper GI tract or nosebleed), red meat, broccoli or turnips (peroxidase activity).

False negatives
- 'Old' sample with bacterial degradation of haemoglobin, presence of ascorbic acid, reduced or absent bleeding.

Hardcastle JD, Chamberlain JO, Robinson MHE, et al. (1996) Randomised controlled trial of faecal-occult-blood screening for colorectal cancer. *Lancet* **348**, 1472–1477.

Serological testing in inflammatory bowel disease

At present, there are no tests which are sufficiently sensitive or specific to confidently diagnose either ulcerative colitis or Crohn's disease.

Perinuclear antineutrophil cytoplasmic antibodies (pANCA)

Occur in the serum of 50–80% of patients with histologically confirmed ulcerative colitis, but only 10% of those with Crohn's disease. This is likely to be genetically determined. These antibodies are particularly associated with primary sclerosing cholangitis in association with ulcerative colitis.

Antibodies to *Saccharomyces cerevisiae* (ASCA)

Found in 60% of patients with Crohn's disease, but only 5% of those with ulcerative colitis. In Crohn's disease, the presence of high titres of ASCA appears to be associated with early age of onset, and both fibrostenosing and fistulating disease types.

Faecal calprotectin

This is a neutrophil granulocyte cytosol protein which acts as a marker of intestinal inflammation. It is positively correlated with inflammation scores in Crohn's disease and ulcerative colitis. However, it is non-specifically elevated in neoplasia and radiation proctitis. At present it is available in few centres and it identifies a group of patients who require further investigation from those with probable irritable bowel syndrome.

Greig ER, Rampton DS. (2003) *Management of Crohn's Disease.* Martin Dunitz Ltd. London, UK.

Tumour markers

Carcinoembryonic antigen (CEA)

- ↑ in 60% of those with localised colorectal carcinoma and 80–100% of those with metastatic disease.
- Non-specific and non-diagnostic—also ↑ in bronchial carcinoma, heavy smokers, inflammatory bowel disease.
- Levels do not relate to tumour load but a rising level which was previously low or normal, may imply recurrence of colorectal carcinoma.

α-fetoprotein

- Normally produced by fetal liver.
- High levels in non-pregnant adults imply hepatocellular carcinoma (raised in over 90% cases).
- ↑ serological concentrations in pregnancy suggest neural-tube defect.
- Blood levels may be ↑ in hepatocyte regeneration, acute viral hepatitis, cirrhosis, choriocarcinoma and teratoma.

Carbohydrate antigen 19-9 (CA 19-9)

- ↑ in pancreaticobiliary obstruction with the highest levels in pancreatic carcinoma.

- Levels >40IU/L have 75–90% sensitivity and 80–95% specificity for ductal pancreatic carcinoma.
- Serum levels may be elevated in jaundice, cholangitis, choledocholithiasis and chronic pancreatitis.

Sakamoto K, Haga Y, Yoshimura R, Egami H, Yokoyama Y, Akagi M. (1987) Comparative effectiveness of the tumour diagnostics, CA 19-9, CA 125 and carcinoembryonic antigen in patients with diseases of the digestive system. *Gut* **28**, 323–329.

Investigations for small bowel pathology

General investigations

Presenting features of small bowel pathology include diarrhoea (or steatorrhoea), abdominal pain, weight loss and nutritional deficiencies. Investigation of diarrhoea is shown in Fig. 7.4. Occasionally, occult GI bleeding may originate in the small bowel and an algorithm for investigation of anaemia is shown in Fig. 7.5.

Serology

Anti-endomysial antibodies (100% sensitivity for coeliac disease but may be false −ve in presence of a low IgA)—this can be confirmed using duodenal or jejunal biopsies which would reveal partial villous atrophy. Now largely replaced by anti-tissue transglutaminase (see p315).

Endoscopy

OGD and enteroscopy allow views of the small intestine to obtain tissue and allow therapeutic possibilities. Wireless capsule endoscopy allows diagnosis but no therapeutic options.

Radiology

Barium follow-through involves ingestion of dilute barium with images taken every 10–30 minutes until barium reaches the caecum. Small bowel enema (enteroclysis) uses insertion of a nasoduodenal tube to infuse barium slowly, with this column followed continuously using fluoroscopy. Both studies define structural abnormalities. Small bowel enema allows more focused views of areas of interest such as the terminal ileum.

Fig. 7.2 Barium follow-through image showing a terminal ileal stricture.

Nuclear medicine

Radiolabelled white cell scintigraphy for inflammation/infection

This uses ^{99m}-technetium-hexamethylpropyleneamine oxide (^{99m}Tc-HMPAO) to show intensity and extent of inflammation or infection one and three hours after injection of autologous, radiolabelled leucocytes and is used in Crohn's disease and ulcerative colitis to delineate disease extent. False negative results occur, particularly with small bowel Crohn' disease. There is a sensitivity of 96% and specificity of 97% for inflammatory bowel disease and a sensitivity of 85–100% and specificity of 100% for detecting abscesses. (See 📖*Nuclear medicine*, p788).

Fig. 7.3 Radiolabelled white cell scintigraphy using ^{99m}-technetium-hexa-propyleneamine oxide (^{99m}-Tc-HMPAO) to show inflammation of the terminal ileum consistent with Crohn's disease (image taken at 3h).

Radionuclide studies to detect Meckel's diverticulum

Intravenous ^{99m}-Tc pertechnate accumulates in gastric mucosa with a time course of 5–60 minutes. Uptake in ectopic mucosa (e.g. Meckel's diverticulum) occurs simultaneously. Imaging at 5–10 minute intervals up to 2 hours after injection allows localisation of the site of ectopic mucosa. False positives are caused by early gastric emptying and duplication cysts. Sensitivities vary from 90% in children to 60% in adults. (See 📖*Nuclear medicine*, p784).

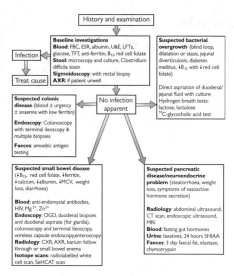

Fig. 7.4 Investigation of diarrhoea.

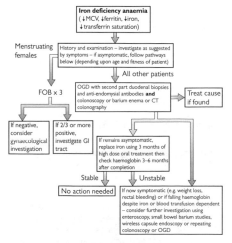

Fig. 7.5 An algorithm for investigation of anaemia.

Cooney DR, Duszynski DO, Gamboa E et al. (1982). The abnormal technetium scan (a decade of experience). J Paediatr Surg **17**, 611–619.

Tests of absorption

Tests of carbohydrate malabsorption

D-xylose tolerance test

Xylose is absorbed from the proximal small bowel, and urinary excretion and blood levels reflect absorption. It is used mainly in paediatric practice and has a low sensitivity.

Lactose tolerance test

Oral administration of 50g lactose is followed by blood sampling every 30 minutes for 2 hours. A rise in blood glucose <1.1mmol/L suggests deficiency of disaccharidases, especially with colicky abdominal pain and diarrhoea.

Lactose-hydrogen test

This is similar to the hydrogen breath test for bacterial overgrowth. Lactase-deficient individuals fail to metabolise lactose which normally undergoes luminal metabolism by lactase-producing colonic bacteria to yield hydrogen.

Tests of fat malabsorption

Patients with fat malabsorption secondary to small bowel diseases such as coeliac disease or tropical sprue may malabsorb between 10 and 20g/d of fat while patients with pancreatic insufficiency may malabsorb 30–50g/24 hours. A normal faecal fat excretion is less than 6g/d (17mmol/day).

3-day faecal fat

- Unpleasant test, fallen into disuse but remains gold standard.
- Fat content measured in a 3-day faecal collection.
- Patient takes standard diet of 100g fat per day.
- Does not differentiate small bowel and pancreatic malabsorption.

Radiolabelled ^{14}C fat breath test

- ^{14}C triolein is ingested and $^{14}CO_2$ measured in breath.
- Small bowel malabsorption shows delayed $^{14}CO_2$ excretion.
- Pancreatic malaborption shows low $^{14}CO_2$ excretion which is corrected using oral pancreatic enzyme supplements such as Creon.

Fat microscopy

- Examines faeces for neutral fat, fatty acid crystals and soaps.
- Limited value as it neither quantifies levels nor suggests a cause.

Bile salt malabsorption

SeHCAT scan

- The labelled bile acid ^{75}selenium homotaurocholate (SeHCAT) is administered orally. Retention is measured at 7 days by whole body counting.
- Retention >15% SeHCAT is normal (less indicates malabsorption).
- Useful second line investigation in patients with diarrhoea of unknown aetiology.

Wildt S, Norby Rasmussen S, Lysgard Madsen J et al. (2003) Bile acid malabsorption in patients with chronic diarrhoea: clinical value of SeHCAT test. *Scand J Gastroenterol* **38**, 826–830.

Tests for bacterial overgrowth

Deep duodenal/jejunal aspiration

- Samples may be collected through the biopsy channel at OGD.
- Scanty bacteria are present in normal upper small bowel.
- Numbers in excess of 10^6/mL of aspirated fluid are pathological.
- This technique may culture Giardia and Strongyloides species.

Hydrogen breath tests

Rationale

In mammals, the only source of breath hydrogen is bacterial fermentation of carbohydrates. Hydrogen is absorbed from the intestinal lumen and expired during breathing. In bacterial overgrowth, hydrogen production can occur in the small intestine as well as in the colon.

Method

- A mouthwash is given beforehand to reduce contamination by oral bacteria.
- Test dose of glucose (50g) and breath hydrogen measured.
- An early peak (e.g. 40 minutes) suggests bacterial overgrowth.

Limitations

- Sensitivity 60–90% with specificity of 80%.
- False negatives result from variations in microflora present in the small intestine or antibiotic administration within 3 weeks.
- False positives occur in patients with impaired glucose tolerance, those with rapid transit to the colon, and smokers.
- Patients should avoid eating pulses for 48 hours prior to the test (normal digestion of pulses liberates excess hydrogen).

Alternative

- Lactulose 10–15g (a non-absorbable disaccharide) which ferments in the small intestine if bacterial overgrowth is present producing hydrogen.
- Rapid transit to the colon will also produce an early peak.

^{14}C-glycocholic acid test

Rationale

- Bacteria act to deconjugate radiolabelled bile salts to produce radioactive glycine which is metabolised in the liver to $^{14}CO_2$.
- An early peak suggests either bacterial overgrowth of the small intestine or rapid transit to the colon.

Method

- The patient is given ^{14}C-labelled bile salts by mouth and breath $^{14}CO_2$ is measured in expired air.
- An early peak suggests bacterial overgrowth (or rapid small intestinal transit).

Limitations
- Difficult to distinguish between small bowel overgrowth and other causes of bile salt malabsorption, e.g. ileal dysfunction, unless faecal bile acid excretion is measured.
- Ileal dysfunction leads to a late peak in $^{14}CO_2$ and high faecal bile acids while bacterial overgrowth results in increased and early breath excretion of $^{14}CO_2$ and low faecal bile acid excretion (<5%).
- It necessitates using radiolabelled bile acids and has few advantages over a hydrogen breath test unless faecal bile acid excretion is measured.

Tests of pancreatic exocrine function

Symptoms of pancreatic exocrine dysfunction include diarrhoea or steatorrhoea and weight loss. Investigations aim to determine the degree of pancreatic insufficiency; however, both biochemical and particularly radiological investigations are unreliable in mild disease. Fat malabsorption may occur in small bowel or pancreatic disease and diagnosis (see p454). A diagnostic algorithm for investigation of diarrhoea is shown on p453.

Faecal testing
Elastase
Elastase is a proteinase produced by pancreatic acinar cells and remains undegraded during gut transit. Immunoassay of faeces allows measurement of elastase in a random faecal sample. Levels of >200µg/g faeces are normal, 100–200 represents mild insufficiency and <100 is diagnostic of severe disease. Sensitivity and specificity are high; however false positives occur with high volume watery stools. This test is not affected by pancreatic enzyme supplements.

Chymotrypsin
This proteinase is cheaper to measure in faeces but is less sensitive than elastase and its use is mainly in children to screen for cystic fibrosis. Result is affected by pancreatic enzyme supplements.

Direct investigations
Secretin test
Direct intubation of the duodenum allows collection of pancreatic juice following intravenous injection of a hormonal secretogogue. Secretin injection allows measurement of volume and bicarbonate content, cholecystokinin (CCK) injection allows measurement of amylase, trypsin and lipase. This test is highly sensitive and specific even with mild pancreatic disease, but is not widely available.

Indirect investigations
Both tests are more sensitive and specific with more advanced pancreatic exocrine dysfunction.

PABA

A synthetic peptide (N-benzoyl-L-tyrosol *p*-aminobenzoic acid) is given orally. In normal patients, pancreatic chymotrypsin hydrolyses this peptide to yield free PABA which is absorbed, metabolised, and excreted in urine. In the presence of pancreatic insufficiency, free PABA levels are reduced and thus absorption and excretion are lower. This results in lower urinary PABA and a lower serum concentration.

Pancreolauryl test

Fluorescein dilaurate (an ester) is taken orally with a set diet. In the presence of normal pancreatic function, arylesterases release fluorescein which is absorbed, partially conjugated in liver, and excreted in urine. A 24h urine collection for excreted levels shows close correlation with pancreatic exocrine function.

Testing for neuroendocrine tumours

Carcinoid and carcinoid syndrome

Urinary 5-hydroxyindole acetic acid (5HIAA)

- 24h collection of urine for 5HIAA.
- High levels imply carcinoid syndrome.
- High specificity but false positives result from serotonin-rich bananas, tomatoes or drugs such as phenothiazines and reserpine.

Further investigations

Abdominal CT scan with biopsy of liver metastases may confirm the diagnosis. The primary tumour is identified in only 50–70%. Radiolabelled octreotide scintigraphy establishes tumour extent in difficult cases as most carcinoid tumours express somatostatin receptors.

Hormone-secreting pancreatic tumours

- Pancreatic islet-cell tumours which produce vasoactive peptide hormones.
- Measured using fasting gut hormone assays.
- Single tumours often secrete more than one type of hormone.
- Up to 50% of these slow-growing tumours are thought to be non-functional.
- Several types of tumour occur as part of the multiple endocrine neoplasia syndrome type 1 (MEN-1).
- Hormones to measure are: *insulin* (paired with a serum glucose sample), *glucagon*, *vasoactive intestinal peptide* (VIP), *pancreatic polypeptide* (PP), *gastrin* and *somatostatin*.
- Concurrent therapy with a proton pump inhibitor will falsely raise serum gastrin levels.

Further investigations

- Abdominal CT scan.
- Endoscopic ultrasound.
- Laparoscopy.

- Radiolabelled octreotide scintigraphy.
- Rarely, selective venous sampling will confirm the diagnosis.

Oberg K. (1999) Neuroendocrine gastrointestinal tumours—a condensed overview of diagnosis and treatment. *Ann Oncol* **10** (suppl 2), S2–8.

Fig. 7.6 Endoscopic image of a rectal carcinoid tumour. **(Colour plate 5.)**

Gastrointestinal physiology

pH monitoring

Indications
- Assessment of gastro-oesophageal reflux disease (GORD).
- Atypical symptoms such as asthma or non-cardiac chest pain.
- Before consideration of anti-reflux surgery.
- Poorly controlled GORD to confirm diagnosis on or off treatment.

Investigation
An ambulatory 24h test which places a pH electrode through the nose to sit 5cm above the lower oesophageal sphincter. This is connected to a portable microprocessor which records episodes where the pH dips below 4. The patient fills in a simultaneous event diary, to correlate symptoms and episodes of low pH. For most patients, H_2 receptor antagonists and proton pump inhibitors are stopped 7 days beforehand. A few patients require testing on medication to establish treatment response.

Results
Several parameters are collected
- Frequency and duration of episodes of pH <4.
- Duration of longest episode.
- Correlation between symptoms and pH.
- Excessive oesophageal acid reflux is defined as a total duration of pH <4 of 4–6% of recording time.

Oesophageal manometry

Indications
- Diagnosis and assessment of motility disorders suggested by symptoms/OGD/barium swallow findings.
- Defining the precise location of the lower oesophageal sphincter prior to 24h pH monitoring.
- Before consideration of anti-reflux surgery.

Investigation
A static test using a nasogastrically-placed multiple channel, water perfused catheter which is gradually withdrawn during a series of wet and dry swallows. Pressure is measured through the length of the oesophagus, at the upper and lower oesophageal sphincter and the duration and frequency of contractions are recorded.

Table 7.3 Results

Non-specific motility disorder	Abnormal and incomplete peristalsis with normal body contractions
Achalasia	Incomplete relaxation and high pressure of lower oesophageal sphincter with aperistalsis of the oesophageal body
Nutcracker oesophagus	High amplitude and duration of contractions, normal peristalsis
Oesophageal spasm	Disordered peristalsis with simultaneous prolonged contractions throughout

Gastric emptying

Scintigraphy using the radioactive tracer ^{99m}technetium displays gastric movements with a range of test meals (liquid to solid) to quantify gastric emptying and intestinal filling over time. This confirms dysmotility although in practice, barium and endoscopic studies provide enough information. (See 📖 *Nuclear medicine*, p.782.)

Intestinal transit studies

Intestinal transit may be established using 50 radioopaque plastic markers inside a pH-sensitive gel capsule, which is designed to release its contents in the terminal ileum. An abdominal radiograph at 100 hours should show less than 20% of markers present in the colon. A rarely used alternative is radioactive indium-labelled polystyrene pellets with gamma camera recording of the pellet's progress through the intestine. These investigations are useful to determine colonic transit in suspected slow transit constipation. Normal transit from mouth to anus is 1–3 days.

Anorectal manometry

A water-perfused catheter measures anorectal pressures to assess voluntary and involuntary sphincter squeeze pressures and reflex responses to balloon distension in the rectum. Readings allow assessment of rectal sensation, spinal reflexes, and internal and external sphincter integrity. These tests are useful for assessment of faecal soiling, incontinence and chronic constipation.

Sphincter of Oddi manometry

A water-perfused pressure catheter is used during ERCP to measure sphincter of Oddi pressures to formally diagnose sphincter of Oddi dysfunction (SOD: a triad of abnormal liver function, biliary type abdominal pain and dilatation of the biliary tree in the absence of a physical cause such as gallstone disease). Diagnosis is confirmed by high resting pressure, retrograde peristalsis and a failure of contrast to drain from the biliary tree within 45 minutes. Although patients with SOD have an increased risk of pancreatitis after ERCP, biliary sphincterotomy may relieve symptoms of pain.

Non-invasive liver investigations

Basic liver function testing

These are basic serological screening tests which establish whether liver inflammation, infection or obstruction is present.

Alanine transaminase
(ALT: cytosol enzyme specific to the liver) and *aspartate transaminase* (AST: mitochondrial enzyme also present in heart, muscle, kidney and brain)—both enzymes are present in hepatocytes and leak into blood with liver cell damage.

Alkaline phosphatase
(ALP: canalicular and sinusoidal membranes of liver but also bone, intestine, placenta)—specific isoenzymes for ALP are produced by different tissues but a simultaneously raised γGT and ALP implies a hepatic origin. Extra- and intrahepatic cholestasis may cause raised ALP and result from benign or malignant disease with or without raised bilirubin. Highest levels result from primary biliary cirrhosis and hepatic metastases.

γ-glutamyl transpeptidase
(γGT: microsomal enzyme)—activity can be induced by drugs such as phenytoin, rifampicin and alcohol. Mild elevation of γGT is common with even a small alcohol intake and isolated elevation does not imply liver disease. It rises in parallel with ALP in cholestasis.

Albumin
A protein which is synthesised in the liver. Plasma concentration partially results from functional capacity within the liver. However, it has a serum half-life of 20 days and may be normal in early phases of acute liver disease. Hypoalbuminaemia may also arise from an increased volume of distribution (sepsis, overhydration, pregnancy); increased excretion or degradation (nephrotic syndrome, protein-losing enteropathy); haemorrhage; or catabolic states such as malignancy or burns.

Prothrombin time (PT)
Test of plasma clotting activity and reflects the activity of vitamin K-dependent clotting factors synthesised by the liver. PT may be elevated in acute or chronic liver disease. In vitamin K deficiency with normal liver function, PT will return to normal within 18 hours of administration of parenteral vitamin K.

Bilirubin
In liver disease, a raised bilirubin is usually associated with other liver function abnormalities. There are many causes of raised serum bilirubin. Bilirubin may be conjugated or unconjugated, although in practice, this conjugation state only differentiates congenital hyperbilirubinaemias. In Gilbert's syndrome (the most common, benign cause of an isolated raised serum bilirubin) an elevated unconjugated bilirubin which rises during fasting and mild illness diagnoses the condition.

Immunoglobulins
- IgG ↑ in viral hepatitis, chronic autoimmune hepatitis and cirrhosis.

- IgM ↑ in primary biliary cirrhosis, non-biliary cirrhosis and acute viral hepatitis.
- IgA is ↑ in alcoholic liver disease with β–γ fusion seen on electrophoresis.

Specific biochemical tests

These are summarised in Table 7.4, with serological tests, diagnosis and definitive investigations required to confirm the diagnosis.

Specific virological tests

Hepatitis A (HAV)

- Acute infection—positive IgM antibodies to HAV.
- Chronic infection—does not occur.
- Markers of clearing virus—positive IgG antibodies to HAV and anti-HAV IgM.

Hepatitis B (HBV)

Acute infection with subsequent clearing of virus

- HBsAg appears in blood from 6–12 weeks after infection then disappears.
- HBeAg appears early then declines rapidly.
- Anti-HBs appears late and indicates immunity.
- Anti-HBc is the first antibody to appear and IgM anti-HBc may persist for many months as the only marker of ongoing viral replication when HBsAg has disappeared and anti-HBs is not yet detectable.
- Anti-HBe appears after anti-HBc and indicates decreased infectivity.

Acute infection leading to chronic hepatitis B

- HBsAg persists and indicates chronic carrier state.
- HBeAg persists, correlating with increased severity and infectivity.
- Anti-HBe indicates seroconversion (if this occurs) with disappearance of HBeAg and a rise in ALT.
- HBV DNA suggests continued viral replication.

Hepatitis C (HCV)

- Acute infection—HCV RNA is positive 1–2 weeks after infection with HCV antibodies developing after ~12 weeks.
- Chronic infection—more than 50% patients with persistent HCV RNA which can be measured as viral load.
- Hepatitis C has 6 genotypes which determine response to treatment.

Hepatitis E (HEV).

- Similar to hepatitis A with no chronic or carrier state.

Investigation of liver disease

Figure 7.7 shows an algorithm for investigation of liver disease. This differentiates obstructive from parenchymal liver disease to suggest further investigation and treatment.

Specific biochemical tests

Advised by history, examination or basic liver screen abnormalities

Table 7.4

Test	Condition	Findings	More specific tests
Serum ferritin Serum iron Transferrin saturation	Haemochromatosis	Serum iron >30µmol/L Serum ferritin >500µg/L Transferrin sat >60%	HFE gene testing (83–90% patients have Cys 282 Tyr mutation; 25% have His 63 Asp; 187G in complete linkage disequilibrium with Cys 282 Tyr)
Urinary copper excretion Serum copper Caeruloplasmin	Wilson's disease	Serum copper and caeruloplasmin levels are usually reduced but can be normal	Liver biopsy—with dry weight of iron Liver biopsy—with dry weight of copper
α1-antitrypsin	α1-antitrypsin def.	Levels of <10% of normal in homozygotes and 60% in heterozygotes	Liver biopsy and lung function testing for emphysema
Anti-mitochondrial antibodies (AMA)	Primary biliary cirrhosis	Antimitochondrial antibodies present in titres >1/160 specific M2 antibody (possible non-specific ↑ ANA/SMA)	Liver biopsy
Anti-nuclear antibodies (ANA)/anti-smooth muscle antibodies (SMA)	Type I autoimmune hepatitis	↑ ANA ± SMA ↑ total IgG	Liver biopsy
Anti-liver/kidney microsomal (anti-LKM1) or anti-liver cytosol anti-bodies	Type II autoimmune hepatitis	↑ antibodies titres ↑ total IgG	Liver biopsy
Fasting cholesterol and glucose, glycosylated haemoglobin	Non-alcoholic fatty liver disease/ non-alcoholic Steatohepatitis	Impaired glucose tolerance	Liver biopsy

Fig. 7.7 An algorithm for investigation of liver disease.

Liver biopsy

- Obtains tissue for diagnosis of diffuse or localised parenchymal disease.
- Severity of histological liver dysfunction cannot be predicted from basic LFTs.
- Consent should be obtained based on risks (see *below*).
- Transjugular liver biopsy overcomes many contraindications (see *below*).

Indications

- Unexplained persistently abnormal LFTs.
- Staging of disease in hepatitis B or C infection, and prior to considering antiviral treatment.
- Acute hepatitis of unknown aetiology.
- Cirrhosis of unknown aetiology.
- Alcohol-related liver disease.
- Primary biliary cirrhosis/chronic active hepatitis.
- Targeted liver biopsy of lesions (not if resection is a possibility).
- Pyrexia of unknown origin.
- Haemochromatosis/Wilson's disease.
- Storage diseases.
- Post-liver transplant to rule out acute or chronic rejection.

Methods for obtaining tissue: (risks and benefits)

Percutaneous with or without ultrasound viewing

- Standard method for obtaining tissue.
- Ultrasonography of liver and biliary tree pre-procedure to identify anatomical variations increasing risk and to rule out obstruction.
- Most complications <2h but can occur up to 24h.
- No evidence that direct ultrasound-guided biopsy is safer and ultrasound should be used only if a targeted biopsy is required.

Contraindications

- An uncooperative or confused patient.
- PT prolonged by >3 seconds, platelets <80 x 10^9/L or bleeding diathesis.
- Ascites.
- Hydatid cysts (risks of anaphylaxis and abdominal seeding).
- Extrahepatic cholestasis.
- Higher risk of bleeding if amyloidosis present.

Minor complications

- Shoulder tip pain, minor intra-abdominal bleeding or mild abdominal pain (up to 30%)—usually settles with analgesia.

Major complications

- Perforation (0.01–0.1%: pneumothorax, gallbladder puncture, kidney, colon).
- Intra-abdominal haemorrhage; haemobilia (0.05%: a triad of biliary colic, jaundice and melaena within 3 days of liver biopsy).
- Mortality varies between 0.01–0.1% and results from intra-peritoneal haemorrhage or biliary peritonitis.
- Risk of tumour seeding if a malignant lesion is biopsied: if curative resection is planned, needle biopsy should be avoided.

Transjugular
- Specialist technique carried out using fluoroscopic guidance.
- Catheter passes from the right internal jugular vein, through the right atrium, inferior vena cava and into the hepatic veins.
- Patient holds his/her breath while the biopsy needle is advanced through the catheter then rapidly pushed forward by 1–2cm into the liver to obtain a small core of liver parenchyma.
- Safe technique with few complications (1.3–20% morbidity and 0.5% mortality) usually performed in higher risk patients.
- Complications range from neck haematoma, puncture of intrathoracic arteries, transient Horner's syndrome, cardiac arrhythmias, infection and perforation of the liver capsule.
- Test of choice in patients excluded from percutaneous biopsy by coagulopathy, bleeding diathesis, ascites, portal hypertension and amyloidosis.
- Transjugular cannulation allows measurement of portal venous pressures.

Laparoscopic
- Allows sampling of the liver when an operation is planned.
- Allows targeted biopsies as well as parenchymal biopsies.
- Bleeding is directly controlled and perforation is avoided.
- Risks of surgery and anaesthesia should be considered.

Grant A, Neuberger J, Day C, Saxseena S. (2004). Guidelines on the use of liver biopsy in clinical practice. *British Society of Gastroenterology* October 2004, 1–15. ⬧ www.bsg.org.uk

Table 7.5 Percutaneous liver biopsy—practical procedure

Procedure	Should be carried out by an experienced doctor using aseptic precautions
Check	Clotting, FBC, and take G&S within 24h before procedure (cancel if platelets <80 x 10^9/L or PT prolonged >3 sec)
Patient	Lies flat on his/her back
Liver margins	Delineated using percussion or ultrasound
1% lignocaine	5mL injected at the point of maximal dullness down to the liver capsule through intercostal space in expiration
Menghini or Trucut needle	Used to obtain sample with patient's breath held in expiration (up to 2 passes may be used) Menghini needles use suction, have a lower rate of complications and allow more rapid biopsy but have a lower yield for tissue than Trucut (a cutting needle)
Sample	Placed into 10% formalin (or into a dry pot to estimate dry weight of iron or copper or for culture)
Patient	Nurse in supine position or right lateral for >6h with regular BP and pulse measurements (every 15min for 2h, every 30min for the next 2h then hourly) with urgent medical review if any sign of deterioration
If stable	At 6 hours, the patient can be discharged home as long as s/he can return to hospital within 30 minutes and have a responsible adult with him/her overnight

Investigations of ascitic fluid

Fluid in the peritoneal cavity has multiple causes.

Investigation requires diagnostic aspiration of 40–50mL fluid

- 10mL is sent for cell count, Gram stain, Ziehl–Neelsen (ZN) stain culture (10mL should be added to a pair of blood culture bottles to increase diagnostic yield).
- 10mL is sent for cytology.
- 10mL for biochemical investigation of protein, glucose, lactate dehydrogenase (LDH), triglycerides (if chylous ascites is suspected), and amylase if pancreatic ascites is suspected.

Results

Cell count
- Polymorphonuclear leucocytes (neutrophils) >250cells/mm^3 suggest underlying spontaneous bacterial peritonitis (or secondary infection).
- Total leucocytes of >500cells/mm^3 imply peritonitis if a specific neutrophil count is not available.
- WBC count >500cells/mm^3 implies tuberculous peritonitis (seen in association with a raised protein, a positive ZN stain or TB culture and a low glucose).

Gram stain and culture
- Gram staining for early identification of bacteria and bacterial culture allows targeting of antimicrobial therapy.

Protein
- Ascitic fluid is divided into transudates (ascitic protein >11g/L below serum albumin concentration) and exudates (levels closer to serum albumin concentration).
- Risk of spontaneous bacterial peritonitis is greatest if ascitic protein concentration <10g/L.

Cytology
- Diagnostic in cases of peritoneal malignancy.

Amylase
- ↑ ascitic amylase (usually in order of 2000 IU/L) is typical of pancreatic ascites.

Triglycerides
- ↑ in chylous ascites.

Table 7.6 Ascitic fluid aspiration—practical procedure

Patient	Lies on his/her back tilting towards one side
Percussion	Used to find shifting dullness in left or right lower quadrant
Chlorhexidine or betadine	Used to clean the site
Lignocaine	2–3mL of 1% used to infiltrate a site in the left or right lower quadrant and below the site where shifting dullness is detected. It should be possible to aspirate ascitic fluid using a standard 19G needle
50mL syringe	With a sterile 19G needle is placed through the same site to obtain the samples required
Rare complications	Include bowel perforation, secondary bacterial peritonitis or haemorrhage

Respiratory medicine

Airway hyperresponsiveness test or histamine/methacholine
    challenge test 472
Arterial blood gas sampling 474
Diagnostic pleural aspiration 476
Epworth test/Epworth sleepiness scale (ESS) 478
Exercise testing 480
Exhaled nitric oxide 482
Fibreoptic bronchoscopy & video bronchoscopy 484
'Fitness to fly' assessment 486
Flow volume loops/maximum expiratory flow-volume curve 488
Nijmegen questionnaire 490
Peak flow charts 492
Pleural needle biopsy 496
Polysomnography 498
Pulse oximetry 500
Skin prick tests 501
Spirometry 502
Sputum microscopy & culture/sputum cytology 504
Static lung volumes/whole body plethysmography 506
Sweat test 510
Medical thoracoscopy 512
Transfer factor 514

Airway hyperresponsiveness test or histamine/methacholine challenge test

Clinical indications
Suspected asthma.

Patient preparation
1. Explain procedure to patient.
2. Obtain informed consent.
3. Warn that wheezing and shortness of breath may occur and that a bronchodilator may be given.
4. Baseline FEV_1 measured.
5. Patient breathes in a nebulised aerosol of histamine (or methacholine) of increasing concentrations. This stimulates bronchoconstriction in a dose-dependent manner.
6. The FEV_1 is measured after each dose.
7. Patient must remain in department for 30min following the procedure to observe any delayed reactions.

Possible results
The % fall in FEV_1 from baseline is plotted against the dose of inhaled histamine on a logarithmic scale. A dose–response curve is constructed and the provocation concentration (PC) of inhaled histamine required to reduce the FEV_1 by 20% (PC_{20}) can be derived by linear extrapolation. This figure has been arbitrarily chosen to assess degrees of bronchial reactivity for ease of comparison and safety.

Interpretation
Asthma suggested by PC_{20} <8mg/mL.

A direct relationship exists between the severity of asthma and requirement for medication and the PC_{20} value as an index of bronchial hyperresponsiveness.

Non-asthmatic subjects almost always have a PC_{20} >8mg/mL.

Advantages over other tests
- Easy to do.
- Cheap.
- Non-invasive.
- Quick.
- Reproducible.
- Safe: bronchoconstriction may be reversed by inhaled β-adrenergic agonist. It is important that personnel performing the test are able to recognise severe bronchospasm and that resuscitation equipment is available.

Contraindications
- Documented cholinergic hypersensitivity, e.g. cholinergic urticaria or angio-oedema or both.
- Allergy to histamine/methacholine.

- Inability to perform acceptable quality spirometry
- Unstable cardiac status, e.g. recent MI, arrhythmia or heart failure.
- Uncontrolled hypertension (systolic BP >200 or diastolic BP >100).
- Pregnancy.
- Severe baseline obstruction with FEV_1 <80% predicted or <1.5 litres.

Ancillary tests

PEFR chart: diurnal variation.

Pitfalls

- Bronchial hyperresponsiveness in asthma is not a static phenomenon and may vary widely from day to day.
- May change quite markedly without any change in symptoms (and vice versa).
- Represents only one component contributing to the symptomatology of asthma:
  - Others include airway oedema and mucus hypersecretion.

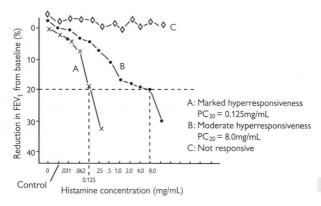

Fig. 8.1 Differing responses to varying concentrations of histamine.

Pratter MR, Irwin S. (1984) The clinical value of pharmacologic bronchoprovocation challenge. *Chest* **85**, 260–265; Lotvall J, Inman M, O'Byrne P. (1998) Measurement of airway hyperresponsiveness: new considerations. *Thorax* **53**, 419–424; Smith CM, Anderson SD. (1989) Inhalation provocation tests using nonisotonic aerosols. *J Allergy Clin Immunol* **84**, 781–790. Crapo RO, Casaburi R, Coates AL et al. (2000) Guidelines for methacholine and exercise challenge testing-1999. *Am J Respir Crit Care Med* **161**, 309–329.

Arterial blood gas sampling

Clinical indications
- Breathlessness (acute or chronic).
- Cardiorespiratory failure.
- Metabolic disturbance.
- Poisoning with drugs.
- Acute asthma with O_2 saturation <92% (on air).

📖OHCM p193.

Patient preparation
Informed consent (verbal usually satisfactory).

Common sites: radial/brachial/femoral arteries.

Contraindications to radial
- Absent ulnar circulation.
- AV fistula for dialysis.
- Fractured wrist.
- Poor peripheral circulation.

Contraindications to brachial
- AV fistula.
- Fractured elbow.
- Poor peripheral circulation.

Contraindications to femoral
- Presence of graft/extensive vascular disease.

Procedure
1. Identify pulse.
2. Clean skin with alcohol swab.
3. Confirm position of maximum pulsation with non-dominant hand.
4. Local anaesthetic reduces pain.
5. Insert 23G needle attached to heparinised syringe.
6. If using low-resistance syringe this will fill automatically, otherwise aspirate gently.
7. Remove needle and apply firm gentle pressure with cotton wool ball for 5min.
8. Label hazardous specimens.
9. Expel air bubbles from sample.

Possible results
- Hypoxia with normal CO_2.
- Hypoxia with ↑ CO_2.
- Normoxia with ↓ CO_2.
- Metabolic acidosis *vs.* compensation.

📖OHCM pp154, 682.

Interpretation
Must be aware of the patient's inspired oxygen concentration (FiO_2) at time of sampling.

Advantages over other tests
- Easy, quick, cheap.
- No real alternative for assessing CO_2 or acid–base balance.
- Greater precision in upper ranges of SaO_2 curve.

Ancillary tests
- Pulse oximetry: gives indication of oxygenation status but not CO_2 levels.
- Arterialised blood sampling.

Complications
- Haematoma.
- Nerve damage.
- Inadvertent venous sampling.

Pitfalls
- If sample is to be analysed in a laboratory with >5min transit time it should be kept in melting ice to slow the metabolic activity of the cells.
- Avoid arterial puncture if possible in patients on anticoagulant therapy, with bleeding disorders or who have received thrombolytics in previous 24h.
- Failure to note FiO_2 will lead to difficulty in interpretation and potential therapeutic errors.

Fig. 8.2 Dissociation curve for oxyhaemoglobin.

Carruthers DM, Harrison BD. (1995) Arterial blood gas analysis or oxygen saturation in the assessment of acute asthma? *Thorax* **50**, 186–188; Syabbalo N. (1997) Measurement and interpretation of arterial blood gases. *Br J Clin Pract* **51**, 173–176.

Diagnostic pleural aspiration

Clinical indications

Pleural effusion detected clinically *and* with imaging, e.g. CXR, USS, CT chest.

Patient preparation

1. Informed consent (verbal usually acceptable).
2. Patient sitting with arms forward supported on table/pillows.
3. Posterior or axillary approach if effusion large (otherwise be guided by USS).
4. Clean skin with iodine solution.
5. Infiltrate area one rib space below upper level of dullness to percussion with local anaesthetic (1% or 5% lignocaine).
6. Insert 19G needle attached to 50mL syringe. *Note*: ensure needle enters immediately above rib to avoid the neurovascular bundle.
7. Aspirate fluid. If no fluid then try adjusting angle of needle.
8. Remove needle and apply plaster.
9. Post-aspiration CXR.

Possible results

- Pleural fluid is normally straw coloured.
- Pleural fluid analysed for protein, glucose, LDH, microbiology, cytology and pH.
- If heavily bloodstained suspect malignancy, pulmonary infarction or trauma. A traumatic tap will become progressively less bloodstained.
- If pus present: empyema.
- If creamy opalescent fluid: chylothorax (lymphoma, trauma to thoracic duct, yellow nail syndrome, lymphangioleiomyomatosis) or pseudo-chylothorax, e.g. in TB or RA.

Interpretation See Table 8.1.

Advantages over other tests

- Quick and easy.
- Cheap.
- Relatively non-invasive.
- Provides cytological, microbiological and biochemical data.

Ancillary tests

- Thoracoscopy.
- Pleural needle biopsy.

Pitfalls

- Traumatic tap.
- Difficult to locate effusion if loculated: use USS chest to guide aspiration attempt.

Complications

- Haemorrhage.
- Pneumothorax.

Table 8.1

Cytology	+ve in ~60% especially carcinoma of lung/breast Increased diagnostic rate with repeated sampling
Protein	Exudate >30g/L protein Transudate <30g/L protein
PH	<7.0: empyema, oesophageal rupture >7.0 and <7.3: collagen disorders, TB, malignancy, empyema
Glucose	↓ in RA, TB, malignancy, infection
Microbiology	Organisms, ZN stain
Eosinophilia	>10% in benign asbestos effusions, parasitic, hydropneumothorax
Neutrophilia	>1.0 × 10⁹/L in acute inflammation, e.g. pneumonia, infarction
Lymphocytosis	Chronic effusions, e.g. TB, malignancy or RA
Amylase	↑↑↑ in pancreatitis ↑ in oesophageal rupture (salivary amylase) ↑ in malignancy
ANF	>1:160 virtually diagnostic of SLE
LDH	↑ in infection
Rheumatoid factor	+ve in RA
Complement	↓ in RA, SLE, malignancy, infection

Epworth test/Epworth sleepiness scale (ESS)

Clinical indications
Screening tool for obstructive sleep apnoea. Measures general level of daytime sleepiness.

Patient preparation
1. Ask patient to fill in questionnaire.
2. Subject rates on a scale of 0–3 the chances that, as part of his usual life in recent times, he would doze in each of 8 different situations.

Use the following scale to choose the most appropriate number for each situation:

0 = Would NEVER doze
1 = SLIGHT chance of dozing
2 = MODERATE chance of dozing
3 = HIGH chance of dozing

Situation
- Sitting and reading.
- Watching TV.
- Sitting inactive in a public place (e.g. theatre or a meeting).
- As a passenger in a car for an hour without a break.
- Lying down to rest in the afternoon when circumstances permit.
- Sitting and talking to someone.
- Sitting quietly after lunch without alcohol.
- In a car, while stopped for a few minutes in the traffic.

Possible results
ESS score is the sum of eight item scores and can range from 0 to 24.

Interpretation
Clinically normal score = 10. Each ESS item gives an estimate of sleep propensity in one of eight specific situations whereas the total ESS score gives a measure of more general average sleep propensity. Does not measure 'subjective' sleepiness.

Advantages over other tests
- Cheap.
- Easily administered.

Ancillary tests
- Polysomnography/Visi-Lab studies.
- Stanford sleepiness scale.

- Multiple sleep latency test.
- Maintenance of wakefulness test.

Pitfalls

Limited by patient's ability to read and comprehend the questionnaire and answer questions honestly.

Exercise testing

Clinical indications
- To confirm that reduced exercise tolerance exists.
- To determine the degree of impairment and disability.
- To investigate which system appears responsible for the reduction.
- To evaluate treatment results.
- To plan rehabilitation.

Patient preparation
1. Evaluate patient's medical history for contraindications to test.
2. Warn patient of cardiovascular complications (e.g. mortality 1:10,000 tests).
3. Obtain written consent.
4. Patient to wear comfortable clothes and shoes.
5. Monitoring: ECG, O_2 saturation, BP.
6. Exercise: treadmill/bike/free run on flat surface.
7. Steady state 5–12min walking test (usually 6min) or stepped stress test.
8. During a maximal exercise test the patient should be able to achieve 85–90% of predicted maximum heart rate.

Contraindications to test
- Unstable myocardium (recent MI, unstable angina, arrhythmias, severe valvular heart disease, congestive heart failure).
- Acute asthma.
- Acute febrile illness.
- Uncontrolled diabetes.
- Systemic hypertension (systolic >200mmHg, diastolic >120mmHg).

Possible results
Cardiac response: ECG, BP, cardiac output and stroke volume response.
Ventilatory response: ventilatory limitation (reduced breathing reserve), pattern of response, V_T, minute volume, respiratory rate.
Gas exchange: arterial blood gases, A–a gradient, P_aCO_2.
Ventilatory (anaerobic) threshold: normal or ↑.
VO₂ max (maximum oxygen uptake): normal or ↑.

Interpretation
Useful in making the distinction between exertional dyspnoea secondary to lung disease or fatigue secondary to cardiac dysfunction. In patients known to have asthma, exercise test is +ve in 75% of cases with a single treadmill run and 97% if the test is repeated in –ve responders. A fall of 10% or more from baseline in PEFR or FEV₁ suggests exercise-induced asthma.

Advantages over other tests

Best assessment of exercise capacity. Adds to diagnostic accuracy quantitatively (measurement of work capacity, maximum VO_2 and sustained work capacity) and qualitatively (identification of the cause of exercise limitation).

Ancillary tests

- Static lung function tests.
- For asthma: histamine/methacholine inhalation challenges and PEFR diary.

Pitfalls

- Dependent on patient effort and compliance.
- Not suitable for patients with severe objective measurement of respiratory impairment.

Complications

▶ Bronchospasm: usually easily reversed with an inhaled adrenergic agent.
▶ Cardiac arrhythmias/arrest: appropriate equipment and drugs should be available in the exercise testing area. Personnel should be trained in basic and advanced cardiopulmonary resuscitation.

Hughes JMB, Pride NB, eds. (1999) *Lung Function Tests. Physiological Principles and Clinical Applications*, WB Saunders Philadelphia pp133–148; König P. (1989) Exercise challenge: indications and techniques. *Allergy Proc* **10**, 345–348; Sue DY. (1994) Exercise testing in the evaluation of impairment and disability. *Clin Chest Med* **15**, 369–387.

Exhaled nitric oxide

Clinical indications

Asthma

- Diagnosis.
- Assessment of severity.
- Assessment of treatment response to β_2 agonists.

Patient preparation

1. Patient breathes directly into the nitric oxide (NO) analyser.
2. With this technique, gas samples from various compartments of the exhaled volume can be selectively analysed. This prevents contamination by nasal NO.
3. Perform three tests each time and record the largest value.

Possible results

- Exhaled NO can be detected by chemiluminescence analysis in the range of 3 to 20 parts per billion (ppb).

Interpretation

- Patients with asthma have higher concentrations of NO in their expirate than do similar nonasthmatic subjects (13.9 vs. 6.2ppb in one study).

Advantages over other tests

- Simple.
- Non-invasive.
- Objective measure of response to treatment.

Ancillary tests for diagnosis of asthma

- PEFR diary.
- Histamine/methacholine inhalation challenges.

Pitfalls

- Exhaled nitric oxide is also elevated in bronchiectasis and upper/lower respiratory tract infections.
- Exhaled nitric oxide levels are reduced by smoking, alcohol and caffeine.

Kharitonov SA, Barnes PJ. (2001) Exhaled markers of pulmonary disease. *Am J Respir Crit Care Med* **163**; 1693–722, Massaro AF, Gaston B, Kita D, Fanta C, Stamler JS, Drazen JM. (1995) Expired nitric oxide levels during treatment of acute asthma. *Am J Respir Crit Care Med* **152**, 800–803.

Fibreoptic bronchoscopy & video bronchoscopy

Clinical indications
- Any patient with persistent/substantial haemoptysis.
- Suspected lung neoplasm:
  - For histology.
  - To assist with staging.
- Infection:
  - To identify organism.
  - To determine course of recurrence/persistence.
- Diffuse parenchymal lung disease (DPLD) to obtain transbronchial biopsies (useful in diagnosis of sarcoidosis, extrinsic allergic alveolitis and lymphangitis carcinomatosa).

Pre-assessment
- CXR.
- FBC.
- Spirometry.
- Clotting.
- Pulse oximetry.
- ABGs on air if hypoxia suggested by oxygen saturation.

Patient preparation
Endoscopy suite
1. Patient informed and consented.
2. Frontal approach with patient lying on couch, trunk at 45°.
3. IV access obtained.
4. Basic monitoring: pulse oximeter and cardiac monitor.
5. Supplementary O_2 via single nasal cannula.
6. IV sedation: midazolam/alfentanil.
7. Topical lignocaine spray to nose and pharynx (30–50mg of 4% or 10%).
8. Bronchoscope lubricated with 2% lignocaine gel and passed via nostril or mouth guard.
9. Further boluses of lignocaine (4%) applied to cords and then bronchial tree (2%).

Possible results
- Direct inspection of nares, nasopharynx and oropharynx.
- Assess movement of vocal cords (ask patient to say 'eee').
- Direct inspection of bronchial tree down to subsegmental level.
- Able to take bronchial/transbronchial biopsies and brushings. Bronchoalveolar lavage (BAL): wedge tip of bronchoscope into a subsegmental bronchus and instil 20mL sterile saline into the distal airway. Aspirate immediately aiming to obtain approximately 50% of instilled volume.

Table 8.2 Interpretation

Histology:	Tumours/DPLD	Biopsy
Cytology:	Tumours	Brush
Microbiology:	Gram stain ZN stain Stain for *Pneumocystis carinii* Fungi Virus	Lavage

Some appearances diagnostic.
Screening: x-ray-guided biopsy of non-visible lesions.

Advantages over other tests

- Well tolerated.
- Quick, cheap.
- Provides histological and immunobiological confirmation (to back up CT/CXR diagnosis).
- Therapeutic: removal of retained secretions, mucus plugs, blood clots.

Ancillary tests

- Rigid bronchoscopy: under GA:
  - Allows therapeutic interventions, e.g. laser therapy, cryotherapy, stent insertion, debulking of large tumours in the major airways and better control of haemorrhage.
  - Preferable for removal of foreign body.

Side effects and complications

- Pneumothorax with transbronchial biopsies.
- Haemorrhage post-biopsy.
- Hypoxia.
- If performed on day case unit patient will not be able to drive home and will need a responsible adult in attendance overnight.

Pitfalls

- Only visualises proximal airways.
- Biopsies may be inadequate or from necrotic areas.
- Not easy to biopsy submucosal tumour.
- Needs good quality cytology preparation.

'Fitness to fly' assessment

Clinical indications

The following groups of patients should be referred to a chest physician for assessment before flying:

- Severe asthma or COPD.
- Severe restrictive disease (including chest wall and respiratory muscle disease).
- Cystic fibrosis.
- Recent pneumothorax.
- Within 6 weeks of discharge for an acute respiratory illness.
- Pre-existing requirement for ventilator support or oxygen therapy.
- Co-morbidities with other conditions worsened by hypoxaemia (e.g. coronary artery disease).

Patient preparation

1. Take a history and examine patient with particular reference to cardiorespiratory disease and previous symptoms during flights.
2. Perform spirometry.
3. Measure SpO_2 by pulse oximeter. Arterial blood gases should be performed if hypercapnia is suspected.
4. A hypoxic challenge test (breathing 15% FiO_2 for 20 minutes via a face mask followed by arterial blood gas sampling) may be necessary depending on the results of the initial assessment.

Possible results

Table 8.3 Results of initial assessment

Screening result	Recommendation
Sea level SpO_2 >95%	Oxygen not required
Sea level SpO_2 92–95% and no risk factor*	Oxygen not required
Sea level SpO_2 92–95% and additional risk factor*	Perform hypoxic challenge and ABGs
Sea level SpO_2 <92%	In-flight oxygen

*Additional risk factors: hypercapnea; FEV_1 <50% predicted; lung cancer; lung fibrosis; kyphoscolosis; respiratory muscle weakness; cerebrovascular or cardiac disease; within 6 weeks of discharge for an exacerbation of chronic lung or cardiac disease.

Table 8.4 Results of hypoxic challenge test

Hypoxic challenge result	Recommendation
P_aO_2 >7.4 kPa (>55mmHg)	Oxygen not required
P_aO_2 6.6–7.4 kPa (50–55mmHg)	Borderline—seek advice
P_aO_2 <6.6 kPa (<50mmHg)	In-flight oxygen (flow rate 2L/min)

Interpretation

- Identifies most patients requiring in-flight oxygen therapy.

Ancillary tests

- Exercise testing.
- In complex cases patients may require testing in a hypobaric chamber.

Pitfalls

- Infectious patients should not fly.
- Even with in-flight oxygen therapy, travel cannot be guaranteed to be safe.

Anon. (2002) Managing passengers with respiratory disease planning air travel: British Thoracic Society recommendations. *Thorax* **57**, 289–304.

Flow volume loops/maximum expiratory flow-volume curve

Clinical indications

Patient in whom COPD/small airways disease or upper airway obstruction is suspected.

Patient preparation

- Advised to wear comfortable, loose clothing.
- Technician explains procedure to patient.
- Mouthpiece in position, patient breathes in maximally and then out as hard and fast as possible.
- 3 acceptable manoeuvres should be performed. Patients must perform the test with maximal effort each time and the results should be similar for each of the 3 attempts.

Interpretation

Particularly useful in recognising patients with narrowing of the central airway (larynx and trachea). Narrowing at this site has greatest effect on maximum expiratory flow and also on maximum inspiratory flow giving rise to a characteristic appearance. Also identifies patients with reduced elastic recoil (bullae, emphysema) or reduced airway lumen (asthma, chronic obstructive pulmonary disease, bronchiolitis).

Oscillation of flow gives a 'saw tooth' pattern. This usually signifies instability of the upper airway and has been observed in obstructive sleep apnoea, thermal injury to the airway, bulbar muscle weakness, extrapyramidal neuromuscular disorders, upper airway stenosis/tracheomalacia and snoring.

Advantages over other tests

- Allows early detection of small airway disease—more sensitive than FEV_1 alone.
- Reproducible.

Ancillary tests

- Spirometry.
- Transfer factor.

Pitfalls

- Dependent on patient understanding and maximal effort.
- Infection control necessary in patients with known or suspected transmissible disease (e.g. active pulmonary tuberculosis).

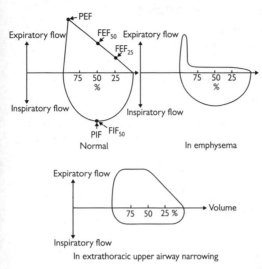

Fig. 8.3 Flow volume loops.

Nijmegen questionnaire

Clinical indications

Hyperventilation syndrome

- Diagnosis.
- Assessment of severity.
- Assessment of response to therapy.

Patient preparation

1. Ask patient to fill in questionnaire.
2. Subject rates on a scale of 0–4 the frequency of 16 different symptoms.

Use the following scale to choose the most appropriate number for each symptom:

0 = Would NEVER experience that symptom
1 = RARELY experience that symptom
2 = SOMETIMES experience that symptom
3 = OFTEN experience that symptom
4 = VERY OFTEN experience that symptom

Symptoms

- Chest pain.
- Feeling tense.
- Blurred vision.
- Dizzy spells.
- Feeling confused.
- Faster or deeper breathing.
- Short of breath.
- Tight feelings in chest.
- Bloated feeling in stomach.
- Tingling fingers.
- Unable to breathe deeply.
- Stiff fingers or arms.
- Tight feelings around mouth.
- Cold hands or feet.
- Heart racing (palpitations).
- Feelings of anxiety.

Possible results

Nijmegen score is the sum of 16 item scores and can range from 0 to 64.

Interpretation

Clinically normal score <23.

Advantages over other tests

- Cheap.
- Easily administered.

Ancillary tests

- Arterial blood gases to identify hypocapnia and respiratory alkalosis.

- Hyperventilation provocation test. (Ask the patient to over-breathe for several minutes to see if it reproduces symptoms).

Pitfalls

Limited by patient's ability to read and comprehend the questionnaire and answer questions honestly.

Van Dixhoorn J, Duivenvoorden HJ. (1985) Efficacy of Nijmegen Questionnaire in recognition of the hyperventilation syndrome. *J Psychosom Res* **29**, 199–206.

Peak flow charts

Clinical indications

Asthma
- Diagnosis.
- Assessment of severity.
- Assessment of treatment response to β_2 agonists.

Occupational asthma
- Diagnosis.

Patient preparation

Patients need to be equipped with a peak flow meter and peak flow and symptom diary and have a thorough understanding of how to use them.

Guidelines to patients should include

1. Perform the test standing (if possible).
2. Hold the meter lightly and do not interfere with the movement of the marker.
3. Perform three tests each time and record the largest value.

Readings should be taken at various times throughout the day. Limiting the patient to two readings in each day may aid compliance. In occupational asthma 2-hourly peak flow readings are required during the day and evening.

Possible results

- Diurnal variability: as measured by the lowest PEFR value (usually on waking) and the highest PEFR value (usually in the afternoon/evening).
- Patient symptoms and PEFR can be examined together.

Interpretation

Diurnal variation is increased in patients with asthma compared to normals (amplitude >20%), i.e. peak flow falls significantly overnight and in the early morning.

Advantages over other tests

- Cheap.
- Saves time of respiratory physician and technician.
- Reproducible.
- Objective measure of response to treatment.

Ancillary tests for diagnosis of asthma

- Bronchoprovocation test.
- Exercise test.

Peak Flow Meter Record

Name: J. Smith   Predicted normal: 240   Personal Best: 280

Peak flow chart of an asthmatic patient showing diurnal variations.
↑ indicates morning dips

Fig. 8.4 An example of a patient's peak flow record.

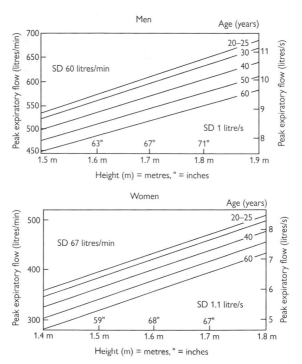

Fig. 8.5 Peak flow readings.

Pitfalls

• Not all asthma exacerbations are associated with increased diurnal variability.
• Calculating diurnal variation can be complicated and tedious.
• Time of recording or recent use of β_2 agonist drugs may result in minor changes in peak flow, but can cause large errors in diurnal variability.
• Dependent on patient understanding, cooperation and accuracy.

Reddel H, Jenkins C, Woolcock A. (1999) Diurnal variability—time to change asthma guidelines? *BMJ* **319**, 45–47; Hetzel MR, Clark TJ. (1980) Comparison of normal and asthmatic circadian rhythms in peak expiratory flow rate. *Thorax* **35**, 732–738.

Pleural needle biopsy

Clinical indications

Pleural effusion of unknown aetiology especially if TB or malignancy suspected. *Note:* may be combined with diagnostic and/or therapeutic pleural aspiration. In which case, obtain diagnostic fluid sample first, then do needle biopsy, then follow with therapeutic aspiration.

Patient preparation

1. Informed written consent.
2. Patient sits with arms forward supported on table/pillows.
3. Posterior or mid-axillary approach.
4. Skin cleaned with iodine solution.
5. Lignocaine (1 or 5%) infiltrated in rib interspace: check pleural fluid aspirated.
6. Stab incision with narrow scalpel.
7. Insert closed Abrams needle (requires firm pressure to be applied until it penetrates parietal pleura: *take care not to apply too much force*).
8. Attach 50mL syringe.
9. Twist open Abrams needle.
10. Aspirate fluid to ensure needle in pleural space.
11. Withdraw needle at angle to chest wall until side hole 'snags' parietal pleura.
12. Maintain lateral pressure and rotate to close hole thereby cutting biopsy. Remove needle and extract biopsy tissue.
13. Repeat with samples taken from 3, 6 and 9 o'clock (avoid the 12 o'clock position to avoid the neurovascular bundle).
14. May require suture to close.
15. Apply dressing.
16. Obtain CXR post-procedure.
17. Place samples in formalin for histological examination and saline for microbiological culture.

Possible results

- Slivers of white pleural tissue.
- Examine histology and culture for AAFBs.

Interpretation

- Malignant mesothelioma may be diagnosed on histology, especially with addition of immunohistochemical methods looking at tumour cell markers.
- More sensitive than pleural fluid aspiration in diagnosing TB.
- Carcinoma cells may arise from direct spread from lung primary or represent secondary carcinoma. In either case, management is palliative.

Advantages over other tests

- Easy, quick, cheap; more reliable than diagnostic pleural aspiration.
- Less invasive than thoracoscopy for diagnosis of TB.

Ancillary tests

- Diagnostic pleural fluid aspiration.
- Thoracoscopy.
- CT-guided pleural biopsy is more sensitive than Abrams' pleural biopsy at diagnosing malignancy.

Complications

- Pneumothorax.
- Haemothorax.

Pitfalls

- Skeletal muscle biopsy: inadequate specimen.
- Damage to neurovascular bundle.
- Diagnosis of mesothelioma may remain equivocal.

Kirsh CM et al. (1995) A modified Abrams needle biopsy technique. *Chest* **108**, 982–986; Kirsh CM et al. (1997) The optimal number of pleural biopsy specimens for a diagnosis of tuberculous pleurisy. *Chest* **112**, 702–706; Prakash UB, Reiman HM. (1985) Comparison of needle biopsy with cytologic analysis for the evaluation of pleural effusion: analysis of 414 cases. *Mayo Clin Proc* **60**, 158–164; Maskell NA, Gleeson FV, Davies RJ. (2003) Standard pleural biopsy versus CT-guided cutting-needle biopsy for diagnosis of malignant disease in pleural effusions: a randomised controlled trial. *Lancet* **361**, 1326–30.

Polysomnography

Clinical indications

Note: symptoms alone do not help predict which patient with sleep disturbance has obstructive sleep apnoea (OSA).

- Patients with low probability sleep disorder, e.g. snores with no other features suggestive of OSA.
- Patients with high probability sleep disorder, e.g. typical symptoms and physiognomy. Need study for diagnosis and assessment of severity.
- Known OSA: assessing treatment response.
- Assessment of nocturnal hypoventilation syndromes, e.g. scoliosis.
- Patients with unexplained sleep–wake disorders.

Patient preparation

The patient is admitted to the sleep laboratory in the early evening. Monitoring is explained and attached, using some combination of the following:

Table 8.5

Sleep	Electroencephalogram	
	Electro-oculogram	
	Electromyogram	
Oxygenation	Oxygen saturation probe (ear or finger)	
Breathing pattern	Airflow by:	Thermocouples
		Thermistor
		End tidal CO_2 pressure
	Thoracoabdominal movement by:	Inductance plethysmo graphy
		Impedance
		Strain gauge
Miscellaneous	Snoring:	Microphone
	Leg movement by:	EMG
		Video
		Movement detector

Possible results

Original diagnosis of OSA based on polysomnography—overnight recording of sleep, breathing patterns and oxygenation. It is relatively expensive and most centres use a combination of video to assess quality of sleep, identify transient arousals and paroxysmal leg movement disorder (PLMD) and oximetry (to detect desaturation) plus some form of measuring the breathing pattern to detect hypopnoea.

Interpretation

Obstructive sleep apnoea diagnosed in the context of multiple (typically >15/h) hypopnoeic/apnoeic events occurring throughout the night and resulting in desaturation.

Advantages over other tests

Demonstrates number of hypopnoeic (reduction in breathing) or apnoeic (absence of breathing) events occurring per hour. May be used to monitor effectiveness of treatment.

Ancillary tests

Epworth sleepiness score.

Pitfalls

- Expensive.
- Time-consuming.
- Most sleep study systems are poorly validated; therefore need expert interpretation of results to consider false positives and negatives.
- Patients need to sleep for >3h/night and have rapid eye movement (REM) sleep.

Pulse oximetry

Clinical indications

- Any acutely unwell patient—avoids repeated blood gas measurements provided that hypercarbia is absent.
- Monitoring of long-term oxygen therapy (LTOT)—but not suitable for initial assessment.
- Assessment of nocturnal FiO_2 and screening for sleep apnoea syndrome—identification of nocturnal desaturations.
- Exercise walk test.

Patient preparation

1. Clean probe site (ear or finger).
2. Ensure good contact of probe with warm well-perfused skin.
3. Avoid nail-varnished fingers.

Possible results

Oxygen saturations expressed as %.

Interpretation

- Respiratory failure unlikely if O_2 saturation >92% on air.
- Provides almost immediate arterial oxygen saturation data.
- Must know the inspired oxygen (FiO_2) concentration the patient is breathing.

Advantages over other tests

- Non-invasive.
- Easy, cheap.
- Instantaneous.
- Sensitive.
- Portable.

Ancillary tests

Arterial blood gas sampling.

Pitfalls

- Does not detect carbon dioxide levels.
- If carboxyhaemoglobin or methaemoglobin are present in the blood in elevated levels the pulse oximeter will give a falsely elevated reading for the arterial oxygen saturation.
- ↑ in jaundice.
- Erroneous information if patient poorly perfused.
- Excessive patient movement can give false readings.

Skin prick tests

Clinical indications

- To evaluate atopy in asthmatic individuals.
- To assess the possible development of allergic broncho-pulmonary aspergillosis (ABPA) in patients with asthma/other long-standing lung disease.

Patient preparation

1. Explain what the test involves.
2. Use a pen to label the patient's forearm with the antigens to be tested, including positive and negative controls.
3. Clean the test area with an alcohol wipe.
4. Place a drop of antigen next to the corresponding label.
5. Use a lancet to puncture the skin.
6. Wipe away any excess antigen taking care not to contaminate other test sites. Repeat with other antigens using a new lancet each time.
7. After 30 minutes measure any resulting wheal and flare reaction using a ruler.

Possible results

- A positive result is indicated by a wheal and flare reaction ≥2mm providing there is a wheal and flare reaction at the positive control site and no reaction at the negative control site.

Interpretation

- A positive result indicates sensitisation to the allergen.

Advantages over other tests

- Cheap, quick.

Ancillary tests

- Total IgE and specific IgE to allergens (e.g. *Aspergillus*).
- *Aspergillus* precipitins (IgG).

Pitfalls

- False negative results if the patient has taken an antihistamine within 5 days of the test.
- False positive results with dermatographism or inflamed skin.

Spirometry

Clinical indications

- To evaluate symptoms, signs or abnormal test results.
- Provide objective, quantifiable measures of lung function.
- Evaluate and monitor disease.
- Assess effects of environmental/occupational/drug exposures both adverse (e.g. amiodarone) and beneficial (e.g. bronchodilators).
- Pre-operative assessment.
- Employment/insurance assessment.
- Early detection of bronchiolitis obliterans in lung transplant patients.

Patient preparation

1. Explain what the test involves. Most respiratory technicians demonstrate technique to ensure maximal effort and cooperation of patient.
2. Patient must fully inhale before test.
3. Exhale into breathing tube. Must be maximal effort with no hesitation.
4. No cough/glottal closure in the first second.
5. Test must last at least 6s (up to 15s with obstruction).
6. No evidence of airflow leak/obstruction of mouthpiece.

Possible results

Table 8.6

FEV_1:	Forced expiratory volume in 1s
	Test of mechanical function of the lungs
	Depends on size and elastic properties of the lungs, calibre of the bronchial tree and collapsibility of airway walls
FVC:	Forced vital capacity

Interpretation

At least three acceptable tracings should be obtained. Examine each tracing to ensure adequate effort made by patient, that it is reproducible, and that there are no artefacts.

Table 8.7

FEV_1/FVC ratio:	Index of the presence/absence of airflow limitation
	Young and middle aged healthy non-smokers rate ≥75%
	Older normal patients ratio 70–75%
FEV/FVC ↓:	Obstructive
	Classify severity using FEV, expressed as % of predicted value, e.g. COPD, asthma
FEV/FVC ↔ or ↑:	Restrictive but need reduced TLC to confirm, e.g. lung fibrosis, chest wall problems, pulmonary effusion and oedema

If used for monitoring purposes need adequate baseline study.

Advantages over other tests
- Cheap, quick.
- Bedside/outpatient test.
- Reproducible.

Ancillary tests
- Total lung capacity to confirm interstitial disease with restrictive spirometry.
- Pre- and post-bronchodilator studies: an increase of 15% in FEV_1 and 20% in FVC suggest reversibility.

Pitfalls
- Need standardisation of normal data for height, weight, age, sex and race.
- Level at which a result may be considered abnormal is contentious, usually accepted to be outside range of 80–120% of mean predicted.
- FEV_1 may remain relatively normal in early stages of generalised lung disease.
- FEV_1/FVC ratio is good guide to presence or significant airway narrowing but as disease progresses, both will fall and correlation with severity of disease is poor.
- Variability (noise) is greater in pulmonary function tests than in most other clinical laboratory tests because of the inconsistency of effort by patients.

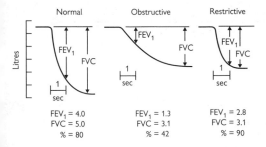

Fig. 8.6 Examples of spirograms.

See examples of spirograms 📖OHCM p329.

Crapo RO. (1994) Pulmonary-function testing. *NEJM* **331**, 25–30.

Sputum microscopy & culture/sputum cytology

Clinical indications

Microbiology
- Productive cough with sputum.
- Infective exacerbations of any chronic lung disease.
- Pneumonia.

Cytology
- Suspected lung cancer, especially in elderly/frail patients.

Patient preparation

- Explain need for the sputum sample.
- Provide suitable sputum pots.
- Early morning samples are best.
- Consider induced sputum—use ultrasonically nebulised hypertonic saline to facilitate sputum production in association with chest physiotherapy.

Possible results

Induced sputum results in successful sputum production in >70% of normal and asthmatic subjects who cannot produce sputum spontaneously.

Table 8.8

Gram stain	Gram +ve or −ve organisms
ZN stain	AAFB
Microscopy	Differential cell count Eosinophils in asthma
Cytology	Malignant cells Small cell, squamous cell, adenocarcinoma cells

Interpretation

- Commensal organisms common.
- *Streptococcus pneumoniae* and *Haemophilus influenzae* likely pathogens in COPD.
- *Streptococcus pneumoniae* commonest organism in community-acquired 1° pneumonia.
- *Staphylococcus aureus* and *Pseudomonas* likely in bronchiectasis.
- Nosocomial infections:
  - *Staphylococcus aureus*.
  - *Pseudomonas*.
  - *Klebsiella*.
- Squamous cell carcinoma on cytology can reflect premalignant change.

Advantages over other tests
- Cheap, easy.
- Non-invasive.

Ancillary tests
- Bronchoscopy and bronchoalveolar lavage.
- Serum serology if atypical pneumonia suspected.
- PCR for drug-resistant TB.

Pitfalls
- Sputum may be diluted by saliva.
- Diagnosis of squamous cell carcinoma is not as robust as for small cell lung cancer or adenocarcinoma. Needs careful cross-referencing to radiology and should be confirmed if possible with biopsies.
- Negative results should not preclude further investigations if malignancy suspected.

Static lung volumes/whole body plethysmography

Clinical indications
- Differentiate between obstructive and restrictive disease patterns.
- Identify and quantify trapped air (shown by ↑RV/TLC ratio).
- Assess response to therapeutic interventions (e.g. drugs, radiation, transplantation).
- Identify presence and amount of unventilated lung.
- Assess chronic lung disease (e.g. sarcoidosis, rheumatoid lung).
- Pre-operative assessment.
- Assessment of pulmonary disability.

Patient preparation
1. Ask patient to wear comfortable clothes.
2. Place mouthpiece securely in mouth with lips tight around it.
3. Breathe in a relaxed manner through spirometer system (nose clips mandatory).
4. After total of 5 tidal breaths with consistent end-expiratory levels, patient asked to maximally inspire to total lung capacity followed by exhalation with encouragement to force out the last 5–15% of air.
5. A minimum of 2 attempts should be obtained.
6. More may be needed in the young and elderly to obtain reproducible results.

Most accurate results are obtained with whole body plethysmography.

Possible results
Total lung capacity
Volume of air in the lungs at the end of full inspiration.

Residual volume
Volume of air remaining in the lungs after maximal expiration.

Vital capacity
The amount of air expired (or inspired) between maximum inspiration and maximum expiration.

Functional residual capacity
The amount of air in the lungs at the end-tidal position.

Inspiratory capacity
The maximum amount of air that can be breathed into the lungs from the end-tidal position.

Tidal volume
The volume of air inspired and expired with each breath.

Inspiratory reserve volume
The volume between the peak inspiratory tidal position and maximum inspiration.

Interpretation

Only interpret if test is reproducible, i.e. if the 2 largest vital capacity values are within 5% or 100mL (whichever is the larger).

VC may remain within normal range in some pulmonary disease, e.g. emphysema.

↓VC: restrictive pulmonary disease, neuromuscular disease, e.g. amyotrophic lateral sclerosis.

During the testing process, the patient is enclosed in a chamber equipped to measure either pressure, flow or volume changes. Because all the gas in the thorax is accounted for, this method is particularly useful in patients with trapped gas, e.g. bullous emphysema.

Advantages over other tests

Reproducible.

Pitfalls

- Patient cooperation essential: they must provide maximal effort and be capable of understanding instructions.
- Calibration should take place on a regular basis.
- Risk of disease transmission between patients and between patient and technician, therefore avoid if pulmonary TB suspected.

Fig. 8.7 Lung volumes: physiological and pathological.

Table 8.9

Causes of ↑ TLC:	Generalised airway obstruction, e.g. COPD
	Emphysema (including bullae)
	Bronchiectasis
	Asthma
	Other, e.g. acromegaly
Causes of ↓ TLC:	*Intrapulmonary*
	– pneumonectomy
	– collapsed lung
	– consolidation
	– oedema
	– fibrosis
	Extrapulmonary
	– pleural disease
	– effusion
	– thickening
	– pneumothorax
	– rib cage deformity
	– scoliosis
	– thoracoplasty
	– respiratory muscle weakness
Causes of ↑ RV:	Generalised airway obstruction
	Pulmonary vascular congestion, e.g. mitral stenosis, ASD
	Expiratory muscle weakness, e.g. spinal injury, myopathies
Causes of ↑ FRC:	Age, lung disease causing air trapping, e.g. asthma, emphysema, COPD
Causes of ↓ FRC:	Restrictive lung diseases, e.g. diffuse interstitial pulmonary disease of any aetiology, pneumonectomy

Sweat test

Clinical indications

Suspected cystic fibrosis (CF) in the context of

- Bronchiectasis/recurrent chest infections.
- Pancreatic insufficiency/diabetes mellitus.
- Family history.
- Fertility problems.

Patient preparation

1. Obtain informed consent: verbal usually sufficient but important to discuss reasons for test and possible implications. Perform two sweat tests simultaneously on each arm for greater accuracy.
2. Induce sweating by pilocarpine iontophoresis; a weak electrical current aids penetration of pilocarpine into skin. Stimulated in this way, the sweat glands of the forearm, previously washed and dried, secrete sweat.
3. Collect sweat on preweighed filter paper (>100mg), then measure eluted Na^+ and Cl^-.

Possible results

- 98–99% of children homozygous for CF have sweat Cl^- and Na^+ levels well >70 and 60mmol/L, respectively.
- Sweat Na^+ concentrations tend to increase with age and show wide variability between individuals.
- Diagnostic accuracy is improved in borderline cases by a suppression test using fludrocortisone.

Interpretation

A +ve test is virtually diagnostic of cystic fibrosis. This should lead to counselling and genetic testing.

Equivocal results are defined as Na^+ or Cl^- concentrations between 50 and 70mmol/L.

The diagnosis should never rest on the sweat test alone and should be considered together with the clinical findings and laboratory evidence of pancreatic insufficiency.

Advantages over other tests

- Cheaper than genetic tests.
- Assesses functional deficit, therefore capable of detecting patients who have rare variants of CF.

Ancillary tests

- Nasal potential difference.
- Pancreatic function tests (3-day faecal collection).
- Genetic studies.

Pitfalls

- A wide discrepancy between the results from each arm suggests a problem with technique.

- Accurate interpretation of sweat tests requires knowledge of the age- related changes in sweat Na^+ and Cl^- concentrations and should be done in a specialised centre.

False negatives

- Inexperience of operator.
- Low rates of sweating.
- Poor skin preparation.
- Poor iontophoretic contact with skin.
- Faulty chemical analysis.

False positives

- Evaporation of sweat secondary to inadequate sealing during collection.
- Untreated adrenal insufficiency.
- Nephrogenic diabetes insipidus.
- Hypothyroidism.
- Glycogen storage disease.
- Nephrotic syndrome.
- Severe malnutrition.
- AIDS (some reports of abnormal sweat electrolytes).
- Faulty chemical analysis.

Hall SK, Stableforth DE, Green A. (1990) Sweat sodium and chloride concentrations—essential criteria for the diagnosis of cystic fibrosis in adults. *Ann Clin Biochem* **27**, 318–320; Heeley AF, Watson D. (1983) Cystic fibrosis—its biochemical detection. *Clin Chem* **29**, 2011–2018; Green A, Dodds P, Pennock C. (1985) A study of sweat sodium and chloride; criteria for the diagnosis of cystic fibrosis. *Ann Clin Biochem* **22**, 171–176.

Medical thoracoscopy

Clinical indications
- Pleural effusions when pleural fluid analysis non-diagnostic.
- Pneumothorax.
- Staging of lung cancer.
- Diagnosis of malignant mesothelioma and other pleural abnormalities, e.g. neurinomas, lipomas, plastocytomas.
- Suspected empyema.

Pre-assessment
- A recent (<1 month) CT scan of the chest is mandatory.
- FBC.
- Clotting.
- Spirometry.
- Pulse oximetry.
- ABGs on air if hypoxia suggested by oxygen saturation.

Patient preparation
Endoscopy suite
1. Patient informed and consented.
2. Intravenous access obtained.
3. Patient lying supine with affected side nearest to operator. Must be able to keep hand behind head in order to prevent arm from obscuring operating field.
4. Basic monitoring: pulse oximeter and cardiac monitor.
5. Supplementary oxygen given via face-mask or nasal cannulae.
6. Intravenous sedation: midazolam.
7. An absolute prerequisite for thoracoscopy is the presence of an adequate pleural space (i.e. at least 6–10cm diameter).
8. If pleural effusion: drain using 3-way tap. Replace with equal quantity atmospheric air.
9. If no effusion: create pneumothorax.
10. Insert needle connected to manometer into pleural space. Introduce 400–1000mL air.
11. Skin incision 5th intercostal space, mid-axillary line 1.5–2cm.
12. Insert 5–10mm pleural trocar and cannula.
13. Introduce thoracoscope via trocar into pleural cavity.
14. After inspection and biopsies remove trocar and insert drain.
15. CXR post-procedure.
16. Commence chest drain suction at rate of 20cmH$_2$O on ward.

Possible results
- Direct inspection of pleural surfaces.
- Biopsy of parietal pleura—histology/culture esp. AAFBs.
- Pleural fluid   → MC&S
                           → cytology.
- Therapeutic options: pleurodesis, coagulation of blebs, resection of fibrinous loculations in empyemas.

- Drainage of large pleural effusions possible without risk of re-expansion pulmonary oedema due to rapid equalisation of pressures by entrance of air into pleural space.

Interpretation

Macroscopic appearance of pleura may be diagnostic, e.g. TB, RA, scleroderma, metastatic disease.

Advantages over other tests

- Better than blind pleural biopsy.
- Able to obtain diagnosis in 70–95% of cases.
- Especially good at diagnosing TB.
- Less invasive than thoracotomy.
- Less expensive than thoracotomy: does not require a theatre or anaesthetist.
- Done under sedation unlike VATS (video-assisted thoracic surgery), which requires a GA and selective one-lung ventilation.

Ancillary tests

Diagnosis of mesothelioma improved with use of immunohistochemical markers.

Pitfalls

Biopsies may be inadequate or non-representative.

Contraindications

- Obliterated pleural space.
- Small pneumothorax.
- Patient short of breath at rest unless secondary to pneumothorax or pleural effusion which can be treated during procedure.
- Disturbed haemostasis:
  - Platelets <40 x 10^9/L.
  - APTT >50% normal.
- Recent MI, arrhythmias, heart failure.

Complications

- Fever 24–36h post-procedure.
- Empyema (<1%).
- Wound infection.
- Subcutaneous emphysema.
- Air embolism.
- Bronchopleural fistula following lung biopsy.
- Seeding of metastases/mesothelioma along trocar wound. (Radiotherapy a few weeks post-thoracoscopy should be carried out to prevent this.)
- Haemorrhage.
- Arrhythmias.
- Mortality rate <0.01%.

Blanc FX, Atassi K, Bignon J, Housset B. (2002) Diagnostic value of medical thoracoscopy in pleural disease: a 6-year retrospective study. Chest 5, 1677–1683; Loddenkemper R. (1998) Thoracoscopy—state of the art. Eur Resp J 11, 213–221; Colt HG. (1999) Thoracoscopy: window to the pleural space. Chest 116, 1409–1415; Buchanan DR, Neville E. (2004) Thoracoscopy for Physicians: a Practical Guide, Arnold.

Transfer factor

Clinical indications
Test for abnormalities of pulmonary gas exchange.

Patient preparation
- Avoid smoking 6h prior and strenuous exercise 2h prior.
- Allow 15–30min for test.
- Usually measured by single breath inhalation technique.
- Patient breathes in air containing a known concentration of CO and holds breath for 10s.

Possible results
- Transfer factor (TLCO).
- Transfer coefficient (KCO).
- May need to correct for anaemia:
  - Result usually standardised to Hb 14.6g/dL.
  - Effect of mild anaemia (Hb >10g/dL) slight but becomes progressively more marked at lower values.

Interpretation
↓ *in DLCO*
- Obstructive lung disease, e.g. COPD, emphysema.
- Diffuse interstitial lung disease, e.g. CFA, amiodarone lung.
- Pulmonary involvement in systemic disease e.g. SLE, RA, Wegener's.
- Cardiovascular disease e.g. pulmonary oedema, mitral stenosis, PE.
- Others: anaemia, cigarette smoking.

↑ *in DLCO*
- Diseases associated with polycythaemia.
- Pulmonary haemorrhage.
- Diseases associated with increased pulmonary blood such as from left to right intracardiac shunts.
- Exercise.
- Asthmatics (reasons not clear).

Advantages over other tests
- Quick.
- Relatively easy to perform.
- Reproducible.

Pitfalls
- Breath holding time may be difficult for some patients to achieve.
- Calculation of TLCO is based on assumption that ventilation and diffusion are homogeneous in the entire lung. With unequal distribution of ventilation and diffusion, the TLCO will be underestimated on the alveolar level.
- With extrapulmonary lung restriction and consequent inability to achieve full inspiration, KCO tends to be higher than normal.

Neurology

Lumbar puncture (LP) *518*
Skull radiograph *524*
Ultrasound *525*
Angiography *526*
Myelography *527*
Radionuclide scans *528*
Computed tomography (CT) *530*
Magnetic resonance imaging (MRI) or nuclear magnetic resonance (NMR) imaging *532*
Nerve conduction studies *534*
EMG *537*
EEG *539*
EEG abnormalities *541*
EEGs in epilepsy *542*
How to use to EEG *542*
Invasive EEG techniques *545*
Polysomnography *545*
Sodium amytal (Wada) test *546*
Sensory evoked potentials or responses (EPs or ERs) *546*
Transcranial magnetic stimulation (TMS) *550*
Neurological investigation of sphincter disturbance *551*
Edrophonium (Tensilon®) test *552*
Biopsies *553*
Oligoclonal bands (OCBs) *555*
Diagnostic & prognostic antibodies & other markers in blood & urine *555*
Biochemical markers *558*
Genetic tests *560*
Neuro-otology *564*

Lumbar puncture (LP)

Indications
- Meningitis.
- Encephalitis.
- Polyradiculitis, polyneuritis.
- Multiple sclerosis.
- Myelitis.
- Vasculitis.
- Suspected subarachnoid haemorrhage (SAH). *Note*: In general, a −ve CT does not exclude a SAH.
- Suspected malignancy with meningeal involvement.
- Assessment of CSF pressure:
  - High (e.g. idiopathic or 'benign' intracranial hypertension, BIH).
  - Low (e.g. 'low pressure' headache).
- Therapeutic trials, e.g.
  - BIH.
  - Normal pressure hydrocephalus, NPH (not particularly helpful).
- To seek specific antibodies/markers in CSF, e.g.
  - HIV.
  - Lyme (*Borrelia*).
  - Syphilis.
  - ACE (for neurosarcoid).
  - Tumour markers.
  - Lactate in mitochondrial cytopathies.

Preparation
- Decide exactly what investigations you want. If necessary, alert the appropriate laboratories and organise transport of samples. In particular, samples for xanthochromia and cytology should be rapidly taken to the laboratory to be spun down.
- If the patient is also due to have a neuroradiological investigation with contrast and LP is not urgent, delay LP until after scan as there may be diffuse meningeal enhancement after the LP.
- If the patient is extremely anxious, s/he may benefit from 5–10mg of oral diazepam prior to the LP.

Procedure
1. Explain to the patient what you are about to do.
2. Arrange all your equipment on a sterile tray, including assembled CSF manometer.
3. Position patient on his side, with back perpendicular to bed, at the edge of a firm bed. Place head on one pillow. Draw knees up and place one pillow between them.
4. Adjust height of bed so that you are comfortable.
5. Identify the bony landmarks. L3/L4 space is in line with the iliac crests, and is most commonly used. L2/L3 to L5/S1 are also. If you like, mark the target space with the imprint of your thumb nail. Take time over these first four stages.

6. The insertion of the needle should be a sterile procedure. Clean the skin over the lower back. Don sterile gloves and mask.
7. Insert a little (0.25–0.5mL) local anaesthetic—too much can obscure the bony landmarks.
8. Pass LP needle horizontally into the space, with tip angled at about 10–15° (toward the umbilicus), in the midline horizontal plane. At all times, stylet should be fully inserted and bevel of needle facing up.
9. Slight resistance should be felt as needle passes through ligamentum flavum and the dura, and then a 'give' as it enters the subarachnoid space.
10. Slowly withdraw the stylet. CSF drops should appear.
11. If CSF does not appear, reinsert the style and slightly rotate the needle—this sometimes frees it of obstructing nerve roots. A gentle cough from the patient can also help.
12. If the needle encounters bone, or the patient complains of pains shooting down the leg, check the position of the needle (is it in the midline? Is it angled correctly?) and then withdraw it entirely.
13. Insert a fresh needle, correcting for any error noted above.
14. If this second pass is unsuccessful, withdraw needle and inform patient. If he is happy for you to proceed, then attempt LP in another space, repeating all steps from 4 down. Use a fresh needle.
15. If you fail again, explain to patient and seek a more experienced operator to perform the LP. Multiple failed attempts are painful and discouraging (to both you and your patient).
16. If a more experienced operator fails, ask your friendly radiologist to do it under x-ray guidance, but give him the help he requests and precise instructions about the samples required.
17. When CSF collection is complete, gently pull out the needle and place a sterile dressing over the insertion site.
18. Allow the patient to mobilise shortly after the LP.

Measuring the CSF pressure

As soon as the CSF starts to flow, attach the pre-assembled manometer. Wait until the CSF stops rising. If the patient is very anxious, or uncomfortable, a falsely raised opening pressure may be recorded. Sometimes having the patient slightly relax his legs will help. Using the 3-way tap, let the CSF run into your first pre-labelled tube (do not waste the CSF!). Having collected all the CSF you require, if the opening pressure was elevated, note the closing pressure. If the opening pressure is expected to be very raised, e.g. in suspected or confirmed idiopathic (benign) intracranial hypertension, then two or more manometers should be pre-assembled, as the pressure may excel 40mm CSF.

Collecting samples

• As always, tailor your investigations to the clinical picture. If you are just checking the CSF pressure, then no samples need necessarily be collected. If you suspect a subarachnoid haemorrhage, collect three samples in sequentially labelled bottles and promptly hand carry to the laboratory for quantitative estimation of xanthochromia and haemoglobin breakdown products. If you are looking for evidence of

malignant cells, then at least one sample should be sent to the
laboratory promptly for cytology.
- To avoid contamination, allow the microbiology lab to split samples
rather than attempting this yourself.
- Collect at least 10 drops in each bottle. The microbiology and cytology
laboratories in particular will thank you for greater volumes.
- As soon as the CSF is collected, a blood sample should be obtained
(if necessary) for glucose and oligoclonal band detection.

Alternative positioning of patient

Sometimes there is a dry tap if the CSF pressure is too low to distend
the lumbar cistern. This can sometimes be overcome by performing the
LP with the patient sitting on a firm reversed chair, leaning forward to
bend over its back. This manoeuvre maximises the separation of the
vertebrae. Again the needle should be angled, slightly (10°) upward relative to the spine at that point. This position does not allow precise
measurement of CSF pressure.

Which needle to use?

22G usually appropriate. Needles with larger bores tend to cause a
greater CSF leak (and thus more headache). Some advocate even finer
needles, but these make the collection of CSF take too long. 'Blunt'
anaesthetists' needles probably also reduce the risk of post-LP headache.

Clinical record keeping

Record what you did in the notes after the procedure (e.g. if more than
one pass was required; which space you used), the opening and closing
CSF pressure, and what investigations you have requested. Note the
appearance of the CSF (if normal, it will be clear and colourless). If the
CSF appears bloody, record this and whether the final bottle collected is
clearer than the first.

When *not* to attempt an LP

- Risk of herniation:
  - Space-occupying lesions.
  - Non-communicating hydrocephalus.
  - Cerebral oedema (if in doubt, cranial imaging should be performed
    first).
- Uncorrected bleeding diathesis/anticoagulant use.
- (Caution) if previous lumbar spine surgery or known anatomical
  abnormalities.
- Local skin sepsis.

Complications and what to do about them

Headache
- Usually starts within 24h of LP.
- May last from a few hours to 2 weeks, but typically several days.
- Probably related to persistent CSF leak via the dural tear; therefore
  tends to have 'low pressure' characteristics (frontal, worse on sitting
  up, better on lying down). There may be mild meningism and nausea.

- Treatment has traditionally involved bedrest, analgesia and the encouragement of plenty of fluids.
- If nausea is a major problem, the patient may require IV fluids.
- Rarely, if the headache is severe and persistent, then an anaesthetist may place an autologous blood patch to 'plug' the dural tear. Surgical intervention is very rarely required.

Low backache

- A variety of causes of post-LP backache exist; these may usually be treated conservatively.

Infection

- Very rare if sterile technique is used. Occasionally may occur if the needle passes through a region of infection. Meningitis typically develops within 12h; very rarely there may be an epidural abscesses or vertebral osteomyelitis. Treat with appropriate antibiotics and if necessary surgery.

Herniation

- Uncal or cerebellar herniation may occur, particularly in the presence of a posterior fossa mass. ►►*An LP should not be performed if there is suspicion of raised intracranial pressure without first obtaining cranial CT or MR imaging.*
- Should the CSF pressure be found to be very high (300mm of CSF), even after relaxing patient, and in the absence of idiopathic (benign) intracranial hypertension, manage as follows: nurse patient prone with no pillow, raise foot of bed, start infusion of 20% mannitol at 1g/kg over 20min, start neurological observation chart, arrange urgent CT of brain and notify neurosurgeons. ►►*Do not instil saline into the subarachnoid space.*

Haemorrhage

A 'traumatic' tap may cause a little local bleeding that is rarely of clinical significance. Patients with impaired clotting (remember warfarin) or platelet function are at risk of more extensive bleeding and LP should not be attempted unless the coagulopathy is corrected. An arachnoiditis or spinal subdural or epidural haemorrhage may develop. A spinal subdural haematoma (SDH) is otherwise rare, and an intracranial SDH very rare.

CSF constituents: normal values

- White cells 0–4/mm^3.
- Red blood cells   ideally none!
- Protein 0.15–0.45g/L.
- Glucose $\sim 1/2$ to $2/3$ of simultaneous blood glucose.
- Opening pressure 8–20cm CSF.

Note: If there is a traumatic 'bloody' tap, there may be hundreds or thousands of red blood cells/mm3. If so, then white cells should be expected in the CSF, but in similar proportions to the peripheral blood.

📖OHCM p752.

Rules of thumb

1. *Pressure*:
   - ↑ by space-occupying lesions within the cranial vault, such as oedema, masses, chronic inflammation.
   - ↑ by increased central venous pressure, e.g. in the anxious patient with tensed abdominal muscles.
   - ↓ if the spinal subarachnoid space is obstructed, thus impeding CSF flow.
2. *Cells*:
   - Polymorphs (neutrophils): suggest acute bacterial infection.
   - Lymphocytes & monocytes: viral and chronic infections or tumours.
   - Eosinophils: tumours, parasites, foreign body reactions.
3. *Glucose*: ↓ by non-viral processes causing meningeal inflammation.
4. *Total protein*: ↑ by breakdown of the blood–brain barrier.
5. Immunoglobulins specific to the CSF, i.e. without matching Igs in a simultaneous blood sample: inflammation within the theca, e.g. MS, infection, tissue damage.

Common patterns

These are shown in Table 9.1.

Table 9.1

Condition	Glucose	Protein	Cells	Comments
Acute bacterial meningitis	↓	↑	Often >300/mm³	Polymorphs; lactate ↑*
Acute viral meningitis	N	N or ↑	<300 mononuclear	Culture, antigen detection may be possible
Fungal meningitis	↓	↑	<300 mononuclear	Culture and antigen detection
Tuberculous meningitis	↓	↑	Mixed pleocytosis <300	ZN stain organisms, culture PCR
Herpes simplex encephalitis	N	Mildly ↑	5–500 lympho	PCR
Guillain–Barré syndrome	N	↑	Normal	
Subarachnoid haemorrhage†	N	May be ↑	Erythrocytes	Look for bilirubin pigments on spectrophotometry; xanthochromia unreliable.
Malignant meningitis	↓	↑	Mononuclear	Rapid cytospin and look for malignant cells
HIV	N	N or ↑	Mononuclear pleocytosis	Culture, antigen detection, antiviral antibodies
Neurosyphilis –early –late	N or ↓	↑ ↑	<300 lymphocytes	VDRL Treponema pallidum Immobilisation tests

†LP should be done >12h after onset of headache; the CSF should be spun down within 45min; decreasing numbers of RBCs in successive bottles are compatible with SAH.

*Kleine TO et al. (2003) New and old diagnostic markers of meningitis in cerebrospinal fluid (CSF). *Brain Research Bulletin* **61**, 287–297.

Skull radiograph

Indications

Usually more modern imaging techniques are much more informative, but there are occasions when these may not be speedily available. However, the plain SXR has quite low specificity and sensitivity for detecting many abnormalities of neurological importance.

Used in (suspected) cases of

- Skull fracture.
- Pituitary fossa abnormalities.
- Tumours involving bone.
- Bone changes related to meningiomata.

Procedure

- Lateral view in the first instance.

Consider

- Occipitofrontal.
- Towne's (half axial).
- Basal (submentovertical).
- Specific views (e.g. orbits).

What to look for (what you see will depend on the pathology)

- Shape and symmetry of vault.
- Pituitary fossa.
- Position of calcified pineal (midline shift?).
- Bone density changes (e.g. tumour, meningioma, Paget's).
- Fractures.
- Evidence of neurosurgical procedures.
- Intracranial air.
- Post-nasal space.
- Craniocervical junction.

Indications for SXR after head injury, (but see section on cranial CT below; in general, CT is the preferred imaging modality)

In an orientated adult patient

- Loss of consciousness or amnesia.
- Fall >60cm.
- Full thickness scalp laceration.
- Scalp haematoma.

If a skull fracture is detected, proceed to CT.

Wasserberg J. (2002) Treating head injuries. *BMJ* **325**, 454–455.

Ultrasound

Ultrasound may be used in a variety of modes.

Mostly commonly used in neuroradiology

- B mode: gives 2-dimensional images.
- Doppler effect is used to assess alterations in the pattern (especially velocity) of flow in vessels.
- Duplex scanning combines B mode and Doppler.

Extracranial vessels

B mode

- Can image from clavicle (common carotid bifurcation), and internal and external carotids to angle of jaw.
- Can image proximal and distal subclavian, and vertebral arteries.
- Supraorbital artery (anterior circulation).
- Fibrofatty plaques and thrombus on plaques not very echogenic therefore missable.
- Fibrous plaques more echogenic.
- Calcification in plaque is highly echogenic.
- Can sometimes detect intraplaque haemorrhage or ulceration.

Note: requires patient cooperation and considerable operator skill. High grade stenosis can appear as total occlusion.

Doppler mode

- Stenosis alters the normal pattern of velocities recorded.

Duplex

- Combination of anatomic and flow imaging more sensitive and specific for clinically significant stenoses.

Comment

Use of carotid ultrasound: most commonly in the assessment of patients with carotid territory ischaemic strokes or TIAs, who might be candidates for carotid endarterectomy. Recent work suggests that there is little value in performing such studies >2 years after a cerebral event. If a patient has neurological signs or symptoms suggestive of posterior circulation events, there is little point in organising carotid (that is, anterior circulation) studies. Both the degree of stenosis and the morphology of the plaque (irregular plaques are more pathogenic) are important.

Intracranial vessels

Transcranial Doppler

- 2mHz to penetrate thinner bone.
- Flow velocity in anterior, middle, and post cerebral, ophthalmic and basilar arteries; carotid siphon.

What it shows

- Intracranial haemodynamics.
- Vasospasm in SAH.

- Monitoring of microemboli.
- This is an area of active research with new clinical indications being described frequently.

Rothwell PM *et al.* (2003) Analysis of pooled data from the randomised controlled trials of endarterectomy for symptomatic carotid stenosis. *Lancet* **361**, 107–116; Tegeler CH. (1995) Ultrasound in cerebrovascular disease, pp577–595 in *Neuroimaging*, ed Greenberg JO, McGraw-Hill, New York.

Angiography

Indications
- Strongly suspected or confirmed SAH.
- Suspected cerebral vasculitis.
- Delineation of other vascular abnormalities (e.g. arteriovenous malformations, AVM).
- Delineation of tumour blood supply (occasionally).

Procedure
1. Catheter passed via femoral artery to carotid or vertebral artery under image intensification.
2. Contrast is given.
3. In digital subtraction angiography, subtraction of pre-contrast from post-contrast images (pixel by pixel) is used to help remove signals from bone density.

Arch angiography (aortography)
- Visualises aorta, major neck vessels and sometimes circle of Willis.
- No venous imaging.

Selective intra-arterial angiography
- Later images show venous system.

Carotid artery
- AP, lateral and oblique views: anterior and middle cerebral and internal carotid arteries.

Vertebral artery
- Towne's and lateral views: vertebral, basilar, posterior cerebral arteries.

What can be demonstrated?
- Occlusion, stenosis, plaques.
- Aneurysms.
- Arteriovenous and other blood vessel abnormalities.
- Abnormal tumour circulation*.
- Displacement or compression of vessels*.
- Experimental role in acute stroke analysis.

Complications
- Sensitivity to the contrast medium.
- Cerebral ischaemia, e.g. secondary to dislodgement of embolic fragments by catheter tip or thrombus in the catheter lumen.

- The rate of transient or permanent neurological defect following angiography depends on the operator.

Osborne AG. (1999) *Diagnostic Cerebral Angiography*, 2nd edition, Lippincott, Williams & Wilkins, New York; Larsen DW, Teitelbaum GP. (2000) Radiological angiography, pp617–643 in Neurology in Clinical Practice, 3rd edition, eds Bradley WG *et al.*, Butterworth-Heinemann, Boston.

*Although CT and MRI give finer spatial details, angiography is still useful, e.g. delineating blood supply of a tumour.

Myelography

Indications
- Largely superseded by CT and especially MRI.
- Still used in subjects in whom MRI is contraindicated (e.g. cardiac pacemaker, metallic implants, claustrophobia).
- Can screen whole spinal cord and cauda equina for compressive or expanding lesions.
- Can visualise roots.
- Spinal vasculature abnormalities.

Procedure
5–25mL of (usually water-soluble) radio-opaque contrast medium is injected via an LP needle in the usual location (occasionally cisternal puncture is used). By tipping the patient on a tilt table, the whole spinal subarachnoid space may be visualised.

Complications
- Those of LP.
- Spinal arachnoiditis (after months or years), now rare with water-soluble contrast.
- Acute deterioration if there is cord/root compression.
- Direct neurotoxicity (3 in 10,000):
  - Seizures, encephalopathy.
  - Usually resolves in 48h.
- Allergic reaction to contrast:
  - Give dexamethasone 4mg 12 and 2h prior to investigation if known allergy.

Note: Send CSF for usual investigations (p519).

📖OHCM p405.

Radionuclide scans

Gamma camera scanning

- Give potassium perchlorate (to stop choroid plexus and salivary gland uptake).
- Then ^{99m}technetium labelled sodium pertechnetate IV.
- Look at intracranial distribution with gamma camera from lateral, anterior and posterior views.

What does it show?

- Areas of increased vascularity.
- Areas of BBB breakdown.

However it has been superseded by CT and MRI and is rarely available.

Positron emission tomography (PET)

Unstable positron-emitting isotopes (produced locally by a cyclotron or linear accelerator) are incorporated into biologically active compounds. The distribution of isotope shortly after IV administration is plotted. A range of compounds may be labelled, such as ligands for specific neurotransmitter receptors, or ^{18}F fluorodeoxyglucose (FDG). Commonly, PET is used to determine regional cerebral blood flow.

Single photon emission computed tomography (SPECT)

- Stable radioactive isotopes are incorporated into biologically active compounds.
- Their distribution after IV administration is plotted.
- These images often lack fine spatial detail.

Although the range of ligands available is limited, SPECT has certain advantages over PET:

- Isotopes are stable and therefore a cyclotron or linear accelerator need not be on site.
- A labelled ligand can be given after a clinically important event, e.g. can give agent and scan within 20min of the occurrence of a seizure.

Uses of PET and SPECT

PET is not widely available as a clinical tool. With the advent of functional MRI (FMRI), the uses of PET in both clinical practice and in neuroscience research may well become more restricted. SPECT is more widely available in clinical centres.

Clinical/research applications of PET and SPECT have included

- Determination of regional cerebral blood flow, glucose metabolism and oxygen utilisation
- Hypometabolism may be seen following a stroke. The affected area may exceed that with a demonstrable lesion on conventional CT or MR imaging.
- The epileptogenic focus may show interictal hypometabolism (ictal hypermetabolism may be demonstrated with SPECT).
- Regional hypometabolism may be seen in Alzheimer's, Parkinson's and related degenerative conditions.

- 'Pseudodementia' secondary to psychiatric disease such as depression (with normal SPECT scans) may sometimes be differentiated from dementia due to 'organic' neurological disease (with regional hypo-perfusion), although psychiatric diseases may themselves be associated with regional hypoperfusion.
- Whole body FDG-PET may be useful in demonstrating occult malignancy in paraneoplastic syndromes.
- Assessment of Parkinsonism.

The functional integrity of the nigrostriatal system can be assessed, e.g. by the use of SPECT ligands for the dopamine transporter (e.g. FP-CIT). Such DAT scans can be used to differentiate true parkinsonism from other causes of movement disorders.

- *In vivo* pharmacology (e.g. distribution of neurotransmitter receptors).

📖*Nuclear medicine*, p754.

Marshall V, Grosset D. (2003) Role of dopamine transporter imaging in routine clinical practice. *Mov Disord* **18**, 1415–1423; Younes-Mhenni S et al. (2004) FDG-PET improves tumour detection in patients with paraneoplastic neurological syndromes. *Brain* **127**, 2331–2338.

Computed tomography (CT)

Cranial CT

Now widely available; it should be considered a basic neurological tool.

Look for

- Disturbances in the normal anatomy of the ventricular system.
- Skull base and vault.
- Width of cortical fissures/sulci.
- Midline shift.
- Areas of abnormal tissue density.
- Opacity or lucency of sinuses.
- Normal flow voids.

High density ('white') signal
- Fresh blood.
- Calcification:
  - Slow growing tumour.
  - AVM/aneurysm.
  - Hamartoma.
  - In pineal/choroid plexus/basal ganglia, may be normal.

Low density ('black') signal
- Infarction.
- Tumour.
- Abscess.
- Oedema.
- Encephalitis.
- Resolving haematoma.

Mixed density
- Tumour.
- Abscess.
- AVM.
- Contusion.
- Haemorrhagic infarct.

After administration of IV contrast medium, areas with a breakdown in the blood–brain barrier may 'enhance' (appear 'white'). This may reveal previously 'invisible' lesions (isodense with the surrounding tissue). Especially useful for tumour and infection.

Common patterns of enhancement include
- Ring enhancement of tumours and abscesses.
- Solid enhancement of meningiomas.
- Meningeal enhancement with meningeal disease involvement.

Indications for head CT after head injury

- GCS <13 at any point after injury.
- GCS =13 or 14 at 2 hours after injury.
- Suspected open or depressed skull fracture.
- Signs of basilar skull fracture.

- Post traumatic seizure.
- Focal neurological deficit.
- 1 episode of vomiting (in adults).
- Pretraumatic amnesia >30min.

Also if some loss of consciousness or amnesia after the injury and one of the following risk factors:

- >64 years old.
- Coagulopathy.
- Dangerous mechanism of injury (pedestrian hit by motor vehicle, occupant ejected from a motor vehicle, or fall from >1m or down >5 stairs; lesser fall if <5 years old).

See NICE guidelines (2003) for further details of the management of head injury, and the use of radiological investigation at 🖰 www.nice.org.uk

CT angiography

Rapid image acquisition with helical CT can allow imaging of the intracranial vasculature. This technique has been particularly used in the detection of aneurysms, but is not widely available.

CT of spine

MRI is usually preferable but plain CT can give information about the discs and bony architecture. After myelography compressive lesions can be demonstrated.

📖OHCM p405.

Vieco PT. (1998) CT angiography of the intracranial circulation. *Neuroimaging Clin N Am* **8**, 577–792.

Magnetic resonance imaging (MRI) or nuclear magnetic resonance (NMR) imaging

For most applications, MRI is superior to CT, but has more restricted availability.

Note: MRI is not safe in the presence of ferromagnetic materials (e.g. certain prostheses, metal filings in the eye).

Most common sequences are T1 and T2, but increasingly other sequences are being used clinically, such as FLAIR, proton density, diffusion-weighted imaging.

In general
- T1 CSF is hypointense ('black'); fat and mature blood clot white.
- T2 CSF is hyperintense ('white').

MRI with enhancement
Intravenously administered gadolinium leaks through areas of damaged blood–brain barrier to give a marked enhancement.
- Ischaemia.
- Infection.
- Tumour (may help differentiate from surrounding oedema).
- Active demyelination.

MR venography and angiography
MR may be used to obtain non-invasive images of blood vessels by using special MRI sequences and image reconstruction. While standard angiography remains a 'gold standard' for many purposes, MR angiography has the advantage of being non-invasive and therefore 'safe'. MRA images flow rather than structure, and therefore may fail to 'pick up' low flow abnormalities such as cavernous angiomas. *Caution*: congenital abnormalities in the venous sinuses may be misinterpreted as thrombosis on MRV.

Uses
- Assessment of patency of major arterial and venous vessels.
- Visualisation of large (~3mm diameter) aneurysms.

Functional MRI (FMRI)
A recent development allows certain (indirect) indices of neural activity (most commonly changes reflecting regional perfusion) to be imaged with sufficient temporal resolution to be useful for both research and clinical applications (although FMRI has been largely a research tool to date). As a conventional MRI machine, albeit with special software, is required, it is likely that FMRI will become a widely used clinical tool.

Clinical and research applications have included
- Demonstration of the language areas prior to epilepsy surgery.
- Demonstration of the functional anatomy of cognitive, sensory and motor processes.

Table 9.2 Comparison of T1 and T2 MRI

T1	T2	Tissue or lesion
Good anatomical detail	Reveals most pathology better than T1	
Hypointense	Hyperintense	CSF
Hyperintense	Iso-intense	Fat, e.g. dermoid, lipoma, some metastases (melanoma), atheroma
Very hypointense	Very hyperintense	Cyst, hygroma
Hypointense	Hyperintense	Ischaemia, oedema, demyelination, many malignant tumours
Hyperintense	Moderately hyperintense	Subacute or chronic haemorrhage
Iso	Hypointense	Acute haemorrhage
Iso	Iso	Meningioma

📖 OHCM p405.

Powell HW et al. (2004) The application of functional MRI of memory in temporal lobe epilepsy: a clinical review. *Epilepsia* **45**, 855–863; White PM et al. (2001) Intracranial aneurysm: CT angiography and MR angiography for detection prospective blinded comparison in a large patient cohort. *Radiology* **219**, 739–749.

Nerve conduction studies

Please give your neurophysiologist as much information as possible about your case, and, if necessary, discuss it with him/her. S/he will then be in the position to organize the most appropriate neurophysiological investigations. In certain circumstances, you may need to specifically ask for unusual investigations, such as repetitive stimulation in suspected LEMS (see p536).

Sensory nerve action potential (SNAP) and sensory conduction velocity

Procedure

Orthodromic conduction velocity: electrically stimulates distal sensory branches (e.g. index finger) and records the evoked sensory nerve action potential (SNAP) proximally (e.g. over median nerve at wrist). The distance between the two sites (D) and the latency (L) of the onset of the SNAP determine the sensory conduction velocity (D/L). The SNAP amplitude is also useful.

Antidromic conduction velocity: supramaximal electrical stimulation proximally; records distally (e.g. by a ring electrode on little finger). By varying the position of the stimulating electrode, the conduction velocity in various portions of the nerve may be ascertained.

Motor velocities are more commonly measured

Table 9.3

Typical values	Latency	Amplitude
Median nerve (index finger to wrist)	2–3ms	9–40mV
Ulnar nerve (little finger to wrist)	2–2.6ms	6–30mV
Sural nerve (midcalf to below med. mall.)	2–4ms	5–40mV

med. mall, medial malleolus.

What does it mean?

- ↓ SNAP amplitude or SNAP absence altogether imply a lesion distal to the dorsal root ganglion.
- ↓ velocity/↑ latency (Table 9.3).

Motor conduction velocity

Procedure

Supramaximally stimulate a peripheral nerve trunk at a proximal (p) and a more distal (d) site. Record the time to the onset of the evoked muscle response (CMAP) from each (Tp and Td), and the distance between them (D). The motor conduction velocity between p and d is therefore D/(Tp–Td).

Typical values

- Median nerve in forearm (to abductor pollicis brevis) >48m/s.
- Ulnar nerve in forearm (to abductor digiti minimi) >48m/s.
- Common peroneal nerve (to extensor digitorum brevis) >40m/s.

What does it mean?
See Table 9.4.

Distal motor latency
Latency from stimulation of most distal site on nerve to CMAP.

Typical values
- Median nerve (wrist to abductor pollicis brevis) <4.1m/s.
- Ulnar nerve (wrist to abductor digiti minimi) <3.8m/s.
- Radial nerve (spiral groove to brachioradialis) <5m/s.

Note: these latencies include time taken for impulses to pass along the most distal (unmyelinated) portion of the nerve, and for transmission at the neuromuscular junction (therefore they may not be used to calculate nerve conduction velocities). Compare with velocities elsewhere in the nerve being studied.

What does it mean?
↑ *DML seen in*
- Conditions in which the very distal segment of a nerve is compromised (most commonly carpal tunnel syndrome).
- Early demyelinating neuropathy (e.g. Guillain–Barré syndrome).
- Chronic demyelinating neuropathy.

Compound motor action potential (CMAP)
The waveform, amplitude and area-under-the-curve of the CMAP reflect the number of depolarised muscle fibres (e.g. reduced in axonal neuropathy and denervated muscle) and the temporal dispersion of conduction velocities in the motor neurones to them (e.g. increased in demyelinating neuropathy).

Table 9.4

	Conduction velocity	AP amplitude	AP dispersion
Axonal neuropathy	Late stage: ↓ distally > proximally (loss of fastest conducting axons)	Late stage: ↓	Not seen
Demyelination	Marked		Greater dispersion, perhaps especially in acquired not inherited demyelination
Ganglionopathies	Slowing proportional to loss of large fibres; often not marked	↓ proportional to loss of large fibres; often not marked	not seen

Note: limbs should be warm; look for asymmetries.
What are your laboratory's current values?

Late responses

F wave

- If a motor nerve is stimulated, there are orthodromically directed action potentials that may cause a response in the muscle (CMAP). However, antidromically directed action potentials will also pass proximally towards the cell body. If these result in sufficient depolarisation of the axon hillock, then a second orthodromic volley will pass down the nerve. This may cause a second motor action potential (the F wave). Therefore the F wave (i) does not involve synapses (other than the neuromuscular junction of course) and (ii) depends on the integrity of the whole axon.
- It may be difficult to elicit.

Delay or absence of the F wave may reflect a lesion proximal to the site of stimulation, in parts of the nerve that may be inaccessible to electrodes, e.g. brachial plexopathy or thoracic outlet syndrome. May also be an early feature in GBD.

H wave

- This is 'an electrical ankle jerk': submaximal stimulation of posterior tibial nerve in the popliteal fossa causes trans-synaptic activation of soleus, recorded as a CMAP.
- Amplitude may be ↓ by afferent or efferent problems, e.g. neuropathy or radiculopathy.

Repetitive stimulation

Procedure

- Stimulate a motor nerve with 3 to 5 supramaximal stimuli at 2–4Hz while recording evoked CMAPs.

Normal response

- No change in CMAP amplitude.

In myasthenia gravis

- >10% decrement in CMAP amplitude after 2 stimuli.

In Lambert–Eaton myasthenic syndrome

- After voluntary contraction, or after rapid stimulation (20–50Hz) for 2–10 seconds, the CMAP amplitude, often initially small, increases by 25% (suggestive) or 100% (diagnostic).
- At a slow (3Hz) rate of stimulation, there is a response decrement.

EMG

Procedure

- A concentric needle electrode is usually used.
- It is inserted into the muscle to be studied.
- The difference in potential between the inner part of the electrode and the outer core is amplified and displayed on an oscilloscope or computer screen.
- It is also 'displayed' as an auditory signal, and experienced electromyographers as much listen to as watch the pattern of electrical activity.

Normal muscle is 'silent' (electrically inactive) at rest (there is no 'spontaneous activity'), although there will be a brief burst of activity when the electrode is first inserted (the 'insertional activity').

The electrode can pick up electrical activity from muscle fibres within about 0.5mm of its tip, therefore muscle fibres from several motor units (each innervated by a different motor neurone) in this volume can contribute to the signal. However, with care, potentials from a single motor unit may be recorded when a cooperative subject tries to exert the muscle a little (the 'motor unit potential'). With increasing muscular effort, more muscle fibres are recruited, giving rise to the 'interference pattern'.

Various nerve and muscle problems cause characteristic alterations to these four patterns of activity

1. Insertional.
2. Spontaneous.
3. Motor unit potential.
4. Recruitment.
5. In addition, certain other patterns may be observed in certain diseases (myotonia).

1. Insertional activity

- Usually there is a brief burst of potentials which lasts <1.
- Insertional activity is normal in upper motor neurone (UMN) lesions and most non-inflammatory myopathies.
- It may be longer lasting in lower motor neurone (LMN) lesions, inflammatory myopathies and acid maltase deficiency.
- In myotonia, myotonic discharges occur (*see below*).

2. Spontaneous activity

- Normal muscles at rest are silent.
- This is also the case in UMN lesions, non-inflammatory myopathies (unless secondary denervation has set in) and myotonia.
- Fibrillation potentials and positive sharp waves are seen in LMN lesions and inflammatory myopathies. They occur in regular bursts of constant amplitude (unlike activity related to voluntary contraction).
- Fibrillation potentials are spontaneous APs in irritable, acutely denervated, muscle fibres. They are low amplitude brief negative potentials.

- Positive sharp waves are brief positive potentials, followed by a negative wave. Typically they can be seen for 2–3 weeks after denervation, but may persist.

3. Motor unit potentials (MUPs)

- If the electrode is positioned quite close to the fibres of a motor unit which is active during slight voluntary contraction, then a motor unit potential may be recorded. In normal muscle (and in UMN lesions), this waveform is triphasic, 5–10ms and has an amplitude of 0.5–1mV (larger muscles have larger motor units).
- In myopathies and muscular dystrophies, the motor units are smaller and polyphasic. They tend to be briefer but in some cases last longer than usual.
- In denervated and then reinnervated muscles (typically LMN lesions), the size of individual motor units increases (as the surviving motor neurones 'take over' the muscle fibres previously innervated by now absent other motor neurones). MUPs therefore are of greater amplitude and duration, and are polyphasic.
- In myotonia, myotonic discharges are seen.

Note: up to 15–20% of MUPs in 'normal' muscle may be polyphasic.

4. Recruitment

- Normally, as the strength of voluntary contraction increases, increasing numbers of motor units are recruited, and these units tend to be larger (Heinneman's size principle). The potentials due to these active units overlap, and become difficult and finally impossible to tell apart—a full 'interference pattern', usually well below maximum voluntary contraction.
- In muscle diseases, a full interference pattern may be produced, but it is of low amplitude. In weak muscles, there may be 'early recruitment' (i.e. recruitment of many motor units at low levels of voluntary contraction).
- In denervated muscles, a full interference pattern may not be achieved, because of the decreased number of motor units.
- In UNM lesions, there is a lower frequency of 'normal' MUPs.

5. Other phenomena: myotonia

High frequency repetitive discharges occurring after voluntary movement or provoked by moving the electrode. The amplitude and the frequency wax and wane, giving the auditory signature likened to the sound of a Second World War dive bomber (or a motor cycle).

Note: following the onset of a neuropathy, it may take at least 10–14 days for evidence of denervation to appear in the EMG, therefore a repeat study after this time is often useful.

Single fibre EMG

A recording electrode with a smaller recording surface than usually used samples a few muscle fibres from a single motor unit (supplied by a single motor neurone). The variability ('jitter') in the timing of action potentials from different muscles should be less than 20–25ms. Conduction block during voluntary contraction may also be shown. These techniques are used to investigate neuromuscular disorders and reinnervation in neuropathies.

EEG

The standard EEG is non-invasive. Electrodes are attached to the scalp with collodion adhesive. Stable recordings may be made for days. Usually they are arranged according to the international 10–20 system. This is a method for positioning electrodes over the scalp in an orderly and reproducible fashion. Additional electrodes can be applied to the scalp, depending on the region of interest.

Standard recording conditions

- *Rest.*
- *Hyperventilation* for 3–5min, can activate generalised epileptiform changes (and precipitate absence seizures):
  - Can ↑ frequency of focal discharge.
  - Can ↑ slow wave abnormalities.
- *Photic stimulation* (a strobe light at 30cm with a frequency of 1–50Hz); this can produce several patterns of activity:
  - *Photoparoxysmal response*: bilateral spike or spike and wave discharges not time-locked to the visual stimulus, which may outlast the visual stimulus by hundreds of milliseconds. Generalised, but may have frontal or occipital predominance.
  - Commonly seen in idiopathic generalised epilepsies.
  - High voltage occipital spikes, time-locked to the stimulus.
  - Weakly associated with epilepsy.
  - *Photomyogenic (photomyoclonic) responses*: non-specific mostly frontal spikes due to muscle activity.
  - Associated with alcohol and some other drug-withdrawal states.
- Sleep studies:
  - Subject either stays awake the night before the recording or is given a small dose of choral prior to the recording (sometimes both).
  - Subjects tend to show the earlier stages of non-REM sleep.
  - These studies increase the yield of EEG abnormalities, including epileptiform ones.
  - By capture of 'natural sleep': certain seizure types are more common in sleep (e.g. juvenile myoclonic epilepsy).
  - Sleep deprivation itself increases the number of seizures and epileptiform changes.

📖 *Polysomnography*, p545.

Table 9.5

Activity	Frequency (Hz)	Amplitude (mV)	Scalp location	Behavioural state
Alpha	8–12	20–60	Usually occipital	Maximum relaxed, awake, eyes close
Beta	>13	10–20	Frontocentral	Wakeful, drowsy; REM and slow wave sleep 1 and 2
Theta	4–8	Variable diffuse	Frontocentral, temporal	Minimally awake, drowsy, sws (slow wave sleep)
Delta	<4	Variable	Diffuse	Awake; drowsy
Mu	8–10	20–60	Central	Awake, suppressed in voluntary movements

The terms alpha, beta, theta and delta are often used to describe the background activity but are also used to describe the frequency of EEG activity. Sharp activity may be a normal phenomenon.

EEG abnormalities

The normal EEG

There is a wide range of normal EEG phenomena. Some of the common patterns in the awake adult are listed in Table 9.5.

EEG abnormalities (not peri- or per-seizure)

- A variety of EEG abnormalities may be seen outside the peri- or per-seizure period.
- Abnormalities in the EEG are not restricted to the appearance of abnormal waveforms.
- The loss, or redistribution in the scalp location, of normal background activities is abnormal.

The classification of EEG abnormalities is complex. Below is a highly simplified guide

1. General excess of slow waves: commonly seen in:
   - Metabolic encephalopathy.
   - Encephalitis.
   - Post-ictal states.
2. Focal slow waves: commonly seen in:
   - Large cerebral lesions (e.g. tumour, haematoma).
   - Post-ictal states.
   - Migraineurs.
3. Localised intermittent rhythmic slow waves: may be seen in:
   - Idiopathic generalised and localisation related epilepsies.
4. Epileptiform abnormalities:
   - Spikes (if last <80ms) or sharp waves (80–200ms) may be associated with slow waves.
   - Consistently focal spikes suggest epilepsy with a focal seizure onset. (*Note*: 2–4% of non-epileptics have occasional spikes or sharps).
5. Repetitive stereotyped 'periodic' complexes.

EEG patterns may show periodicity. These patterns may be epileptiform or not, and may be focal or generalised. They are an abnormal EEG feature, the interpretation of which depends on the clinical context.

Examples include

- Burst suppression: bursts of generalised high voltage mixed waveforms, alternating with generalised voltage suppression:
  - Coma.
  - Late stage status epilepticus (both convulsive and non-convulsive).
- Triphasic waves over one or both temporal lobes:
  - Common in herpes simplex encephalitis.
- Periodic lateralised epileptiform discharges (PLEDs) are localised sharp or slow wave complexes 0.2–1s long, every 1–5s.
  - Non-specific but suggest localised cerebral insult (stroke, haematoma, tumour).
  - Occasionally seen in migraine and focal epilepsies.
- BIPLEDs are bihemispheric PLEDs.
  - Suggest more widespread insults, e.g. anoxia, encephalitis.

- Bilateral or generalised high voltage complexes for 0.5–2s every 4–15s:
  - Characteristic of subacute sclerosing panencephalitis.
- Triangular waves:
  - Characteristic of Creutzfeldt–Jakob disease (CJD).
  - Not seen in vCJD; may see a 'disorganised' EEG without repetitive complexes).
- Runs of broad triphasic waves (1.5–3Hz).
  - Severe metabolic encephalopathy (e.g. renal or hepatic failure).
- Periodic spikes or sharp waves; bi- or multiphasic morphology (0.5–2Hz); usually generalised—suggest severe encephalopathy, e.g.
  - Herpes encephalitis.
  - CJD (in setting of rapid dementia and myoclonus).
  - Lithium intoxication.
  - Post-anoxic brain injury.
  - Tricyclic antidepressant overdose.

EEGs in epilepsy

Idiopathic (primary) generalised epilepsy (IGE)
- Generalised, bilaterally synchronous epileptiform discharges with virtually normal background.
- Absence epilepsy: 3Hz spike and wave.
- Juvenile myoclonic epilepsy (JME): 6Hz multiple spike and wave.

Symptomatic (secondary) generalised epilepsy
- More variable.
- Interictal background activity: excess slow.
- Interictal epileptiform activity: irregular spikes or sharp and slow waves 1.5–4Hz. Usually generalised, but may show asymmetry or (multi) focal features.

Localisation-related partial epilepsy
- Interictal EEG is often normal, particularly if the focus is located deeply (especially common with frontal foci).
- There may be lateralised or localised spikes or sharp waves.

How to use the EEG

In suspected epilepsy
- Routine EEG with photic stimulation and hyperventilation gives about up to a 50% detection rate for interictal epileptiform abnormalities in a subject with epilepsy (higher 'yield' in primary generalised epilepsies than in localisation-related epilepsies).
- Sleep-deprived or choral-induced sleep recording: this may increase the yield of EEG abnormalities to up to 60–70%.

- Consider 24h or longer ambulatory EEG, ideally with audio/video monitoring. Most useful in helping to determine the nature of the seizure in a subject with frequent (e.g. daily) attacks.

In general, avoid reduction in anti-epileptic drugs or drugs such as pentylenetrazole to induce seizures, except in exceptional circumstances, e.g. videotelemetry as part of workup for epilepsy surgery.

Note:
- No interictal spikes does not imply no epilepsy.
- Similarly, interictal spikes do not always imply epilepsy.
- A negative ictal EEG does not necessarily imply a non-epileptic ('pseudo') seizure, especially in simple partial and some brief complex partial seizures. Scalp electrodes may fail to record deep, especially frontal, activity.
- However, a tonic-clonic seizure with loss of consciousness should be associated with an epileptiform EEG during the ictus. This EEG activity may be obscured by muscle artefact, but post-ictal slowing may be seen (*see below*).
- The EEG may be slow after a tonic-clonic seizure for many tens of minutes.

Note: the diagnosis of epilepsy is mainly clinical! Remember that most episodes of altered consciousness are not epileptic in origin. In many cases, cardiological investigations are appropriate. Have a low threshold for ordering a 12-lead ECG. Ambulatory ECG monitoring, particularly with cardiac memo devices, can be very useful.

In established epilepsy
- Classification (e.g. complex partial seizure (CPS) *vs.* absence).
- Assessment of frequency of seizures (e.g. ambulatory EEG to assess frequency of absence seizures).
- Reduction in interictal discharges in some syndromes (e.g. absence, photosensitive epilepsy) correlates with AED efficacy.

In focal cerebral dysfunction
Often not particularly helpful. Modern imaging studies usually provide more information.
- Small, deep or slow growing lesions often cause no effects.
- Asymmetric voltage attenuation may be caused by a subdural haematoma (or other fluid collection) overlying the cortex.
- Direct grey matter involvement may cause alteration/loss of normal EEG, or cause epileptiform discharges.
- Subcortical white matter changes can cause localised polymorphic slow waves.
- Deeper subcortical lesions tend to produce more widespread slow wave disturbances.

In CNS infections
- CJD and subacute sclerosing panencephalilits (SSPE) have relatively characteristic EEG associations.

- Meningitis and encephalitis cases may show diffuse background disturbances and polymorphic or bilateral intermittent slow wave abnormalities.
- Encephalitis usually causes more changes than meningitis.
- Focal changes may be seen over abscesses and in cases of herpes simplex encephalitis.

In dementia

- To exclude some conditions such as toxic encephalopathy, non-convulsive status epilepticus (NCSE).
- A few dementing conditions have characteristic EEGs (CJD, SSPE).
- Slowing of background frequency occurs in Alzheimer's disease, but values may overlap with those of the normal aged; therefore not very helpful clinically.

In confusional states

- Helpful in diagnosing NCSE (absence and complex partial status).
- To exclude cerebral dysfunction.
- Not very useful in psychiatric diagnosis *per se*, but an abnormal EEG in a confusional state may help exclude psychogenic causes for an apparent reduction in level of consciousness.

In toxic-metabolic encephalopathies

- EEG always abnormal.
- Diffuse slowing in mild cases.
- Other abnormalities may develop in later stages.
- Specific patterns may be seen in certain aetiologies.
- Excess fast activity: barbiturate and benzodiazepine toxicity.
- Triphasic waves: hepatic and renal failure, anoxia, hypoglycaemia, hyperosmolality, lithium toxicity.
- Periodic spikes or sharp waves: anoxia, renal failure, lithium and tricyclic antidepressant toxicity.

In coma

- EEG, especially serial EEGs, provides an indication of degree of cerebral dysfunction.
- In general, any 'normal'-looking EEG, spontaneous variability, sleep–wake changes, and reaction to external stimuli are relatively good prognostic signs.
- An invariant, unreactive EEG is a poor prognostic sign; the pattern however is not uniform, it may include periodic spikes of sharp waves, episodic voltage attenuation, alpha coma, burst suppression.
- May give some diagnostic clues, e.g. localised abnormality—supratentorial mass lesion; persistent epileptiform discharges—status epilepticus.
- 'Alpha coma': monotonous unresponsive alpha with anterior distribution seen after cardio/respiratory arrest is a poor prognostic feature.
- Monotonous but partially reactive alpha may follow brainstem infarcts.

Invasive EEG techniques

These are generally restricted to specialist centres, most commonly used in the pre-surgical workup of patients.

Foramen ovale electrodes, corticography (usually done by laying strips of electrodes on the surface of the brain) and depth EEG (electrodes implanted into the parenchyma of the brain) may be used, depending on the region of interest. Sphenoidal electrodes are rarely used today, but can give useful EEG information about the medial temporal structures.

Polysomnography

- This is the multimodal recording used in the analysis of sleep-related disorders.
- There is concurrent recording of EMG, EEG and EOG (electro-oculography—eye movements), often with audiovisual channels. Other physiological parameters may also be recorded, e.g. nasal air flow, chest expansion.

Sleep is classically divided into 4 stages (1–4), of progressively 'deeper' slow wave sleep (SWS), and a fifth stage of rapid eye movement (REM) sleep, characterised physiologically by bursts of rapid eye movements (saccades).

Table 9.6

Stage	Behaviour	Main EEG pattern	Comments
1	Drowsy	Diffuse alpha → theta	Flat to medium
2	Light sleep	High theta	K complexes
3	Medium sleep	Delta	Broad K complexes delta activation
4	Deep sleep	Continuous delta	None

REM: rapid eye movements.

There is progression through stages 1 to 4, and several episodes of REM during a typical night's sleep. Polysomnography can be important in understanding the pathophysiology of the insomnias, parasomnias and other sleep patterns.

Multiple sleep latency test

This is a diagnostic test for narcolepsy. Following a good night's sleep, normal subjects typically enter REM sleep with a latency of >>10min (usually ~90min). In narcolepsy the latency is <10min.

Sodium amytal (Wada) test

Sodium amytal is injected into the R or L internal carotid artery. It is a short-acting barbiturate, and temporarily causes hemispheric dysfunction on the injected side. If injected into the left in most right-handers, the ability to speak and continue to hold up the R arm is temporally impaired. If speech is preserved following R-sided injection, it suggests normal left-lateralisation for language function. More complex testing may also be undertaken during the period of hemispheric dysfunction, but it is usually used to determine language dominance prior to certain neurosurgical procedures.

Sensory evoked potentials or responses (EPs or ERs)

While many techniques and protocols have been developed in research laboratories, there are only a few techniques in widespread clinical use. A stimulus is delivered to the periphery, thus activating a sensory system and evoking an electrical response over a more central, often cortical, area. Multiple surface electrode recordings time-locked to the peripheral stimulus are recorded and averaged, to help eliminate ongoing random background 'noise' from the sensory stimulus-evoked 'signal'. Deviations of this evoked potential or response (EP or ER) from the norm (especially in latency and waveform) suggest pathology in the sensory pathway tested.

Visual EPs

Pattern-evoked VEP

An alternating chequerboard pattern (temporal frequency 1–2Hz) is presented to each eye individually (Fig. 9.1). The EP is recorded over the occipital (primary visual) cortex. Most commonly the first large positive wave, called P1 or P100 (as it typically occurs at about 100ms), is studied.

A delayed, smaller or dispersed VEP indicates disease in the retino-geniculo-striate pathway (if severe refractive errors or cataracts have been excluded), but most commonly affecting the optic nerve (a uniocular deficit implies a lesion anterior to the optic chiasm) or at the chiasm.

Flash-evoked VEP

In subjects with very poor vision or fixation, and in the very young, a bright flash may be used as the stimulus. This gives less reproducible results, particularly in the P100 latency.

Common uses

The VEP is used in general to document intrinsic, inflammatory or compressive lesions of the optic nerve (or chiasm).
1. Suspected optic or retrobulbar neuritis.
2. In a patient with suspected MS, evidence of a VEP abnormality in an asymptomatic eye would suggest a previous episode of an optic neuritis.
3. Evaluation of hysterical blindness (may need to use a strobe light stimulus if patient non-cooperative).

4. Evaluation of optic nerve function in compressive lesions such as dysthyroid eye disease, optic nerve glioma.
5. Follow-up after surgery to decompress the optic nerve or chiasm.
6. Assessment of poor visual acuity in patients unable to cooperate with usual testing. Vary the size of the chequerboard squares; subjects with poor acuity will only have a VEP to the coarser patterns.

Somatosensory EPs

- Stimulation site over a peripheral nerve, e.g. ulnar or median at wrist, common peroneal at knee, posterior tibial at ankle (Fig. 9.2).
- Record over Erb's point (above the medial end of the clavicle), C7 or C2 vertebra, parietal cortex for arm stimulation; L1, C7, C2 or vertex for leg stimulation.
- Calculate absolute and interpeak latencies.
- Need to show with nerve conduction studies (NCS) that distal parts of the somatosensory pathways are conducting normally.
- Assesses dorsal column not anterolateral (spinothalamic) tract pathways:
  - E.g. stimulate median nerve at wrist, prolonged latency to Erb's point; suggests brachial plexus (or more distal) lesion.
  - Prolonged Erb's point to C2 latency suggests spinal cord lesion.

Uses
- Diagnosis of plexopathies.
- Evaluation of subclinical myelopathy in possible MS.
- Evaluation of hysterical sensory loss.
- Per-operative monitoring (e.g. during scoliosis surgery).

Brainstem auditory evoked potentials (BAEPs, BAERs, BSAEPs, Fig. 9.3)

- Stimulus: rarefaction clicks of 50 or 100ms duration, presented mono-aurally at 10Hz at 60–70DB above threshold (masking noise to other ear).
- Record over mastoid and vertex of skull.
- Classic waveform has seven peaks, said to be generated by sequential auditory nuclei:

I VIIIth nerve (must be present to interpret subsequent waves)
II Cochlear nucleus (may be absent in normals)
III Superior olive
IV Lateral lemniscus (may be absent in normals)
V Interior colliculus (should be 50% or more of wave I's amplitude)
VI Medial geniculate (too variable for regular clinical use)
VII Auditory thalamocortical radiation (too variable for regular clinical use)

Latency I to V (central conduction time) should be no more than 4.75ms. The difference between left and right central conduction times should be <0.4ms.

Uses
- Hearing assessment, especially in children.
- Evaluation in suspected MS and other myelinopathies (e.g. adreno-leukodystrophy; MRI more important now).

- Evaluation and detection of posterior fossa lesions (e.g. acoustic neuromas; MRI more important now).
- Evaluation of brainstem function (e.g. tumour, CVAs).
- Evaluation of brainstem function in coma and brain death.
- Per-operative, e.g. acoustic neuroma excision.

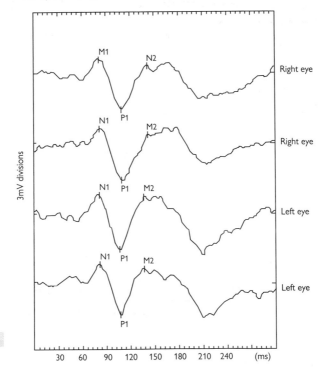

Fig. 9.1 Visual evoked potential (to chequerboard stimulus).

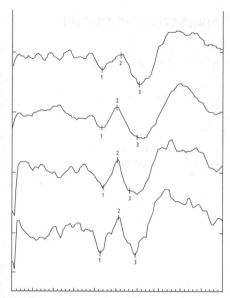

Fig. 9.2 Leg somatosensory potentials.

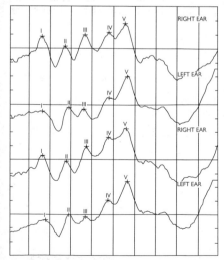

Fig. 9.3 Brainstem auditory evoked potentials.

Transcranial magnetic stimulation (TMS)

- Brief, high-current pulse produced in a circular or figure-of-eight-shaped coil held over the scalp.
- This induces a magnetic field with flux perpendicular to the coil.
- This in turn produces an electric field perpendicular to the magnetic field.
- The result is excitation or inhibition of the subjacent cortex (depending on stimulus parameters).

Measurement of central motor conduction time

- TMS over the motor cortex indirectly (presumably via synaptic activation of corticospinal neurones) causes a volley of activity in the corticospinal tracts. The latency of the EMG in, say, the abductor digiti minimi may be measured.
- May be used in cervical myelopathy and MS to show increased latency of EMG in hand muscles evoked by TMS over the motor cortex. If the EMG latency to more distal stimulation (e.g. at C7 over the spinal cord and in the ulnar nerve) is normal, then an increased central motor conduction time may be inferred.
- Latency may also be increased in other neurogenerative conditions.

Psychogenic limb weakness

Some authorities have used TMS to evoke muscle activity in 'paralysed' limbs in patients with psychogenic paralysis. This needs to be done in the context of an 'holistic' approach to the patient, aimed at dealing with any psychological pathology.

Potential clinical applications

There have been many TMS studies; some that may prove useful as clinical tests, e.g.

- Determination of lateralisation of language function by repetitive TMS (rTMS) prior to surgery for epilepsy.
- Assessment of cortical excitability in certain epilepsy syndromes.
- Assessment of decreased intracortical inhibition in dystonia.

Curra A et al. (2002) Transcranial magnetic stimulation techniques in clinical investigation. Neurology **59**, 1851–1859.

Neurological investigation of sphincter disturbance

EMG

- Of pelvic floor muscles may be helpful in faecal incontinence, stress urinary incontinence and cauda equina syndrome.
- Pelvic floor and sphincter muscle EMGs may reflect pudendal nerve damage.
- Anal sphincter EMG abnormalities may reflect damage to Onuf's nucleus, e.g. in multi-system atrophy. It is characteristically unaffected in motor neurone disease.

MRI

- In suspected sacral spinal cord, conus medullaris and equina equina lesions.

Urodynamics

Flowmetry

- Measurement of rate and amount of urine flow over time.
- Allows calculation of parameters such as time to maximal flow, maximum and mean flow rate, volume voided.
- Post-micturition ultrasound can determine residual volume.

Cystometry (needs urinary catheterisation)

- Measurement of intravesicular pressure during filling (usually at 50mL/min) or emptying. Typically bladder filling sensation starts at about 100mL, and the bladder is full at 400–600mL (with no more than a 15cm of water rise in pressure). Detrusor instability may cause sharp rises in the pressure during filling.
- During voiding, flow rate should be >15mL/min (♂) or >20mL/min (♀) with pressures of <50cmH$_2$O (♂) or 30 cmH$_2$O (♀).

Fowler CJ. (1998) Investigational techniques. *Eur Urol* **34** suppl 10–12.

Edrophonium (Tensilon®) test

Procedure

- Explain the test to patient.
- Select weak and/or fatiguable muscles to be assessed.
- Attach ECG monitor.
- Draw up 0.6mg atropine (for use if extreme bradycardia develops), 10mg of edrophonium in 5mL normal saline (A), 5mL normal saline (B) and saline flush.
- Administer 1mL of test solution (A or B, ideally patient and administrating physician should be blinded to the nature of the solution).
- If no adverse reaction, administer remaining 4mL.
- Repeat with other solution (B or A).

Note: if the diagnosis of MG is clinically obvious, and the patient has responded to pyridostigmine given empirically, there is little point in stopping this and performing an edrophonium test.

Interpretation

- In myasthenia gravis, there should be a response within 30–60s, which should wear off in 2–4min.
- There may be a response in LEMS, polymyositis and motor neurone disease (MND).

Biopsies

- Always liaise with those taking the biopsy and those processing it!
- A biopsy should be undertaken to answer specific questions, in the light of a differential diagnosis formulated following history, examination and other investigations.

Skeletal muscle

Indications

- Primary muscle disease, e.g. metabolic myopathy, polymyositis, muscular dystrophy.
- Neurogenic atrophy.
- Mitochondrial cytopathies (even in the absence of clinical muscle involvement).
- Multi-organ disease, e.g. vasculitides.

Which muscle to biopsy?

- An involved but not endstage muscle.
- One that has not been used for EMG recording or had an injection for >1 month.
- Quadriceps and deltoid often used.

Open or needle biopsy?

Open biopsy

- Larger specimen.
- Can fix specimen at *in situ* length.
- Especially for inflammatory myopathy and in vasculitis.

Needle biopsy

- Smaller scar.
- Multiple biopsies possible.
- But:
  - Smaller biopsies.
  - Difficulties in orientating the sample.

What may be done to the tissue?

- Routine histology.
- Examination of small blood vessels.
- Histochemistry.
- Electron microscopy.
- Tests of muscle metabolism.
- Mitochondrial DNA studies.

Nerve

Indications

- Distinction between segmental demyelination and axonal degeneration (if not already determined).
- Certain neuropathies with characteristic histological features, e.g. due to amyloid deposition, sarcoid, vasculitis, neoplastic involvement.
- Certain myelinopathies (e.g. leukodystrophies) with PNS and CNS involvement.

Which nerve to biopsy?
- The cutaneous branch of the sural nerve at the ankle (usually).
- Superficial peroneal (sometimes).
- Superficial radial (occasionally).
- Occasionally small motor nerve twigs are obtained in muscle biopsy.
- Overlying skin may be co-biopsied.

What is done?
- 2–3cm of full-thickness nerve or fascicle.

What may be done to the tissue?
- Routine light microscopy (morphometry, structural survey; amyloidosis).
- Frozen section light microscopy (immunochemistry).
- Electron microscopy (ultrastructure).
- Teased out single fibres (to examine sequential myelin internodes).

Brain/meningeal biopsy
Indications
- Diagnosis and management of suspected primary and some metastatic brain tumours.
- Differential diagnosis of other mass lesions (inflammatory and infective).
- Differentiation of radiation necrosis and tumour regrowth.
- Differentiation of neoplastic and non-neoplastic cysts (and their drainage).
- Diagnostic biopsy of a suspected infectious lesion that has not responded to a trial of therapy.
- Diagnosis of cerebral vasculitis or vasculopathy.

What is done?
- High quality cranial CT/MRI, possibly with contrast, to delineate lesion.
- If no discrete lesion, generally an area of non-dominant, non-eloquent cerebrum is taken.
- Stereotactic needle biopsy with image guidance:
  - Deep, small, lesions in 'eloquent' areas.
  - Multiple biopsies along needle track (useful in heterogeneous lesions such as some gliomas).
- And/or open biopsy:
  - Accessible lesions.
  - When resection considered during procedure.
- Intra-operative evaluation of frozen samples:
  - E.g. can a biopsy be made?
  - E.g. is the sample adequate?

Note: caution in suspected CJD!!

Skin
- Some storage diseases:
  - Lafora body.
  - Batten's disease.
- Mitochondrial cytopathies.

Bone marrow
- Niemann–Pick type C.
- Haematological and other malignancies.

Rectal and appendicectomy
- Most neuronal storage diseases affect the autonomic nervous system, so evidence can be sought in neurones of the gut's intrinsic plexi.
- Amyloid in rectal biopsy.

Tonsillar biopsy
- Research tool in vCJD.

Oligoclonal bands (OCBs)

- Electrophoresis of serum and CSF separates protein components by size and charge.
- OCBs may be present in serum and CSF. Bands in the CSF not seen in the serum suggest intrathecal-specific synthesis of immunoglobulins.
- This pattern is seen in most (95%) cases of established MS but may also occur in other conditions such as chronic meningitis, neurosyphilis, SSPE and neurosarcoid (although uncommonly).

Thompson EJ. (1997) Cerebrospinal fluid, pp443–466 in *Neurological Investigations*, ed Hughes RAC, BMJ Publications, London.

Diagnostic & prognostic antibodies & other markers in blood & urine

Multi-system disorders

PNS and CNS are affected in many multi-system disorders; markers in blood and other fluids and tissues for these are therefore commonly requested in neurology patients.

Vasculitides, e.g.
- Extractable nuclear antigens in SLE.
- ANCA in Wegener's.
- Rheumatoid factor in RA.

Enteropathies, e.g.
- Gliadin and endomysial antibodies in coeliac disease (an area of controversy).

Systemic infections, e.g.
- Serology for many diseases e.g. *Borrelia* in Lyme disease; HIV.
- PCR for TB.

Disorders of coagulation: thrombophilia screen currently commonly includes
- Protein S and C levels.
- Antithrombin III levels.

- Screening for the Leiden mutation in factor V.
- Lupus anticoagulant.

Tumour markers, e.g.
- CEA for gut neoplasia.
- Serum and urinary paraproteins in haematological disorders like myeloma.

Sarcoid
- ACE and ACE genotype.

Endocrinopathies, e.g.
- TSH, FT4 and FT3, thyroid autoantibodies in thyroid dysfunction.

Other metabolic disorders, e.g.
- Wilson's disease: blood copper and caeruloplasmin; some authorities also request 24h urinary copper excretion. *Note*: slit lamp examination performed by an experienced ophthalmologist reveals Kayser–Fleischer rings in most cases of Wilson's disease with neurological involvement.
- Phaeochromocytoma: catecholamine metabolites in three 24h urine collections.

Disease-specific markers
- Myasthenia gravis: anti-acetylcholine receptor and MuSK antibodies.

Paraneoplastic antibodies

Certain neurological syndromes are 'paraneoplastic', i.e. due to remote but non-metastatic effects of non-nervous system cancers. These paraneoplastic syndromes are rare, but important to recognise. In perhaps 50% of cases, the neurological symptoms may predate those of the cancer. This is an area of intensive research. Antibody tests that are well-described include those in Table 9.7.

Table 9.7

Antibody	Paraneoplastic syndrome	Associated tumour
Anti Hu (ANNA1)	Encephalomyelitis Sensory neuronopathy Cerebellar degeneration Chronic GI pseudo-obstruction Limbic encephalitis	Small cell lung cancer (SCLC)
Anti Yo (PCA1)	Cerebellar degeneration	Breast, ovary
Anti Ri (ANNA2)	Brainstem encephalitis	Breast, SCLC
CV2 (CRMP5)	Encephalomyelitis Chorea Sensory neuronopathy Sensorimotor neuropathy Cerebellar degeneration Limbic encephalitis Chronic GI pseudo-obstruction	Thymoma, SCLC
Anti Ma2 (Ta)	Limbic/diencephalic encephalitis Cerebellar degeneration Brainstem encephalitis	Testis, lung
Anti-amphiphysin	tiff person syndrome Other syndromes	Breast, SCLC

Graus F et al. (2004) Recommended diagnostic criteria for paraneoplastic neurological syndromes. J Neurol Neurosurg Psychiatry **75**, 1135–1140.

Biochemical markers

Many 'inborn errors of metabolism' cause neurological disease. A variety of investigations, including tests on blood, urine and csf, biopsies and genetic analyses, is used in their diagnosis (*see previous and next sections*, and for an accessible review *see reference* p679).

Biochemical tests

Some basic principles

Many autosomal recessive and X-linked metabolic diseases are caused by reduced or absent activity of a specific enzyme, in turn due to a single gene defect.

In some there is a tissue-specific deficit:

- E.g. McArdle's (glycogen storage disease V): demonstrates absence of phosphorylase activity in muscle biopsy (as only the myophosphorylase isozyme is affected).

In other conditions, notably the lipidoses, the enzyme is deficient in many tissues

- E.g. in Niemann–Pick diseases A and B, sphingomyelinase is deficient in brain and spinal cord, but also in the gastrointestinal tract, liver, spleen and bone marrow. Abnormal lipid metabolism can therefore be demonstrated in relatively easily accessible tissue such as fibroblasts.

Not only may the absence or lower activity of an enzyme reduce the amount of the product of the reaction it catalyses, it may lead to the accumulation of precursors in the metabolic pathway:

$$A \text{ —}(1) \rightarrow B \text{ —}(2) \rightarrow C\text{—}(3) \rightarrow D$$

If enzyme (3) is reduced, A, B and C may accumulate, with lower levels of D than usual being produced

- E.g. in acute intermittent porphyria, there is increased urinary excretion of δ haeminolevulinic acid and porphobilinogen (intermediates in the heme synthetic pathway) during an acute attack.
- Decreased levels of porphobilinogen deaminase may be demonstrated in erythrocytes, leucocytes and cultured fibroblasts.

Ischaemic forearm exercise test (ischaemic lactate test)

Procedure

1. Rest patient supine for 30min.
2. Draw a baseline lactate sample from a catheter in an antecubital vein.
3. Inflate sphygmomanometer cuff on that arm to above arterial pressure.
4. Subject squeezes a rubber ball in that hand until exhaustion.
5. Rapidly deflate cuff.
6. Take further venous samples at 30, 60 and 240s.

Results

Normally the venous lactate will rise by 2, 3 or even 4-fold; if it fails to rise by 1.5-fold, then there is likely to be a glycogenolysis or glycolysis defect (or the patient has not exercised sufficiently!):

- E.g. in disorders of glycolysis and glycogenolysis the venous lactate fails to rise in the ischaemic forearm exercise test.

Gray RG *et al.* (2000) Inborn errors of metabolism as a cause of neurological disease in adults: an approach to investigation. *J Neurol Neurosurg Psychiatry* **69**, 5–12.

Genetic tests

The list of diseases for which we have specific genetic tests grows each month. Rather than give a necessarily incomplete compendium, we discuss some general principles.

Several important neurological conditions may today be diagnosed by (relatively) simple genetic tests, whereas in the past biopsy was necessary. For example, Duchenne, Becker and oculopharyngeal muscular dystrophies are associated with well defined genetic abnormalities. Similarly, several mitochondrial cytopathies (such as myoclonic epilepsy and ragged red fibres—MERRF, and mitochondrial myopathy, lactic acidosis and stroke-like episodes—MELAS) may now often be diagnosed by finding common mutations or deletions in mitochondrial DNA.

When might a neurologist refer to a clinical geneticist?
- Genetic counselling of an index patient and his family.
- Cytogenetic or molecular diagnosis.
- Long-term follow up of family:
  - Notification of advances.
  - Counselling family members as they become adult.
  - Coordinating care with paediatric and adult neurologists.

Cytogenetics: when to do it
- Female with an X-linked disorder.
- Unexplained mental retardation.
- Unexplained major CNS malformation.
- The coexistence of two genetic diseases in a patient.

What is done?
- Conventional karyotype.
- Fluorescent *in situ* hybridisation (FISH) for suspected submicroscopic chromosomal aberrations:
  - E.g. a p13.3 deletion may cause lissencephaly.

Molecular genetics: when to do it
- Confirming a clinical diagnosis.
- Identify carriers in the family.

What is done?
An ever-increasing range of diseases may be tested for. Some of these tests may be routinely available at your local clinical genetics lab; others at regional, national or even supranational centres. Other tests may be available on a 'research' basis. It is clear, however, that tests for genetic 'lesions' or risk factors will become increasingly available. Rather than give an, at best, partial list of readily available tests, we give a few examples below of the kinds of tests that are available. The astute reader will spot that different mutations within a given gene can give rise to different clinical phenotypes. Indeed, recent work has shown that the same mutation in some genes can give rise to more than one phenotype: we clearly have a great deal yet to learn about the genetics of neurological diseases!

Detection of deletions
- E.g. in mitochondrial (mt)DNA in MELAS and MERRF.
- E.g. of dystrophin gene in Duchenne and Becker muscular dystrophies.

Detection of DNA rearrangement
- E.g. PMP22 gene duplication in some cases of Charcot–Marie–Tooth disease type 1 (or hereditary motor-sensory neuropathy type 1, (HMSN1); deletions within this gene cause hereditary neuropathy with liability to pressure palsies (HNPP).

Detection of trinucleotide repeats
- Found in >10 neurological diseases.
- So far, there in no overlap in the number of repeats in controls and affected patients (except rarely in Huntington's, in the region of 33 to 36 repeats).
- Anticipation (more severe phenotype and earlier onset) often reflects in increased number of repeats in the most recent generations (especially myotonic dystrophy).

Table 9.8

Disease	Gene	Triplet repeats	Transmission
Fragile X	FMR1	CGG	X-linked
Myotonic dystrophy	DM	CTG	AD
Friedreich's ataxia	FRDA	GAA	AR
Spinobulbar muscular atrophy	androgen receptor	CAG	X-linked
Huntington's disease	IT15	CAG	AD
Spinocerebellar atrophy			
SCA 1	SCA 1	CAG	AD
SCA 2	SCA 2	CAG	AD
SCA 3	SCA 3	CAG	AD
SCA 6	SCA 6	CAG	AD
SCA 7	SCA 7	CAG	AD
Dentorubropalli-doluysian atrophy	DRPLA	CAG	AD

Note: SCA 6 is a CAG triplet expansion in the CACNL1A4 calcium channel gene. Other (non triplet repeat) mutations in the gene cause other conditions: episodic ataxia type 2 and familial hemiplegic migraine.

Detection of single base mutations
This involves fragmenting the DNA of the gene into manageable pieces, then amplifying these so that there are multiple copies. Subsequently, various methods may be used to detect fragments with abnormal sequences, even if only differing at a single base from 'wild type'. There are several such techniques, constantly being refined, and many are restricted to research laboratories.

- However, molecular genetics is proceeding at a tremendous pace, both in terms of the number of conditions with identified genetic lesions, and the laboratory techniques for analysis.
- High speed DNA sequencing will facilitate sequencing large pieces of DNA.
- E.g. point mutations in the MPZ gene, which encodes for P0, a component of the myelin sheath, have been found in some families with Charcot–Marie–Tooth disease type 1B.

Genetic risk factors

Another area of clinical genetics which is likely to become more important is the detection of genetic 'risk factors' for diseases. Certain allelic variants, whilst not 'causing' a disease in the traditional sense, may predispose an individual to exhibiting a certain clinical phenotype, or alter the age at which it might become apparent.

- E.g. there are three allelic variants in the apolipoprotein E (APOE4) gene, e2, e3, e4. Homozygosity for e4 is likely to be a risk factor for developing Alzheimer's disease, and for developing it at an earlier age. However, the majority of e4 homozygotes do not develop the condition (therefore it is not 'causative').

Detection of the presence of abnormal protein or altered levels of normal protein

Immunocytochemistry and immunoblotting (Western blots) on tissue samples from the patient allow direct visualisation of the presence of abnormal protein, or absence or reduced levels of normal protein, in a variety of conditions. (These techniques are not genetic in the strictest sense, but are often useful in 'genetic' conditions.)

- E.g. Duchenne and Becker muscular dystrophies have absent or reduced levels of dystrophin in muscle biopsy samples.

Useful website

Online Mendelian Inheritance in Man (OMIM) is a continually updated catalogue of 'genetic' diseases in man, giving data about the genotype, mode of inheritance and the clinical phenotype of thousands of disorders (not just neurological).

🖱 http://www.ncbi.nim.nih.gov/Omim/

Young AB. (1998) Huntington's disease and other trinucleotide repeat disorders, pp35–54 in *Scientific American Molecular Neurology*, ed Martin JB, Scientific American, New York.

Neuro-otology

Pure tone audiometry

Measure threshold for air and bone conduction at frequencies from 250 to 8000Hz.

Typical patterns

- Conduction deafness BC > AC at all frequencies.
- Sensorineural deafness AC = BC at all frequencies, but increasing deafness as frequency rises.

(AC = air conduction; BC = bone conduction)

More specialised tests

- Tone decay.
- Loudness discomfort.
- Speech audiometry.
- Acoustic impedance.

Caloric testing

Procedure

1. Inspect eardrum; if intact, proceed.
2. Place patient supine with neck flexed 30° (on pillow).
3. Irrigate external auditory meatus with 30°C water (ice water if testing for brain death).
4. Observe for (or record*) nystagmus.
5. Repeat after 5min with 44°C water.

What should happen

1. Cold water induces convection of fluid in ipsilateral lateral semicircular canal (LSCC).
2. There is less output from ipsilateral LSCC.
3. Imbalance of signals from the two LSCCs results in eye drift towards the irrigated ear.
4. Fast phase contraversive movements correct for eye drift (hence nystamus with fast phase away from irrigated ear).
5. This nystagmus starts in about 20s and persists for 1min.
6. Warm water reverses the nystagmus.

Common pathological responses

Canal paresis

1. Reduced duration of nystagmus following irrigation on one side (with cold or warm water).
2. Suggests ipsilateral peripheral or central lesion.

Directional preponderance

1. Prolonged nystagmus in one direction.
2. Suggests central lesion on side of preponderance or contralateral peripheral lesion.

Combination of clinical examination, audiometry and caloric testing of the vestibulo-ocular reflex will help localise a lesion (peripheral vs. central; L vs. R).

Brainstem auditory evoked responses

📖p547.

---

*There are various techniques for recording eye movements. Although quite crude, electronystography has the advantage that it requires no instrumentation of the eyeball directly, allows recordings in the dark or with closed eyes (thus abolishing visual fixation and other responses that can interfere with the vestibulo-ocular reflex) and is relatively cheap.

Troost BT, Arguello LC. (2000) Neuro-otology, in *Neurology in Clinical Practice*, 3rd edition, eds Bradley WG et al., Butterworth-Heinemann, Boston.

Renal medicine

Estimation of kidney function 568
Classification of kidney disease 570
Assessment of proteinuria 574
Assessment of renal tubular function 576
Assessment of acid–base balance 578
Assessment of urinary acidification 581
Plasma potassium 582
Urinary potassium & chloride measurements 584
Urine sodium concentration 586
Urine dipstick testing 588
Urine culture 590
Urine microscopy 592
Investigations in patients with renal or bladder stones 594
Renal biopsy 596
Renal imaging 598
Renal bone disease 600
Immunological test in renal medicine 602

Estimation of kidney function

Estimates based on serum creatinine

Measurement of serum creatinine concentration is the most commonly used way of assessing the excretory function of the kidneys, which is mostly dependent on glomerular filtration rate (GFR). Creatinine is the non-enzymatic breakdown product of creatine and phosphocreatine (almost exclusively found in skeletal muscle). Its production rate is proportional to muscle mass—the average individual produces around 10mmol per day. Its production rate is usually constant, but ingestion of cooked meat and severe exercise cause a rapid, temporary rise in production of creatinine and thus in creatinine concentration. It is excreted mainly by glomerular filtration, but tubular secretion of creatinine also occurs, and contributes a significant proportion of overall excretion when GFR falls, resulting in overestimation of GFR at low GFR. Drugs, e.g. cimetidine, trimethoprim, can block the secretory component and elevate serum creatinine without any change in true GFR.

Because of the reciprocal relationship between clearance and serum creatinine, serum creatinine does not rise outside the normal range until there has been a substantial fall in GFR, particularly in patients with low muscle mass (Fig. 10.1). However, in an individual patient, a progressive increase in serum creatinine over time, even within the normal range, indicates declining GFR. Wide variation between individuals based on muscle mass, sex and age makes serum creatinine an imperfect screening test for renal failure. Estimation of 24h urine creatinine excretion allows measurement of creatinine clearance, but is beset with difficulties largely related to the timing and completeness of urine collections. For these reasons, use of creatinine clearance in clinical practice has been superseded by the use of prediction formulae.

The Cockcroft and Gault formula gives an estimate of creatinine clearance:

> **Creatinine clearance** = $\{(140 - \text{age (years)}) \times \text{weight (kg)}/\text{serum creatinine (mmol/L)}\} \times .04$ if ♀ or 1.23 if ♂

The 4-variable ('abbreviated') MDRD formula is the simplest of several formulae derived from the Modification of Diet in Renal Disease dataset and gives an estimate of GFR normalized to a body surface area of 1.73 m²:

> **GFR** (mL/min/1.73m²) = $186 \times \{[\text{serum creatinine (mmol/L)}/88.4]^{-1.154}\} \times \text{age (years)}^{-0.203} \times 0.742$ if ♀ and $\times 1.21$ if Afro-Caribbean

See ⌖ http://www.kidney.org/professionals/kdoqi/guidelines_ckd/p5_lab_g4.htm for a discussion of these and other formulae, including those that can be used to estimate GFR in children. The MDRD formula can be downloaded for use on PDAs. Note that there is also a 6-variable MDRD equation in use that also requires urea and albumin values: because of interlaboratory differences in albumin estimations, *this equation is not recommended.*

One of these formulae should be used to estimate GFR each time serum creatinine concentration is measured, and the formula used should be specified. The choice of which formula to use is controversial, and there are important differences between the two estimates, particularly as GFR declines at extremes of body size, but either formula is a major advance on the use of serum creatinine alone.

A: daily creatinine production 15mmoL
B: daily creatinine production 10mmoL
C: daily creatinine production 5mmoL

Fig. 10.1 Creatinine production is dependent on muscle mass which varies widely. Graph illustrates the theoretical relationship between GFR and plasma creatinine, ignoring effects of tubular secretion of creatinine, which results in overestimation of GFR from plasma creatinine or measurement of creatinine clearance. Note that in a patient with low muscle mass, creatinine does not rise outside the normal range until the GFR has fallen <30mL/min, whereas a patient with higher muscle mass will reach the same level of creatinine at a GFR of 90mL/min.

Classification of kidney disease

The classification proposed by the National Kidney Foundation Kidney Disease Outcomes Quality Initiative (K-DOQI) should be used (⁂http://www.kidney.org/professionals/kdoqi/guidelines_ckd/p4_class_g1.htm). This classification has been adopted in the UK (full guidelines available on ⁂www.renal.org).

Stage 1: Normal GFR; GFR >90mL/min with other evidence of chronic kidney damage*

Stage 2: Mild impairment; GFR 60–89mL/min with other evidence of chronic kidney damage*

Stage 3: Moderate impairment; GFR 30–59mL/min

Stage 4: Severe impairment: GFR 15–29mL/min

Stage 5: Established renal failure (ERF): GFR <15mL/min or on dialysis

*Other evidence of chronic kidney damage includes proteinuria, haematuria (after exclusion of other causes), biopsy-proven kidney disease, and structural abnormalities (e.g. reflux nephropathy, polycystic kidney disease).

Serum urea

Urea is the product of protein catabolism in the liver. Production is ↑ by high protein intake, catabolic states, breakdown of blood in the gut lumen in GI bleeding and tetracycline, and may ↓ in liver disease. Urea is freely filtered at the glomerulus with variable reabsorption, which is influenced by extracellular volume status. Intravascular volume depletion, diuretics, CCF, GI bleeding, tetracyclines and renal failure cause elevated levels. Disproportionate rise in serum urea compared to creatinine occurs in hypovolaemia and GI bleeding. Reduced levels are seen in chronic liver disease and alcohol abuse. By itself, serum urea is a very poor marker of excretory kidney function.

Cystatin C

Cystatin C, a 13kDa protein of the cystatin superfamily of cysteine protease inhibitors, is produced by all nucleated cells at a relatively constant rate. It can be assayed using efficient, enzyme-linked immunoassays. Preliminary studies suggest serum cystatin C may be a more sensitive and specific marker than creatinine for assessing impaired excretory renal function. Minor reductions in GFR cause cystatin C levels to rise above normal when serum creatinine is still within normal range.

Measurement of glomerular filtration rate

Occasionally it is necessary to measure renal excretory function accurately, e.g. in clinical research; when using drugs with a narrow therapeutic index and which are excreted by the kidney; when accurate measurement of kidney function is required in patients with abnormal muscle mass, e.g. paraplegics with bilateral lower limb muscle wasting.

The 'gold standard' for measurement of GFR is measurement of inulin clearance: inulin is freely filtered, not protein bound, and not reabsorbed or secreted. However, measurement of inulin is difficult.

Radionuclide studies

Radionuclide studies are contraindicated during pregnancy and women of childbearing age need to have a negative pregnancy test before proceeding with the test.

A variety of radioisotope markers are available for estimating GFR. An ideal marker should be safe, not extensively protein-bound, be freely filtered but not secreted or reabsorbed by the tubule and should be excreted only by the kidney.

- The commonly used markers are ^{51}Cr EDTA, ^{99m}Tc DTPA and ^{125}I iothalamate. Iothalamate is also available without radiolabelling and can be measured by fluorimetry.
- These substances are injected intravenously (SC in ^{125}I iothalamate) and after allowing for equilibration, plasma levels are measured at pre-determined intervals. Plasma clearance and hence renal elimination is calculated from the rate of fall of the substance from circulation.
- ^{51}Cr EDTA has been the most extensively studied marker and is extensively used in Europe as a single injection technique followed by plasma sampling at 0, 90, 120, 150 and 240min. ^{51}Cr EDTA is reliable even at low levels of renal function. Studies in humans suggest renal clearance estimated by this method is ~10% lower than that of inulin.
- ^{125}I iothalamate is only slightly protein-bound and studies suggest clearance values similar to that of inulin. Unlike other markers it can also be administered SC, and this allows for slow equilibration with stable plasma concentrations. It is considered safe, but potential problems of thyroid uptake necessitate pre-treatment with oral iodine.
- ^{99m}Tc DTPA is also widely available. There is some evidence that renal clearance can be estimated with a gamma camera placed over the patient, without the need for plasma sampling. Also anatomical correlation to renal function, such as information on relative contribution from each kidney, can be obtained. ^{99m}Tc has a very short half-life, and radiation exposure is minimized. Protein binding can result in diminished renal clearance.

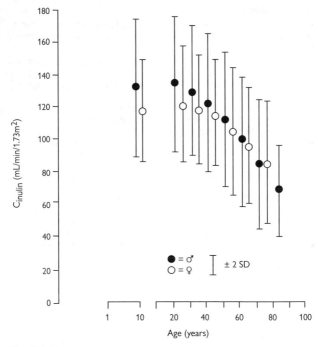

Fig. 10.2 Glomerular filtration rate, measured by inulin clearance (C_{inulin}), in normal individuals according to age.

Assessment of proteinuria

Proteinuria may result from ↑ glomerular permeability or tubular disease, causing ↓ reabsorption of filtered protein or ↑ excretion of tubular enzymes. Glomerular proteinuria is commoner and more likely to signal potentially progressive kidney damage. Disease states influence the absolute amount of protein excreted, so protein excretion should be assessed either by measurement of excretion over 24h (the 'gold standard', but highly inconvenient), or after correction for the degree of urine concentration. Because total daily urine creatinine excretion is constant, the ratio of protein:creatinine in the urine can allow correction for urine concentration. Although dipstick tests are useful, they can be misleading, with false +ve (concentrated urine) and false −ve (dilute urine) results.

Indications for quantitation of proteinuria

Diagnosis of nephrotic syndrome

Nephrotic syndrome is defined as triad of **oedema, hypoalbuminaemia** and **proteinuria** >3g/24h.

Prognosis of progressive renal disease

Proteinuria is one of the most potent risk markers for progressive loss of renal function in renal disease, e.g. diabetic nephropathy, chronic glomerulonephritis and reflux nephropathy. In addition, treatments that reduce proteinuria (e.g. antihypertensive drugs, particularly ACE inhibitors) ↓ rate of progression. Presence of significant proteinuria should result in adoption of lower blood pressure targets and preferential use of ACE inhibitors or ARB drugs. Because reduction of proteinuria is an important therapeutic aim, regular assessment of the severity of proteinuria is also important in monitoring the effects of treatment.

Diagnosis of early diabetic nephropathy

Diabetic nephropathy is most treatable in its early stages—characterised by an ↑ in GFR, ↑ albumin excretion, and then by hypertension. 'Microalbuminuria' is the term for pathologically increased albumin excretion below the limit of detection of standard dipstick tests for proteinuria. Microalbuminuria without diabetic retinopathy should raise suspicion of non-diabetic kidney disease.

Quantitation of proteinuria

Urine protein and creatinine concentrations should be measured in an early morning urine sample (because protein excretion ↑ with activity—see below). Assuming an average creatinine production of 10mmol/day (ignoring inter-individual variation due to variation in muscle mass), a protein:creatinine ratio of $n$mg/mmol allows estimation of the daily protein excretion as 10 × $n$mg/24h.

Protein measurement is cheap but does not differentiate between the various proteins present in urine. Proteinuria >30mg/mmol creatinine is usually defined as pathological, but patients with early diabetic nephropathy have total protein excretions below this limit. Only when proteinuria >100mg/mmol creatinine is there a high suspicion of underlying renal disease.

Detection of 'microalbuminuria'

Albumin measurement is more expensive but justified when the detection of 'microalbuminuria' would alter management—either in the diagnosis of diabetic nephropathy or, possibly, in the early detection of other forms of glomerular disease. The role of screening for microalbuminuria in patients in other situations remains controversial, and is not currently recommended in the UK. Microalbuminuria is present if urine albumin:creatinine ratio is ≥2.5mg/mmol (in ♂) or >3.5mg/mmol (in ♀) in repeated samples. See URLs for NICE guidelines on type 2[1] and type 1[2] diabetes.

1 ⏿www.nice.org.uk/pdf/diabetesrenalguideline.pdf
2 ⏿www.nice.org.uk/pdf/CG015_fullguideline_adults_development_section.pdf

Diagnosis of postural proteinuria

Protein excretion ↑ with activity and upright posture. In some individuals increase is exaggerated, resulting in +ve dipstick tests for proteinuria and even ↑ 24h urine protein excretion. This 'postural proteinuria' has a nearly completely benign prognosis. In patients with proteinuria who have no other evidence of renal disease it is worth quantitating proteinuria separately in urine collected while the patient has been recumbent overnight and in a daytime specimen. This can be done by measuring protein:creatinine (or albumin:creatinine ratio for even greater accuracy) on both an early morning urine and one taken after period of activity. Normal protein excretion during the night with increased protein excretion during the day indicates postural proteinuria.

Assessment of tubular proteinuria

Occasionally of value to detect the relatively low grade proteinuria that results from tubular disease, e.g. Dent's disease (rare genetic disorder caused by mutation in a tubular chloride channel), which causes calcium stone formation and tubular proteinuria. Other examples include screening for generalised tubular dysfunction and for drug toxicity, e.g during treatment with platinum derivatives. Tubular proteinuria is best diagnosed by measurement of specific proteins whose presence in the urine result from tubular disease, e.g. retinol binding protein (RBP), N-acetyl-β-D-glucosaminidase (NAG) or α1-microglobulin, either in 24h urine specimens or as ratios between the protein concentration and creatinine concentration.

Assessment of selectivity of proteinuria

The more severe the damage to glomerular permeability, the larger the protein molecules that pass through the glomerulus in glomerular disease. Measurement of the ratio of clearance of transferrin or albumin (a small molecule) to immunoglobulin G (a large molecule) can therefore be used as a measure of selectivity, and is calculated as follows:

Albumin/IgG clearance = {(urine [IgG] × serum [albumin])/ (serum IgG × urine [albumin])} × 100%

Transferrin/IgG clearance is calculated similarly.

A ratio of <0.16 indicates highly selective proteinuria.

In children, minimal change nephropathy causes selective proteinuria, whereas non-selective proteinuria raises the possibility of an alternative type of renal disease and might lead to a recommendation of renal biopsy to avoid steroid treatment when this would be unlikely to be of benefit. Measurement of selectivity in adults is of very limited use.

Detection and quantitation of urinary light chains (Bence Jones protein)
Measurement of urinary light chains requires specific immunoassays for light chains and is performed on 24h urine samples as part of the regular assessment of disease activity in multiple myeloma. These tests are probably a less reliable marker of disease activity in the presence of severe renal impairment.

Assessment of renal tubular function

There are two main types of renal tubular diseases: those due to a single defect, usually genetic, in solute secretion or reabsorption, and those due to generalised tubular damage.

Screening tests for generalised tubular dysfunction test for
- Renal glycosuria (dipstick or lab test for glucose in urine plus normal plasma glucose).
- Hypophosphataemia (can be followed by estimation of phosphate reabsorption, *see below*).
- Low molecular weight proteinuria (due to failure of tubular reabsorption plus increased release of proteins derived from tubular cells).
- Normal anion gap metabolic acidosis—serum bicarbonate, plus sodium potassium and chloride to permit calculation of the anion gap (followed by tests to confirm renal tubular acidosis, *see below*).
- Aminoaciduria—detected by amino acid electrophoresis on a random urine sample.
- Hypouricaemia—plasma urate may be low due to decreased tubular reabsorption. (This can be followed by measurement of fractional urate excretion; *see below*).

Assessment of phosphate reabsorption
Occasionally useful in the differential diagnosis of hypophosphataemia, e.g. in confirming the diagnosis of X-linked hypophosphataemic rickets.

Procedure
- The patient is asked to fast overnight.
- The overnight urine is discarded.
- The next urine sample is obtained, together with a blood sample.
- Both are analysed for phosphate and creatinine.

Fractional phosphate excretion is calculated as:

$FE_{PO_4} = C_P/C_{Cr} =$ [serum creatinine × urine phosphate]/[urine creatinine × serum phosphate]
—this is the fraction of filtered phosphate which appears in the urine

Fractional tubular reabsorption of phosphate (TRP) is calculated as

$1 - FE_{PO_4}$

TmP/GFR, the tubular maximum for phosphate reabsorption can be read off a nomogram[1], or can be calculated as follows:

If TRP <0.86, TmP/GFR = TRP × plasma phosphate
If TRP >0.86, TmP = {0.3 × TRP/[1−(0.8 × TRP)]} × plasma phosphate

Interpretation
The adult reference range for TmP/GFR is 0.80–1.35mmol/L. Higher values of normal are seen in infancy and childhood[2]. Low values are seen in X-linked hypophosphataemic rickets and in osteogenic osteomalacia, both of which are thought to be due to overproduction or failure of inactivation of phosphatonins (a group of phosphaturic hormones including FG-23 and FRP4). TmP/GFR is raised in hypoparathyroidism and reduced in hyperparathyroidism and by PTH-related peptide secretion.

Reduced phosphate reabsorption may also be seen in hypercalciuric stone formers, but it remains difficult to be certain whether this is the primary disorder, causing increased production of 1, 25-$(OH)_2$ vitamin D, or secondary to tubular damage as a result of renal stones.

Reduced phosphate reabsorption is also seen in a number of primary and secondary disorders of renal tubular function.

Assessment of tubular urate handling
The relative contributions of production rate, glomerular filtration, pre-secretory reabsorption, secretion and post-secretory reabsorption to control plasma urate concentration cannot be dissected out without complex tests involving selective pharmacological blockade of some of these processes. However, it is possible to determine whether an abnormal plasma urate concentration is due to abnormal production or abnormal renal handling.

24h urinary urate excretion is increased in overproduction but normal in patients whose hyperuricaemia is due to decreased excretion. (*Note*: it is not decreased, because in underexcretion the steady state is maintained at the expense of a raised plasma level.) If 24h urinary urate is raised, the collection should be repeated on a low purine diet.

Fractional excretion of urate is calculated as:

$$\{(\text{urinary [urate]} \times \text{plasma [creatinine]})/(\text{plasma [urate]} \times \text{urinary [creatinine]})\} \times 100\%$$

Normal values are dependent on age and sex but in adults are of the order of 10%. High fractional excretion is a cause of hypouricaemia in SIADH and several other conditions; low fractional excretion occurs in primary gout but also in a familial syndrome of hypouricaemia with early-onset gout and progressive renal failure.

1 Walton RJ, Bijvoet OLM. (1975) Nomogram for derivation of renal threshold phosphate concentration *Lancet* **ii**, 309–310; **2** Payne RB. (1998) Renal tubular reabsorption of phosphate (TmP/GFR): indications and interpretation *Ann Clin Biochem* **35**, 201–206.

Assessment of acid–base balance

Plasma HCO_3^- and Cl^- are the two major anions in extracellular fluid. The major reason for measuring them is to assess acid–base status. Changes in serum $[HCO_3^-]$ concentration reflect changes in acid–base balance, with a $\downarrow$ in $[HCO_3^-]$ reflecting metabolic acidosis and an $\uparrow$ reflecting alkalosis. Plasma Cl^- is helpful in assessing the cause of acidosis or alkalosis.

▶There is no justification at all for performing an arterial puncture to measure arterial pH as part of the assessment of metabolic acidosis or alkalosis—it can be adequately assessed from serum $[HCO_3^-]$. Arterial samples are needed when it is unclear whether the acid–base disturbance is respiratory or metabolic in origin, or in mixed disturbances.

Plasma bicarbonate

The most reliable way to interpret plasma HCO_3^- is to use the acid–base diagram (Fig. 10.3), which allows assessment of how much the change in $[HCO_3^-]$ concentration is due to changes in CO_2 excretion via the lungs and how much to changes in $[H^+]$ or HCO_3^- wasting. In the absence of significant respiratory disease it can often safely be assumed that any change is due to metabolic causes, in which case low plasma HCO_3^- indicates increased H^+ production (or, occasionally, increased HCO_3^- loss) and vice versa. If arterial blood gases are obtained, the 'standard bicarbonate' is a calculated value which indicates what the plasma HCO_3^- would be if CO_2 excretion were normal, and is thus a way of allowing assessment of whether there is a metabolic component to an abnormal HCO_3^- concentration or whether it is solely due to the respiratory disturbance.

Remember that the kidneys compensate for respiratory disease and the lungs for metabolic disease: for instance, metabolic acidosis causes hyperventilation, resulting in lower PCO_2 and lessening the acidosis seen. However, overcompensation does not occur.

Plasma chloride

Many laboratories omit plasma Cl⁻ assays from 'routine' serum chemistry measurements, but this measurement is helpful if a systemic acid–base disturbance is suspected. As a useful oversimplification, low bicarbonate with high chloride can be seen as accumulation of hydrochloric acid, which can only result from altered renal handling of acid, as in renal tubular acidosis. If HCO_3^- is low with a normal or low Cl⁻, some other acid must be accumulating. More precision in deciding the cause of metabolic acidosis can be obtained by calculating the anion gap.

The anion gap

The anion gap is the difference between the sum of the concentrations of the positively charged ions routinely measured in plasma and the negatively charged ions:

$$\text{Anion gap} = \{[Na^+] + [K^+]\} - \{[Cl^-] + [HCO_3^-]\}$$

Obviously, the total positive charges in plasma must be balanced by the same number of negative charges. The normal anion gap is caused by the fact that there are more unmeasured anions in plasma (mostly albumin, but including lactate, sulphate and others) than cations (including calcium and magnesium). The concentrations of all of these ummeasured ions can vary, so the normal range for the anion gap is wide, e.g. hypoalbuminaemia reduces the anion gap by 2.5mEq per 1g/dL fall in serum albumin.

The main use of calculation of the anion gap is in the differential diagnosis of metabolic acidosis.

A high anion gap acidosis is caused by an abnormally high concentration of an unmeasured anion, such as

- L-lactate (reflecting anaerobic metabolism or hepatic dysfunction).
- Salicylate (in aspirin poisoning).
- β-hydroxybutyrate (in diabetic ketoacidosis).
- Glycolate and oxalate (in methanol poisoning).
- Hippurate (in toluene poisoning, e.g. glue-sniffing).
- D-lactate (from gut bacterial fermentation in blind-loop syndrome).

A normal anion gap acidosis may be caused by loss of bicarbonate or failure of renal H^+ excretion, for instance

- Renal tubular acidosis.
- High ileostomy losses (bicarbonate wasting).
- Carbonic anhydrase inhibitors.
- Urinary diversions, e.g. ureterosigmoidostomy (Cl⁻/ HCO_3^-) exchange and NH_4^+ reabsorption in the colonic segment).

Beware: in North America the anion gap is usually calculated as $[Na^+]$ – $\{[Cl^-] + [HCO_3^-]\}$, not including $[K^+]$ in the measured cations. This results in a lower reference range for the anion gap. In addition, different laboratories use different assays for chloride. For these reasons, the local laboratory reference range for anion gap should be used.

In general, the anion gap is only useful when very high, confirming high concentrations of an unmeasured anion. If the diagnosis is not already obvious, this then justifies further investigation, including assay of plasma lactate concentration.

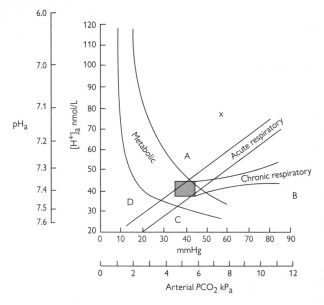

Fig. 10.3 Acid base diagram.

Assessment of urinary acidification

Indications

Unexplained hyperchloraemic metabolic acidosis.

Defects in the kidneys' ability to excrete acid in the urine may lead to permanent systemic acidosis, or to systemic acidosis at times of increased acid generation, depending on the severity of the defect. Acidification defects may occur as part of generalised tubular disease or as isolated, often genetically determined, alterations in function, most commonly of cell surface ion pumps.

Ammonium chloride loading test

This test is regarded as the 'gold standard' for the diagnosis of distal ('type 1') renal tubular acidosis, where there is impaired excretion of 'fixed acid' into the distal tubule.

Procedure

- The patient attends after an overnight fast, but is allowed to drink water.
- At the start of the test, a urine sample is sent to the laboratory for measurement of pH and a plasma or serum sample is sent for measurement of bicarbonate. Because pH changes rapidly in urine exposed to the air, the urine container should be filled to the top or the urine sent in a stoppered syringe, and sent to the laboratory without any delay.
- If the urine pH is <5.4, this indicates normal acidifying ability, and there is no need to continue with the test.
- If the venous blood bicarbonate is low, with a urine pH >5.4, the diagnosis of renal tubular acidosis is confirmed.
- If neither of these conditions is met, then proceed to give the patient ammonium chloride, 0.1g/kg body weight, PO. Ammonium chloride is given as capsules, is unpalatable, and frequently causes nausea and vomiting, but this can be reduced if the capsules are taken slowly, or with bread and honey. It is worth proceeding with the test even if the patient vomits, as acidosis is often achieved; no more ammonium chloride should be given.
- Urine samples are then collected hourly for the next 6–8h and sent, protected from the air (as above), for pH analysis in the laboratory. If any sample has a pH of ≤5.4 the test can be stopped, as this indicates normal acidifying ability of the distal tubule.
- At 3h after ingestion of ammonium chloride, a venous sample should be sent for plasma bicarbonate measurement to ensure that acidaemia has occurred.

Alternative tests of distal acidification

Rationale

The distal tubule reabsorbs sodium ions in exchange for hydrogen ions. Furosemide, by increasing delivery of sodium to the distal tubule, therefore causes a fall in urine pH. A fall in urine pH to <5.5 after furosemide confirms normal distal acidification ability, and may spare the patient the unpleasantness of the ammonium chloride test. The sensitivity of the test is increased in 'salt-avid' states produced by sodium restriction or fludrocortisone.

- The patient attends after a light breakfast without caffeine.
- Fludrocortisone 1mg is given, followed by furosemide 40mg an hour later.
- Drinking is discouraged unless the patient is very thirsty (very dilute urine can invalidate the test).
- Urine samples are collected for laboratory analysis of pH hourly, if possible, for 4–5h. A fall in urine pH to <5.5 excludes a distal acidification defect.

Bicarbonate infusion test

This is the 'gold standard' for the diagnosis of proximal ('type 2') renal tubular acidosis, which is characterised by impaired bicarbonate reabsorption. In this condition, urine pH may be <5.5 in untreated patients, because at steady state serum bicarbonate levels fall to the point at which filtered bicarbonate is reabsorbed, and distal acidification mechanisms are intact.

Procedure
- Sodium bicarbonate is infused IV at 0.5–1.0mmol/kg per hour. After 60min plasma bicarbonate is measured to confirm that this has risen to >20mmol/L. Urine pH is measured hourly and urine bicarbonate measured, to allow calculation of the fractional excretion of bicarbonate:

$$FE_{HCO3} = \{(\text{urine } [HCO_3^-] \times \text{plasma } [\text{creatinine}])/(\text{plasma } [HCO_3^-] \times \text{urine } [\text{creatinine}])\} \times 100\%$$

- Fractional excretion of bicarbonate is normally <15%.
- A level of >20% confirms type 2 renal tubular acidosis.

Plasma potassium

Although most of the body's potassium is intracellular, small changes in extracellular potassium concentration can have major changes in membrane excitability. *Hypokalaemia* causes increased excitability, causing atrial and ventricular cardiac arrhythmias; *hyperkalaemia* decreases excitability, causing a characteristic pattern of ECG changes and eventually causing asystole. Both hypokalaemia and hyperkalaemia may be associated with skeletal muscle paralysis.

Plasma K^+ concentration ($[K^+]$) is influenced both by distribution across cell membranes and by the balance between intake and excretion. Renal excretion is dependent on renal function, urine flow rate and aldosterone.

Pseudohyperkalaemia

Caused by excessive release of K^+ from cells after venepuncture, and should be considered when hyperkalaemia 'doesn't fit' with the clinical picture. The laboratory should report the presence of visible haemolysis

(usually due to RBC trauma during difficult venepuncture), but pseudo-hyperkalaemia can also occur in the absence of visible haemolysis, e.g.:
• Haematological malignancies causing a high white cell or platelet count.
• Other causes of leucocytosis and thrombocytosis, e.g. leukaemoid reactions, rheumatoid arthritis.
• Familial pseudohyperkalaemia: rare disorder of RBC cation transport leading to an increased rate of release of K^+ from red cells at low temperatures.

Diagnosis can be confirmed by showing that plasma $[K^+]$ is normal in a heparinised sample analysed immediately, and then by demonstrating that delayed separation results in higher values being obtained. Pseudohyperkalaemia with a normal WBC and platelet count can be further investigated by measuring the rate of rise of plasma $[K^+]$ in samples incubated at $37°C$ and at $22°C$, and studying the effects of drugs that affect cation exchange, e.g. thiazide diuretics and quinine. Artefactual hyperkalaemia can be caused by fist clenching plus a venous tourniquet during phlebotomy: plasma K^+ can rise by as much as 2mmol/L.

Hyperkalaemia due to redistribution across cell membranes

Hyperkalaemic periodic paralysis is an autosomal dominant genetic muscle disorder caused by mutations in the voltage-gated sodium channel. It presents in early infancy with attacks of paralysis associated with hyperkalaemia.

Other causes of release of potassium from tissues (including muscle) include
• Exercise.
• Acidosis (particularly inorganic acidosis).
• Muscle damage (rhabdomyolysis), e.g. crush injury, revascularisation of ischaemic limb, prolonged unconsciousness following drug intoxication.
• Burns.
• Tumour lysis, e.g. after initiation of chemotherapy for haematological malignancy.
• Drugs, e.g. digoxin, depolarising muscle relaxants, β-blockers.
• Malignant hyperthermia.

Hyperkalaemia due to altered external balance
• ↑ ingestion is seldom able to cause hyperkalaemia on its own, but can contribute to hyperkalaemia when combined with impaired excretion of a potassium load.
• ↓ excretion may be due to decreased glomerular filtration rate, ↓ urine flow rate, ↓ aldosterone production, drugs which inhibit renal tubular K^+ excretion, or genetic defects in renal potassium excretion (pseudohypoaldosteronism, Liddle's syndrome).
• In most cases the cause is obvious.

Investigation of unexplained hyperkalaemia
• Serum creatinine, creatine kinase, bicarbonate.
• Urine K^+, creatinine, osmolality, allowing calculation of transtubular K^+ gradient (⎕*Urine potassium & chloride measurements* p584): occasionally useful, for instance in confirming trimethoprim-induced inhibition of K^+ secretion.

- Tests for type IV renal tubular acidosis:
  - Normal synacthen test (to exclude Addison's disease).
  - 24h urinary aldosterone (low in type IV RTA).
  - Plasma renin and aldosterone response to upright posture and 40mg furosemide (subnormal levels of both suggest hyporeninaemic hypoaldosteronism).
  - Correction of hyperkalaemia with oral fludrocortisone 0.1mg/day.

Pseudohypokalaemia

Can be caused by delayed separation of samples kept at warm ambient temperatures, and is caused by continued uptake of K^+ into cells. This occurs more in heparinised samples than in those allowed to clot.

Hypokalaemia due to redistribution across cell membranes

- Alkalosis.
- Insulin treatment.
- β_2-adrenergic stimulation (e.g. high dose nebulisers).
- B_{12} therapy of pernicious anaemia.
- Rapid cell division, e.g. acute leukaemia.
- Hypokalaemic periodic paralysis (precipitated by carbohydrate intake, rest after exercise):
  - Confirm diagnosis (under strict supervision) by infusing 2g/kg glucose and 0.1u/kg insulin; consider referral for mutation analysis of $\alpha 1$-subunit of calcium channel.
  - Consider thyrotoxic hypokalaemic periodic paralysis in non-familial patients, particularly of oriental background: check thyroid function tests.

Hypokalaemia due to increased renal loss
p140.

Urine potassium & chloride measurements

Measurement of urine potassium concentration is occasionally useful in the differential diagnosis of hyperkalaemia. The proportion of potassium filtered at the glomerulus which is excreted in the urine is extremely variable, and is modulated by the distal tubule in response to aldosterone, plasma potassium concentration, acid–base balance, urine flow rate, sodium status and other factors. The final concentration of potassium in the urine also depends on urine dilution, controlled independently by factors (e.g. ADH) controlling water excretion.

Low urinary K^+ (<20mmol/L) with hypokalaemia is seen in

- Gastrointestinal potassium loss, e.g. diarrhoea, laxative abuse, villous adenoma, high ileostomy output, enterocutaneous fistula, ureterosigmoidostomy.
- Dietary deficiency
- Skin losses, e.g. burns, severe eczema.

High urinary K$^+$ (>20mmol/L) with hypokalaemia and normal blood pressure is seen in

- Vomiting (K$^+$ is exchanged for hydrogen ions: acid–base preservation takes precedence)—*note*: urinary chloride will be low.
- Diuretic use, abuse and conditions which mimic diuretic use, e.g. Bartter's syndrome, Gitelman's syndrome.
- Tubular damage causing potassium wasting, e.g. renal tubular acidosis types 1 and 2.
- Diabetic ketoacidosis.

High urinary K$^+$ (>20mmol/L) with hypokalaemia and high blood pressure is seen in

- Hyperaldosteronism—adrenal adenomas, bilateral adrenal hyperplasia.
- Apparent mineralocorticoid excess.
- Liddle's syndrome.

Transtubular potassium gradient

This is a calculation that is promoted in the USA, but not widely used in the UK or Europe. The main purpose is to distinguish hyperkalaemia caused by decreased aldosterone action from hyperkalaemia due to effective volume depletion. The principle is that correcting for urine dilution, by using the ratio of plasma and urine osmolality, allows estimation of the urine potassium gradient in the cortical collecting duct, after the main site of potassium secretion (which is influenced by aldosterone) but before the main site of urine dilution or concentration (which is influenced by ADH). The index is only valid when the urine is concentrated, i.e. the urine osmolality exceeds the plasma osmolality, and when urine sodium concentration is >25mmol/L. It is calculated as follows:

$$TTKG = \{urine\ [K^+]/(urine\ osmolality/plasma\ osmolality)\}/plasma\ [K^+]$$

TTKG can vary widely in healthy subjects, but is commonly around 7–9

- Values <7 in a patient with hyperkalaemia suggest hypoaldosteronism.
- Values >7 in a hyperkalaemic patient suggest that aldosterone is acting normally, and that hyperkalaemia is due to low urine flow, limiting the rate at which potassium can be excreted.
- Values <7 in hypokalaemic patients suggest extrarenal potassium loss.
- Values >9 in hypokalaemic patients suggest renal potassium loss.

Urine chloride

This measurement is helpful in the differential diagnosis of otherwise unexplained normotensive hypokalaemia. Urine chloride is low if hypokalaemia is being caused by extrarenal sodium chloride or hydrogen chloride losses, as seen in diarrhoea or vomiting, respectively: in these conditions potassium is exchanged in the distal tubule for sodium or hydrogen respectively, but chloride is conserved. Urine chloride is high when the cause of hypokalaemia is inappropriate loss of potassium chloride, as in diuretic use and in Bartter's syndrome (the genetic equivalent of being on permanent high dose loop diuretics) and Gitelman's syndrome (the genetic equivalent of being on permanent high dose thiazide diuretics).

The distinction between the drug-induced and genetic causes can be very difficult to make, but temporary withdrawal from diuretics causes intense chloride retention and a very low urinary chloride concentration, which is never seen in Bartter's or Gitelman's syndromes. Repeated measurements of urine chloride are therefore helpful in this situation, together with screens for the presence of diuretics in the urine when urine chloride is high.

Urine sodium concentration

In health, serum electrolyte concentrations are kept constant because intake of electrolytes is balanced by excretion in the faeces and urine. Renal excretion is tightly regulated to achieve this balance. These basic principles imply that the urinary excretion of, for instance, sodium, is nearly totally dependent on dietary intake of sodium. Because this is very variable, there is no 'normal range' of urinary sodium, or any other urinary electrolyte. Measurements of urinary electrolytes therefore have to be interpreted with great caution.

24h urine sodium excretion is a good marker, at steady state, for dietary intake, and has been used in epidemiological studies of the relationship of salt intake to blood pressure. Dietary sodium intake varies from as little as 10mmol/day in the Amazon rainforest to >400mmol/day in Westerners living on processed foods. Current UK advice is to restrict sodium intake to around 100mmol/day.

In clinical practice there are several reasons for measuring sodium output, including

- *Calcium stone formers*. Sodium and calcium excretion are linked, and reduction of excessive salt intake results in a reduction in calcium excretion.
- *Cystine stone formers*. Similarly, cystine excretion is reduced by reduction of dietary salt intake.
- *During antihypertensive and antiproteinuric treatment*. Salt restriction amplifies the effects of ACE inhibitors in reducing not only systemic blood pressure but also protein excretion in renal disease, and may be more tolerable than diuretic treatment.

24h urine sodium is usually measured on a sample collected in a plain container. However, it can also be measured, by flame photometry, in a sample collected into an acid container, and this is useful if calcium and oxalate excretion are also being measured, for instance in stone formers.

Spot urine sodium concentration is of very limited value, because sodium excretion varies considerably through the day and because it is normally influenced by urine dilution and hence by recent water intake. However, there are two situations in which it may be of value:

Acute renal failure
The normal response of the kidneys to underperfusion from hypovolaemia or hypotension is to retain salt avidly, urine sodium concentration

dropping to <10mmol/L. If urinary sodium concentration is this low in acute renal failure, this indicates normal ability of the renal tubules to retain salt. Low urine sodium concentration is seen in 'pre-renal' renal failure; acute tubular necrosis results in loss of tubular salt reabsorption and a higher urine sodium concentration. The problem is that conditions other than underperfusion cause low urine sodium (e.g. contrast nephropathy, rhabdomyolysis) and a high urine sodium does not necessarily indicate acute tubular necrosis—indeed, it is seen in normal people. In any case, the measurement seldom has a useful impact on management, which both in pre-renal failure and in acute tubular necrosis is to restore renal perfusion by correcting hypovolaemia, hypotension and sepsis as quickly as possible.

Syndrome of inappropriate ADH

This diagnosis cannot be made in a hypovolaemic patient, because hypovolaemia is a physiological stimulus to ADH secretion. For this reason, the diagnosis cannot be made if the urine sodium concentration is low (p122).

Fractional excretion of sodium is calculated as

$$\{(\text{urine [sodium]} \times \text{plasma [creatinine]})/(\text{plasma [sodium]} \times \text{urine [creatinine]})\} \times 100\%$$

This gives an index of avidity of sodium reabsorption independent of changes in overall renal function. An FE_{Na} of <1% is seen in pre-renal failure and >1% in acute tubular necrosis. However, this measurement is prone to the same criticisms as that of urine sodium excretion.

Sodium wasting and sodium retaining states

Sodium wasting is caused by diuretics, Bartter's syndrome, Gitelman's syndrome, and occasionally by renal tubular disease. It cannot be diagnosed by measurement of urine sodium excretion alone, as at steady state this equals sodium intake, but is diagnosed by finding clinical evidence of hypovolaemia without avid renal sodium retention.

Sodium retention is caused by diseases causing effective hypovolaemia (e.g. congestive cardiac failure), in which case the diagnosis is suggested by oedema and the clinical signs of the underlying disease. However, sodium retention can also cause hypertension without oedema, as in hyperaldosteronism, pseudohyperaldosteronism, chronic renal failure and inherited disorders of renal tubular sodium excretion (e.g. Liddle's syndrome). Again, measurement of sodium excretion alone is not helpful in the diagnosis of these conditions.

Urine dipstick testing

Urine analysis is useful for screening patients with potential renal disease and for serial assessment of patients with known renal pathology.

Many commercially available dipsticks rapidly test the urine for multiple chemical contents. The sticks use reagent strips, which change colour following a chemical reaction with an active constituent depending on the presence (or absence) of a particular component.

Depending on the type of dipstick used, urine can be tested for

- pH.
- Specific gravity.
- Haemoglobin.
- Leucocyte esterases and nitrites.
- Glucose.
- Ketones.
- Protein.
- Urobilinogen.

The reagent strip is fully immersed in urine obtained by voiding or, if warranted, by urethral catheterisation, and the excess shaken off. The change in colour, if any, is read after the time specified by the manufacturer—usually 30s.

pH

Dipstick testing only gives a rough estimate of pH, because of the effects of storage and reaction on exposure to atmospheric air on urine pH *in vitro*. The dipstick contains a polyionic polymer bound with H^+, which is released on reaction with the cations in urine. Release of H^+ causes change in colour of a pH-sensitive dye. Normal pH varies between 4.5 and 8.0, depending on diet: vegetarians, in whom fixed acid ingestion is low, commonly have alkaline urine. Urine infection with urease-producing organisms also causes alkaline urine. Urine pH >5.5 in spite of metabolic acidosis is seen in renal tubular acidosis. Urine pH is important in some recurrent stone formers. For instance, uric acid solubility in urine is critically dependent on urine pH, and many uric acid stone formers are found to have normal 24h urinary urate but highly acidic and concentrated urine (e.g. as a result of high losses from an ileostomy). In patients with triple phosphate stones, alkaline urine is commonly seen due to infection with urea splitting organisms.

Specific gravity

Not accurate on dipstick testing. Non-ionic constituents including albumin, glucose and urea are also estimated. Normal values: between 1003 and 1030, vary with the patient's hydration status and hence urinary concentration. SG ↓ with age as the kidney loses its concentrating ability. Fixed SG of 1010 is seen in chronic renal failure.

Haemoglobin

Reagent strips use peroxidase-like activity of haemoglobin to induce a colour change in a dye linked to organic peroxide. Does not distinguish haemoglobinuria from erythrocyturia and myoglobin. False +ve results are obtained with myoglobin, contamination with menstrual blood and iodine. Positive dipsticks for blood with absence of RBC on microscopy suggest lysis of RBCs due to prolonged storage, myoglobinuria or haemoglobinuria. False −ve results are seen with high dose vitamin C and rifampicin.

Leucocyte esterases and nitrites

The esterase method relies on esterases released from lysed WBC. Esterases release pyrroles, which react with a diazonium salt on the dipstick resulting in a colour change. False +ve results seen in vaginal contamination. Presence of glucose, albumin, ketones, tetracyclines and cephalosporins in the urine can give false −ve results.

Most, but not all, uropathogenic bacteria convert nitrates to nitrites, which react with a diazonium compound resulting in a colour change. False −ve results are due to frequent bladder emptying, prolonged external storage and ascorbic acid. Some bacteria including *N. gonorrhoea* and *Mycobacterium tuberculosis* do not convert nitrates.

Sensitivity and specificity of the above tests vary, and are not useful for screening low-risk populations. However a −ve test is useful in excluding UTI in a patient with a high pre-test probability of infection. Further guidance on diagnosis of urinary tract infections is available at
⌨www.prodigy.nhs.uk/ClinicalGuidance/

Glucose

Most strips use the glucose oxidase/peroxidase method and can estimate levels as low as 50mg/dL. Ketones, salicylate and ascorbic acid can interfere with results. Estimates all reducing sugars including fructose and lactose. In the absence of concomitant hyperglycaemia, glycosuria is suggestive of proximal tubular disorders or, rarely, reduced renal threshold for glucose.

Ketones

Acetoacetic acid is detected by the nitroprusside test. Ascorbic acid results in false +ve result. Dipsticks do not detect beta hydroxybutyrate, which comprises the largest ketone fraction in blood.

Protein

Binding of proteins to the dye indicators is highly pH dependent and the indicators undergo a sequential colour change based on the concentration of protein in the sample. Albumin binds at a pH of 5–8 and has the highest affinity, so most commercially available dipsticks almost exclusively detect only albumin. Sticks with sensitivity as low as 250mg/L are available currently. Dipsticks are thus cheap, reliable and give rapid semi-quantitative assessment of proteinuric renal disease. However, remember that these tests measure concentration of protein, rather than absolute excretion; false negative tests are therefore possible in dilute urine caused by a high fluid intake, and false positive tests may be obtained in highly concentrated urine. At pH <5 or >8 results obtained by dipsticks are not accurate. Immunoglobulin light chains (Bence Jones proteins) do not result in positive dipstick tests for proteinuria even when present in high concentrations.

Urine culture

There are numerous situations in which accurate diagnosis of UTI is important. 'Sending an MSU' is not, however, quite as simple as it sounds and is not always the most appropriate test.

Obtaining a mid-stream urine sample

The aim is to obtain a sample of bladder urine, avoiding contamination by cells or organisms on perineal skin. Men should retract the foreskin prior to micturition; women should hold the labia well apart with the parted fingers of one hand to allow the urine to exit directly from the urethral meatus. The patient should be asked to begin to pass urine, and then, without stopping passing urine, pass a sterile container into the path of the urinary stream and collect a sample, before finishing passing urine normally. If a sterile foil container has been used to catch the specimen, the specimen is then transferred into a specimen container and sent to the laboratory.

Suprapubic aspiration of urine

In patients suspected of having bladder infection but in whom the results of culture of mid-stream urines are equivocal, it may be necessary to proceed to suprapubic aspiration (widely performed in paediatrics, but not in adults). After skin preparation a fine needle (e.g. a lumbar puncture needle) is introduced into the bladder by direct puncture just above the symphysis pubis, and urine aspirated. Ultrasound can be used to confirm that the bladder is full prior to the procedure.

'In–out' catheter urine specimens

Although bladder catheterisation carries a small (1–2%) risk of introducing new infection into the bladder, this risk is sometimes justified by the importance of obtaining urine direct from the bladder. A urethral catheter is passed into the bladder, the first few millilitres discarded, and sample collected.

Obtaining urine specimens from ileal conduits

Urine in ileal conduit bags is always contaminated by skin organisms, and the culture of 'bag urine' is not a useful way of diagnosing upper urinary tract infection in patients with conduits. In patients suspected of having ascending infection, a urine specimen should be obtained by passing a catheter as far into the conduit as it will go.

'Two glass test'

This is a test for urethritis, and is performed when a patient presents with dysuria or urethral discharge and a sexual history suggesting possible recent infection. Culture of a urethral swab or of the urethral discharge should also be obtained and sent for gonorrhoea testing (requires attendance at a sexual health clinic). Two urine samples are collected; the first 10mL passed and a mid-stream sample. Each is sent for culture; urethritis is diagnosed when the bacterial count is highest in the first sample. The first sample should also be sent for *Chlamydia* testing.

'Stamey–Mears test'

This test is performed for the diagnosis of prostatitis. A MSU sample is obtained, and then the patient is asked to stop passing urine. The prostate gland is massaged per rectum and 'expressed prostatic secretions' collected, followed by a final urine sample. In prostatitis, bacterial counts are higher in the expressed prostatic secretions or the post-massage urine sample than in the mid-stream sample.

Indwelling catheter urine specimens

Colonisation of the bladder is nearly inevitable within a fortnight of insertion of an indwelling urethral or suprapubic catheter. Unnecessary antibiotic treatment increases the selective pressure for the emergence of antibiotic-resistant organisms and must be reserved for symptomatic infection. There is no point in sending catheter specimens unless there is a suspicion of symptomatic infection at the time. 'Surveillance' samples sent to predict which antibiotics should be used if the patient becomes symptomatic at a later time are unjustified, because the colonising organisms may change over time. A fresh specimen of urine is obtained from the collection port into the collection pot. Samples should NOT be collected from the reservoir into which the catheter drains.

Localisation tests

- Occasionally it is justified to attempt to localise the site of infection to the bladder or to one or other kidney.
- The 'gold standard' is to obtain samples from each ureter and from the bladder during rigid cystoscopy under general anaesthesia.
- The 'Fairley test' requires passage of a urethral catheter followed by a bladder washout with a wide spectrum antibacterial and a fibrinolytic enzyme. Sequential samples of urine are then obtained. If infection is present in the upper tracts, this will not have been affected by the bladder washout, and organisms will be detected in the first specimen obtained after washout, whereas if infection was confined to the bladder, subsequent samples will be sterile.
- Infection may be confined to one or other kidney as a result of ureteric obstruction, or may be present within a renal cyst. In these situations, direct aspiration of urine under ultrasound control in the radiology department is necessary.

Microscopy and culture of urine

Once a sample has been obtained it is sent to a microbiology laboratory for microscopy and culture.

Microscopy is required to assess pyuria (WBCs in the urine) and contamination.

- Significant pyuria indicates inflammation within the urinary tract; if this persists despite negative urine cultures the patient has 'sterile pyuria', for which there are a number of causes, including infection with an organism which does not grow on conventional culture media, e.g. *Chlamydia*.
- Pyuria plus a positive culture confirm the diagnosis of urinary tract infection.

- The absence of pyuria makes a urinary tract infection less likely, but can occur in the early stages of infection or in the presence of a very high fluid intake.
- Contamination (in the female) is indicated by the presence of large numbers of squamous cells, which usually come from the vaginal wall; however squamous cells can occasionally come from the bladder.

Culture and sensitivity are necessary to decide what treatment is necessary and to differentiate contamination of the urine sample by organisms outside the bladder from true infection.

- A 'pure growth' of a single organism to >10^5 colony-forming units (cfu)/mL is the conventional criterion for urinary tract infection. However:
- Low counts of 10^2–10^4 cfu/mL can be associated with early infection, and should be taken seriously in the presence of suggestive symptoms in women.
- Low counts in men are likely to represent true infection, because contamination is uncommon.
- Genuine mixed growth may occur, in the presence of impaired urinary drainage or a foreign body within the urinary tract.

Urine microscopy

Urine microscopy is a useful, quick, reliable, cheap and underused investigation—the 'liquid renal biopsy'! Far more information can be obtained by careful microscopy than is usually obtained in the microbiology laboratory, where the priority is detection of significant urine infection.

Indications

- Suspected urinary tract infection (📖p590).
- Suspected acute glomerulonephritis.
- Suspected acute interstitial nephritis (requires staining for eosinophils).
- Unexplained acute or chronic renal failure.
- Haematuria (with or without proteinuria) on urine dipstick test.
- Suspected urinary tract malignancy.

Procedure

A freshly voided, clean catch, mid-stream, early morning specimen is ideal. The sample should be centrifuged and re-suspended in a small volume. Although bright field microscopy will allow identification of most formed elements in the urine sediment, phase contrast microscopy is useful for detection of red cell ghosts, 'glomerular' red cells and some other constituents. Staining of the urine sediment is not necessary for most purposes, but is useful for identification of eosinophils and malignant cells—this is usually performed in the cytology laboratory.

Haematuria

RBCs appear as non-nucleated biconcave discs. Even when urine is red in colour or dipsticks positive for blood it should be examined for the presence of red cells. The differential diagnosis of haematuria is broad, but it is broadly classified into glomerular (renal) and infrarenal causes. Transit of red cells through the renal tubules causes osmotic changes in their shape and size; 'dysmorphic' or 'crenated' red cells are best seen using phase contrast microscopy, and may be missed altogether if bright field microscopy is used. In experienced hands, detection of these glomerular red cells strongly suggests a glomerular origin for haematuria, although failure to detect these changes does not reliably indicate a lower urinary tract cause of bleeding—heavy haematuria in IgA nephropathy, for instance, can result in large numbers of normal red cells in the urine. Urine pH, concentration and storage can affect red cell morphology.

Leucocyturia

The presence of significant numbers of polymorphs (pyuria) in urine is highly suggestive of urinary tract infection ([] p590) but can also occur in glomerulonephritis, interstitial nephritis, and peri-ureteric inflammation, for instance in acute appendicitis. The presence of leucocyte casts is diagnostic of renal parenchymal infection ('acute pyelonephritis'). Eosinophiluria is associated with acute allergic interstitial nephritis and athero-embolic renal disease.

Other cells

Squamous epithelial cells are usually taken as indicative of vaginal contamination, but may also derive from the bladder and urethra. Occasionally malignant cells arising from the lower urinary tract are picked up on routine microscopy. Spermatozoa are also rarely seen.

Microorganisms

Identification of bacteriuria, in association with leucocyturia is very suggestive of infection. Organisms may be in chains or clusters and some are motile. Fungi including yeast and protozoans including *Trichomonas* can also be readily identified.

Casts

Casts are cylindrical bodies, which usually form in the distal tubule and collecting duct. They consist of cells or cell debris held together by Tamm–Horsfall protein. Staining and phase contrast microscopy improves identification and characterisation of casts, but results are operator dependent. Extreme shaking or agitation can disintegrate casts.

Hyaline casts appear translucent and homogeneous and are present in normal urine. Number may be increased in dehydration and proteinuria.

Cellular casts especially red cell casts, always indicate significant parenchymal renal disease. Red cell casts are strongly suggestive of acute glomerulonephritis, but may occur in interstitial nephritis and acute tubular necrosis as well.

White cell casts are seen in acute pyelonephritis and acute interstitial nephritis.

Granular casts are formed from cell debris and are seen in a wide variety of renal diseases.

Waxy broad casts form in atrophic renal tubules and are seen in chronic renal failure.

Crystals

A variety of crystals can be visualised and are of importance in stone formers. A freshly voided sample should be examined as storage and temperature changes can affect type and number of crystals found. A large number of calcium oxalate crystals are seen in hypercalciuria, hyperoxaluria and ethylene glycol poisoning. Presence of a single crystal of cystine is diagnostic of cystinuria as cystine is not a constituent of normal urine. Phosphate crystals can form in normal urine as it cools, and are of no pathological significance.

Investigations in patients with renal or bladder stones

Not all renal tract stones are formed because of abnormal urine chemistry. They may also be formed because of stasis, e.g. in calyceal or bladder diverticula. Infection ('struvite') stones are the result of chronic infection in the urinary tract with urease-producing organisms, which metabolise urea to form an alkaline urine in which struvite readily precipitates.

Indications

Although up to 75% of patients who present with renal stones eventually form a second stone, this may not be for 20 years. Most urologists therefore only refer patients for metabolic evaluation if there is a heightened suspicion of an underlying metabolic cause.

Situations in which evaluation is definitely indicated include

- Formation of stones in childhood or adolescence.
- Recurrent stone formation.
- Nephrocalcinosis (calcification in the renal parenchyma) as well as stone formation in the collecting systems.

Radiology

Intravenous urography will usually have been performed during the patient's presentation with stone disease, but the films should be reviewed to look for evidence of any cause of stasis within the collecting systems, and in particular for medullary sponge kidney. Radiolucent stones can be detected using ultrasound, intravenous urography or CT scanning, and can be made of cystine, uric acid or xanthine. 'Staghorn' calculi filling the collecting systems are most often struvite (infection) stones, but not always—calcium oxalate stones can grow to similar size and shape, particularly in hyperoxaluria.

Stone analysis

Depending on the facilities in the laboratory, this may be qualitative or semi-quantitative. The purpose of analysis is to distinguish calcium stones from cystine, urate and struvite stones, to pick up the rare types of stone, and in addition to distinguish calcium oxalate from calcium phosphate stones. The result of stone analysis should be used to guide further investigation. Stones can be obtained for analysis either at surgery, including percutaneous nephrolithotomy, or by asking a patient to pass urine through a fine sieve.

'Spot' urine tests

Amino acid analysis on a random sample of urine shows increased excretion of cystine, ornithine, lysine and arginine in cystinuria, and this finding is sufficient to confirm a suspected diagnosis. However, measurement of 24h urinary cystine excretion is necessary for optimal management of this condition.

Random urine calcium:creatinine and oxalate:creatinine ratios are used in children to diagnose hypercalciuria and hyperoxaluria, but are not as reliable as 24h urine collections, which are preferred in adults.

24h urine collections

Collections must be made into an acidified container for measurement of calcium and oxalate, and into a plain container for measurement of urate (because acidification is necessary to prevent calcium binding to the plastic surface of the urine container and to prevent *in vitro* generation of oxalate, and because acidification precipitates uric acid crystals). Measurement of sodium and citrate excretion can be made on either type of collection.

Calcium excretion is not a good predictor of stone formation (calcium activity is less than concentration due to the presence in urine of anions that form soluble complexes with calcium). However, marked ↑ of urinary calcium is a risk factor for stone formation.

Oxalate excretion correlates well with the risk of recurrent calcium oxalate stone formation, even within the normal range. Marked hyperoxaluria may result from enteric hyperoxaluria (↑ colonic oxalate absorption resulting from small bowel resection, jejunoileal bypass or malabsorption), ethylene glycol toxicity (acutely), from excess dietary oxalate, or as a result of primary hyperoxaluria (one of several metabolic defects causing increased endogenous oxalate production).

Glycollate and L-glycerate should be measured in patients suspected of having primary hyperoxaluria to allow differentiation between type 1 and type 2 hyperoxaluria. This investigation is only available in a few laboratories.

Citrate excretion should be measured because citrate is a potent inhibitor of calcium stone formation; correction of hypocitraturia with, for instance, oral potassium citrate, reduces stone recurrence rate.

Sodium excretion (a good marker for dietary sodium intake) should be measured in calcium stone formers and in patients with cystinuria, because reduction of dietary sodium intake results in decreased excretion of calcium and cystine, respectively.

Cystine excretion should be measured in cystine stone formers. The aim of treatment is to maintain the cystine concentration well below the solubility limit for cystine (~1mmol/L at urine pH of 7). Worth asking the patient to split the urine collection into day-time and night-time aliquots to ensure that this target is met at night, when urine tends to become more concentrated, as well as during the day.

Urinary phosphate measurement is of no proven value in the management even of calcium phosphate stone formers.

Tests of urinary calcium excretion

Tests performed after calcium restriction and following a high calcium test meal have been used widely in the USA to differentiate 'absorptive' from 'renal' hypercalciuria. These tests are necessary to define different phenotypes associated with hypercalciuria for research studies, but there is no evidence that management strategies based on them have any advantage over those based on simpler tests of urine chemistry.

Renal biopsy

Percutaneous renal biopsy is a valuable tool to establish diagnosis, suggest prognosis and guide therapy in renal diseases. It also has a major role in the management of a renal transplant recipient.

Definite indications (result likely to change management)
- Nephrotic syndrome (in adults).
- Steroid-unresponsive nephrotic syndrome in children.
- Acute nephritic syndrome.
- Rapidly progressive glomerulonephritis.
- Unexplained renal failure with normal-sized kidneys relative to body size and age.
- Renal involvement in multi-system disorders.
- Diagnosis of renal transplant dysfunction.

Relative indications (result may change management or help to define prognosis)
- Non-nephrotic range proteinuria with or without haematuria.
- Isolated haematuria.
- Unexplained chronic renal failure.
- Diabetic patient with renal dysfunction, particularly with features not typical of diabetic nephropathy.

▶▶Absolute contraindications
- Uncontrolled severe hypertension.
- Bleeding diathesis including platelets $<50 \times 10^9$/L, uncorrected familial bleeding/clotting disorders and patient on anticoagulation with prolonged clotting times.

Relative contraindications
- Single kidney.
- Kidney size small compared to patient's body size and age.
- Renal tumour/mass for fear of abdominal seeding.
- Uncooperative patient (can be done under sedation or under GA).
- Multiple renal cysts.

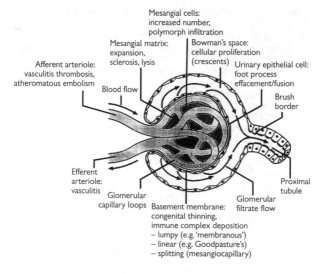

Fig. 10.4 The normal glomerulus and its repertoire of response to injury. Reprinted from Tomson CRV (1998) Essential Medicine, 2nd edition, p220, by permission of the publisher Churchill Livingstone.

For an excellent patient information sheet on renal biopsy see:
http://renux.dmed.ed.ac.uk/EdREN/EdRenINFObits/RenalBiopsyShort.html

Procedure

1. Recent imaging of kidneys to document size and rule out obstruction is mandatory. A recent normal platelet count, clotting profile and informed consent is necessary.
2. The procedure is performed where proper ultrasound facilities are available and usually done under local anaesthesia. Sedation can be given to an uncooperative or tense patient.
3. An attending pathologist or technician at the time of sampling to comment on adequacy of tissue is very useful.
4. Biopsy with automated spring-loaded devices or a biopsy gun, under ultrasound visualisation is considered ideal but techniques vary based on availability of local expertise.
5. The patient lies prone and the kidney is identified with ultrasound.
6. The skin over the target area is prepared and anaesthetised with lignocaine.
7. A small cut in the skin is made using a scalpel. The kidney is localised with a fine bore 21G lumbar puncture needle and local anaesthetic

infiltrated up to the level of the renal capsule. Either kidney can be biopsied: all parenchymal renal diseases are bilateral. After suitably protecting the ultrasound probe, the biopsy needle/gun is inserted along the anaesthetised track under ultrasound guidance to the level of the renal capsule, aiming to obtain a sample from the cortex of the lower pole. The patient is asked to hold their breath while the biopsy is taken.

8. The needle/gun is fired and subsequently withdrawn. The patient is then allowed to breathe normally.

9. Two cores of tissue are usually taken; this may require three or four 'passes' with the biopsy needle. If an attending pathologist or technician is present, they can comment on the adequacy of tissue by examining the core for glomeruli using a hand held magnifying glass or a simple microscope. If immunofluorescence is to be performed, part of one core is placed in saline; the remainder is placed in formalin.

10. Following the biopsy the patient is turned supine and strict bed rest enforced for a minimum of 6h. Vital signs are monitored every 15min for 2h, every 30min for 2h and hourly thereafter. If no complications are encountered at 6h the patient is allowed to mobilise. Most bleeding complications occur within the first 8h, but bleeding can start up to 72h after the biopsy. If macroscopic haematuria is present and does not resolve within the observation period, discharge should be delayed.

📖OHCM p261.

Renal imaging

Contrast nephropathy

Renal toxicity due to radiocontrast agents may cause or exacerbate renal impairment. Nephrotoxicity is due to a combination of local vasoconstriction and direct tubular injury. There is an increased risk in patients with pre-existing renal impairment, diabetes, myeloma, hypovolaemia or effective hypovolaemia (e.g. congestive cardiac failure), and concurrent administration of nephrotoxic medication including non-steroidal anti-inflammatory drugs and angiotensin converting enzyme inhibitors. The Royal College of Radiologists also recommends discontinuation of Metformin prior to investigation with intravascular contrast media. (🖱www.rcr. ac.uk/pubtop.asp?PublicationID=70). Although usually reversible, contrast nephropathy can precipitate the need for dialysis in patients whose renal function is already seriously impaired. Non-ionic media, adequate hydration and acetylcysteine (given by mouth) administered prior to the examination can reduce the risk in high-risk patients.

Details of the radiological investigation of the urinary tract appear on pp598, 684, 774, 776, 778.

Choice of investigation

Unexplained renal impairment

When a patient first presents with renal impairment it is important to decide whether this is acute—and therefore potentially reversible—or chronic. Although the history, examination and blood tests may give some clues, considerable doubt may remain.

All patients presenting with renal impairment should therefore undergo

- Ultrasound:
  - Hydronephrosis suggests obstructive nephropathy.
  - Small, smooth, kidneys with increased echogenicity and decreased corticomedullary differentiation suggests chronic parenchymal renal disease, e.g. chronic glomerulonephritis.
  - Irregular cortical scarring can be caused by reflux nephropathy, previous obstructive nephropathy (e.g. complicating renal stones) and renal infarction from vascular disease or embolism.
  - Renal asymmetry, particularly in a patient with known atherosclerosis elsewhere, suggests renal artery stenosis, although this can just as commonly be bilateral.
  - Renal enlargement can occur in acute tubular necrosis, renal vein thrombosis and renal infiltration, e.g. in haematological malignancy.
- Plain abdominal film (KUB—kidneys, ureters, bladder):
  - Nephrocalcinosis and urinary tract stones, particularly if outside the renal pelvis can be missed on ultrasound.

Further radiological investigations, including renal angiography and isotope scanning, are sometimes helpful.

Suspected nephrolithiasis

IVU is the investigation of first choice: CT may be necessary, particularly for radiolucent stones.

Investigation of haematuria

In patients over 40, and possibly in some younger patients, it is important to exclude urinary tract malignancy. Ultrasound is the investigation of choice for the detection of renal cell carcinoma, but will miss some transitional cell carcinomas of the renal pelvis, which are best detected using IVU.

Investigation of suspected renal artery stenosis

In younger patients in whom fibromuscular dysplasia is suspected, conventional angiography should be performed. Atherosclerotic renal artery stenosis can be reasonably assessed by contrast CT angiography or by gadolinium-enhanced MR angiography. The Royal College of Radiologists webpage ⌐Ⓑwww.rcr.ac.uk/patradio.asp?pageID=223 provides information for patients undergoing interventional radiological procedures including angiography and angioplasty.

Reflux nephropathy

Confirming this diagnosis can be important in counselling patients, as reflux nephropathy is often inherited as an autosomal dominant trait. Cortical scarring is best detected using a static DMSA renal scan. However, there are other causes of cortical scarring. The diagnosis is best confirmed by showing the combination of cortical scarring with underlying calyceal deformity on IVU. Demonstration of vesicoureteric reflux on direct or indirect micturating cystourethrography is useful in infants and small children, but reflux commonly resolves with growth, so these tests are seldom used in adults.

Obstructive uropathy

Although hydronephrosis demonstrated on IVU or ultrasound is usually sufficient to confirm obstruction, it is possible to have obstruction without much dilatation (e.g. complicating encasement by tumour). More commonly, there is uncertainty over whether dilatation of the collecting system and pelvis is due to previous obstruction, now resolved, or continuing obstruction. In these situations the options are diuretic MAG3 renography, insertion of nephrostomy, or retrograde insertion of ureteric stents. If doubt persists, a Whitaker test may be performed: this involves infusion of saline at a constant rate through a nephrostomy tube and measuring the relationship between pressure and flow down the ureter.

Renal transplant dysfunction

The differential diagnosis usually lies between obstruction, ureteric leak, rejection, acute tubular necrosis, nephrotoxicity and renal vein thrombosis. Depending on the centre, ultrasound with Doppler assessment of renal blood flow (giving resistance index) or isotope renography may be the investigation of first choice.

Renal bone disease

Parathyroid hormone (PTH)

Indications
Diagnosis of primary, secondary or tertiary hyperparathyroidism.

Procedure
A serum sample is sent and separated within 4h of venepuncture. Alternatively, PTH remains stable for 24h if the sample is taken into EDTA, allowing samples to be sent from primary care. (Check with local laboratory).

Other markers of bone biochemistry

Serum calcium is often normal even in patients with significant renal disease, because a fall in serum calcium caused by reduced $1,25-(OH)_2$ vitamin D production results in an increase in parathyroid hormone secretion, returning serum calcium towards normal. Hypocalcaemia occurs after parathyroidectomy or after treatment with bisphosphonates. Hypercalcaemia occurs when the parathyroid hormone release loses sensitivity to serum calcium in tertiary hyperparathyroidism.

If PTH is raised in the presence of stage 3 CKD, check $25-(OH)$ vitamin D; vitamin D deficiency should be corrected before treatment of hyperparathyroidism.

Serum phosphate is often increased in patients with renal impairment due to impaired renal excretion of phosphate.

Serum total alkaline phosphatase rises in severe hyperparathyroidism and in osteomalacia.

Serum bone alkaline phosphatase is a more sensitive marker of bone turnover, but quantitative measurement is not widely available. If total alkaline phosphatase is raised, alkaline phosphatase isoenzymes can be measured as an indicator of whether the increase is of bone origin.

Serum aluminium and the desferrioxamine test

Patients with renal disease may be exposed to aluminium from contaminated water used for preparation of dialysate or by ingesting aluminium hydroxide as an antacid or, rarely nowadays, as a phosphate binder taken with meals. Because of the effects of aluminium on the brain, bone marrow and bones it is important to monitor patients at risk for evidence of aluminium accumulation.

Serum aluminium has to be taken into an aluminium-free glass tube. Serum aluminium levels reflect current exposure, and do not give any information about cumulative exposure. Serum aluminium levels may be increased by iron deficiency. Levels above 60μg/L (2.2μmol/L) are considered indicative of a dangerous level of exposure and should lead to a review of treatment.

The increment in serum aluminium 24 or 48h after IV desferrioxamine is a marker of aluminium 'load'. The original protocol requires the use of 40mg/kg desferrioxamine; a rise in serum aluminium of >200μg/L correlates well with the presence of aluminium-related bone disease on bone biopsy. Low dose protocols have also been described and validated.

Skeletal survey

Severe hyperparathyroidism causes erosion of the terminal phalanges, subperiosteal erosions and, in rare cases, brown tumours and pathological fractures. Severe osteomalacia causes loss of bone density and Looser zones (pseudo-fractures). These radiological signs are not commonly seen in modern renal patients because biochemical monitoring allows earlier detection of bone disease.

Transiliac bone biopsy

This is the 'gold standard' for the diagnosis of renal bone disease, but is not commonly used in clinical (as opposed to research) settings. However, it can be useful particularly for the confirmation of aluminium-related bone disease. For the maximum information to be gained from this invasive test, double tetracycline labelling should be performed.

Procedure

14 and 13 days before the procedure the patient takes a tetracycline antibiotic, e.g. oxytetracycline 250mg qds, and 4 and 3 days before the procedure a different tetracycline, e.g. demeclocycline 300mg bd. Under general anaesthetic a transiliac core of bone, including both cortical surfaces, is taken and placed in absolute alcohol. The sample should be sent

to a laboratory specialising in the interpretation of bone biopsies in patients with metabolic bone disease.

Immunological tests in renal medicine

Immune-mediated diseases can affect the kidney in isolation or as part of a systemic disorder. Immunological tests commonly used to diagnose or monitor progress of renal disease are discussed here.

Complement
Indications

Acute nephritic syndrome, renal failure with skin ± neurological involvement and suspected SLE, endocarditis or cryoglobulinaemia. The normal complement system, its activation pathways and assay methods are discussed elsewhere (p300). In relation to renal disease, hypocomplementaemia is important and relative deficiencies of various components can point to certain disorders.

Table 10.1

	C3	C4
Post-streptococcal GN	Low	Normal
SLE	Low	Low
Cryoglobulinaemia	Low/normal	Very low
Membranoproliferative GN	Low	Low/normal
Subacute endocarditis	Normal/low	Low

GN, glomerulonephritis

Successful treatment normalises complement levels in endocarditis, and in SLE except when SLE results from congenital complement deficiency.

C3 nephritic factor (C3Nef) is an IgG autoantibody that binds to and stabilises alternative pathway C3 convertase—C3bBb. This results in continuous activation of the alternative pathway with C3 depletion. It is detected by ELISA. C3Nef is classically associated with type 2 membranoproliferative glomerulonephritis.

Immunoglobulins and serum electrophoresis for paraproteins
Indications

- Suspected myeloma or other clonal B cell disorders.
- Unexplained renal failure, with or without proteinuria, particularly in patients >50 years.
- Renal failure in association with hypercalcaemia.

Serum electrophoresis to identify a monoclonal immunoglobulin band is useful, but should always be combined with tests for urinary light chains (Bence–Jones protein), as some types of myeloma cause light chain proteinuria without a monoclonal band in the serum.

Measurement of serum immunoglobulin concentrations is of value in patients with known myeloma, but is otherwise not useful in the assessment of patients with renal disease. Polyclonal hypergammaglobulinaemia is seen in chronic infections, connective tissue disorders (e.g. rheumatoid arthritis, Sjögren's syndrome), neoplasms and chronic liver disease. Measurement of serum IgA concentration is of no value in the diagnosis of IgA nephropathy.

Paraproteins are products of abnormal B cell clones and can be detected in serum as monoclonal bands on immunoglobulin electrophoresis or in urine as Bence–Jones proteins. Paraproteins may be whole immunoglobulins or heavy or light chains in isolation. Light chains are sufficiently small to be filtered at the glomerulus, are not reabsorbed and are not picked up on routine dipsticks. Bence–Jones proteins are light chains excreted in the urine. Bence–Jones proteins precipitate on heating to 45°C and redissolve on boiling but are now detected by electrophoretic techniques.

Paraproteins can cause a number of different renal lesions, including
- Myeloma cast nephropathy.
- Light chain nephropathy.
- AL amyloidosis.
- Fibrillary/immunotactoid glomerulopathy (although this appearance is more frequently not associated with a plasma cell dyscrasia).

Cryoglobulins

Cryoglobulins are immunoglobulins, which precipitate on cooling and redissolve on warming.

Cryoglobulinaemia should be suspected in
- Renal failure with otherwise unexplained hypocomplementaemia or positive rheumatoid factor.
- Renal failure in association with skin and neurological involvement.
- Unexplained proteinuria/renal failure in patients with clonal B cell disorders.

Meticulous attention to collection, transportation and assessment of the sample is required: a serum sample must be kept at 37°C and sent to the laboratory for analysis immediately, having warned the lab that the sample is on the way. False negative results are common due to improper handling of the specimen.

Once a cryoglobulin has been found, further electrophoresis and immunofixation allows identification of three distinct types:
- Type 1 has a single monoclonal immunoglobulin (IgG, IgA or IgM) and is associated with monoclonal B cell disorders.
- Type 2 has a monoclonal IgM directed against the Fc portion of IgG, and the cryoprotein therefore consists of monoclonal IgM with polyclonal IgG. Tests for rheumatoid factor (i.e. anti-IgG antibodies) are positive. This may be associated with haematological malignancy, chronic hepatitis C infection or may be unexplained ('essential').
- Type 3 has polyclonal IgG and polyclonal IgM and occurs in chronic infections (e.g. bacterial endocarditis, viral hepatitis), autoimmune disorders (e.g. rheumatoid arthritis, SLE) or may be unexplained ('essential').

Hypocomplementaemia, especially very low C4 levels due to classical complement pathway activation, is characteristic and helpful in diagnosing active cryoglobulinaemic disorder. Renal disease can present as an acute nephritic disorder or as nephrotic syndrome and is usually seen in association with skin and systemic involvement.

Antineutrophil cytoplasmic antibody (ANCA)

These are autoantibodies directed against enzymes present in the cytoplasm of human neutrophils. They are present in nearly all patients with small vessel vasculitis (including Wegener's granulomatosis, microscopic polyangitis, renal limited crescentic GN and Churg–Strauss syndrome), and changing titres can reflect changing disease activity. However, a negative ANCA does not rule out vasculitis, and false positive tests occur, so the test is not a substitute for renal biopsy.

Poisoning & overdose

General principles *608*
Samples of medicolegal importance *610*
Methods used in analytical toxicology *610*
Brainstem death testing & organ donation *611*
Interpretation of arterial blood gases in poisoned patients *612*
Amphetamines & derivatives *614*
Anticonvulsants *615*
Benzodiazepines *616*
Carbon monoxide *616*
Cocaine *617*
Cyanide *618*
Digoxin *619*
Ethylene glycol, ethanol & methanol poisoning *620*
Iron *622*
Lead poisoning *624*
Lithium *624*
Methaemoglobinaemia *625*
Opioids *626*
Organophosphorus insecticides *627*
Paracetamol (acetaminophen) poisoning *628*
Salicylate poisoning *633*
Theophylline *634*
Tricyclic antidepressants *635*
Table of conversion factors between mass & molar units *636*

General principles

Many poisoned patients recover without specific management other than supportive care. A minority have life-threatening toxicity. In assessing the poisoned patient it is important to ensure adequate *Airway, Breathing* and *Circulation*, take an adequate history and undertake a full clinical examination. Tablets, bottles, syringes, aerosol containers and other items found with or near the patient should be retained, although it is usually best to analyse biological specimens (usually blood and/or urine) if analytical confirmation of exposure is required.

The role of blood and urine tests in toxicology

Close collaboration between analytical staff and clinicians is required if anything other than the simplest toxicological analysis is to be useful.

Toxicological analysis using blood or urine is used to confirm the diagnosis of poisoning when this is in doubt or for medicolegal purposes, to help the management, in the diagnosis of brain death, or to work out the time to restart chronic drug therapy. Few centres have full analytical toxicology services and a 'toxicology screen' rarely influences inpatient management, with the exception of paracetamol, salicylate, lithium, digoxin and iron poisoning, and on occasions a drugs of abuse screen. Toxicological analysis of blood plasma or serum is also of value if an extracorporeal method of elimination such as haemodialysis or MARS® (Molecular Absorbance Recirculating Systems ⤷http://www.teraklin.com/eng/mars.html) is being contemplated. Any toxicology should be tailored to that patient's circumstances and the poisons commonly encountered in that country. In Western Europe and North America, most patients will have taken drugs, but pesticide poisoning, for example, is common in less well developed countries.

Plasma paracetamol, salicylate, lithium, digoxin and iron measurements in blood are usually available on an urgent basis. For other patients, particularly those who present a complex clinical picture or who are unconscious, a 50mL sample of urine and a 10mL sample of heparinised blood should be collected on admission and stored at 4°C (→ refrigerator). This can be analysed later if it is felt the result will influence your management, or is needed for medicolegal purposes (*see below*). Urine is useful for screening, especially for drugs of abuse, as it is often available in large volumes and often contains higher concentrations of poisons and their metabolites than blood. The samples should be obtained as soon as possible after admission, ideally before any therapeutic drugs are administered. Urine samples usually provide qualitative results, e.g. detect the presence of amphetamines or benzodiazepines. Quantitative measurements in urine are of little use because some compounds, such as benzodiazepines, are extensively metabolised prior to excretion in urine.

Sample requirements

Plasma or serum is normally used for quantitative assays for drugs and drug metabolites and in general there are no marked significant differences in concentration between these fluids. Evacuated blood tubes and containers containing gel separators or soft rubber stoppers are not recommended if a toxicological analysis is to be performed as the plasticisers (phosphates and phthalates) used in many such tubes may interfere with chromatographic methods, and volatile compounds such as carbon monoxide or ethanol may be lost.

EDTA tubes are preferred for carboxyhaemoglobin assays and for measurement of lead, and some other metals as these are concentrated in red blood cells. A fluoride/oxalate tube should be used if ethanol, cocaine or benzodiazepines are being assayed, although special tubes containing 1% (w/v) fluoride are needed if enzymic hydrolysis of these and other compounds is to be completely prevented.

The use of disinfectant swabs containing alcohols should be avoided, as should heparin, which contains phenolic preservatives (chlorbutol, cresol) and preservatives containing mercury salts (see Table 11.1).

Sample requirements for metals/trace elements analysis

Table 11.1

Metal	Sample needed
Aluminium	10mL whole blood in plastic (not glass) tube —no anticoagulant/ beads*
Antimony	5mL heparinised whole blood; 20mL urine
Arsenic	5mL heparinised whole blood; 20mL urine
Bismuth	5mL heparinised whole blood
Cadmium	2mL EDTA whole blood*; 10mL urine*
Chromium	2mL heparinised whole blood*; 20mL urine*
Copper	2mL heparinised or clotted whole blood, or 1mL plasma; 10mL urine
Iron	5mL clotted blood or 2mL serum (avoid haemolysis)
Lead	2mL EDTA whole blood
Lithium	5mL clotted blood or 2mL serum (NOT lithium heparin tube!)
Manganese	1mL heparinised whole blood or 0.5mL plasma*
Mercury	5mL heparinised whole blood; 20mL urine
Selenium	2mL heparinised whole blood or 1mL plasma/serum
Thallium	5mL heparinised whole blood; 20mL urine
Zinc	2mL whole blood (not EDTA) or 1mL plasma/serum

*Send unused container from the same batch to check for possible contamination.

Samples of medicolegal importance

A toxicology screen is helpful if murder, assault or child abuse is suspected. Samples collected in such cases are often so important that they should be kept securely at $-20°C$ or below, until investigation of the incident is concluded. Legal requirements mean that all specimens should be clearly labelled with the patient's family or last name and any forenames, the date and time of collection and the nature of the specimen, if this is not obvious. Strict chain of custody procedures should be implemented and the doctor or nurse taking the sample should seal the bag with a tamper-proof device and sign and date the seal. A chain of custody form must accompany the sample and should be signed and dated by every person taking possession of the sample. The sample should be secured in a locked container or refrigerator if left unattended before arrival at the laboratory.

Methods used in analytical toxicology

A range of chromatographic and other methods such as radioligand immunoassays are available for toxicological analyses. Plasma concentrations associated with serious toxicity range from micrograms per litre (mcg/L $\equiv$ µg/L) in the case of drugs such as digoxin to grams per litre (g/L) in the case of ethanol. Specialised labs use use a combination of solvent extraction and thin layer chromatography (TLC) together with gas–liquid chromatography (GLC) using either flame-ionisation or selective detectors such as nitrogen/phosphorus detectors or mass spectroscopy (MS) as the basis for a poison screen. It is unwise to use TLC without corroboration of results by another method, e.g. GLC, because the resolution power of TLC is limited and interpretation of chromatograms is subjective. A commercial kit for TLC (Toxi-lab, Marion Laboratories) is supplied with a compendium of colour plates but even so problems can arise in differentiation of compounds with similar mobility and colour reactions. The kit is aimed at the US market and some common UK drugs are not included.

Spectrophotometry is commonly used to measure salicylates, iron and carboxyhaemoglobin. However, UV spectrophotometry and spectrophotofluorimetry are often used as detectors for high-performance liquid chromatography (HPLC) and in immunoassays. Spectrophotometric methods and immunoassays often suffer from interference from metabolites or other drugs. Immunoassays have the advantage of long shelf life and simplicity, but all require confirmation with a chromatographic method if the results are to stand scrutiny. This is because immunoassays for small molecules are often not specific, e.g. some urine amphetamine immunoassays give positive results with proguanil, isoxuprine, labetalol, tranylcypromine and phenylethylamine. The Syva Emit antidepressant assay cross-reacts with phenothiazines after overdose. Chromatographic methods have the advantage of selectivity and sensitivity and ability to perform quantitative measurements, but are expensive. Generally, GLC is still used to measure basic drugs and HPLC is used to analyse specific compounds/groups of compounds.

Modern methods of assay for heavy metals vary enormously. Isotope dilution mass spectrometry is a reference method. Atomic absorption spectrophotometry, with either flame or electrothermal atomisation is used most widely. In the case of iron, reliable kits based on the formation of a coloured complex are available.

There is wide variation in the units that various laboratories use to report results. This has caused confusion and errors in treatment and *great care* is needed to ensure that clinical interpretation is undertaken in full knowledge of the units used.

Flanagan RJ. (1995) The poisoned patient; the role of the laboratory. *Br J Biomed Sci* **52**, 202–213; Baselt RC, Cravey RH. (2002) *Disposition of Toxic Drugs and Chemicals in Man*, 6th edition, Chemical Toxicology Institute, California.

Brainstem death testing & organ donation

Brain death cannot be diagnosed in the presence of drugs that mask central nervous system (CNS) activity. There is a rule of thumb, based on the pharmacological principle that most drugs need five half-lives to be effectively eliminated from the circulation, to allow four half-lives of any drug to elapse before declaring death, or to allow at least 2–3 days for drug effects to wear off. Whether this is satisfactory for patients with organ failure and hence impaired drug elimination is unclear and often in such patients measurement of plasma concentrations of residual drugs is required to determine whether brainstem death tests are valid or whether a drug could be interfering with the results.

Selected donor organs from those who have died from poisoning by tricyclic antidepressants, benzodiazepines, barbiturates, insulin, carbon monoxide, cocaine, methanol and paracetamol have been used in transplantation. It is important to identify which organs act as reservoirs for drugs and either not consider such organs, e.g. a liver from a paracetamol-poisoned patient, or take prophylactic precautions like N-acetylcysteine administration in the case of donation of a heart from a paracetamol-poisoned patient.

Jones AL, Simpson KJ. (1998) Drug abusers and poisoned patients: a potential source of organs for transplantation? *Q J Med* **91**, 589–592.

Interpretation of arterial blood gases in poisoned patients

Interpretation of blood gas values may be found in ☐OHCM pp168, 682. Essentially four patterns emerge, which may be mixed together.

Respiratory acidosis

Hypoventilation results in retention of carbon dioxide. This can occur after an overdose with any drugs that depress the CNS, e.g. tricyclic antidepressants, opioids and barbiturates.

Respiratory alkalosis

Hyperventilation with respiratory alkalosis is classically caused by aspirin (commonly measured as salicylate). It can also occur in response to hypoxia, drugs and CNS injury.

Metabolic alkalosis

Metabolic alkalosis is very uncommon in poisoning. Rarely it may result from excess administration of alkali, e.g. deliberate alkali ingestion.

Metabolic acidosis

This is the commonest metabolic abnormality in poisoning. If acidosis is particularly severe (e.g. pH <7.2), this should raise the question of poisoning by ethanol, methanol or ethylene glycol. Measuring the anion gap and osmolal gaps are helpful in further differentiation (☐*Ethylene glycol, ethanol & methanol,* p620).

Amphetamines & derivatives

E.g.: MDMA (ecstasy), MDEA, MDA (adam)

The following investigations should be considered in patients presenting to hospital with acute amphetamine(s) intoxication.

Plasma urea and electrolytes and glucose

It is critical that at least one set of U&E are checked in every patient. Most are profoundly dehydrated and require vigorous rehydration. Some patients develop hyponatraemia, often after drinking excess water and antidiuretic hormone secretion may be responsible for this (☐OHCM p692). Hypoglycaemia may occur.

Dipstick test of urine for myoglobin and subsequent serum creatine kinase

A hyperthermic (serotonin-like) syndrome with autonomic instability and rigidity, can develop leading to rhabdomyolysis. Dipstick testing of urine is positive for blood as myoglobin is detected by the haemoglobin assay. This is an indication that serum CK should be then be measured. If found to be elevated, adequate rehydration is needed to avoid deposition in renal tubules and incipient renal failure.

Full blood count

Rarely, aplastic anaemia (☐OHCM p662) has been reported after ecstasy (MDMA) ingestion.

Clotting studies

Disseminated intravascular coagulation (☐OHCM p650) can occur, often in the context of hyperthermia. Once liver damage ensues the INR/PT (☐OHCM p646) will rise.

Temperature

Hyperpyrexia can lead to rhabdomyolysis, disseminated intravascular coagulation and hepatocellular necrosis. Risks relate to the time in hours spent above 39°C. A rectal thermometer is the most accurate measure of temperature.

Liver function tests

Acute liver injury can occur with a rise in aspartate aminotransferase (AST) or alanine aminotransferase (ALT), often of several thousands.

▶▶Note: don't miss a hidden paracetamol overdose—check paracetamol levels in blood, from the earliest sample you have on that patient!

ECG

Cardiac arrhythmias are common and deaths, which occur soon after ingestion, may be due to these. Arrhythmias are often supraventricular, though ventricular arrythmias also occur.

Urine tests

Urine tests, e.g. EMIT dipstick system or by immunoassay in the laboratory, are sensitive and group-specific for amphetamines and can confirm an amphetamine has been ingested if that is in doubt, e.g. agitated patient in A&E. *Note*: amphetamine, MDMA, MDEA and MDA concentrations in blood are of no value in determining management.

Anticonvulsants

These can be assayed in blood by gas–liquid chromatographic (GLC) methods and in urine by thin layer chromatography (TLC) methods.

Carbamazepine toxicity

Plasma concentrations of carbamazepine and its active metabolite 10, 11-epoxide can be measured by HPLC but do not correlate well with the degree of toxicity. They are seldom performed unless the diagnosis is in doubt or there is concern about a therapeutic excess. The therapeutic range is between 8 and 12mg/L. Toxicity has been seen with carbamazepine concentrations above 20mg/L (85mmol/L). Coma, fits, respiratory failure and conduction abnormalities have been seen with concentrations in excess of 40mg/L (170mmol/L).

An ECG should be performed in all but the most trivial carbamazepine overdosage

The U&E should be checked as hyponatraemia and SIADH (📖OHCM p690) have been reported. Hypoglycaemia has also been reported.

Lamotrigine toxicity

Plasma concentrations of lamotrigine can be measured for compliance purposes (therapeutic range 1–4mg/L; upper limit may be as high as 10mg/L) but are not of value in the overdose situation.

An ECG should be performed in all but the most trivial lamotrigine overdosage.

Valproate toxicity

Plasma concentrations of sodium valproate can be measured by HPLC but do not correlate well with either with depth of coma or risk of seizures after overdose. The therapeutic range is 40–100mg/L. U&E and glucose should be measured as hypernatraemia, hypoglycaemia and hypocalcaemia have been reported after overdosage.

Phenytoin toxicity

Most patients with acute phenytoin poisoning do not require measurement of the plasma phenytoin concentration. An urgent phenytoin measurement may help in severe phenytoin poisoning where charcoal haemoperfusion is contemplated if the plasma phenytoin concentration is rapidly rising towards or exceeds 100mg/L.

Patients with suspected chronic phenytoin toxicity as a result of therapeutic dosing should have their plasma phenytoin concentration measured. The 'therapeutic range' is 10–20mg/L. Routine measurements may be useful to monitor anticonvulsant therapy or to time re-institution of chronic therapy after overdose.

Benzodiazepines

Most patients who have taken an overdose with benzodiazepines just sleep off the drug without sequelae within 24h. However, more severe effects can occur when benzodiazepines are mixed with other drugs such as tricyclic antidepressants, especially in patients with pre-existing cardiovascular or respiratory disease. Pulse oximetry is useful for monitoring the adequacy of ventilation if significant CNS depression is present.

Generally, measuring benzodiazepine concentrations in blood or urine is not of value in the management of benzodiazepine overdose patients. Rarely a urine screen by EMIT (immunoassay) is undertaken to confirm ingestion. Liquid chromatography simultaneously assays diazepam and its polar metabolites, and postmortem blood concentrations of 5mg/L and 19mg/L have been found in fatalities.

Carbon monoxide

Carbon monoxide is the commonest cause of death by poisoning in the UK. Those particularly at risk include patients with pre-existing cardiac or respiratory disease.

Carboxyhaemoglobin (COHb)

A carboxyhaemoglobin concentration in blood confirms exposure and should be measured urgently in all patients with suspected carbon monoxide poisoning, including those with smoke inhalation. The space above the blood in the sample tube (headspace) should be minimised. Normally expected values for COHb are up to 5% in non-smokers and up to 10% in smokers. However, after acute exposure the blood COHb concentration does not indicate the severity of poisoning because COHb begins to dissociate from the moment of removal from the source of exposure, and the rate of dissociation is also dependent on factors such as oxygen administration in the ambulance. Thus the use of nomograms to 'back-extrapolate' to find the initial highest COHb is meaningless. Management of the patient is determined by the clinical condition and also on circumstantial evidence such as the intensity and duration of exposure, rather than a COHb concentration *per se*, although a level of >40% has been used as one criterion to guide the use of hyperbaric oxygen. A patient should be administered high flow oxygen (e.g. 12L/min through a tightfitting, e.g. CPAP, mask) until the COHb is <5% and clinical signs of carbon monoxide poisoning such as impaired heel–toe walking and finger–nose incoordination have resolved.

Arterial blood gases

Any patient with suspected poisoning by carbon monoxide requires arterial blood gas analysis. Oxygen saturation monitors are misleading as they read carboxyhaemoglobin as oxyhaemoglobin (HbO) and the true oxygen saturation of the patient can only be determined by arterial blood gas analysis.

ECG

An ECG should be performed in anyone severely poisoned (e.g. drowsiness or any neurological abnormality, chest pain or breathlessness) or with pre-existing heart disease. ECG changes such as ST segment depression, T-wave abnormalities, ventricular tachycardia or fibrillation and arrest can occur. If ischaemia/infarction is seen on the ECG or suspected clinically, the patient should also have cardiac enzymes sent.

Cocaine

Cocaine is snorted into the nose or injected intravenously.

Blood pressure monitoring

Patients with cocaine intoxication should have frequent measurements of their blood pressure, as hypertension is a significant risk, and strokes or myocardial infarcts have been widely reported. A Dynamap or equivalent advice for repeated measurements is suitable.

ECG and cardiac enzymes

Cocaine-induced angina and myocardial infarction are common. ECG monitoring is advised for all but the most trivial exposure to cocaine. Appropriate cardiac enzyme activity, i.e. CK, AST, LDH, and troponin T should also be performed in any patient with chest pain or ECG abnormalities.

Urine or blood testing

Cocaine can be detected in urine by simple 'drugs of abuse' screening tests, e.g. EMIT testing. This may help identify if a bodypacker (who has swallowed packets containing cocaine) is either a pre-existing cocaine user or is leaking cocaine from the packets. Gas chromatography-mass spectroscopy is more specific and can be carried out on blood or urine. Metabolites of cocaine (benzoylecgonine) can be detected in urine 2–3 days after exposure. Cocaine is unstable in blood and samples are best taken into 1% w/v fluoride oxalate tubes if medicolegal sequelae are a possibility. Nasal insufflation of 106mg of the drug to 6 volunteers produced mean peak plasma concentrations of 0.22mg/L at 0.5h and 0.61mg/L for the metabolite benzoylecgonine at 3h. Smoking 50mg in 6 volunteers produced mean peak plasma concentrations of 0.2mg/L at 0.08h and 0.15mg/L for bezoylecgonine at 1.5h. Patients have survived plasma concentrations of 5.2mg/L but usually fatalities are associated with cocaine/benzoylecgonine concentrations in excess of 5mg/L, depending on the route of use. The IV route is the most dangerous.

Cyanide

Cyanide poisoning can occur by deliberate inhalation of gas, ingestion of salts or by exposure in industrial fires.

Arterial blood gas estimation

Such measurements are essential to determine the oxygen saturation and acid–base status of the patient.

Serum lactate

This is helpful in confirming suspected toxicity. It is likely to exceed 7mmol/L in cases of significant exposure.

ECG

All patients should have an ECG. It should be examined for evidence of ischaemic damage, e.g. ST depression, ST elevation, T-wave inversion.

Cyanide assay

Blood cyanide concentrations are rarely of use in emergency management because they cannot be measured quickly enough. However, a sample should be taken before antidote administration for assay at a later stage. Cyanide concentrations of <0.2mg/L are 'normal'; 1.0–2.5mg/L causes obtundation and coma; and more than 2.5mg/L is potentially fatal.

▶▶*Note*: the dicobalt edetate antidote should only be given if cyanide poisoning is certain, i.e. a proper history is available; otherwise you may kill your patient with cardiotoxicity of the antidote. Otherwise give oxygen, sodium thiosulphate and sodium nitrite and/or hydroxocobalamin; these are antidotes that can safely be given without certainty of cyanide ingestion. Excessive administration of sodium nitrite, however, can cause significant methaemoglobinaemia.

Jones AL, Dargan Pl. (2001) *Churchill's Pocketbook of Toxicology*, Churchill-Livingstone, Edinburgh.

Digoxin

Patients who are already taking digoxin and those with pre-existing cardiovascular disease are more susceptible to digoxin toxicity after overdosage. Digoxin toxicity can also result from progressive renal impairment or due to interactions with other drugs, as well as overdoses.

ECG

All patients with suspected digoxin poisoning should have a 12-lead ECG and all symptomatic patients should be attached to a cardiac monitor. Digoxin poisoning can cause virtually any type of cardiac arrhythmia. The combination of heart block with tachyarrhythmia is very common.

Plasma digoxin concentration

Absorption of digoxin often peaks at 4–6h after ingestion. Its half-life is in excess of 30h. Digitoxin is a structurally-related drug that has an even longer plasma half-life (6 days). A digoxin measurement is a useful, but not absolute, guide to toxicity as plasma digoxin concentrations correlate poorly with the severity of poisoning, particularly early in the course of acute poisoning. However it is desirable (though not essential) if anti-digoxin Fab antibody fragments are to be used, as it is useful in calculating the dose of fragments (*see below*), as well as confirming exposure. Plasma digoxin concentrations cannot be interpreted after administration of digoxin antibody fragments using normal assay procedures. Samples taken to investigate probable chronic digoxin intoxication should be taken at least 6h after dosing. They are not normally analysed urgently unless life-threatening features of toxicity are present and use of antibody fragments (Fab) is being considered. The therapeutic range for digoxin is 0.8–2.0mg/L.

Urea and electrolytes

It is important to ascertain if the patient has any renal impairment and plasma creatinine and urea are helpful, though of course do not exclude renal impairment completely. Hyperkalaemia is common in acute digoxin overdose and may be severe, e.g. >7mmol/L. If possible a magnesium level is helpful to exclude hypomagnesaemia, which contributes to risk of cardiotoxicity and is easily corrected.

Indications for Fab fragments and doses of Fab fragments

- Severe hyperkalaemia (>6.0mmol/L) resistant to treatment with insulin/dextrose infusion.
- Bradycardia or heart block associated with hypotension.
- Tachyarrhythmias associated with hypotension, especially ventricular arrhythmias.

Fab antibody fragment administration should be considered in less severe stages of poisoning in older patients and those with pre-existing cardio-vascular disease.

The dose of Fab fragments to give can be calculated from either the dose of digoxin ingested or the plasma digoxin concentrations. Or if in doubt 10 ampoules of 'Digibind' can be given.

> *Number of 40mg vials of Fab =*
>
> plasma digoxin concentration (ng/mL) × body weight × 0.0084
>
> **OR**
>
> ingested dose (mg) × 1.2
>
> **OR**
>
> best guess of 10–20 vials

📖OHCM p830.

Ethylene glycol, ethanol & methanol poisoning

A history of ingestion or the presence of a metabolic acidosis raises suspicion of poisoning with these substances. Calculation of the anion gap and osmolal gaps is helpful in the assessment of such patients.

Anion gap

> *Calculating the anion gap =*
> $$([Na^+] + [K^+]) - ([Cl^-] + [HCO_3^-])$$
> The normal anion gap is 12 ± 2

Many toxins cause a high anion gap acidosis and these include
- Ethanol.
- Methanol (*Note*: the high anion gap is due to metabolites and may take several hours to develop).
- Ethylene glycol (*Note*: the high anion gap is due to the metabolites and may take 6–24h to develop).
- Metformin.
- Cyanide.
- Isoniazid.
- Salicylates (aspirin).

This list can be further reduced by measuring the osmolal gap.

Osmolal gap
This is the difference between the laboratory estimation of osmolality (Om) and calculated osmolality (Oc).

> *Calculating the osmolal gap =*
> $$Oc = 2([Na^+] + [K^+]) + [urea] + [glucose]$$
> The osmolal gap is normally <10

Toxic causes of a raised osmolal gap include
- Methanol.
- Ethylene glycol.
- Diethylene glycol.
- Isopropanol.
- Ethanol.

The acronym 'MEDIE' can be a helpful mnemonic.

Ethylene glycol and methanol plasma concentrations
Often the diagnosis of ethylene glycol or methanol poisoning can be difficult because assays for these substances are not widely available. If possible, their measurement can help manage severe intoxication. Other parameters may have to be used, i.e. anion gap, osmolal gap and arterial blood gas analysis. A normal osmolal gap does not exclude poisoning with ethylene glycol or methanol, but if the osmolal gaps and anion gaps are both normal and the patient is not symptomatic, then significant ingestion is unlikely to have occurred. In general, ethylene glycol or methanol measurements should not be carried out unless metabolic acidosis is present and there is an anion gap.

Ethylene glycol and methanol concentrations in blood are useful to confirm ingestion, and indicate when to stop antidotal treatment (with ethanol or 4-methylpyrazole) and/or haemodialysis (>500mg/L, *see below*). However, a low concentration may just mean that most of the parent compound has been metabolised. Formate (i.e. the methanol metabolite) levels can also be checked in patients who may have taken methanol.

Microscopy of urine for oxalate crystals
In suspected ethylene glycol poisoning, microscopy should be performed to look for oxalate crystals; however they are only present in 50% of cases, and often only many hours after ingestion. Treatment of a patient should not be delayed or dependent upon looking for crystals.

Plasma ethanol concentrations
Plasma ethanol concentrations are usually not needed in patients who are drunk unless there is doubt about the diagnosis, e.g. patients with a widening osmolar gap or the patient is so severely poisoned that haemodialysis is being considered for the ethanol poisoning. They are, however, essential to guide appropriate use of ethanol as an antidote in ethylene glycol or methanol poisoning (*see below*). Rarely, a plasma ethanol measurement will be needed in child protection cases and such sampling will need chain of custody and a specific (GLC) method by a specialist laboratory.

Antidotal therapy with ethanol

The dose of ethanol for treatment of ethylene glycol and methanol poisoning can be very difficult to predict because ethanol metabolism is variable and unpredictable. It is therefore important to frequently recheck the blood ethanol concentrations on patients receiving an ethanol infusion. The dose should be adjusted to achieve a blood ethanol concentration of 1–1.5g/L.

Indications for continued ethanol therapy are
- Methanol or ethylene glycol poisoning with blood concentrations >200mg/L.
- Metabolic acidosis with pH <7.3.
- Osmolal gap >10mOsmol/kg water.
- Formate concentration >10mg/L.
- Urinary oxalate crystals.
- Severe symptoms.

Indications for haemodialysis in methanol or ethylene glycol poisoning are

- Methanol or ethylene glycol concentration >500mg/L.
- Severe metabolic acidosis (pH <7.3) unresponsive to therapy, i.e. arterial blood gases are needed in all cases of high anion gap poisoning.
- Renal failure—hence it is essential to check plasma urea and electrolytes in all patients.
- Presence of visual problems in methanol poisoning.
- Formate concentration >500mg/L in methanol poisoning.

▶Haemodialysis should be continued until the methanol/ethylene glycol concentration is well below 200mg/L.

Iron

Serum iron concentrations

Serum iron concentrations should be measured urgently in all patients who may have ingested more than 30mg/kg of elemental iron. One 200mg tablet of ferrous sulphate contains 60mg elemental iron. If a sustained-release preparation of iron has been taken, a later serum iron concentration should be taken. A blood sample taken late after ingestion may underestimate the iron as it may have already started distributing to tissues, i.e. in a late presenting patient a low concentration cannot be interpreted, but a high one indicates toxicity. If the antidote desferrioxamine is given before 4h have elapsed, it interferes with the colorimetric assay for iron and so a serum sample for iron should be taken off before it is given. If atomic absorption spectrophotometry is available for measurement of serum iron, there is no interference from desferrioxamine.

It is essential to interpret the serum iron concentration result in the context of the clinical state of the patient. If <55µmol/L (<300mg/dL), mild toxicity is expected. If above 90µmol/L (500mg/dL), severe toxicity is expected and treatment with desferrioxamine is necessary. Antidotal treatment is also indicated for patients with iron concentrations

>55µmol/L if there is additional clinical evidence of toxicity, e.g. gastrointestinal symptoms, leucocytosis or hyperglycaemia. Antidotal therapy with desferrioxamine is indicated without waiting for the serum iron concentration in patents with severe features (e.g. fitting, unconscious or hypotensive). Desferrioxamine is usually continued until the urine has returned to a normal colour, symptoms have abated and all radio-opacities of iron tablets on abdominal x-ray have disappeared. Urine free iron estimation is the best test of when to stop chelation therapy with desferrioxamine, but is not widely available.

Working out if the patient needs a serum iron level checked

If a patient has ingested <30mg/kg body weight of elemental iron (a 200mg ferrous sulphate tablet ≡ 60mg elemental iron) then no serum iron level is required. If in doubt a plain abdominal x-ray will usually indicate if lots of tablets are present. A serum concentration of <55µmol/L (<300mg/dL) also indicates low risk (see *above*).

Abdominal x-ray

This is required in patients who have ingested in excess of 30mg elemental iron/kg body weight. The AXR determines the need for gut decontamination either by gastric lavage or whole bowel irrigation with polyethylene glycol. Undissolved tablets appear radio-opaque but they disappear once dissolved, so the absence of radio-opacities does not exclude the possibility of toxicity.

Full blood count

This is needed in all cases of iron poisoning. A leucocytosis (>15 × 10^9/L) is common with significant toxicity.

Blood glucose

Hyperglycaemia is common in serious poisoning.

Arterial blood gases

These should be checked in symptomatic or severely poisoned patients. Metabolic acidosis is common.

Total iron binding capacity

This has no role in the assessment of acute iron poisoning.

What to do if estimation of serum iron concentration is unavailable

If serum iron assay is not available, the presence of nausea, vomiting, leucocytosis (>15 × 10^9/L) and hyperglycaemia (>8.3mmol/L) suggests significant ingestion and the need for treatment with desferrioxamine.
📖OHCM p830.

Lead poisoning

Blood lead concentrations

Blood lead concentrations are used to confirm the diagnosis and decide on whether chelation therapy is required. Samples are not 'urgent' (except in the case of suspected acute lead encephalopathy) and must be taken into an EDTA tube. 'Normal' concentrations are <100µg/L. Lead causes changes in red cell and urinary porphyrins, but these are not measured routinely. A plain AXR should be performed in all children, particularly if there is a history of pica, to exclude ingested paint or lead foreign bodies such as curtain pulls. Long bone x-rays in children may show lead lines.

There are two agents used for chelation therapy in lead poisoning: (1) intravenous EDTA (disodium calcium edetate) and (2) oral DMSA (2,3-dimercaptosuccinic acid). Before use, chelation therapy should be discussed with a poisons centre. In general patients with a blood lead concentration >450µmg/L should be treated with chelation therapy and removal from further exposure. Children with encephalopathy or a blood lead concentration of >750µg/L require admission to hospital for urgent chelation therapy.

Other essential investigations

Patients should also have a full blood count and blood film (for basophilic stippling), urea and electrolytes, liver function tests and serum calcium measured.

Lithium

Blood lithium concentration

Lithium is available as sustained-release, non-sustained-release tablets and liquid. After ingestion of liquid preparations, plasma lithium concentrations peak at 30min. With sustained-release preparations peak concentrations occur at 4–5h. The plasma half-life is often in excess of 24h. Interpretation of plasma lithium concentrations depends on the clinical circumstances of exposure (see below). Do not take blood for lithium levels into a lithium heparin tube!

Acute overdose in lithium naïve patient

A single overdose in a lithium naïve patient is of low risk. However, onset of toxicity may be delayed for as much as 24h. Samples for lithium assay should be taken at 6h post-ingestion and measured urgently. Consider haemodialysis if plasma lithium concentration is >7.5mmol/L.

Chronic excess of lithium

Lithium toxicity can occur if the patient has been taking too high a dose, is dehydrated, or if an interaction with thiazide diuretics, NSAIDs, ACE inhibitors or tetracycline has occurred. Risk of toxicity is further enhanced by the presence of hypertension, diabetes, cardiac failure, renal failure or schizophrenia. Blood for plasma lithium assay should be taken at presentation. Consider haemodialysis if the plasma lithium exceeds 2.5mmol/L.

Acute on chronic lithium poisoning

A patient taking lithium chronically who takes an acute overdose is at risk of serious toxicity, because tissue binding of lithium is already high. The plasma lithium levels should be measured urgently at 6h post-ingestion. Lithium measurements should be repeated 6–12 hourly in symptomatic patients until clinical improvement occurs. Consider haemodialysis if plasma concentrations exceed 4mmol/L.

Indications for haemodialysis

Lithium is effectively removed by haemodialysis. It is indicated in all patients with severe lithium poisoning, i.e. coma, convulsions, respiratory failure or acute renal failure. Plasma lithium concentrations can also guide the need for haemodialysis. Each hour of dialysis will reduce the plasma lithium by 1mmol/L, but plasma lithium often rebounds after haemodialysis so the assay should be repeated at the end of dialysis and again 6–12h later.

Urea and electrolytes

Hyponatraemia is common in lithium toxicity. It is also important to check the serum potassium concentration and urea, as lithium is renally excreted and renal failure delays its elimination.

Methaemoglobinaemia

Oxidising agents convert haemoglobin to methaemoglobin (MetHb) and this renders it incapable of carrying oxygen. Common agents causing methaemoglobinaemia include: dapsone, sulphonamides, chlorates, nitrites, nitrates and local anaesthetic including lignocaine. The onset and duration of symptoms will depend on the agent. Nitrites cause breathlessness and flushing within minutes of exposure but dapsone may cause a methaemoglobinaemia several hours after ingestion and the methaemoglobinaemia may then persist for days.

Essential investigations

Patients with suspected methaemoglobinaemia should have the following
- Arterial blood gases.
- BC (especially if dapsone has been taken → haemolytic anaemia).
- Blood methaemoglobin concentration.

Methaemoglobin can produce a normal PO_2 in the presence of reduced oxygen saturation. Pulse oximetry measures both methaemoglobin and oxygenated haemoglobin, so can give false results.

Methaemoglobin estimation in blood

Measurement of blood methaemoglobin is required to confirm the diagnosis and assess the severity of poisoning. The measurement must be done urgently when administration of the antidote (methylene blue) is contemplated. Samples for methaemoglobin estimation need to be analysed as soon as possible after collection, as if left to stand around the methaemoglobin will be falsely low owing to a reduction by endogenous methaemoglobin reductase. The severity of symptoms correlates roughly with the measured methaemoglobin concentrations. Anaemia, cardiac or pulmonary disease will lead to more severe symptoms at a lower methaemoglobin level.

Table 11.2

MetHb conc. (%)	Clinical effects
0–15	None
15–30	Mild: cyanosis, tiredness, headache, nausea
30–50	Moderate: marked cyanosis, tachycardia, dyspnoea
50–70	Severe: coma, fits, respiratory depression, metabolic acidosis, arrhythmias
>70%	Potentially fatal

If the patient has severe clinical features of toxicity or if the blood methaemoglobin concentration is >30% the patient should be given methylene blue. Methylene blue can be given at lower blood methaemoglobin concentrations in those who are symptomatic.

Opioids

Classic features of opioid poisoning
- Depressed respiration.
- Pin-point pupils.
- Coma.
- Signs of parenteral drug use, e.g. needlemarks.

Toxicity can be prolonged for 24–48h, particularly after ingestion of methadone, which has a long half-life. The life-saving measure is prompt administration of adequate doses of naloxone, before waiting for results of any investigations.

Adequacy of ventilation
Oxygen saturation monitoring and/or arterial blood gas analysis demonstrates the adequacy of ventilation in those whose respiration is depressed.

Drug screening
Qualitative screening of the urine (group-specific immunoassay) confirms recent use. This may not detect fentanyl derivatives, tramadol and other synthetic opioids.

Measuring opioids in blood with gas chromatography-mass spectroscopy
This is sometimes required for medicolegal purposes, particularly where a fatality or a child-care issue is involved. Plasma morphine levels as high as 0.3mg/L were observed in addicts taking IV doses of heroin (diamorphine) of 150–200mg. Postmortem morphine levels in heroin overdose

deaths vary depending on prior narcotic history but in general exceed 0.3mg/L. Following a single oral dose of 15mg of methadone, plasma concentrations peaked at 4h at 0.075mg/L and declined slowly (t½ = 15h) until 24h when the concentration was still 0.03mg/L. Plasma methadone concentrations in maintenance patients increase by approximately 0.26mg/L for every 1mg/kg increase in oral dose. Deaths are due largely to reduced tolerance and blood concentrations of 0.4–1.8mg/L have been found postmortem, though live patients with tolerance exceed these values. 8.75mg/70kg IV morphine given to adults produces mean serum concentrations of 0.44mg/L at 0.5min, with rapid decline to 0.02mg/L by 2h. Average morphine concentrations in fatalities range from 0.2 to 2.3mg/L, depending on tolerance.

Paracetamol screening
Opioid tablets are frequently combined with paracetamol. All unconscious patients should therefore have a plasma paracetamol measured.

Organophosphorus insecticides

Measurement and interpretation of AChE
Measurement of red cell cholinesterase (AChE) is useful in confirmation of exposure to organophosphorus compounds such as insecticides or nerve warfare agents, where this is suspected, e.g. restlessness, tiredness, headache, nausea, vomiting, diarrhoea, sweating, hypersalivation, chest tightness, miosis, muscle weakness and fasciculation. In general, clinical features are more helpful than red cell cholinesterase measurements in determining the severity of intoxication and hence the prognosis. There is a wide degree of intersubject variation in cholinesterase activity and clinical effects (see Table 11.3).

Table 11.3

Cholinesterase activity	Clinical effects
Approx. 50% of normal	Subclinical poisoning
20–50% of normal	Mild poisoning
<10% of normal	Severe poisoning

The need for treatment with cholinesterase reactivators such as pralidoxime is largely judged by the occurrence of convulsions, fasciculation, flaccid paralysis and coma. Such features rapidly reverse within 20–30min of pralidoxime administration, together with atropine. The need for further therapy is guided by clinical improvement, together with monitoring of cholinesterase activity. It may take 90–120 days for red blood cell cholinesterase to recover to normal values.

Other vital investigations
An ECG should be carried out in all organophosphorus poisoned patients, and urea and electrolytes and glucose should also be monitored. In those with respiratory embarrassment or muscular paralysis, frequent assessment of tidal volume/peak flow rates and oxygen saturations is essential in anticipating the need for intubation.
📖OHCM p831.

Paracetamol (acetaminophen) poisoning

Overview
▶▶Paracetamol is the commonest drug taken in overdose in the UK. Measurement of a plasma paracetamol concentration is essential for assessing the need for antidotal treatment within 16h of a paracetamol overdose and should be performed urgently in all patients with known or suspected paracetamol overdose. It can be measured by a variety of assay methods but HPLC is less susceptible to interference than some enzyme-based assays. It should also be done urgently in patients with undiagnosed coma, or where a history is unreliable. Routine measurement of paracetamol concentrations in awake patients who deny taking paracetamol is unnecessary. For most patients, only a single measurement of paracetamol concentration is indicated. It is important to err on the side of caution and to give the antidote N-acetylcysteine if the blood paracetamol concentration lies near or just below the treatment line (Fig. 11.1) as stated timing of the overdose may be inaccurate and other agents such as opioids may slow gastric emptying.

If N-acetylcysteine is given within 12h of the overdose, it provides complete protection against liver injury and renal failure. Beyond 12h after ingestion the protection is less complete and assessment of liver damage is required. Paracetamol poisoning can be deceptive, as there is a latent phase of many hours, where the patient remains well before liver damage develops.

INR/PT
The most sensitive marker of prognosis in paracetamol poisoning is the prothrombin time (PT) or INR. This often starts to increase within 24–36h of the overdose and peaks at 48–72h. Once the INR/PT starts to improve, this is a sign that hepatotoxicity is starting to improve and the patient will not go on to develop acute liver failure. Approximately half of patients with a PT of 36s at 36h post-ingestion will develop acute liver failure.

Plasma alanine and aspartate aminotransferases (ALT and AST)
These may begin to rise as early as 12h post-ingestion but usually peak at 72–96h. AST or ALT values in excess of 10,000IU/L are not unusual and a plasma ALT>5000IU/L is very suggestive of paracetamol poisoning (Fig. 11.2). Serum bilirubin may peak after the aminotransferase and this should not lead to concern for patients in whom the INR or PT have begun to fall.

▶▶*Do not correct abnormalities in PT or INR with FFP or cryoprecipi-tate unless life-threatening bleeding is taking place; otherwise the most sensitive marker of how the patient is progressing will be lost.*

Other blood test abnormalities in paracetamol poisoning

Hypoglycaemia and metabolic acidosis are common. Early metabolic acidosis is often associated with very high plasma paracetamol concentra-tions, e.g. >400mg/L. Later, development of acidosis indicates incipient acute liver failure and the need to urgently check ABGs, liver function tests and INR/PT.

Pancreatitis with ↑ serum amylase has been reported. Five cases of thrombocytopenia have been reported.

Renal failure can occur in the context of hepatic failure, but also in its absence (in 1 in 100 patients). It is treated with N-acetylcysteine and supportive measures, e.g. haemodialysis, if needed. Full recovery with supportive care is common.

Investigating the patient who has taken a paracetamol overdose <4h ago

Ingestion of >150mg/kg paracetamol or a paracetamol-containing product should be recognised as a hepatotoxic dose for most people. If ingestion of this amount or more has occurred within the last 1h, activated char-coal should be given orally (50g for an adult). Chronic alcohol ingestion (>14 units per week for ♀, >21 units per week for ♂), regular use of enzyme- inducing drugs (e.g. anticonvulsants) or the presence of eating disorders have been reported to reduce the ceiling of toxicity of paracetamol to 75mg/kg.

A plasma paracetamol should then be checked at 4h from the time of ingestion, to determine the need for N-acetylcysteine treatment from the treatment curve (Fig. 11.1). Very rarely, e.g. after ingestion of 4 × 500mg tablets by an adult, a confirmatory plasma paracetamol level is not needed, but in general it is cheap (approx £1) and safer to be certain by checking a blood concentration.

Investigating the patient who has taken a paracetamol overdose between 4 and 8h ago

A plasma paracetamol level should be checked as soon as possible to determine the need for N-acetylcysteine antidote treatment from the treatment curve (Fig. 11.1). ▶▶Use high-risk treatment line for patient with induced enzymes (e.g. anticonvulsants) or glutathione depletion (e.g. eating disorders).

Investigating the patient who has taken a paracetamol overdose between 8 and 24h ago

Start treatment with N-acetylcysteine straight away. Take blood for a paracetamol level, INR/PT, creatinine and plasma venous bicarbonate (if plasma venous bicarbonate is abnormal, check arterial blood gases). Check results and refer to graph to determine whether treatment with N-acetylcysteine needs to be continued (i.e. is the plasma level above the treatment line?) or can be stopped (below the line). ▶▶Beyond 16h after ingestion the sensitivity of the assay for paracetamol may be too low to detect a treatable level—check and, if in doubt, treat the patient with N-acetylcysteine! On completion of N-acetylcysteine, check blood INR/PT, creatinine and plasma venous bicarbonate (if abnormal check ABGs). If the patient is asymptomatic and the INR or creatinine is normal or falling discontinue the N-acetylcysteine. If the patient has symptoms (abdominal pain or vomiting) or the INR or creatinine is rising, continue maintenance N-acetylcysteine (50mg/kg in 500mL dextrose every 4h) until the INR improves. ▶▶Contact a poisons centre/liver unit.

Fig. 11.1 N-acetylcysteine treatment graph. Patients whose plasma paracetamol concentrations are above the **normal treatment line** should be treated with acetylcysteine by IVI (or, provided the overdose has been taken **within 10–12h**, with methionine by mouth). Patients on enzyme-inducing drugs (e.g. carbamazepine, phenobarbitone, phenytoin, rifampicin and alcohol) or who are malnourished (e.g. in anorexia, in alcoholism, or those who are HIV-positive) should be treated if their plasma paracetamol concentrations are above the **high-risk treatment line**. *Note:* if paracetamol ingestion has been staggered (over some hours) serum levels may mislead: treat regardless, if significant amounts have been taken. Reproduced with permission from Dr Alun Hutchings and the *Oxford Handbook of Clinical Medicine*, 5th edition, Oxford University Press.

Investigating the patient who has taken a paracetamol overdose >24h ago

It is too late for plasma paracetamol level estimation to be of any value. Start treatment with the antidote N-acetylcysteine straight away, unless a trivial amount has been taken. Take blood for baseline INR/PT, creatinine and venous bicarbonate (if abnormal check ABGs).

If the patient is asymptomatic and the lab tests normal, discharge the patient and advise to return if vomiting/abdominal pain develops. If the blood results are abnormal, phone a liver unit/poisons centre for advice.

Investigating the patient in whom the timing of overdose is unknown

Err on the side of treating the patient with the antidote N-acetylcysteine, checking an INR/PT, creatinine, plasma venous bicarbonate (ABGs if abnormal) at baseline and at the end of the first full course of treatment. If abnormal contact liver unit/poisons centre for further advice.

Investigating the patient who has taken a staggered overdose

Determine if the patient is in an at-risk group (i.e. enzyme induction or glutathione depletion) as discussed above. If the patient is not in an at-risk group but has ingested >150mg/kg body weight over 24h they should receive a full course of IV N-acetylcysteine. If they are in an 'at-risk' group and have ingested more than 75mg/kg body weight of paracetamol over 24h, they should receive a full course of N-acetylcysteine. There is no point measuring a plasma paracetamol level in this group of patients, unless the substance ingested is in doubt, and a 'not detected' result may be falsely reassuring. At admission and at the end of the course of N-acetylcystine a blood INR/PT, creatinine and venous bicarbonate should be checked. If abnormal at any stage, consult the poisons centre/liver unit. 📖OHCM pp830–831.

Fig. 11.2 Time course of liver function tests in paracetamol poisoning.

Salicylate[*] poisoning

Features of severe poisoning

Ingestion of >150, 250 and 500mg/kg body weight of aspirin, respectively, produces mild, moderate and severe poisoning, respectively. Signs of serious salicylate poisoning include metabolic acidosis, renal failure and CNS effects such as agitation, confusion, coma and convulsions. Death may occur as a result of CNS depression and cardiovascular collapse.

▶▶ The development of metabolic acidosis is a bad prognostic sign as it also indicates increased CSF transfer of salicylate.

Plasma salicylate concentration

Plasma salicylate should be measured urgently in all but the most trivial overdose, i.e. all those thought to have ingested >150mg/kg of aspirin or any amount of oil of wintergreen. It should be performed at 4h post-ingestion, because delayed absorption of the drug renders such levels uninterpretable before this time. As salicylates form concretions in the stomach, which delay absorption, it is recommended that a salicylate level is rechecked 3–4h after the first sample, to catch the peak salicylate concentration. There is no evidence for indiscriminate requesting of salicylate concentrations in every unconscious patient (unlike paraceta-mol) or in conscious patients who deny taking aspirin and who have no features suggesting salicylate toxicity. The plasma salicylate concentration is not an absolute guide to toxicity, as paracetamol levels are in paracetamol poisoning, but should be interpreted together with clinical features and acid–base status of the patient.

Urinary alkalinisation (📖OHCM p832) is indicated for patients with salicylate concentrations of 600–800mg/L in adults and 450–700mg/L in children and the elderly. Metabolic alkalosis is not a contraindication to bicarbonate therapy as patients may have high base deficit in spite of an elevated serum pH.

Haemodialysis is very effective at salicylate removal and correction of acid–base and electrolyte abnormalities. It should be considered if the plasma salicylate levels are >700mg/L in children and >800mg/L in adults. Other indications for haemodialysis include resistant metabolic acidosis, severe CNS effects such as coma or convulsions, pulmonary oedema and acute renal failure.

Arterial blood gases

Acid–base problems are common in salicylate poisoning. Respiratory centre stimulation causes respiratory alkalosis. Uncoupled oxidative phosphorylation and interruption of glucose and fatty acid metabolism by salicylates often causes a concurrent metabolic acidosis. Serial ABGs are needed in severe salicylate poisoning.

---

[*]Aspirin, oil of Wintergreen.

Theophylline

Acute theophylline poisoning can carry a high mortality and its management is best guided by the Shannon severity grading scheme (see reference below), bearing in mind that delayed effects tend to occur after sustained-release formulations have been ingested. The adult therapeutic range is 10–20mg/L. Serious toxicity occurs at >100mg/L (770mmol/L).

Urea and electrolytes
It is vital to check the plasma K^+ concentration frequently, as hypokalaemia is a life-threatening complication and the serum K^+ concentration is a useful guide to severity. If >2.5mmol/L the patient is less severely poisoned (grade 1) than if it falls <2.5mmol/L (grade 2). Check blood glucose since hyperglycaemia is a common complication.

Arterial blood gases
In potentially serious poisoning (e.g. ingestion of >20mg/kg body weight) ABG analysis is helpful in optimising the acid–base status of the patient. An initial phase of hyperventilation with respiratory alkalosis can be followed by a further stage of metabolic acidosis.

Plasma theophylline concentrations
Measuring plasma theophylline concentrations confirms theophylline ingestion where this is in doubt and is usually undertaken by HPLC. It is also helpful in deciding when to employ charcoal haemoperfusion in seriously poisoned patients, particularly if plasma concentrations are >100mg/L (770mmol/L). Charcoal haemoperfusion can be considered at lower concentration, e.g. 80mg/L, in the elderly or those with pre-existing ischaemic heart disease. Charcoal haemoperfusion can also be decided on the basis of grade 3 or 4 severity grading alone, especially if administration of multiple doses of activated charcoal is not possible. However, for the vast majority of poisoned patients, obtaining a plasma theophylline concentration does not guide their management.

Therapeutic levels rarely exceed 20mg/L (155mmol/L). Theophylline peak concentration in plasma may occur at 1–3h after ingestion of a standard-release formulation. However, overdose is often with sustained-release products and delayed absorption can result in delayed peak plasma concentration and toxicity, often 12–24h later.

Urine testing for myoglobinuria & measuring serum creatine kinase
Theophylline poisoning can be accompanied by rhabdomyolysis. Hence the urine should be dipsticked and if found positive for blood a serum CK should be obtained. This will then indicate that renal function should be closely monitored and the urine should undergo alkalinisation.

Shannon M. (1993) Predictors of major toxicity after theophylline overdose. *Ann Intern Med* **119**, 1161–1167.

Tricyclic antidepressants

The main risks of overdose with these drugs are CVS and CNS toxicity.

ECG

An ECG should be performed in all but the most trivial cases of overdose.

ECG abnormalities are common in moderate–severe poisoning and include

- QRS prolongation: >110ms in adults predicts the risk of ventricular cardiac arrhythmias (and the need for IV sodium bicarbonate) and QRS >160ms predicts the risk of fits. In children a QRS >110ms is predictive of the risk of arrhythmias but not fits.
- *Note*: ECG criteria are not the only factors assessing risk of arrhythmias, fits and acidosis—electrolyte disturbances contribute. Supraventricular and potentially fatal ventricular arrhythmias can occur.

Cardiac monitoring

This is essential if ingestion of >10mg/kg body weight has taken place. It is seldom necessary beyond 24h after ingestion.

Arterial blood gas analyses

These should be done on all patients with marked symptoms and signs, particularly those with a reduced Glasgow Coma Score. It should also be performed on those with widened QRS or seizures, not least because such patients are receiving intravenous sodium bicarbonate therapy and a pH of 7.5 should not be exceeded.

Plasma concentrations

This is of no value as plasma concentrations of tricyclic antidepressants correlate poorly with clinical features of toxicity.

Table of conversion factors between mass & molar units

Table 11.4

Drug	Mass units	Molar (SI) units	Conversion factor
Carbamazepine	mg/L	μmol/L	4.23
Digoxin	mg/L or ng/mL	nmol/L	1.28
Ethanol	g/L	mmol/L	1.28
Iron	mg/L	mmol/L	0.179
Lead	mg/L	mmol/L	0.0048
Paracetamol	mg/L	mmol/L	0.0066
Phenytoin	mg/L	mmol/L	3.96
Salicylate (aspirin)	mg/L	mmol/L	0.0072
Theophylline	mg/L	mmol/L	7.7

Rheumatology

Rheumatological investigations *640*
Inflammatory markers: ESR and CRP *641*
Biochemistry tests *642*
Urine testing *643*
Immunology *643*
Autoantibodies in connective tissue disease *645*
Arthrocentesis *646*
Electromyography (EMG) *647*
DEXA scan *647*
Diagnostic imaging *648*

Rheumatological investigations

Rheumatological investigations are likely to be useful only if performed in the background of appropriate clinical indication. Investigations should only be complementary to careful history taking and physical examination. No investigations should be requested unless the results are likely to influence the outcome of clinical management.

Haematology

Haemoglobin (Hb)

Anaemia (↓Hb) is a common manifestation of many primary rheumatological disorders as well as rheumatological manifestations of a primary (non-rheumatological) systemic disease. It is therefore important to assess the type and degree of anaemia in the background of the global clinical picture of the patient.

Microcytic hypochromic anaemia

The major differential diagnoses are (1) thalassaemia trait, (2) chronic iron deficiency anaemia, and (3) anaemia of chronic disease (typically associated with normal MCV but if *chronic* the MCV will ↓): iron deficiency related to acute or chronic blood loss (e.g. due to NSAID ingestion) nutritional or primary bowel disease such as coeliac-related arthritis. Inflammatory bone disease should be considered.

Macrocytic anaemia

Vitamin B_{12} or folate deficiency related to nutritional deficiency, e.g. scleroderma causing jejunal diverticulosis, Whipple's disease causing malabsorption, or due to drug therapy such as methotrexate and azathioprine. Excessive alcohol consumption may also cause macrocytosis without significant anaemia.

Normocytic

Usually a reflection of chronic disease (*but see above*) and the degree of anaemia may vary with severity of the disease. In inflammatory polyarteritis such as RA, ankylosing spondylitis, polymyalgia rheumatica (PMR).

Dimorphic anaemia (large and small red cells)

This picture is seen in mixed deficiency, e.g. iron deficiency + vitamin B_{12} or folate deficiency, post-transfusion or during iron replacement therapy in a patient with iron deficiency. A feature of malabsorption associated with coeliac related arthritis, scleroderma of the gut and jejunal bypass arthritis.

White cell count

Increased: a common finding in patients with septic arthritis and crystal arthritis with or without sepsis.

Decreased: SLE, drug induced such as methotrexate, azathioprine or other cause of bone marrow failure or cytotoxic therapy.

Neutrophilia: sepsis, crystal arthritis (gout and pseudogout) and systemic corticosteroid administration.

Neutropenia: SLE, Felty's syndrome, drug-induced (e.g. salazopyrin, methotrexate, azathioprine and other cytotoxics).

Lymphocytosis: chronic lymphocytic leukaemia with joint symptoms.

Lymphopenia: SLE, rheumatoid arthritis, immunosuppressive therapy.

Eosinophilia: primary vasculitis such as ANCA-associated vasculitis, polyarteritis, eosinophilic fasciitis and also Addison's disease (can complicate rheumatological diseases).

Platelet count
Thrombocytosis: active rheumatoid arthritis, polycythaemia rubra vera can be associated with gout.

Thrombocytopenia: connective tissue disease such as SLE, therapy with drugs such as salazopyrin, azathioprine, methotrexate and other cytotoxics, Felty's syndrome and primary antiphospholipid syndrome (APS).

Inflammatory markers: ESR and CRP

ESR
A useful, but non-specific, indicator of inflammation or infection. However, the ESR is dependent on many variables such as the serum immunoglobulin concentration, fibrinogen level, and haematocrit and may not truly reflect the degree of inflammation. In some centres plasma viscosity is preferred as a screening for acute phase response rather than ESR. 📖p216.

Elevated ESR: commonly associated with active rheumatoid arthritis, septic or crystal arthritis and also polymyalgia rheumatica. Acute inflammatory muscle disease such as polymyositis/dermatomyositis and giant cell arteritis (temporal arteritis) and other vasculitides such as Wegener's granulomatosis, polyarteritis or Churg–Strauss syndrome may also result in an elevated ESR.

Normal or low ESR: found in inactive rheumatoid arthritis or other connective tissue diseases. It is usually low in gout associated with polycythaemia rubra vera or sickle cell disease.

C-reactive protein (CRP)
The CRP is a arguably more acute reflection of any acute or chronic inflammatory or infective process. CRP production is driven by interleukin-1 (IL-1) and IL-6 on hepatocytes and is independent of variables that normally complicate ESR measurement such as hyperglobulinaemia and anaemia.

Elevated C-reactive protein: active inflammatory or infective arthritis, active sero-negative spondyloarthritis (ankylosing spondylitis, Reiter's disease, enteropathic arthritis, Whipple's disease), polymyalgia rheumatica, polymyositis and dermatomyositis, amyloidosis, SLE with serositis.

Normal or low CRP: found in active SLE without serositis.

The CRP is always a better marker than ESR of active disease in rheumatoid arthritis, polymyalgia rheumatica as it is not influenced by other variable parameters of blood. It is also a better marker for assessing response to treatment, particularly when steroids are used as in polymyalgia rheumatica or giant cell arteritis.

Other acute phase proteins may also increase in acute inflammation such as serum caeruloplasmin, serum ferritin and plasma fibrinogen.

Serum ferritin
This is primarily used as a surrogate marker to assess body iron stores but as an acute phase reactant is useful in the diagnosis of adult-onset Still's disease. *Note:* in the presence of active inflammation or infection a normal or high serum ferritin may be found even if the patient has true iron deficiency. p211.

Biochemistry tests

It is important to perform regular assessments of biochemical analytes such as urea and electrolytes, liver function tests, uric acid, and bone panels (alkaline phosphatase, serum calcium and serum phosphate).

Systemic diseases such as rheumatoid arthritis, SLE, systemic amyloidosis and the vasculitides are associated with renal function abnormalities and it is important to detect such organ involvement at an early stage.

Renal function
Urea may be elevated due to dehydration or drug therapy. However, the serum urea concentration should be judged in conjunction with the serum creatinine. An increased creatinine may be early manifestation of renal impairment in diseases such as rheumatoid arthritis, complicated by drug therapy or complications such as amyloidosis, SLE or vasculitis such as polyangiitis, Wegener's granulomatosis or pulmonary/renal syndromes. In addition, renal impairment may be due to non-steroidal anti-inflammatory drugs or other drug therapies such as cyclophosphamide or methotrexate.

Alkaline phosphatase
May be elevated as a result of either hepatic impairment e.g. hepatic cholestasis (primary biliary cirrhosis—associated with other autoimmune diseases) or Paget's disease of bone. An isolated rise in alkaline phosphatase may be found in bone secondaries as well as Paget's disease with or without sarcomatous changes.

Serum calcium
Hypercalcaemia may be found in 10–15% cases of sarcoidosis and also in hyperparathyroidism.

Uric acid

May be elevated in some cases of acute gout, particularly in males—but elevation of uric acid in women is usually related to diuretic therapy. However, increased cell turnover from psoriatic skin disease can also be a cause of raised uric acid as is often found in the treatment of various high cell turnover malignant (e.g. leukaemias, lymphomas) and non-malignant (e.g. myeloproliferative disorders such as polycythaemia vera) conditions.

Urine testing

This is a valuable tool for assessing kidney function in many rheumatological diseases. It is an important tool for assessment of renal function in systemic vasculitides and the presence of red blood cells, protein casts are useful indicators for renal involvement by disease. Proteinuria may be the only early feature of amyloidosis in longstanding rheumatoid arthritis or in cases of drug-induced renal disease. Assessment of 24h urinary protein collection is a useful tool for assessment of renal lesion in these diseases.

Immunology

Assessment of immunological function is important in autoimmune diseases such as rheumatoid arthritis, SLE, scleroderma and its variants and the vasculitides. Detection of antibodies against specific antigens is useful for diagnostic and prognostic purposes. Some of the autoantibodies, which are often used in daily rheumatological practice, are shown in Table 12.1.

Rheumatoid factor

Rheumatoid arthritis particle agglutination test (RAPA) is useful in confirming a diagnosis of rheumatoid disease, if supported by the appropriate clinical picture of symmetrical inflammatory polyarthritis. The presence of rheumatoid factor in isolation does not necessarily suggest rheumatoid disease. It may be falsely positive in chronic infection, malignancy and other non-organ specific autoimmune diseases. Rheumatoid factor may also be found in healthy individuals in a small proportion of cases.

Antinuclear factor

A positive antinuclear factor is a useful indicator of an underlying connective tissue disease. It is usually positive in SLE and many other autoimmune disease such as lupoid hepatitis, autoimmune thyroiditis as well as scleroderma and other connective tissue diseases with overlapping features (overlap symptoms).

Anti-DNA antibody

The presence of this antibody is useful in confirming a diagnosis of SLE and also assessing the activity of the disease.

ENA antibodies
Antibodies to extractable nuclear antigen such as anti-Ro (SSA), anti-La (SSB), anti Jo-1, anti-MRNP, anti-Scl70 and anti-centromeric antibodies are useful markers in diseases such as Sjögren's syndrome, SLE, scleroderma and CREST syndrome (calcinosis, Raynaud's, esophageal involvement, sclerodactyly and telangiectasia). Anti-Ro antibodies may be a particularly important prognostic marker for patients with SLE as presence of these antibodies may be associated with congenital heart block in a small proportion of children born of such patients.

Antiphospholipid antibody (ACL)
The antibodies to a variety of phospholipids can be found in patients with connective tissue diseases such as SLE but can also be found in pathological concentrations in the background of no systemic disease such as primary antiphospholipid syndrome. The common association of primary antiphospholipid syndrome is with thrombocytopenia. The antibodies are usually of IgG and IgM class but other classes of immunoglobulins may also be associated, such IgA.

The presence of high titres of ACL is important in patients with SLE/lupus with recurrent miscarriages and thrombocytopenia. Such patients may also have another abnormality of clotting cascade such as lupus anticoagulant. The term lupus anticoagulant is a misnomer since the presence of such abnormality of clotting is commonly associated with increased thrombosis. The detection of such abnormality involves specialised clotting assays such as the dilute Russel viper venom test (dRVVT, see p309).

Antineutrophil cytoplasmic antibody (ANCA)
This antibody was first described in 1985 in patients with crescenteric glomerulonephritis and particularly its presence has been confirmed in many patients with primary systemic vasculitides such as Wegener's granulomatosis, microscopic polyangitis and in some patients of Churg–Strauss syndrome. Detection of ANCA involves an ELISA assay and the staining pattern may be peripheral (P-ANCA) or cytoplasmic (C-ANCA). The latter is usually specific for Wegener's granulomatosis and it reflects antigen specificity to proteinase 3. The presence of P-ANCA reflects antigen specificity to myeloperoxidase. Occasionally ANCA can be positive without antigen specificity in some diseases such as inflammatory bowel disease and malignancy.

Complement
The presence of low levels of complement (C4) can be a useful indicator of complement fixation in lupus nephritis. Low levels of C1 can be associated with development of SLE.

HLA B27
This is a genetic test often done to clarify the association with ankylosing spondylitis. It is present in more than 90% of patients with classical ankylosing spondylitis but reverse is not true. HLA B27 can also be present in other associated diseases in the group of seronegative spondyloarthritis

such as psoriatic arthritis, reactive arthritis or enteropathic arthritis. HLA B27 is also present in some patients with idiopathic uveitis who may later develop features of ankylosing spondylitis.

Autoantibodies in connective tissue disease

Table 12.1

Target	Clinical associations
ANA	Sensitive for SLE (not specific)
DNA	Specificity high for SLE
Sm antibody	Specificity high for SLE
U1RNP antibody	Overlap syndrome/MCTD
Anti-Ro & La	Primary Sjögren's syndrome Neonatal lupus Subacute cutaneous lupus
Anti-Ku	Specificity high for SLE
Anti-B2 glycoprotein-1	Anti-phospholipid syndrome
Antisynthetase (Anti-Jo-1)	Associated with polymyositis (Anti-synthetase syndrome)
Anti-Mi2	Classical dermatomyositis
Anti-Scl-70	Diffuse scleroderma
Anti-centromere	Limited scleroderma (CREST syndrome)
Cryoglobulins	Cryoglobulinaemic vasculitis
ANCA	Systemic vasculitides

Arthrocentesis

This refers to a procedure where joint is punctured aseptically for the sake of aspiration of synovial fluid and/or injection of drugs. It is an essential skill and tool for all rheumatologists and often used for diagnostic and therapeutic purposes.

Indications

Acute monoarthritis: to assess the joint fluid for sepsis or crystal arthritis. In suspected cases of septic arthritis fluid should be sent immediately for microscopy, (Gram stain) culture and crystal analysis.

In absence of sepsis the joint can be injected with steroid (Depomedrone or triamicinolone) to induce remission of acute inflammation.

Arthrocentesis is normally be performed under aseptic technique but may be carried out in the outpatient clinic with simple procedures for maintenance of asepsis. In children it is always performed under general anaesthesia in the operating theatre. Arthrocentesis is a relatively safe technique in skilled hands and complications are uncommon although the following complications have been noted.

1 Infection (iatrogenic)
2 Crystal synovitis due to steroid.
3 Theoretical risk of osteonecrosis due to repeated steroid injections in any one joint—usually more than 3–4 injections per year per joint.

Synovial fluid examination is paramount in all cases of monoarthritis and in some cases of polyarthritis where sepsis or crystal arthritis cannot be excluded. Synovial fluid should be assessed for physical characteristics (naked eye examination) such as colour and viscosity. The presence of turbid fluid can be associated with sepsis or crystal arthritis, and a straw coloured fluid of high viscosity is generally associated with degenerative arthritis such as osteoarthritis. However, inflammatory arthritides generally produce a straw coloured but less viscous fluid.

Microscopical examination of synovial fluid is important to assess the cell count and cell type. A significantly elevated white cell count may be found in septic and crystal arthritis. Microbiological investigations including Gram stain and culture are essential to exclude septic arthritis, particularly associated with indolent infections such as tuberculosis. Examination of synovial fluid under polarised microscopy is also essential to detect presence of crystals such as uric acid or calcium pyrophosphate. Occasionally, other varieties of crystals can be detected such as hydroxyapatite or cholesterol.

Arthroscopy

Arthroscopy and synovial biopsy may occasionally be required for the diagnosis of chronic indolent infections such as tuberculosis or unusual slow growing organisms such as *Coxiella* (fever polyarthritis). Arthroscopy is essentially a diagnostic procedure used by orthopaedic surgeons where direct visualisation of the affected joint is required.

⌖ www.orthoinfo.aaos.org/

Electromyography (EMG)

This is a very useful tool for detecting involvement of the nerves in certain rheumatological disorders such as carpal tunnel syndrome and axonal neuropathy secondary to vasculitides or amyloidosis. It may also help to identify the site of the problem in obscure neuropathies and provides clues as to the possible underlying aetiology. EMG should not be performed without a thorough clinical examination of the patient.

EMG is useful in the following circumstances
1 Assessment of entrapment neuropathy such as carpal tunnel and tarsal tunnel syndromes.
2 Assessment of neurological symptoms related to cervical spine disorders.
3 Acute mononeuritis multiplex due to vasculitis or inflammatory disorders such as amyloidosis.
4 Acute onset of polymyositis/dermatomyositis.

The presence of fibrillations with polyphasic potential are very useful indicators for early detection of inflammatory primary muscle disorder.

DEXA scan

This is a non-invasive assessment of bone density for patients at risk of developing osteoporosis. The latter can occur at a number of sites at various age groups, such as the wrist, neck of femur and the spine, temporally related to the age of the patient. This scan is predominantly performed at two sites, e.g. spine and neck of femur, as they are the common sites for development of fracture in at-risk populations although other varieties of scans are available, e.g. ones that can scan at the wrist.

The DEXA scan predicts fracture in almost 30% of cases but when associated with other risk factors in addition to the scan it has a much higher predictive value for fracture.

Diagnostic imaging

Imaging techniques are essential tools in the management of rheumatological conditions and are useful if performed under appropriate indications. It is not a substitute for clinical examination and findings should be interpreted in the context of clinical abnormalities. It is important to follow the guidelines for radiological investigations published by the Royal College of Radiologists.

Plain radiographs

These may be a useful for confirmation of structural damage of a joint but often detection of such changes depends on the duration and severity of a particular joint disease. In an established case of rheumatoid arthritis, osteoarthritis or osteoporosis radiographs may show the classical changes, but in early cases plain radiographs may not be as informative as other modalities of imaging. Figures 12.1–12.4 show the use of plain radiology in a variety of rheumatological disorders.

Fig. 12.1 Hands in rheumatoid disease.

Fig. 12.2 Hands showing calcinosis, especially prominent distally.

Fig.12.3 Plain CXR showing pulmonary fibrosis in rheumatoid disease.

Fig.12.4 X-ray of pelvis showing avascular necrosis of the femoral heads.

Ultrasound

Ultrasound scanning is a useful 'x-ray free' technique for detecting soft tissue lesions, particularly enthesopathy such as plantar fasciitis, Achilles tendonitis and epicondylitis or rotator cuff tendonitis of the shoulder. It also has a useful role in providing information about the dynamic state of the joint such as assessment of the shoulder pain. Ultrasound can also be used therapeutically to treat musculoskeletal conditions such as joint or soft tissue by identifying the appropriate area of inflammation prior to injection with e.g. steroids.

CT (computerised tomography) scans

These are much less frequently used in assessment of the musculoskeletal system. CT scanning can, however, be useful at a particular cross sectional level when assessing back disorders.

Nuclear medicine imaging

Radionuclide imaging with ^{99m}technetium or ^{67}gallium is often used in detection of certain primary bone and joint disorders, as well as musculo-skeletal manifestation of a primary systemic illness such as bony secondaries from a primary malignant lesion elsewhere.

Such scanning is of use in detecting osteomyelitis and minor fractures undetectable on x-rays, bone tumours (primary or secondary) and also inflammatory lesions such as chronic multi-focal osteomyelitis or sacroiliitis in a case of ankylosing spondylitis.

Fig. 12.5 PET scanning in aortitis pre (L) and post (R) treatment.

Recent scanning techniques such as single photon emission CT (SPECT) or positron emission tomography (PET) are useful for detecting early pathology, particularly in vasculitic disorders such as aortitis (Fig. 12.5) or Takayasu's arthritis. They are also useful in detecting neoplastic lesions. It is always important to interpret the findings in the context of clinical features as well as plain x-ray findings. One can expect a disproportionate increase in uptake of the radionuclide in cases of degenerative arthritis unless plain radiographs are performed to define the latter.

Magnetic resonance imaging (MRI)

This is a more recent method for assessing musculoskeletal systems without exposure to radiation.

Indications

Assessment of back pain particularly disc disease or disease associated with infection or malignancy. It can be used with contrast (Gadolinium) in post operative patients.

Assessment of specific joints such as hips e.g. for early detection of avascular necrosis of the hip.

Non-invasive diagnosis of polymyositis where it can be used to assess response to treatment.

Chapter 13

Radiology

Radiology & the role of imaging 652
Plain x-rays 654
Digital radiology 654
Chest x-ray: useful landmarks 656
Chest radiograph 658
Patterns of lobar collapse 662
Cardiac enlargement 664
Computed tomography of the thorax 666
Abdominal x-ray: useful landmarks 668
Plain abdominal x-ray (AXR) 670
Barium studies 672
Barium swallow 674
Barium meal 676
Small intestine 678
Cholangiography 680
Barium enema 682
Radiology of the urinary tract 684
Breast imaging 688
Ultrasound 690
Computed tomography (CT) 694
Magnetic resonance imaging (MRI) 698
Spinal imaging 704
Pelvis 706
Vascular intervention 708
Interventional radiology 710
Hands 716
Neuroradiology 718
Skull x-ray 720
Reference section 722
Internet resources 724

Radiology & the role of imaging

The effective use of the radiology department relies on good communication between radiologists and their clinical colleagues. The overall aim must be to target investigations efficiently in order to provide answers to clinical dilemmas at minimal cost and radiation dose. The investigation of neurological problems has been transformed by the advent of CT and MRI. Local availability varies and CT in particular can add considerably to the radiation burden. Conversely, if a CT is likely to provide the best answer and minimize overall costs by resulting in an early discharge then it should be the investigation of choice. It is helpful to consider plain films, contrast studies, ultrasound and then CT/MRI as a hierarchy where plain films are requested as an initial investigation. This hierarchy may be circumvented if a more expensive investigation is likely to produce the definitive result.

The following are important points to consider:

1. Will the investigation alter patient management? i.e. is the expected outcome clinically relevant? *Do you need it?*
2. Investigating too often or repeating investigations before there has been an adequate lapse of time to allow resolution or to allow treatment to take effect. *Do I need it now?* Especially relevant when investigations may have been performed elsewhere. Make every effort possible to obtain prior studies.
3. Would an investigation that does not use ionising radiation be more appropriate, e.g. USS/MRI?
4. Failure to provide accurate clinical information and questions that you are hoping will be answered by the investigation may result in an unsatisfactory outcome. Have I explained the problem?
5. Would another technique be more appropriate? The advances in radiology mean that discussion with a radiologist may be helpful in determining the best possible test. *Is this the best investigation?*
6. Overinvestigating: are you taking comfort in too many tests or providing reassurance to the patient in this way?

Table 13.1 Typical effective doses from diagnostic medical exposures

Procedure	Typical effective dose (mSv)	Equivalent number CXRs	Equivalent period background radiation
Chest (PA)	0.02	1	3 days
Lumbar spine	1.0	50	5 months
Abdomen	0.7	35	4 months
IVU	2.4	120	14 months
Barium enema	7.2	360	3.2 years
CT head	2.0	100	10 months
CT abdomen	10.0	500	4.5 years
Bone scan (Tc-99m)	4.0	200	1.8 years
PET head (F-18 FDG)	5.0	250	2.3 years

UK average background radiation = 2.2mSv per year.

Royal College of Radiologists (2003) Guidelines for Doctors. Making the Best Use of a Department of Clinical Radiology, fifth edition.

Plain x-rays

Wilhelm Roentgen discovered x-rays in 1895. X-rays form part of the electromagnetic spectrum with microwaves and radio waves lying at the low energy end, visible light in the middle and x-rays at the high energy end. They are energetic enough to ionise atoms and break molecular bonds as they penetrate tissues, and are therefore called ionising radiation. Diagnostic x-rays are produced when high energy electrons strike a high atomic number material. This interaction is produced within an x-ray tube. A high voltage is passed across two tungsten terminals. One terminal (cathode) is heated until it liberates free electrons. When a high voltage is applied across the terminals the electrons accelerate towards the anode at high speed. On hitting the anode target x-rays are produced.

The x-ray picture is a result of the interaction of the ionising radiation with tissues as it passes through the body. Tissues of different densities are displayed as distinct areas depending on the amount of radiation absorbed. There are 4 basic densities in conventional radiography: *gas* (air), *fat, soft tissue* and *fluid*, and calcified structures. Air absorbs the least amount of x-rays and therefore appears black on the radiograph, whereas calcified structures and bone absorb the most, resulting in a white density. Soft tissues and fluid have a similar absorptive capacity and therefore appear grey on a radiograph.

Digital radiology

X-ray film is exposed by light photons emitted by intensifying screens sensitive to radiation transmitted through the patient. Storage phosphor technology uses photo-stimulable phosphor screens to convert x-ray energy directly into digital signals. The increased dynamic range and image contrast of digital radiography compared with conventional film screen combinations and the facility to manipulate signal intensity after image capture reduce the number of repeat exposures. This increases efficiency and minimises patient radiation dose. Digital images can be made available on a local network for reporting by a radiologist or for review on a ward-based computer. Picture archiving and communication systems (PACS) are efficient at image production and manipulation and in the storage, retrieval and transmission of data. PACS facilitates remote radiology reporting and alleviates workflow pressures. Currently 10% of NHS acute trusts have PACS capability. The government is investing millions to ensure national coverage within 3 years.

Chest x-ray: useful landmarks

In order to interpret a plain PA or lateral CXR some knowledge of chest anatomy and the major landmarks on the film is required. We have highlighted the major bony and soft tissue structures visible on the plain film in order to make it easier to spot abnormalities.

Fig. 13.1 Patient position for PA CXR.

Fig. 13.2 PA CXR.

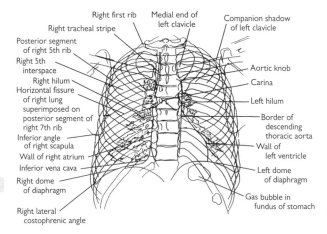

Fig. 13.3 PA CXR landmarks.

Labels (clockwise from top left):
Right first rib
Right tracheal stripe
Posterior segment of right 5th rib
Right 5th interspace
Right hilum
Horizontal fissure of right lung superimposed on posterior segment of right 7th rib
Inferior angle of right scapula
Wall of right atrium
Inferior vena cava
Right dome of diaphragm
Right lateral costophrenic angle
Medial end of left clavicle
Companion shadow of left clavicle
Aortic knob
Carina
Left hilum
Border of descending thoracic aorta
Wall of left ventricle
Left dome of diaphragm
Gas bubble in fundus of stomach

Fig. 13.4 Patient position for lateral CXR.

Fig. 13.5 Lateral CXR.

Fig. 13.6 Lateral CXR landmarks.

Manubriosternal joint

Retrosternal area
Body of sternum

Horizontal fissure
of right lung

Oblique fissure

Gas bubble in fundus
of stomach

Shadow of aortic arch
superimposed on
tracheal lumen

Lumen of
a bronchus

Bodies of lower
thoracic vertebrae
Retrocardiac area
Left dome
of diaphragm
Right dome
of diaphragm
Right posterior sulcus

Chest radiograph

The chest film is the most widely requested, yet most easy to misinterpret, investigation. Using a logical approach will avoid most pitfalls. This should be the initial imaging modality in all patients with suspected thoracic pathology.

Points to consider

- Always obtain prior imaging if available; temporal changes assist greatly in image interpretation and differential diagnosis.
- Standard projections of the chest are posteroanterior (PA) vs. antero-posterior (AP, see *below*) and left lateral (minimize cardiac distortion by positioning heart closer to the film.
- Additional views to aid problem-solving include lordotic, oblique and decubitus projections.
- Initially assess technical quality.

Projection

PA vs. AP will determine whether assessment of cardiac size is reliable.

Posture

Erect films enable a more accurate assessment of the mediastinum since the lungs are more expanded, and allow detection of air–fluid levels, pleural thickening and comment on the size of pulmonary vasculature.

Rotation

Look for the relationship of the medial ends of the clavicles to spinous process at the same level; a common cause of unilateral transradiancy is rotation.

Degree of inspiration

Ideally 6 ribs should be seen anteriorly and 10 ribs posteriorly. If more, this suggests hyperinflation (does the patient have asthma or COPD?). If less (e.g. poor inspiratory effort, obesity or restrictive chest disorders) there will be apparent cardiomegaly, increased basal shadowing and less commonly tracheal deviation.

Quality of image can be assessed by degree of penetration: the thoracic disc spaces should be just visible through the heart. Absence of respiratory or motion artifact.

The heart and mediastinum

Sequentially consider the heart, mediastinum, lungs, diaphragms, soft tissues (breast shadows) and bones. Remember to assess your review areas: the lung apices, behind the heart, under the diaphragm and the costophrenic angles.

Diaphragm: this should lie between the 5th to 7th ribs. If flattened, consider hyperinflation. In 90% of cases the right is higher than the left by 3–4cm. Effacement of the interface between lung and diaphragm suggests pleural or pulmonary pathology. Loss of smooth contour suggests localised herniation (eventration). Peaks laterally may be due to subpulmonary effusion.

Root of neck and trachea: the upper trachea is central with slight displacement to the right inferiorly due to the oesophagus. Thickening of the paratracheal line (>5mm) may imply nodal enlargement.

Mediastinum: the mediastinum should be central. The heart is normally <50% of thoracic width. Mediastinal enlargement or widening is a non-specific finding. The silhouette sign may help but a lateral film is helpful for localisation. Based on location of mediastinal abnormality, possible pathologies include:
- *Superior mediastinum*: thymoma, retrosternal thyroid and lymphoma.
- *Anterior mediastinum*: lymphoma (HD & NHL), germ cell tumours, thymoma, retrosternal goitres and Morgagni hernias (low).
- *Middle mediastinum*: aortic aneurysm, bronchial carcinoma, foregut duplication cysts (including bronchogenic/oesophageal) and hiatus hernia.

Posterior mediastinum: neurogenic tumours, Bochdalek hernia, dilated oesophagus or aorta.

Enlarged lymph nodes: may be seen in any compartment.

Pleural disease
- Pleural and extra-pleural masses generally form obtuse angles with adjacent pleura.
- Pulmonary or intra-parenchymal masses form acute angles with the pleura.

Common pleural abnormalities

Effusion
- The lateral view is more sensitive as accumulation of fluid occurs first in the posterior recess.
- May cause mediastinal/tracheal shift to the contralateral side or adjacent atelectasis.
- Ultrasound invaluable (and better than plain film) in evaluation of small effusions and guiding thoracocentesis.
- If blunting of the costophrenic angles is present it indicates the presence of fluid of at least 200mL (PA) or 75mL (lateral view) or may be secondary to thickening of pleura.
- Pleural thickening most commonly a sequela of inflammatory change.
- Asbestos exposure results in a spectrum of pleural abnormality ranging from benign plaques to fibrosis, and malignant mesothelioma (obtain occupational history).

Pneumothorax
- On an erect film the partially collapsed lung is delineated from pleural air as a curvilinear line (visceral pleura) paralleling the chest wall.
- Subtle pneumothorax will be more readily apparent on an expiratory film or lateral decubitus film (accumulation of air superiorly).
- If the air is under tension there may be mediastinal shift (tension pneumothorax).

Hila: density should be equal, left is higher than the right by 5–15mm. If more disparity consider elevation due to fibrosis (e.g. TB, radiotherapy) or depression by lobar or segmental collapse. Hilar enlargement may be vascular (e.g. pulmonary arterial or venous hypertension) or due to lymphadenopathy (e.g. sarcoidosis, lymphoma or TB). Hilar calcification is seen in silicosis, sarcoidosis and treated lymphoma.

Lung disease

Lung opacities may be subdivided into several basic patterns.

Alveolar (air space) shadowing—ill-defined, non-segmental and with air bronchograms. Large variety of causes:
- Fluid → pulmonary oedema (cardiogenic and non-cardiogenic).
- Fat → fat embolism.
- Haemorrhage → trauma, coagulopathies, pulmonary haemosiderosis.
- Cells → pulmonary alveolar proteinosis, sarcoidosis, alveolar cell carcinoma and infection (bacterial, fungal and viral).

Reticular (linear opacities)—associated obscuration of vessels and late appearance of chest x-ray signs:
- Collagen disorders.
- Extrinsic allergic alveolitis.
- Sarcoidosis, pneumoconiosis.
- Cryptogenic fibrosing alveolitis.
- Early left ventricular failure (LVF).
- Malignancy (lymphangitis carcinomatosis).

Nodular shadows: characterise according to their size and distribution:
- If solitary exclude tumour.
- Multiple:
  - Granulomas (TB, histoplasmosis, hydatid).
  - Immunological (Wegener's, rheumatoid arthritis).
  - Vascular (arteriovenous malformations).
  - Inhalational (PMF, Caplan's syndrome).

Hansell, DM, Armstrong P, Lynch DA, McAdams P. (2005) *Imaging of Diseases of the Chest*, 4th edition, Mosby, London; Corne J, Carroll M, Delaney D. (2002) *Chest X-ray Made Easy*, 2nd edition, Churchill Livingstone, Edinburgh.

Patterns of lobar collapse

Lobar collapse may be complete or incomplete. The commonest cause is obstruction of a central bronchus. The primary signs are opacification due to lack of aeration and displacement of the interlobar fissures.

Secondary signs include

- Elevation of the hemi-diaphragm (more prominent in lower lobe atelectasis than upper).
- Mediastinal displacement (tracheal displacement with upper lobe and cardiac displacement with lower lobe atelectasis).
- Hilar displacement: more prominent with upper lobe atelectasis than lower.
- Crowded vessels in the affected lobe.
- Compensatory hyperinflation of remaining lung.

Silhouette sign

- In a normal CXR the interface between the diaphragm and the mediastinum are visible due to a difference in density between the lung and these structures.
- The silhouette sign refers to loss of normal interfaces implying there is opacification due to consolidation (the most common cause), atelectasis or a mass in the adjacent lung.
- Silhouetting helps to localise the site of the pathology and both pleural and mediastinal disease produce the silhouette sign.

Table 13.2 Localisation using the silhouette sign

Interface lost	Location of lung pathology
Superior vena cava	Right upper lobe
Right heart border	Right middle lobe
Right hemi-diaphragm	Right lower lobe
Aortic knob/left superior mediastinum	Left upper lobe
Left heart border	Lingula
Left hemi-diaphragm	Left lower lobe

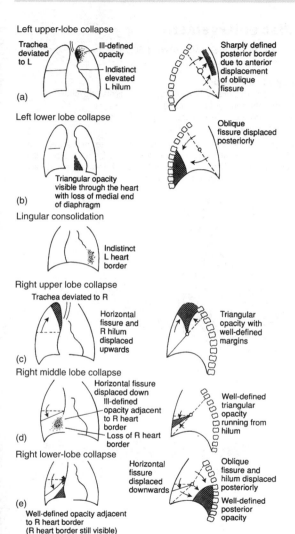

Left upper-lobe collapse

Trachea deviated to L

Ill-defined opacity

Indistinct elevated L hilum

(a)

Sharply defined posterior border due to anterior displacement of oblique fissure

Left lower lobe collapse

Triangular opacity visible through the heart with loss of medial end of diaphragm

(b)

Oblique fissure displaced posteriorly

Lingular consolidation

Indistinct L heart border

Right upper lobe collapse

Trachea deviated to R

Horizontal fissure and R hilum displaced upwards

(c)

Triangular opacity with well-defined margins

Right middle lobe collapse

Horizontal fissure displaced down
Ill-defined opacity adjacent to R heart border
Loss of R heart border

(d)

Well-defined triangular opacity running from hilum

Right lower-lobe collapse

Horizontal fissure displaced downwards

(e)

Well-defined opacity adjacent to R heart border (R heart border still visible)

Oblique fissure and hilum displaced posteriorly
Well-defined posterior opacity

Fig. 13.7 (a) Left upper lobe collapse. (b) Left lower lobe collapse. (c) Right upper lobe collapse. (d) Right middle lobe collapse. (e) Right lower lobe collapse.

Cardiac enlargement

Increase of cardiothoracic ratio beyond 50% is considered abnormal if the PA film is of good quality.

Aetiologies to consider
- Cardiomegaly (hypertrophy or dilatation of cardiac chambers).
- Pericardial effusion (globular heart).
- Poor inspiratory effort/decreased lung volumes.
- Pectus excavatum.

Location of cardiac valves may be relevant when determining the location of calcification. On a lateral projection draw a line from the xiphisternum to the carina and divide the heart into thirds. The location of the cardiac valves will be as demonstrated in Fig. 13.8.

P = pulmonary valve Ao = aortic valve
M = mitral valve   T = tricuspid valve

Fig. 13.8 Schematic diagram showing the relations of the cardiac valves on a lateral film of the chest.

Computed tomography of the thorax

Indications include
- Evaluation of an abnormal finding on plain film.
- Staging of primary or metastatic malignancies.
- Detection of thromboembolic disease (CTPA = CT pulmonary angiography).
- Detection and assessment of aortic dissection.
- Distinguishing empyema from lung abscess.
- Providing guidance for biopsy.

High resolution CT (HRCT) comprises thin section images which are reconstructed using a special algorithm.

Indications include
- Evaluation of a diffuse lung disease.
- Characterisation of a solitary pulmonary nodule.
- Haemoptysis.
- Lung disease in a patient with abnormal pulmonary function tests but apparently normal CXR.
- Assessment of emphysema.

Fig. 13.9 Single slice from CT pulmonary angiogram showing the presence of thrombus within the lower lobe pulmonary artery.

Fig. 13.10 Sagittal reformatted image confirms the extent of the thrombus and its relationship to the lumen.

Fig. 13.11 High resolution CT (HRCT) image of the chest in a patient with cystic lung disease due to tuberose sclerosis.

Abdominal x-ray: useful landmarks

Interpretation of the AXR, like the CXR, requires experience. In order to make things slightly easier we have provided a rough guide to the various bony, soft tissue and gas shadows seen on a 'typical' AXR.

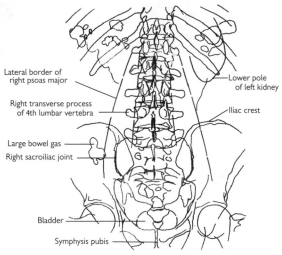

Lateral border of right psoas major

Right transverse process of 4th lumbar vertebra

Large bowel gas

Right sacroiliac joint

Bladder

Symphysis pubis

Lower pole of left kidney

Iliac crest

Fig. 13.12 PA AXR landmarks.

Fig. 13.13 PA AXR.

Fig. 13.14 Diffuse sclerotic metastases in a patient with a prostatic carcinoma. Note the presence of bilateral ureteric stents.

Plain abdominal x-ray (AXR)

The standard plain film is a supine AXR. Erect views have largely been superseded and in the acute setting have been replaced by the erect chest to show free subphrenic air. Furthermore, chest diseases such as myocardial infarction or pneumonia may simulate an acute abdomen. If there is doubt regarding the presence of a pneumoperitoneum, consider a lateral decubitus film (displays as little as 1mL of air).

Indications
Suspected obstruction, perforation, renal colic and toxic megacolon.

Contraindications
None but where abdominal pain is non-specific and not attributable to the conditions listed above, an AXR is unlikely to be helpful.

Interpretation of the plain AXR
A normal patient will have variable amounts of gas in the stomach, small bowel and colon. You can identify the stomach, as it lies above the transverse colon, has an air/fluid level in the erect view and has rugae in its lumen. Large bowel calibre is variable; 5.5cm is considered the upper limit for the transverse colon in toxic megacolon and 9cm for the caecum in obstruction. Short fluid levels are normal. Fluid levels are abnormal when seen in dilated bowel or if numerous. If the bowel is dilated distinguish between small and large bowel by the features listed below. Thickening of the bowel wall may be seen in a variety of aetiologies most notably ischaemia but also in inflammatory bowel disease.

Table 13.3

	Small bowel	**Large bowel**
Haustrae	Absent	Present
Valvulae conniventes	Present in jejunum	Absent
Number of loops	Many	Few
Distribution of loops	Central	Peripheral
Diameter of loops	30–50mm	>50mm
Solid faeces	Absent	May be present

Causes of bowel dilatation include mechanical obstruction, paralytic ileus or a localised peritonitis (meteorism), e.g. adjacent to pancreatitis or appendicitis.

Look for extraluminal gas

Gas in the peritoneal cavity: look for air under the hemidiaphragm, outlining the falciform ligament or both sides of the bowel wall (Rigler's sign). If there is any doubt consider a lateral decubitus film. Causes include perforation (ulcer, neoplasm), post-operative, following peritoneal dialysis or tracking down from the mediastinum.

Air in the biliary tree: following sphincterotomy, gallstone ileus or following anastomosis of CBD to bowel.

Portal vein gas: pre-morbid sign in the context of bowel infarction but less sinister in neonates with NEC (necrotising enterocolitis) or following umbilical catheterisation.

Intramural gas: linear streaks of air in the bowel wall again usually a sinister finding implying ischaemia but may be seen due to benign causes such as in patients with COPD.

Air in the retroperitoenum: delineates the renal shadows and the psoas muscle; common causes are trauma, iatrogenic (e.g. after colonoscopic perforation) and after perforation of a duodenal ulcer.

Gas in an abscess: look for displacement of adjacent bowel and an air/fluid level. Other causes include air in the urinary tract, and within necrotic tumours.

Look for any soft tissue masses or ascites: the latter is detectable on plain films if gross. There will be displacement of the ascending and descending colon from the side walls with loops of small bowel seen centrally.

Look for abdominal or pelvic calcification: first localise the site. This may require another view. The vast majority are clinically insignificant, i.e. vascular calcification, pelvic phleboliths and calcified mesenteric nodes. In the abdomen there may be pancreatic calcification (chronic pancreatitis) or hepatic calcification (old granulomas, abscesses or less commonly hepatomas and metastases from mucinous primaries). Gallstones are less commonly calcified and may contain central lucency (e.g. Mercedes Benz sign), while renal and ureteric calculi commonly calcify. Renal tumours and cysts rarely calcify and more widespread renal calcifications may be seen in nephrocalcinosis due to a wide variety of causes. In the pelvis, ovarian calcification (less common with malignant masses and seen more often in association with benign pathologies such as dermoids) is uncommon whilst uterine calcifications due to fibroids commonly occur. Bladder wall calcifications may be seen with bladder tumours, TB and schistosomiasis. Prostatic calculi and calcifications are common and of no significance. Vas deferens calcifications are seen in patients with diabetes.

Soft tissues: look at renal outlines (normally smooth and parallel to psoas, should be between 2–3 vertebral bodies). Absence of psoas margins may indicate retroperitoneal disease and haemorrhage.

Bones of the pelvis and lumbar spine: look for osteoarthritis, metabolic bone disease (hyperparathyroidism, sickle cell anaemia), the rugger jersey spine of osteomalacia and Paget's disease (📖*Lumbar spine & pelvis*, pp704, 706). Bony metastases may be lytic or sclerotic.

Barium studies

Barium suspension is made up of small particles of barium sulphate in a solution. Due to its high atomic number it is highly visible on x-rays. The constituents of individual suspensions vary depending on the part of the GI tract being examined. The particles are coated to improve flow and aid mucosal adhesion. When made up it comprises a chalky (sometimes unpalatable!) suspension. Advantages include low cost, easy availability and good assessment of mucosal surface.

Risks are more common in the context of

- *Perforation*: if leakage occurs into the peritoneal cavity it can produce pain and hypovolaemic shock (50% mortality). Long-term sequelae include peritoneal adhesions.
- *Aspiration*: in small amounts unlikely to have any clinical significance but if pre-existing respiratory impairment or aspiration of larger amounts (i.e. more than a few mouthfuls) the patient will need physiotherapy.
- *Obscuration*: CT examination in the presence of a recent barium examination will result in a poorly diagnostic study as high density barium results in streak artefacts.
- *Barium impaction*: rarely may exacerbate obstruction if barium collects and is concentrated above a point of obstruction.

Water-soluble contrast media

These are more expensive and provide inferior coating and contrast. They include iodinated agents gastromiro and gastrograffin.

Indications for their use include
- Suspected perforation especially into the peritoneal cavity.
- Meconium ileus.
- To opacify bowel during CT examinations.

Risks include pulmonary oedema if aspirated and hypovolaemia, especially in children. Both are a result of hyperosmolar effects. If aspiration is likely use water-soluble non-ionic contrast which causes less shift of body fluid compartments. Non-ionic contrast should be used in all infants (especially neonates) and pre-operative patients requiring water-soluble contrast.

Contrast agents

For studies other than when barium is being utilised the contrast media are non-ionic iodinated agents that are given orally, endo-luminally or intravenously. Non-ionic contrast agents are higher in cost than their ionic counterparts but have a lower incidence of adverse reactions (by a factor of 9 for severe reactions). They are typically excreted by glomerular filtration. Half-life is dependent on the dose given, distribution, and renal function. Contrast reactions can be idiosyncratic or anaphylactoid or non-idiosyncratic.

High risk patients are those with prior contrast reactions, a history of allergy or atopy, sickle cell disease, phaeochromocytoma and multiple myeloma (to name a few). Contrast induced nephropathy is more common as creatinine is elevated at time of administration or if the patient has a pre-existing renal impairment e.g. diabetes mellitus.

Pre-medication can be administered to patients with prior contrast reactions. Protocols vary but typically include a corticosteroid and antihistamine. Consider use of alternate modalities if risk is high e.g. USS or MRI instead of CT with contrast.

Gadolinium is a MR-based contrast agent that is paramagnetic. Its safety profile is highly favourable in that it does not have any of the nephrotoxicity associated with the iodinated contrast media and is more commonly associated with minor reactions such as headaches. It is also excreted by glomerular filtration.

Table 13.4 Pharmacological agents used in barium studies

Agent	Dose	Advantages	Disadvantages
Buscopan	20mg IV	Reduced bowel peristalsis due to smooth muscle relaxant action. Immediate onset. Short duration of action (15min)	Anticholinergic side-effects Contraindicated with cardio-vascular disease and glaucoma
Glucagon	0.3mg IV for barium meal. 1.0mg IV for barium enema	More potent smooth muscle relaxant than buscopan. Short duration of action, no interference with small bowel transit	Contraindicated with insulinomas or phaeochromocytomas Relatively expensive
Meto-clopramide	20mg PO or IV	↑ gastric peristalsis enhances barium transit during a follow-through study	Possible extra-pyramidal side-effects

Barium swallow

Plain films do not usually demonstrate the oesophagus unless it is very distended, e.g. achalasia. They may be useful in identifying an opaque foreign body within the lumen. The barium swallow is the usual contrast examination to visualise the oesophagus. Rapid sequence films are taken with a fluoroscopy unit while the patient swallows barium (usually in the erect position). Films are taken in an AP and oblique projection (to throw the oesophagus clear of the spine) with the oesophagus distended with barium (to demonstrate its outline) and empty to show the mucosal folds.

Normal anatomy
The oesophagus commences at C5/6. There are normal indentations on its outline by the cricoid cartilage, the aortic arch, left main bronchus and left heart.

Indications
These include the assessment of dysphagia, pain, reflux disease, tracheo-oesophageal fistulae (in children) and post-operative assessment where there has been gastric or oesophageal surgery.

Contraindications
No absolute contraindications exist, but in all barium studies the quality of the study relies heavily on patient cooperation and therefore immobile patients who are unable to weight bear may only be suitable for limited studies. The post-operative oesophagus is usually assessed with gas-tromiro or a non-ionic contrast.

Common disorders and patterns

Diverticulae: these include pharyngeal pouches (a midline diverticulum), traction diverticulae (due to adhesions) or pseudodiverticulae; dilated mucous glands seen in reflux or infective oesophagitis.

Luminal narrowing: strictures may be benign (e.g. oesophagitis, shown in Fig. 13.15, scleroderma, pemphigus, corrosives or infection) or malignant.

Webs: seen with skin lesions, e.g. epidermolysis or pemphigus, graft-versus-host disease and the Plummer Vinson syndrome.

Mega-oesophagus: can be with associated obstruction as in malignant strictures or without as in achalasia, diabetic neuropathy or Chagas' disease (Fig. 13.16a–c).

Ulceration/oesophagitis: may be due to gastro-oesophageal reflux disease, infection, corrosives or iatrogenic. Findings include lack of distensibility, fold thickening and mucosal irregularity.

Oesophageal tears: spontaneous, neoplastic, post-traumatic, iatrogenic and following prolonged emesis. Look for pneumomediastinum, left pleural effusion and features of mediastinitis.

Filling defects: foreign bodies, varices (proximal due to SVC obstruction), distal (in association with portal hypertension), neoplasms which may be benign as in leiomyoma or malignant. Most commonly squamous cell carcinoma (95%).

Fold thickening: may be due to oesophagitis, varices or infiltration by lymphoma.

Air/fluid level: commonest in hiatal hernias but also seen with a pharyngeal pouch.

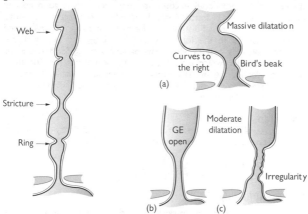

Fig. 13.15 Benign strictures.

Fig. 13.16 Obstruction in: (a) achalasia, (b) scleroderma, and (c) cancer.

Fig. 13.17 Lateral oblique projection during a barium swallow series shows a feline oesophagus. This can be a normal variant but is often associated with reflux disease (GORD).

Barium meal

About 200mL of a high density (250% weight/volume), low viscosity barium is used for a double contrast study which gives good coating without obscuration of mucosal detail. An effervescent agent is given to provide adequate luminal distension. The gastric mucosa is characterised by rugae (parallel to the long axis, 3–5mm thick) and area gastricae (nodular elevations 2–3mm wide). The patient is fasted for about 6h to avoid food residue which may cause diagnostic uncertainty. The techniques for coating the stomach and projections are variable. A smooth muscle relaxant may be given as part of the routine, particularly to assess the pylorus and duodenum.

Indications

Dyspepsia, weight loss, abdominal masses, iron deficiency anaemia of uncertain cause, partial outlet obstruction and previous GI haemorrhage.

Contraindications

Complete large bowel obstruction.

Abnormal findings

Filling defects: these may be intrinsic or extrinsic. Carcinoma remains the commonest cause of a filling defect in an adult (irregular, shouldered with overhanging edges). If there is antral involvement there may be associated outlet obstruction. Diffuse mucosal thickening and failure to distend is seen with linitis plastica. Other causes include gastric lymphoma, polyps (histology difficult to predict) and bezoars. Smooth filling defects are seen in conjunction with leiomyomas, lipomas and metastases. Extrinsic indentation by pancreatic tumours or an enlarged spleen may cause an apparent filling defect.

Fold thickening: (>5mm) is seen in association with hypersecretion states such as Zollinger-Ellison syndrome, gastritis and Crohn's disease. It may also be secondary to infiltration by carcinomas, lymphomas or eosinophilia.

Outlet obstruction: may be diagnosed by failure of the stomach to empty <50% of the barium ingested at 4h. This may be seen in carcinomas but also in scarring caused by chronic duodenal ulceration.

Hiatal hernia: herniation of the stomach into the chest occurs via the oesophageal hiatus in the diaphragm. There are two types: in a sliding hernia (more common) there is incompetence of the sphincter at the cardia, often associated with reflux. Other sequelae include oesophagitis, ulceration or stricture. In a rolling hernia the fundus herniates through the diaphragm but the gastro-oesophageal junction remains competent.

Gastritis and ulceration: gastritis is characterised by small shallow barium pools with surrounding lucent rings due to oedema. There are features which may be used to distinguish benign from malignant ulcers on barium studies. Ulcers are seen either as a crater or as a projection from the luminal surface. Benign ulcers are commonly seen on the lesser curve with smooth radiating folds which reach the edge of the ulcer crater. Malignant lesions may have an associated mass, have a shallow crater and an irregular contour. With the ease of availability of endoscopy, the use of barium meals in diagnosing ulceration has declined. Endoscopy has the advantage of being able to diagnose gastritis more accurately, assess ulcer healing, make a histological diagnosis and more accurately assess the post-operative stomach. However, early assessment of the post-operative stomach is radiologically performed to exclude complications such as anastomotic leaks. A water-soluble contrast agent is preferred in the early post-operative phase.

Fig. 13.18 Double contrast barium meal shows an ulcer crater.

Small intestine

Small bowel follow-through: the patient drinks 200–300mL of barium (with metoclopramide to speed transit time). The single contrast column is followed by films at regular intervals until the barium reaches the colon. Transit time is variable but the entire process may take 1–6h depending on adequacy of bowel preparation. Films are taken at intervals of approximately 20min initially, in the prone position which aids separation of the loops. When the barium reaches the caecum spot views of the terminal ileum are taken.

Small bowel enema (enteroclysis): this technique provides better demonstration and mucosal detail, as there is rapid infusion of a continuous column of barium directly into the jejunum. Methyl cellulose is administered following the barium to provide double contrast. This is achieved via a weighted nasogastric tube which is positioned at, or distal to, the duodendojejunal (DJ) flexure. Disadvantages include poor patient tolerance (related to intubation) and a relatively high screening dose.

Both techniques require the patient to be on a low residue diet beforehand.

Indications
The indications are the same for both techniques and include pain, diarrhoea, bleeding, partial obstruction, malabsorption, overgrowth syndromes, assessment of Crohn's disease activity and extent, and suspected masses. The small bowel enema may be preferred for assessment of recurrent Crohn's disease or complex post-operative problems but the small bowel follow-through is otherwise routinely used.

Contraindications
Complete obstruction and suspected perforation.

Normal findings
The small intestine measures ~5m and extends from the DJ flexure to the ileocaecal valve. The proximal two-fifths is the jejunum, the distal three-fifths is the ileum. Normal calibre is 3.5cm for the jejunum and 2.5cm for the ileum (up to 1cm more on enteroclysis). The valvulae conniventes are circular in configuration and ~2mm thick in the jejunum and 1mm thick in the ileum.

Abnormal findings
Dilatation is indicative of malabsorption, small bowel obstruction (SBO) or paralytic ileus. There may be accompanying effacement of the mucosal pattern. When seen with fold thickening it may be due to Crohn's, ischaemia or radiotherapy. Mucosal thickening may be due to infiltration by lymphoma or eosinophilia, adhesions, ischaemia or radiotherapy.

Strictures are seen in Crohn's disease and in lymphoma. There is usually dilatation of the bowel proximally. Crohn's disease causes skip lesions, ulceration, strictures of variable length and a high incidence of terminal ileal involvement. There may be associated ulceration, fold thickening and fistulation.

Malabsorption: radiological investigation may reveal an underlying structural abnormality. The findings in malabsorption include dilatation, fold thickening and flocculation of barium.

Fig. 13.19 30 minute film in a small bowel follow-through series shows a normal mucosal fold pattern.

Fig. 13.20 Small bowel enema shows at least 2 strictures (arrows) in this patient with Crohn's disease. Compare the mucosal detail with the SBFT.

Cholangiography

Ultrasound
This is the primary modality for assessment of the biliary tree and for exclusion of pancreatic pathology. With current scanner resolution the sensitivity for stone disease is in the range of >95% for stones exceeding 2mm in diameter. For choledocholithiasis(stones in the common duct) the sensitivity falls to around 50% and MRCP or ERCP is more helpful.

Intravenous cholangiography
This is rarely performed but may be useful in patients with biliary symptoms post-cholecystectomy or with a non-functional gallbladder. It is contraindicated in the presence of severe hepatorenal disease, as the side effects related to the contrast media are considerable.

ERCP (endoscopic retrograde cholangiopancreatography)
The biliary and pancreatic ducts are directly filled with contrast following endoscopic cannulation and during x-ray screening. This has both a diagnostic and therapeutic role. It is particularly of value in the demonstration of ampullary lesions and to delineate the level of biliary tree obstruction in patients with obstructive jaundice. It allows sphincterotomy to be performed to facilitate the passage of stones lodged in the common bile duct.

PTC (percutaneous transhepatic cholangiography)
The biliary tree is directly injected with contrast following percutaneous puncture of the liver. This is both diagnostic in defining a level of obstruction and therapeutic in biliary duct obstruction, as it may be used as a precursor to a biliary drainage procedure or prior to insertion of a stent. Contraindications include bleeding diatheses and ascites.

Other cholangiographic techniques
- Per-operative cholangiogram in which the common bile duct (CBD) is filled with contrast during cholecystectomy to exclude the presence of CBD stones.
- T-tube cholangiogram: after operative exploration a T-tube is left in the CBD for a post-operative contrast study to exclude the presence of retained stones.
- MRCP (magnetic resonance cholangiopancreatography): this is a non-invasive, technique where heavily T2-weighted images are obtained without contrast administration. The bile acts as an intrinsic contrast agent and stones are visualised as filling defects. The entire biliary and pancreatic ductal system can be visualised. Common indications for this technique include unsuccessful ERCP, a contraindication to ERCP as well as evaluation of the post surgical biliary tree.

MRCP
- Non-invasive.
- Cheaper.
- Uses no radiation.
- Requires no anaesthesia.

- Less operator-dependent.
- Allows better visualisation of the ducts proximal to the level of obstruction.
- When combined with conventional sequences allows detection of extra ductal disease.

Disadvantages:
- Inability to perform therapeutic endoscopic or percutaneous intervention of obstructing bile duct lesions.
- MRCP is comparable with ERCP in detection of obstruction with a sensitivity and specificity of 91% and 100% respectively.
- Causes of filling defects are usually stones, air, tumours, blood or sludge.

Fig. 13.21 Heavily T2-weighted slab image shows an irregular beaded pancreatic duct in this patient with chronic pancreatitis. There is a small pseudocyst in the tail (arrowhead).

Barium enema

This is the technique of choice for evaluation of the large bowel. Barium is run into the colon under gravity via a tube inserted into the rectum. The column of barium is followed by air to achieve double contrast. Buscopan (a smooth muscle relaxant) may be given to minimise spasm and optimise mucosal relief. Bowel preparation prior to the examination (low residue diet and aperients) is vital to ensure that there is no faecal material which may mask mucosal abnormalities or be mistaken for small polyps. Remember the examination is uncomfortable and requires reasonably good patient cooperation and mobility. ▶ *Do not request this in frail or elderly patients unless there is a good clinical indication.* A rectal examination or sigmoidoscopy is essential to avoid abnormalities being missed.

Single *vs.* double contrast

If evaluation of the colonic mucosa is not the primary aim then a single contrast technique will suffice. This is applicable in children, where the patient is uncooperative and where gross pathology is being excluded, and in the evaluation of obstruction/volvulus or in the reduction of an intussusception.

Indications

Change in bowel habit, iron deficiency anaemia, abdominal pain, palpable mass of suspected colonic origin, and weight loss of unknown cause.

Contraindications

Recent rectal biopsy, toxic megacolon or pseudo-membranous colitis.

Common findings

Solitary filling defect: polyps are classified according to histology. The commonest are hyperplastic (no malignant potential, adenomatous polyps are premalignant with the risk of malignancy increasing with size (<5mm = 0%, >2cm = 20–40%). Also found are adenocarcinoma (increased risk in ulcerative colitis, polyposis syndromes, villous adenoma), and less commonly metastases and lymphoma.

Multiple filling defects: polyps (polyposis syndromes or post-inflammatory pseudopolyps), pneumatosis coli, metastases and lymphoma.

Ulceration: inflammatory bowel disease (IBD), ischaemia, infection, radiation and neoplasia.

Colonic narrowing: neoplasms (apple core lesion), metastases, lymphoma, diverticular disease, IBD, ischaemia and radiation.

Dilatation: mechanical, e.g. proximal to neoplasm, volvulus or non-mechanical, post-operative ileus, metabolic and toxic megacolon.

Diminished haustration: cathartic colon, IBD and scleroderma.

Increased haustration (thumbprinting): ischaemia, haemorrhage, neoplasm and IBD.

Widening of the pre-sacral space (>1.5cm at S2): normal in up to 40% but also seen in association with IBD, neoplasms, infection and sacral/pelvic lipomatosis.

Colonoscopy

Remains a complementary technique and has the advantage of being both therapeutic and diagnostic (e.g. biopsy, polypectomy, etc.). In elderly patients CT with prior bowel preparation and air insufflation is less invasive and less arduous. Virtual colonoscopy: Helical CT images of distended colon taken during a breath hold are used to obtain 2-D or 3-D images of the colon. Images are acquired in the supine and prone position to assess lesional mobility (and thus distinguish stool from polyps). Recent studies using primary 3-D interpretation have shown sensitivity in the range of 94% for polyps at least 1cm in diameter and around 88% for lesions measuring at least 6mm. Current refinements in this technique include use of computer assisted detection (CAD) to improve performance as well as use of prepless techniques (i.e. the patient does not have to undergo prior bowel cleansing).

Fig. 13.22 Standard supine projection from a double contrast barium enema (DCBE) showing a normal large bowel.

Fig. 13.23 Supine DCBE showing a tight stricture in the transverse colon in this patient with inflammatory bowel disease.

Pickhardt PJ, Choi JR *et al.* (2003) Computed tomographic virtual colonoscopy to screen for colorectal neoplasia in asymptomatic adults. *NEJM* **349**, 2191–2200.

Radiology of the urinary tract

Plain abdominal film

Look for any urinary tract calcification: 90% stones are radio-opaque. Other causes include hyperparathyroidism, medullary sponge kidney and renal tubular acidosis.

Renal outline: between T12 and L3 and 10–15cm. Left bigger and higher than the right.

Assess bones of spine and sacrum: for bony metastases or spina bifida (may be relevant in enuresis).

IVU

This provides a good overview of the urinary tract and in particular the pelvicalyceal anatomy. Fluid restriction and laxatives are no longer necessary and in particular the former is to be avoided in diabetics, renal failure and myeloma. Following the preliminary plain film, 300mg/kg of contrast media is injected IV. The film sequence is varied according to the clinical scenario. An immediate film shows the nephrogram phase and displays the renal outlines. An increasingly dense delayed nephrogram is seen in acute obstruction, acute hypotension, acute tubular necrosis (ATN) and renal vein thrombosis. A faint persistent nephrogram is seen with acute glomerulonephritis and it may be delayed in renal artery stenosis (RAS). Later films show the pelvicalyceal systems (pyelogram), ureters and bladder.

Common abnormalities

Loss of renal outline: congenital absence, ectopic kidney, tumour, abscess or post-nephrectomy (look for absent 12th rib).

Small kidney (unilateral): ischaemia (RAS), radiation or congenital hypoplasia.

Small kidney (bilateral): atheroma, papillary necrosis or glomerulonephritis.

Large kidney (unilateral): duplex, acute pyelonephritis, tumour or hydronephrosis.

Large kidney (bilateral): polycystic kidneys and infiltrative disease such as myeloma, amyloid and lymphoma.

Pelvicalyceal filling defect: smoothly marginated (clot, papilloma), irregular margins (tumour, e.g. renal cell or transitional carcinoma), intraluminal (sloughed papilla, calculus or clot), extrinsic (vascular impression or cyst), irregular renal outline (scarring, e.g. in ischaemia, TB, pyelonephritis or reflux nephropathy).

Ultrasound

May be used as an alternative or complementary examination with the IVU and may be used to:

• Demonstrate or exclude hydronephrosis especially in acute renal failure (ARF).
• Evaluate renal tumours, cysts and abscesses.
• Follow-up of transplant kidneys and chronic renal disease.
• Assess renal blood flow using Doppler.
• Serial scanning in children with recurrent urinary tract infections.
• Assess bladder morphology and volume, and the prostate.
• Provide guidance for interventional techniques, e.g. renal biopsy and nephrostomy placement.

CT and MRI

CT is more accurate for staging renal tumours, assessing retroperitoneal pathology, staging bladder and prostatic tumours and for assessment of renal vascular pathology (such as renal artery stenosis). In many centres unenhanced CT is replacing IVU as a gold standard for assessment of renal stone disease. It is more accurate at depicting stone burden than IVU and precisely demonstrating the level and cause of obstruction in the acute setting.

Evaluation of ureteric pathology in the context of haematuria is also being performed with contrast enhanced CT.

MRI is valuable in staging vascular involvement by renal carcinomas. Dedicated pelvic coils and endoluminal coils show excellent results in staging pelvic and gynaecological malignancies.

Micturating cystourethrogram (MCUG)

Following catheterisation of the bladder, contrast is introduced. This is the technique of choice for defining urethral anatomy and gauging the presence/degree of vesicoureteric reflux in children.

Ascending urethrography

Contrast is injected directly into the urethra in males in the assessment of urethral trauma, strictures and congenital anomalies such as hypospadias.

Retrograde pyelography

The ureters are catheterised (usually following cystoscopy in theatre) and contrast injected under x-ray screening. Of value in urothelial tumours and to define the site of obstruction, e.g. non-opaque calculi.

Angiography

A femoral approach with selective catheterisation of renal vessels. Main uses include haematuria (look for AVMs), hypertension (RAS), in transplant donors (to define anatomy) and in renal cell carcinoma (where embolisation is being contemplated).

Nephrostomy

📖*Interventional radiology*, p710.

Renal cyst

Multiple renal cysts
(elongation & distortion
of calyces – polycystic
disease)

Renal tumour

Duplex kidney with
hydronephrotic
upper, moiety.
('drooping flower')

Dilatation of a
single calyx
(may be due to
vascular compression)

Fig. 13.24 Common pattern of abnormalities seen on IVU.

Breast imaging

Breast cancer is a common problem (1 in 12 women). An NHS breast screening programme is in place following the Forrest report. Its aim is to use imaging to detect early clinically occult carcinomas. It screens women aged 50–64 years on a 3-yearly basis (the detection rate is 50 cancers for every 10,000 women screened). There are plans to extend the programme to women up to and including the age of 70. Current research estimates that by 2010 the programme will allow a 25% reduction in mortality.

Mammography

Technical factors: breast tissue has a narrow spectrum of inherent densities and in order to display these optimally a low kilovoltage (kVp) beam is used. It enhances the differential absorption of fatty, glandular and calcific tissues. Dedicated mammographic units provide low energy x-ray beams with short exposure times. The breast is compressed to minimise motion and geometric unsharpness. High resolution is paramount in order to detect microcalcification (as small as 0.1mm). The breast is a radio-sensitive organ so doses need to be kept to a minimum.

Standard projections: these are the mediolateral oblique and craniocaudal views. Adequacy of the lateral oblique view may be gauged by the pectoralis major muscle which should be visible to the level of the nipple, inclusion of the axillary tail, and inclusion of the inframammary fold. Additional projections such as true lateral and magnification views may be used to clarify abnormalities.

Mammographic signs: the breast parenchyma is made up of glandular tissue in a fibro-fatty stroma. Cooper's ligaments form a connective tissue network. The amount of glandular tissue decreases with age; as it is dense on mammography the suitability of the technique for detecting pathology increases with age.

Primary signs of a malignancy
- A mass with ill-defined or spiculate borders.
- Clustered, linear or irregular calcification (which may occur in the absence of a mass).
- Secondary signs include distortion of adjacent stroma, skin thickening and nipple retraction.

94% of breast carcinoma is ductal in origin.

Breast ultrasound: this largely forms a modality for assessment not diagnosis or detection. It can, however, be used to evaluate non-palpable masses, to determine internal architecture (solid vs. cystic), to assess asymmetric density and as a primary imaging modality in young women (<35 years). It is also used as a tool to guide intervention, i.e. drainage of cysts and biopsy of suspicious lesions.

MRI: MRI remains a problem-solving tool in breast imaging. Wide spread implementation of MRI (for instance for screening) is hampered by its low specificity (37–97%). It can increase the number of benign biopsies that are performed. This clearly has resource implications as well as generating unnecessary patient anxiety. Both MRI and ultrasound may be used to evaluate implants and their integrity but MRI is the only modality that is sensitive in the evaluation of intra-capsular implant rupture. Contrast-enhanced MRI of the breast is also a sensitive method for detection of malignancy with reported sensitivities in the region of 93%. It is especially useful to detect recurrent breast carcinoma and where conventional techniques are unable to help in the distinction from more benign lesions. Breast MRI is also being advocated for screening young patients with a family history/genetic risk of breast carcinoma.

Fig. 13.25 Craniocaudal mammographic view of the breast. The arrows depict a stellate mass consistent with a carcinoma.

Fig. 13.26 Subtraction sagittal MR image of the breast following gadolinium showing an enhancing spiculated mass consistent with malignancy.

Ultrasound

Ultrasound is a high frequency mechanical vibration produced by piezo-electric materials, which have the property of changing thickness when a voltage is applied across them. It is an important tomographic modality and has widespread applications in the abdomen, neck, pelvis and extremities. At diagnostic levels there are no known damaging sequelae to tissues and therefore it is safe for use in obstetrics providing invaluable imaging of the developing fetus. Doppler USS is based on the principle that sound reflected by a moving target has a different frequency to the incident sound wave. The frequency shift is proportional to the velocity of the flowing material. Doppler therefore not only enables detection but quantification of velocity.

Indications

USS is cheap, readily available, non-invasive and has high patient acceptability. It has a wide range of applications as listed below. There are also no radiation implications. Again, advances in technology have resulted in vast improvements in the resolution of this modality such that subtle pathology is more readily identifiable.

Contraindications

None, but remember that USS is operator- and patient-dependent and should be used as a problem-orientated modality, not as a total body survey. It cannot be used to image air-containing structures or bone. The resolution of the USS image is inversely related to the depth of penetration. Therefore image quality in obese patients is sub-optimal.

Applications

Head and neck: may be used for evaluation of the salivary glands, thyroid, lymph nodes and palpable or clinically suspected masses. Doppler is used to assess the carotid vessels and quantify degree of stenosis/occlusion.

Chest (excluding breast): the use here is limited to palpable chest wall lesions, assessment of pleural abnormalities, biopsy and drainage of pleural effusions and is occasionally of use in directing a biopsy of peripheral lung or mediastinal masses.

Abdomen & pelvis: this is the main use of USS. Useful for assessment of solid organs, e.g. liver, kidneys, spleen, gallbladder, pancreas, uterus/adnexae and bladder. A full bladder is used as an acoustic window in the pelvis. Retroperitoneal masses and lymph nodes may be visible depending on patient habitus. USS is useful for directing biopsy of solid organs/masses and for drainage of ascites, abscesses and collections.

Limbs: musculoskeletal USS has been revolutionised by advances in high frequency probes which enable characterisation of soft tissue masses, tendon-related pathology, rotator cuff lesions, masses, effusions and collections. It is also used for vascular assessment and the diagnosis of deep vein thrombosis.

Intracavitary transducers: these place the transducer as close as possible to the area of interest. They include transvaginal, transrectal, urethral, oesophageal and intravascular probes. They are usually high frequency transducers that produce detailed high resolution images. Transvaginal USS is more invasive than transabdominal scanning but is used in the routine assessment of gynaecological disorders. It can also be used for infertility monitoring, egg retrieval and the exclusion of suspected ectopic pregnancy. Transrectal scanning is used for screening, assessment and biopsy of suspected prostatic pathology as well as rectal pathology including staging rectal cancers. Endo-anal probes may be used to assess morphology and characterise tears of the anal sphincter.

Contrast agents: ultrasound contrast agents are available as an additional tool in diagnosis, although are currently used primarily in academic centres. These are micro-bubbles which are stable over a period of time and may be used to improve anatomical detail, assess tubal patency (hysterosalpingography), assess tumour vascularity, characterise focal masses (e.g. within the liver) and contrast enhancement.

Fig. 13.27 Trans-axial view of the gallbladder on ultrasound demonstrates a soft tissue mass in the lumen suspicious for carcinoma. There is cholelithiasis, a common coexistent entity. The arrow shows an abnormal interface with the liver parenchyma suggestive of local infiltration.

Fig. 13.28 Colour Doppler image in the same patient shows abnormal vascularity in the wall of the gallbladder. **(Colour plate 6.)**

Fig. 13.29 Dilated intrahepatic ducts are seen in this axial view of the liver.

Computed tomography (CT)

This technique differs from conventional radiography in that it is able to visualise a vast spectrum of absorption values and therefore tissue densities. Furthermore, being a tomographic technique, the resultant image is essentially 2-D and overcomes the problem of confusing overlap of 3-D structures on plain film. The image is a grey scale representation of the density of tissues (attenuation) as depicted by x-rays. Each image is made up of a matrix of squares (pixels) which collectively represent the attenuation values of tissues within that volume (voxel). With conventional CT separate exposures are made for each slice. Current scanners can acquire data in a continuous helical or spiral fashion, shortening acquisition time and reducing artefacts caused by patient movement. This improves overall throughput and increases the likelihood of a diagnostic scan, particularly in uncooperative patients. The volumetric data that is acquired may be manipulated by image processing and displayed in a variety of techniques including 3-D reformats and 'virtual' endoscopy.

The attenuation values are expressed on an arbitrary scale (Hounsfield units) with water being 0, air being −1000 units and bone +1000 units. The range of densities displayed on a particular image can be manipulated by altering the window width and level.

Prior to scanning the abdomen or pelvis dilute oral contrast is given to opacify the bowel. Intravenous contrast is given to aid the problem-solving process and differentiates vascular-enhancing lesions from surrounding tissue.

Multi-slice CT scanners are third generation scanners with helical capabilities and low-voltage slip rings which acquire anywhere between 16–64 slices (and counting!) slices per x-ray tube rotation.

Indications
There are a wide variety as detailed below. CT is often the most diagnostic cross-sectional examination and more definitive than USS in many instances.

Contraindications
Due to the relatively high radiation dose, CT should be avoided in pregnancy. Artefact from indwelling, high density foreign material, e.g. hip prosthesis, dental amalgam and barium, may limit the diagnostic quality of the examination. Claustrophobia is less of a problem compared to MRI.

Applications
CNS/spine: CT remains the tool for primary diagnosis, pre-surgical assessment, treatment monitoring and detection of relapse in many CNS disease conditions. MRI is superior in the posterior fossa and parasellar region and for assessment in multiple sclerosis, epilepsy and tumours. Where MRI is not available it is useful for assessment of degenerative spinal and disc disease. It is superior to MRI in the assessment of head injury. CT is also used as the primary modality in evaluation of acute stroke and in the emergency settling prior to lumbar puncture of patients suspected of CNS infection such as meningitis.

Orthopaedics/trauma: uses include diagnosis and staging of bony and soft tissue neoplasms, and assessment of vertebral, pelvic and complex extremity trauma (e.g. tibial plateau fractures). It is also used in the detection of loose bodies, assessment of acetabular dysplasia and providing an answer in joint instability (especially in shoulders, wrists and elbows where it may be performed as an adjunct to/in conjunction with conventional arthrography).

Oncology/radiotherapy: staging of solid tumours, treatment planning and the detection of relapse. CT is of particular value in obtaining whole body scans in oncology due to the speed and ease of use with the advent of spiral CT. CT is used for radiotherapy treatment planning to allow more precise targeting of treatment.

Chest: indications include the staging of bronchogenic carcinomas, characterisation of solitary nodules, diffuse infiltrative lung disease, widened mediastinum/mediastinal masses and pleural abnormalities. With spiral CT, pulmonary angiography has advanced the diagnosis of pulmonary emboli particularly when V/Q scanning is indeterminate or equivocal. Helical CT is equivalent to formal angiography in detection of emboli within proximal arteries of <5th/6th generation. Sensitivity (80–100%, specificity 78–100%).

Abdomen: applications include the diagnosis of abdominal pathology which may be of traumatic, neoplastic, inflammatory or infective origin. CT is particularly useful for masses, pancreatic and hepatic disease, detection of the site and nature of obstructive jaundice and the assessment of abdominal trauma. It is also used in the pre-surgical assessment of abdominal aneurysms and as an aid to interventional techniques (p710).

Fig. 13.30 Direct coronal reformat through the liver shows findings consistent with primary sclerosing cholangitis. Note the markedly thickened bile duct wall (arrows).

Fig. 13.31 Free intra-peritoneal air secondary to perforation of a gastric ulcer. Note the thickened antrum of the stomach.

Fig. 13.32 Virtual barium enema image reconstructed from CT colonoscopy. The arrow shows the location of the polyps.

Fig. 13.33 Reformat of a CT angiogram to assess the extent of renal artery stenosis in this patient who has bilateral common iliac stents.

Fig. 13.34 Reformatted MIP image of an abdominal CT shows small bowel obstruction due to the presence of a caecal carcinoma (arrows).

Magnetic resonance imaging (MRI)

This is a non-invasive technique which displays internal structure whilst avoiding the use of ionising radiation. The nuclei of certain elements align with the magnetic force when placed in a strong magnetic field. These are usually hydrogen nuclei in water and lipid (at clinical field strengths) which resonate to produce a signal when a radiofrequency pulse is applied and display anatomical information. Further discussion of the physics is beyond the scope of this chapter.

T1-weighted images
- Contrast is due to inherent T1 relaxation.
- Provides good anatomical information.
- Fat is displayed as high signal (white).
- Distinction between cystic (black) and solid structures is possible.
- Good evaluation of marrow signal.
- The sequence of choice when evaluating enhancement, as gadolinium administration makes structures of even higher signal intensity on T1-weighted images.

T2-weighted images
- Technique of choice for evaluating pathology.
- Fluid is of high signal and therefore optimally displays oedema.
- Improved soft tissue contrast allows evaluation of zonal anatomy of organs such as the uterus and prostate.

Table 13.5 MR signal intensity of common tissues

Tissue or body fluid	T1 signal	T2 signal
Air	Nil	Nil
Bone or calculi	Nil	Nil
Fat	High (bright)	Medium to high
Proteinaceous fluid(e.g. abscess or complex cyst)	Medium	High
Muscle	Low	Low to medium
CSF, urine, bile or oedema	Low	High
Blood (*depends on age*) Hyperacute (oxyHb) Chronic (haemosiderin)	Low Low	High Low

MRA (magnetic resonance angiography)

MRI principles are used to exploit the properties of flowing blood. Images generated display structures containing flowing blood with suppression of all other structures. These principles can be further modified so that only vessels with flow in a specific direction (i.e. arteries *vs.* veins are visualised). MRA is currently being used in the evaluation of suspected cerebrovascular disease, renovascular disease and peripheral vascular disease.

Functional imaging

MRI techniques have evolved such that diffusion imaging utilises the diffusion of water protons in diagnosis of evolving ischaemia. This technique shows how movement of water molecules is impeded by cytotoxic oedema of ischaemic cells. These are manifested by signal changes that show early evidence of cerebral ischaemia prior to structural changes becoming apparent. Similarly early ischaemia of the myocardium is detectable on MRI. This has great therapeutic potential as early treatment may prevent establishment of ischaemia and result in overall improvement of ventricular function and survival. MRA is also being used to depict coronary vessel disease non invasively.

Indications

The indications are legion and continue to grow. There is a wide variety of indications which are summarised below. MR is especially useful in imaging the brain, spine, peripheral limbs and joints, neck and pelvis. Again improvements in scanner hardware and software have had huge impact on clinical practice. The prior limitations of long scan times have been overcome by robust sequences that can be performed in a breath-hold. This means that respiratory and peristaltic artifacts are no longer an issue when imaging in the chest and abdomen.

Contraindications

These largely apply to patients with magnetically susceptible devices or materials whose movement or loss of function can have deleterious consequences. These include cardiac pacemakers, metallic fragments and prosthetic heart valves. Relative contraindications include pregnancy (especially the 1st trimester) and claustrophobia. MRI magnets are relatively confined and even those who are not normally claustrophobic may be provoked.

Applications

The spine: MR imaging is superior to other techniques in displaying anatomy and is the technique of choice in assessing disc disease, the postoperative back, evaluating neural compression (benign or malignant), in imaging acute myelitis, infection (such as discitis or osteomyelitis) and excluding marrow infiltration.

CNS: imaging of the CNS is used to evaluate mass lesions, hydrocephalus, white matter disease, leptomeningeal pathology, cerebrovascular disease, degenerative disorders, and visual and endocrine disorders such as pituitary dysfunction. In trauma/acute haemorrhage CT is the preferred technique.

Paediatric: the uses here include assessment of perinatal trauma/anoxic injury, congenital anomalies and developmental delay. Within the spine it is invaluable in the assessment of spinal dysraphism and progressive scoliosis.

Musculoskeletal: along with CNS disease this is a major component of the MRI workload. It has revolutionised musculoskeletal imaging and is used to characterise meniscal pathology, ligamentous injury, degeneration and the sequelae of trauma in the knee, shoulder, wrist and ankle. Further uses include imaging mass lesions, assessing the extent of infection and diagnosing early avascular necrosis.

Chest/cardiac: within the thorax MRI is useful for assessment of apical lesions such as Pancoast's tumours, chest wall and brachial plexus lesions and mediastinal masses. Cardiac applications are legion and fast evolving; they include imaging of the great vessels to exclude congenital/acquired aortic disease (including dissection) and the diagnosis of pulmonary embolus.

Abdominal/pelvic MRI: within the abdomen MR is often a problem-solving tool and can be used to more confidently characterise focal liver and pancreatic lesions as well as assess diffuse liver disease. It is also of use in evaluating indeterminate adrenal masses. Within the pelvis uses include the imaging of congenital anomalies as well as staging tumours such as cervical, prostate and rectal tumours. There have been rapid advances in techniques for imaging bowel-related pathology.

Interventional MRI: open MRI units image the patients in large bore or C-shaped units rather than the closed narrow tunnel used in conventional units. They can therefore be used for claustrophobic patients and to provide imaging guidance for interventional procedures. Disadvantages include a low magnetic field strength (0.1–0.3T *vs.* 1.5T) and a limited anatomical and spatial resolution due to their basic construct.

Recently, short bore magnets have been developed that combine the accuracy of a tunnel scanner and the comfort of an open MRI scan. Although they are not completely open, they are much less constrictive because of the short bore magnet (shorter tunnels), but can produce a high-field.

Fig. 13.35 Axial T2W sequence showing bilateral parametrial infiltration in this patient with a cervical mass.

Fig. 13.36 Saggital and axial T2W images show a large cervical carcinoma. MRI is the modality of choice for local staging.

Fig. 13.37 Axial T2W shows acute infarction in the right cerebellar hemisphere.

Fig. 13.38 Coronal reformatted MRI image shows a tight stenosis of the distal vertebral artery on the right.

Fig. 13.39 AP coronal MRA showing mild irregularity of the carotid siphon on the left. The images are examined in multiple projections to exclude anomalies such as stenosis or small aneurysms.

Fig. 13.40 Sagittal T2W MRI image in patient with superior sulcus (Pancoast) tumour showing invasion into the chest wall.

Spinal imaging

Basic principles of bony trauma imaging

- Obtain 2 films at right angles to one another (most commonly an AP and lateral to rule out fracture).
- Image proximal and distal joints.
- Bone scanning is more sensitive but less specific than plain films to rule out a fracture. (*Not useful in acute setting.*)
- CT is invaluable for complex injuries (e.g. spine, calcaenus, and sacrum).
- MRI is used to assess ligaments, tendons, joint capsules, menisci and cartilage.

In each case evaluate the following

- Site of fracture: assess if proximal/distal and intra *vs.* extra-articular.
- Type of fracture: simple (transverse, oblique, spiral) *vs.* comminuted.
- Degree of displacement: usually described with reference to the distal fragment.
- Soft tissue involvement: exclude foreign bodies, presence of gas. Open (compound) *vs.* closed.

Cervical spine

Trauma: obtain a cross-table lateral first (this has the highest yield) and then perform the remainder of the cervical spine series (AP and open mouth peg views), if patient mobility allows and high index of suspicion. All 7 cervical vertebral bodies should be visualised (a large number of cervicothoracic injuries are missed because of inadequate views). If not seen request a specialised lateral view (swimmers). Then sequentially evaluate:

Alignment: assess the following lines (Fig.13.41). They should be parallel with no step-offs.

Bones: inspect C1 and C2. The anterior arch of C1 should be 3mm from the dens in adults (5mm in children). The vertebral bodies should be intact and they should be uniform in size and shape. Check disc spaces for any inordinate narrowing or widening which may be post-traumatic.

Cartilage

- *Soft tissues:* look for abnormal widening or a localized bulge. 50% of patients with a bony injury will have soft tissue thickening. The soft tissues should be no more than one-third of a vertebral body until C4 and a vertebral body width thereafter.
- *The peg views:* do not mistake a superimposed arch of C1 or the incisors as a fracture. Important points to remember are:
  - The lateral margins of C1 and C2 should align.
  - The spaces on either side of the peg should be equal (Fig. 13.41).

Remember: normal plain films do not exclude ligamentous injury.

In the routine setting cervical spine films are taken to exclude spondylosis (disc space narrowing and osteophytes) and atlantoaxial subluxation which results in long tract signs and cord compression (rheumatoid arthritis, ankylosing spondylitis, Down's syndrome).

Thoracic and lumbar spine

Degenerative disease is common with disc space narrowing, end plate sclerosis and osteophyte formation. Wedge compression fractures are common in the osteoporotic spine and need to be distinguished from the more sinister causes (absence of paraspinal mass, posterior elements spared). Multiple collapsed vertebrae are found in osteoporosis, neoplastic disease, trauma and histiocytosis X. Bone density may help narrow the differential which includes increased (sclerotic metastases, lymphoma) and decreased (acute infection, osteoporosis)

Spondylolisthesis is the subluxation of one vertebral body on another and may be degenerative or due to bilateral pars defects (spondylosis). This is a fracture/defect of the posterior elements of the vertebrae. On an oblique view the posterior elements form a Scottie dog (with the pars making up the collar). This may be a purely incidental finding; however if severe it can result in neuroforaminal stenosis. Plain films are insensitive in the evaluation of disc disease. MRI is the investigation of choice for disc disease and its neurological complications.

1 – Soft tissue line closely applied to posterior aspect of the airway widens at level of laryngeal cartilage
2 – Anterior border of vertebral bodies
3 – Posterior border of vertebral bodies
4 – Spino laminar line = posterior limit of spinal canal
5 – Tips of the spinous processes

Fig. 13.41 Schematic diagram depicting the lines that need to be assessed when looking at a lateral film of the cervical spine.

Fig. 13.42 Saggital T2W image shows a large osteophyte at the C6/7 level.

Pelvis

Pelvic fractures are complex and there are many classification systems around. The pelvis should be regarded as being made up of three bony rings. The SI joints and pubic symphysis are part of the main bony ring. A fracture of one ring is frequently associated with a second ring fracture (Fig. 13.43).

- SI joints should be equal in width.
- The superior surfaces of the pubic rami should align. The joint width should be no more than 5mm.
- The sacral foramina should form a smooth arc.
- Acetabular fractures are subtle—look for symmetry.

Bone texture: the pelvis is a common site for metastatic involvement especially with urological malignancies, e.g. prostate (sclerotic metastases) and myeloma (multiple lytic lesions). Paget's disease of the pelvis may mimic sclerotic metastases but tends to be confined to one hemipelvis and may expand or thicken bone.

Sacroiliitis: SI joint involvement is common in the seronegative arthropathies and is usually symmetrical in conditions such as inflammatory bowel disease, ankylosing spondylitis and hyperparathyroidism. More asymmetrical change is seen in Reiter's disease and rheumatoid arthritis. It is characterised by initial erosion and widening of the joint resulting in chronic sclerosis which has a preferential involvement of the lower one-third of the joint (iliac >sacral side).

Avascular necrosis (AVN) of the femoral heads is an important finding but is often advanced when plain film findings are seen. Radiographically occult AVN may be detected on MRI or a bone scan. On plain x-ray it is characterised by sclerosis, flattening and fragmentation of the femoral head. Subchondral crescents are pathognomonic. AVN can also be a sequel of trauma, but bilateral AVN is seen in conjunction with steroid therapy, sickle cell disease and as part of Perthe's disease.

Fig. 13.43 The pelvis is made up of bony rings: the main pelvic ring and two smaller rings made up of the pubic and ischial bones.

Vascular intervention

Angiography is catheterisation of a vessel followed by subsequent opacification with a water-soluble iodine-containing contrast medium. Catheterisation is usually performed using the Seldinger technique.

Indications include

- Demonstration of arterial anatomy prior to surgery where this is likely to influence surgical management.
- To elucidate the nature of arterial disease, e.g. occlusions, stenoses, thrombi, aneurysms and vascular malformations.
- To identify the source of bleeding in the gastrointestinal tract.
- To demonstrate tumour circulation (often prior to embolisation).

Contrast

Volumes used are variable depending on the area being imaged. The contrast agents are iodinated, non-ionic and of low osmolarity, resulting in reduced toxicity. Nevertheless potential side effects include anaphylaxis, hypotension, urticaria and bronchospasm. Patients particularly at risk include those with a history of a previous reaction, iodine allergy and atopy. Nephrotoxicity is a potential risk and may be exacerbated by dehydration. Contrast reactions are seen in 1/1000 patients. Risk of anaphylaxis is 1/40,0000. Pre-medication with corticosteroids may reduce the incidence of reactions if contrast administration is essential, but this is not universally accepted.

Specific applications

These include pulmonary angiography (gold standard for detection of pulmonary emboli) which is highly invasive and therefore reserved for when thrombolysis or embolectomy are being considered. Cerebral angiography is useful in the diagnosis of aneurysms, AVMs, tumour vascularity and both intra- and extracranial vascular disease. Renal angiography is selectively performed to diagnose renal artery stenosis and prior to embolisation of tumours.

DSA (digital subtraction angiography) is a technique whereby there is subtraction of the contrast-containing shadows from the initial plain films (mask) resulting in an image containing opacified structures only. The resulting images may be digitised and manipulated. The overall advantage is smaller doses of contrast and smaller catheters may be used.

Therapeutic embolisation is used to selectively occlude arteries by introducing a variety of materials via a catheter. Materials used include metallic coil, gelatin foam and cyanoacrylate glue. This technique is used at active bleeding sites, and to reduce tumour vascularity pre-operatively in resectable tumours.

Vascular catheterisation is also used to selectively infuse vessels as with thrombolytic treatment or rarely with cytotoxics. Vascular stenting is of increasing use in coronary and peripheral vascular disease. IVC filters are percutaneously placed via the femoral vein in the treatment of patients with recurrent pulmonary emboli despite anticoagulation or where anticoagulation is contraindicated.

Fig. 13.44 Cavogram showing infra renal deployment of an IVC filter (Gunther–Tulip).

Interventional radiology

Interventional radiology is a sub-speciality where a variety of imaging modalities are used to guide percutaneous procedures. This may obviate alternative surgical procedures and consequently result in lower morbidity. Interventional procedures are usually carried out under local anaesthesia and on an outpatient basis, thereby considerably reducing bed occupancy. There is a huge range of procedures that are currently performed. The following is a limited list of some of them.

Percutaneous biopsy: biopsy needle placement may be done under fluoroscopy, CT, MRI and ultrasound. This provides non-operative confirmation of suspected malignancy and with the aid of a tissue diagnosis it is possible to accurately plan treatment. For histology a 14–18G needle is used. With a fine aspiration needle (20–22G) material may be obtained for cytology. Using imaging guidance, there is avoidance of damage to vital structures such as blood vessels, solid organs and bowel loops. With chest biopsy there is a small risk of pneumothorax.

Percutaneous drainage: with image guidance, surgical intervention may be avoided by accurate placement of a drainage catheter. Calibre varies from 8 to 14F depending on the nature of the underlying fluid. Regular irrigation of the catheter may be necessary to ensure successful drainage. Successful resolution may be impeded in the more complex and multiloculated collections.

Drainage of the urinary system can be via double J stents which are placed into an obstructed collecting system with the distal catheter tip lying in the bladder. More short-term drainage is achieved via a percutaneous nephrostomy. Here the obstructed kidney is punctured under fluoroscopic or ultrasound guidance and a catheter placed in the renal calyx (preferably lower pole). This is the technique of choice in the acutely obstructed or infected kidney.

Biliary system drainage: surgical outcome in patients with malignant bile duct obstruction is often poor. This may be due to carcinoma of the pancreas or cholangiocarcinoma. Biliary stenting alleviates obstruction and improves quality of life. Stenting may be performed at ERCP or percutaneously via antegrade puncture through the liver (PTC to delineate the anatomy being performed first). Other GI interventions include stenting/balloon dilatation of oesophageal strictures and percutaneous gastrostomy insertion.

TIPS (transjugular intrahepatic portosystemic stent shunt) is a procedure whereby a connection is made between the hepatic and portal veins to reduce portal pressure in patients with portal hypertension. The mortality is considerably lower than in acute shunt surgery, particularly in the context of an acute variceal bleed which has failed to respond to sclerotherapy.

Table 13.6

Established techniques	Newer interventional applications
Arterial and venous sampling	Arteriovenous malformation embolisation
Biliary drainage, stenting, angioplasty, biopsy, and stone extraction	Chemoembolisation
Diagnostic angiography	Cryoablation of liver tumours
Embolisation	
Oesophageal dilatation	Endovascular repair of abdominal aortic aneurysms with stent grafts
Fallopian tube recanalisation	Radiofrequency ablation of tumours
Feeding tube placement	Uterine artery embolisation for symptomatic fibroids
Inferior vena cava filter placement	Varicocoele embolisation
Nephrostomy placement	Vertebroplasty
Pain management (e.g. coeliac ganglion block, selective and nonselective nerve block)	
Percutaneous biopsy, cholecystostomy, and drainage of fluid collections	
Primary gastrostomy, gastrojejunostomy or jejunostomy tube placement	
Thrombolysis	
Transjugular intrahepatic portosystemic shunt insertion	
Ureteral stent placement	
Vascular angioplasty and stent placement	
Venous access and foreign body retrieval	

Endovascular repair of abdominal aortic aneurysms with stent grafts is a new image-guided, catheter-based approach that provides a valuable alternative to standard open surgical repair. Radiologic imaging plays an essential role in preprocedure evaluation, the procedure itself and patient follow-up. The ultimate goal remains the same—complete exclusion of the aneurysm sac to prevent rupture.

Radiofrequency ablation: not all patients with tumours are eligible for surgical intervention because of unfavourable location of the tumour, adverse clinical conditions or advanced disease. In addition, the cost, morbidity and mortality associated with surgical resection have led to the search for other forms of therapy. Newer, minimally invasive treatments include intra-arterial chemoembolisation, injection of ethanol and radiofrequency ablation. Among the thermal ablative procedures, radiofrequency ablation is one of the newest and most promising. For this procedure, ultrasound, CT scanning or magnetic resonance imaging (MRI) is used by the radiologist to guide percutaneous placement of long, thin (usually less than 18-gauge), insulated needles into the tumor. The distal end (1 to 3cm) of each needle is not insulated and emits radio waves. Electrodes are attached to a generator, and the electrical energy is converted to heat that kills cells through coagulation necrosis. The radiologist can vary the amount of current used, thereby tightly controlling the treatment radius. The entire treatment session usually lasts 1 hour and can be performed in the outpatient setting. The procedure is typically performed with conscious sedation and local anaesthesia.

Fig. 13.45 Obstructing sigmoid carcinoma has been decompressed with a colonic stent.

Fig. 13.46 Contrast-enhanced CT showing several high attenuation metastases overlying the dome of the liver.

Fig. 13.47 Radiofrequency ablation of the metastasis shows the electrode *in situ*.

Fig. 13.48 Pre-uterine artery embolisation (UFE). Selective catherisation shows the supply to a large left sided fibroid.

Fig. 13.49 Post-embolisation with PVA shows no flow in the previously demonstrated fibroid.

Hands

There are specific patterns that may be seen in the hand as an indicator of the underlying disorder. Some patterns are pathognomonic whereas others are more non-specific.

1. Generalised osteopenia: osteoporosis, multiple myeloma and rheumatoid arthritis.
2. Coarsening of the trabecular pattern is common in haemoglobinopathies especially thalassaemia and Gaucher's disease.
3. Periosteal reaction: (i) HPOA (hypertrophic pulmonary osteoarthropathy) associations include carcinoma of the bronchus, inflammatory bowel disease and coeliac disease, (ii) thyroid acropachy, most common on the radial side of the thumbs, and (iii) juvenile chronic arthritis seen in about 25%.
4. Carpal abnormalities include short metacarpals (Turner's syndrome, pseudo- and pseudopseudohypoparathyroidism), carpal fusion (inflammatory arthritis, RA and JCA, post-trauma), and look for syndactyly and polydactyly.
5. Soft tissue changes, e.g. increase in soft tissue thickness/size seen in acromegaly, localised increase seen in gouty tophi, nodes as in OA, soft tissue calcification seen in CREST and scleroderma.
6. Joint disease: the hand x-ray above all may help in sorting out the type of arthropathy and aid rheumatological management. The ABCS approach is invaluable (see Table 13.7).

Fig. 13.50 Asymmetric oligoarthritis with dominant involvement of the DIP joints. The pencil in cup appearance is typical.

Table 13.7

A: Alignment	Subluxation/dislocation common in rheumatoid arthritis and SLE
B: Bone	Osteoporosis: mineralisation is usually normal except in acute RA Erosions: – Aggressive (i.e. no sclerosis of margins) seen in RA and psoriasis – Non-aggressive (with sclerotic margins) seen in gout; inflammatory erosions are marginal (OA erosions are central); distinguish from subperiosteal resorption (radial border, seen in hyperparathyroidism) Bone production: periosteal new bone formation, psoriasis, Reiter's syndrome: – Ankylosis (bony bridging) in inflammatory arthropathies – Overhanging cortex (typical of gout) – Osteophyte formation, OA
C: Cartilage	Joint space has uniform narrowing in all arthritis except OA which is eccentric Wide joint space in early arthritis, gout and PVNS
S: Soft tissues	*Swelling* Symmetric around joint space commonest in RA Asymmetric usually due to osteophytes and therefore commonest in OA Lumpy bumpy soft tissue swelling: gouty tophi Diffuse swelling of digits: psoriasis, Reiter's *Calcification* Soft tissues: gouty tophi Cartilage: pseudogout, pyrophosphate arthropathy Subcutaneous tissue: scleroderma

Trauma

Two views are essential for ensuring no subtle injuries are missed. On a PA view the spaces between the carpal bones and the carpometacarpal articulations should be roughly equal (1–2mm). If a dislocation is present then there is obliteration/overlap. Common injuries include Bennett's fracture, a first metacarpal base injury extending into the joint surface with dislocation at the carpometacarpal joint. Scaphoid fractures are the most common (75–90%) of carpal injuries. Because of the blood supply there is a potential risk of osteonecrosis of the proximal pole.

Neuroradiology

- CT is the initial study for evaluation of neuropathology due to its speed, availability and lower cost.
- Excellent for evaluation of bony abnormality.
- Done both with and without intravenous contrast depending on clinical indication. The use of contrast delineates vascular structures and anomalies.
- Visualisation of the posterior fossa is inferior to MRI.

Logical approach to interpretation

- Soft tissues.
- Bone.
- Cortical parenchyma.
- Ventricular system.
- Symmetry.
- Falx shift.

Rule out skull fracture, extradural haematoma (lentiform shape), subdural haematoma (crescentic shape), subarachnoid haemorrhage, space occupying lesions, hydrocephalus and cerebral oedema. Look for target lesions (when contrast given): metastases, abscesses and fungal infections.

Cerebral angiography

Evaluation of vascular lesions including atherosclerotic disease, aneurysms, vascular malformations. Supplements information obtained on CT/MRI regarding tumour vascularity. Used for guidance of interventional procedures such as embolisation.

CVA

Imaging may be negative in the first 6 hours. Thereafter look for
- Oedema (loss of grey—white differentiation, sulcal effacement and mass effect).
- Within 24 hours there will be a low density wedge shaped area corresponding to the vascular territory and extending to the cortical surface.
- Acute haemorrhage seen if there is haemorrhagic transformation (white = acute blood).

Multiple sclerosis

MRI is the modality of choice and is highly sensitive. There can be overlap with other entities such as ischaemia and confluent disease may simulate neoplastic mass lesions. T2W MRI shows ovoid high signal lesions in a peri ventricular distribution. Active lesions show enhancement following gadolinium.

Fig. 13.51 Non-contrast CT head showing extensive subarachnoid haemorrhage in patient with underlying cerebral aneurysm (not shown).

Fig. 13.52 Axial T2W MRI showing multiple high signal lesions iin the deep white matter of the right frontal lobe in patient with lung carcinoma. The anterior lesion is cystic. These are consistent with metastases. Note the surrounding oedema.

Skull x-ray

Indications
The main indication is acute trauma although SXRs are of limited use. Occasionally the SXR is obtained as part of a skeletal survey in evaluation of metabolic bone disease, endocrine disorders and in the assessment of metastatic disease. It is still used in assessment of sinus disease and in evaluation of the post-operative skull.

Contraindications
None, but if there is suspicion of underlying intracranial injury plain films are unnecessary (see *below*).

Normal findings
The bones of the skull vault have an inner and outer table of compact bone with spongy diploe between the two. Sutures are visible even after fusion and should not be mistaken for fractures. Blood vessels may cause impressions, as can small lucencies in the inner table near the vertex caused by normal arachnoid granulations which can be mistaken for small lytic lesions.

Trauma: skull x-rays are basic, widely available and yet potentially yield the least information in the context of trauma. The presence or absence of a skull fracture does not correlate with the presence or extent of any intracranial injury. Up to 50% of films may be technically unsatisfactory due to factors such as poor patient cooperation. With the advent of CT this is the technique of choice for evaluation in acute injury and neuro-logical deficit. It allows a firm diagnosis to be made and excludes other alternate diagnoses.

Fractures and associated findings: basic radiographs include a lateral projection (obtained with a horizontal beam) and a further tangential projection, depending on the site of injury.

Findings include
- A linear fracture: well-defined margins, no branching and no sclerosis (*cf.* vascular markings or sutures which have an undulating course and sclerotic margins).
- A depressed fracture: increased density due to overlapping bone; those that are depressed by >5mm may lacerate the dura or cause parenchymal injury and therefore need elevation.
- A fluid level/pneumocephalus: implies an associated basal skull fracture or dural tear.

Note: pineal displacement is an inconstant finding and is not a reliable method of assessing the presence of intracranial injury.

Abnormal findings
Look for intracranial calcification, then examine the pituitary fossa, review bony density and look for focal areas of lysis and sclerosis.
- Intracranial calcification: the majority is normal and of no clinical signifi-cance. However it may be of pathological significance; causes include

primary tumours such as meningiomas, craniopharyngiomas,
arteriovenous malformations, tuberose sclerosis and infections such
as toxoplasmosis.

- Raised intracranial pressure: in practice plain film changes are only seen
  if the condition is long standing. These include sutural widening
  (diastasis) and erosion of the lamina dura of the pituitary fossa.
- Enlargement of the pituitary fossa (normal dimensions: height 6–11mm,
  length 9–16mm). Expansion will result in a double floor, loss of the
  lamina dura and elevation/destruction of the clinoid processes. The
  vast majority of the lesions will be pituitary adenomas; other causes
  include meningiomas and aneurysms.
- Bone lysis: may be diffuse as in metastasis or myeloma. Large areas of
  bone destruction are seen in histiocytosis X and in the active phase of
  Paget's disease (osteoporosis circumscripta).
- Bone sclerosis: may be localised as in meningiomas, depressed skull
  fractures or generalised as in Paget's sclerotic metastases, myeloma
  and fluorosis.
- Sutural widening: may be due to raised intracranial pressure, infiltration
  by malignancy (neuroblastoma or lymphoma) or defective ossification
  as in rickets.

Fig. 13.53 Lateral SXR showing 'hair on end' appearance in thalassaemia major.

Reference section

Table 13.8 Abbreviations used in radiology

AP	Anteroposterior
AXR	Abdominal x-ray
CT	Computed tomography
CXR	Chest x-ray
IVU	Intravenous urogram
MRI	Magnetic resonance imaging
PA	Posteroanterior
USS	Ultrasound scan
V/Q	Ventilation perfusion scan

Management of adverse reactions to intravascular contrast agents

Table 13.9

Symptoms	Treatment
Nausea/vomiting	Reassurance
Urticaria	Antihistamine chlorpheniramine maleate 10–20mg by slow IV injection (0.2mg/kg body weight paediatric dose)
Angio-oedema	Adrenaline(epinephrine) 0.5–1mL 1:10,000 IV
Bronchospasm	IV hydrocortisone 100mg
Hypotension	β_2-agonist by nebuliser O_2, IV access and IV fluids

Order of appearance of ossification centres of the elbow

The order of appearance is more important than the absolute age of appearance which varies widely. Remember 'CRITOE'.

Table 13.10

	Approximate average age (years)
Capitellum	1
Radial head	3–6
Internal (medial) epicondyle	4
Trochlea	8
Olecranon	9
External (lateral) epicondyle	10

Epiphyseal plate fractures: the Salter Harris classification (SALTR)

- *Type I*: epiphyseal slip separates it from physis (5–6%). S = slip of physis.
- *Type II*: fracture line extends into metaphysis (50–75%). A = above physis.
- *Type III*: the epiphysis is vertically split, i.e. the equivalent of an intra-articular fracture (8%). L = lower than physis.
- *Type IV*: fracture involves the metaphysis, epiphysis and physis (8–12%). T = through physis.
- *Type V*: crush injury with vascular compromise, i.e. poor prognosis for growth (1%). R = rammed physis.

Internet resources

National Radiological Protection Board
For issues regarding radiation safety:
⌁🖰www.nrpb.org

Royal College of Radiologists
For information relating to radiological issues, guidelines in clinical management, training and publications:
⌁🖰www.rcr.ac.uk

MRI safety and compatibility
⌁🖰www.mrisafety.com

Radiological Society of North America
⌁🖰www.rsna.org

American College of Radiology
Incorporates guidelines for use of contrast media, practice guidelines as well as information on technical standards (e.g. teleradiology):
⌁🖰www.acr.org

British Institute of Radiology
⌁🖰www.bir.org

Nuclear medicine

Introduction to nuclear medicine 728
Bone scintigraphy: bone scan 730
Reticuloendothelial system: bone marrow scintigraphy 732
Cerebral blood flow imaging 734
Brain receptor imaging 736
CSF shunt patency 738
Thyroid scintigraphy 740
Parathyroid scintigraphy 742
MIBG (meta iodobenzylguanidine) imaging 744
Somatostatin receptor scintigraphy 746
Radioiodine thyroid cancer imaging 748
Sentinel node imaging 750
Scintimammography 752
Positron emission tomography (PET) 754
Myocardial perfusion imaging: MPI 758
Radionuclide ventriculography: MUGA scans 762
Radionuclide first pass cardiac studies 764
Lung scan: ventilation/perfusion imaging 766
Lung shunt studies 770
Lung permeability studies 771
Lymphoscintigraphy 772
Static cortical renography: DMSA imaging 774
Dynamic renography 776
Captopril renography 778
Gastrointestinal bleeding: labelled red cell imaging 780
Gastric emptying studies 782
Meckel's scan: ectopic gastric mucosa localisation 784
Hepatobiliary scintigraphy 785
Splenunculus detection: heat-damaged red cell imaging 786
Hepatosplenic scintigraphy 787
Labelled leucocyte imaging 788
Gallium scintigraphy 790
Dacroscintigraphy 791
Glomerular filtration rate measurement 792
Urea breath test 793
B_{12} absorption studies 794
Ferrokinetic studies 795
Red cell survival studies 796
Red cell volume/plasma volume measurement 797
Bile salt deconjugation studies 798

Introduction to nuclear medicine

Nuclear medicine techniques employ a carrier molecule, selected to target the organ/tissue of interest, tagged with a gamma-emitting radio-isotope. The labelled drug (radiopharmaceutical) is given PO or IV. Its distribution is mapped *in vivo* using a gamma camera or, for non-imaging tests, *in vitro* using a radiation counter.

Nuclear medicine procedures detect the earliest physiological response to disease processes, generally before structural changes have taken place. Scintigraphy is often more sensitive than conventional radiology in early disease. Specificity varies depending on the radiopharmaceutical used and characterisation of abnormalities relies upon pattern recognition within a particular clinical setting. Anatomical detail is poor compared with conventional radiology, although tomographic cameras generate high resolution 3D images.

Nuclear medicine procedures are non-invasive and allow the whole body to be imaged during a single examination. Absorbed radiation doses depend on the radiopharmaceutical used but are usually in the same range as diagnostic radiology. Pregnancy is an absolute contraindication to nuclear medicine examinations except where likely clinical benefit far outweighs potential risk—e.g. lung perfusion imaging. Some radiopharmaceuticals are excreted in breast milk and additional precautions may be advisable for lactating women.

Diagnostic radiopharmaceuticals are used in tracer quantities and toxicity is negligible. Individual hypersensitivity reactions are rare.

Specific information required when requesting nuclear medicine tests includes
- Patient identification details.
- Examination requested.
- Relevant clinical history including results of other investigations.
- Pregnancy/lactation details where relevant.
- Special needs—visual/hearing/learning difficulties; needle phobia.

Bone scintigraphy: bone scan

Background
Nuclear medicine investigations supplement the anatomical information obtained from radiology. Bone scintigraphy is sensitive, with changes frequently detected earlier than on plain film, but non-specific. It plays a pivotal role in the staging of patients with malignant disease and in difficult orthopaedic cases. May be restricted to 'local views' only, e.g. loose hip prosthesis, or 'whole body imaging' in metastatic screening. Can include a dynamic phase image at the time of isotope administration in addition to the delayed, bone phase image 2–4h post-injection. Dynamic phase reflects blood flow to the site of interest—useful when there is concern over vascularity, infection or recent trauma. Helps to differentiate soft-tissue from bone pathology e.g. cellulitis *vs*. osteomyelitis.

The ^{99m}Tc-polyphosphonate complex used to target the skeleton is renally excreted. Patients with poor renal function may need delayed imaging to improve the bone:soft tissue ratio.

Indications
- Tumour staging—assess skeletal metastases.
- Bone pain.
- Trauma—when radiographs unhelpful.
- Prosthetic loosening, e.g. THR.
- Infection.
- Avascular necrosis (AVN).
- Paget's disease to assess extent.

Patient preparation
Should be well-hydrated and continent.

Procedure
Inject ^{99m}Tc-phosphate complex IV. For suspected AVN or sepsis, image immediately to assess vascularity. Otherwise, image 2–4h later. Whole body views are required for metastatic screening. Tomography improves anatomical definition and detection of small lesions e.g. osteoid osteoma.

Results
- Radiopharmaceutical uptake reflects osteoblastic activity.
- Focal ↑ uptake in sclerotic metastases, trauma or infection.
- Diffuse ↑ uptake associated with advanced metastases, Paget's and metabolic bone disease.
- ↑ uptake in acute AVN and lytic bone metastases.

Interpretation
Sensitive but non-specific. Interpretation relies on pattern recognition in the clinical setting.

Advantages
Sensitive—detects early changes in bone physiology, often before abnormal plain radiographs, e.g. occult trauma, metastases and sepsis.

Pitfalls
False −ves in multiple myeloma. Artefacts due to urine contamination.

Fig. 14.1 Normal whole body ^{99m}Tc phosphate bone scan.

Fig. 14.2 Bone scan showing extensive metastases.

Fig. 14.3 Bone scan showing Paget's disease affecting the right hemipelvis and distal femur.

Reticuloendothelial system: bone marrow scintigraphy

Background
Largely superseded by magnetic resonance imaging (MRI). Colloid particles are cleared from the circulating blood pool by reticuloendothelial tissue—larger particles → liver and spleen; smaller particles → bone marrow. Abnormal uptake pattern where bone marrow is replaced, e.g. by tumour infiltration.

Indications
- Suspected malignant marrow infiltration.
- Equivocal conventional bone imaging.
- Osteomyelitis (rarely used).

Patient preparation
None.

Procedure
- ^{99m}Tc nanocolloid injected IV.
- Whole body gamma camera imaging at 30–45min.

Results
Normal marrow distribution in thoracic cage, spine, pelvis and proximal long bones. Homogeneous uptake in liver and spleen.

Interpretation
- Focal or generalised ↓ skeletal uptake indicates marrow replacement or infiltration with marrow displacement to distal femora and humeri.
- Heterogeneous hepatic uptake is abnormal but non-specific.

Advantages
Non-invasive. Avoids sampling errors compared with bone marrow biopsy.

Pitfalls
False −ves in early malignancy. Liver and spleen uptake may obscure abnormalities in the mid spine.

Smith FW. (1998) The skeletal system, *Practical Nuclear Medicine*, 2nd edition, eds Sharp PF, Gemmel HG, Smith FW, Oxford University Press, Oxford.

Cerebral blood flow imaging

Background
Used to study acute and chronic cerebrovascular disease, dementias and epilepsy using a radiolabelled lipophilic amine hexamethyl-propylene-amine-oxime or exametazine (HMPAO) which crosses the blood–brain barrier and fixes in the cerebral cortex and basal ganglia. Uptake is proportional to blood flow, with high accumulation in cortical grey matter, compared to white matter. Images reported with CT/MRI correlation to ensure appropriate interpretation *cf.* normal variants of cerebral asymmetry.

Indications
- Dementia characterisation.
- Epilepsy for localisation of epileptogenic focus.

Patient preparation
Secure venous access under resting conditions. Allow the patient to relax before injection of the radiopharmaceutical. Ensure that the patient can cooperate with the imaging procedure.

Procedure
- ^{99m}Tc-HMPAO (exametazine) injected IV in quiet, darkened room, with patient's eyes closed.
- Tomographic brain imaging undertaken immediately and again 4h later.

Results
Cortical grey matter uptake is proportional to blood flow.

Interpretation
- Characteristic patterns of abnormal uptake recognised in different dementias and in cerebrovascular disease.
- ↑ uptake at epileptogenic focus on interictal scans—often changing to ↑ uptake on ictal imaging.

Advantages
Abnormalities on functional imaging should predate structural atrophy on anatomical imaging.

Pitfalls
- Tomographic image analysis degraded by movement artefact and asymmetric positioning.
- Data processing is operator-dependent.

(a)

(b)

Fig. 14.4 ^{99m}Tc-HMPAO brain imaging. Transaxial tomographic slices: (a) normal and (b) dementia. (**Colour plate 7**.)

Brain receptor imaging

Background
Reflect role of dopamine and dopamine receptors in movement disorders, e.g. Parkinsonian syndromes, essential tremor. Post-synaptic receptor imaging agents are necessary to differentiate between the various Parkinsonian syndromes.

Indications
Movement disorders: distinguishes Parkinson's syndrome (PS) from benign essential tremor.

Patient preparation
- Block thyroid—potassium iodate/iodide.
- Multiple potential drug interactions—*stop*:
  - Amphetamine.
  - Benztropine.
  - Biperidin.
  - Citalopram.
  - Cocaine.
  - Fluoxetine.
  - Fluvoxamine.
  - Mazindol.
  - Methylphenidate.
  - Orphenadrine.
  - Phentermine.
  - Procyclidine.
  - Sertraline.

Procedure
^{123}I-labelled radiotracer, e.g. ioflupane injected IV. Tomographic gamma camera imaging 3–6h later.

Results
Intense, symmetric uptake in basal ganglia receptors—striatum, caudate and putamen.

Interpretation
↓ basal ganglia uptake in PS.

Advantages
Sensitive and specific for PS, differentiating PS from essential tremor. No other imaging technique currently available to demonstrate receptor status.

Pitfalls
Drug interactions (*above*).

(a)

(b)

Fig. 14.5 ^{123}I-ioflupane brain receptor imaging: (a) normal dopamine receptors and (b) in Parkinson's disease. (**Colour plate 8**.)

Booij J, Harbraken JBA, Bergmans P et al. (1998) Imaging of dopamine transporters with I[-123] FP CIT in healthy controls and patients with Parkinson's disease. J Nucl Med **40**, 1091–1097; Benamer H et al. (2000) Accurate differentiation of parkinsonism and essential tremor using visual assessment of ^{123}I FP CIT spect imaging. The ^{123}I FP CIT Study Group Writing Committee. Movement Disorders **15**, 503–510.

CSF shunt patency

Background
Ventricular shunts are routinely used to manage hydrocephalus. Symptoms of shunt obstruction may be non-specific and do not indicate the level of obstruction. Nuclear medicine offers a straightforward means of determining shunt patency.

Indications
Suspected VP shunt obstruction.

Patient preparation
None.

Procedure
Inject ^{99m}Tc-DTPA or ^{111}In-DTPA into shunt reservoir using strict aseptic technique. Image head and abdomen immediately and 30–60min post injection.

Results
Normally, rapid reservoir emptying and shunt visualisation within 2–3min of injection. Free activity within abdominal cavity by 30min.

Interpretation
Delayed clearance implies obstruction—level usually at reservoir/proximal shunt or due to intra-abdominal kinking.

Advantages
Sensitive, simple, rapid results.

Pitfalls
Infection risk.

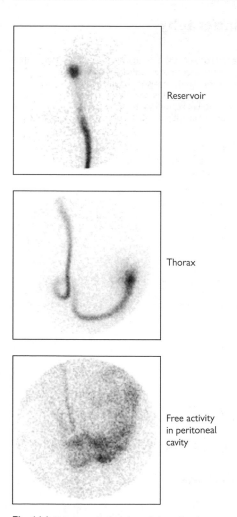

Reservoir

Thorax

Free activity
in peritoneal
cavity

Fig. 14.6 Patent ventriculoperitoneal shunt showing reservoir, shunt and
free activity within the peritoneal cavity.

Thyroid scintigraphy

Background

Used to investigate thyrotoxicosis and thyroid ectopia. Thyroid mass or suspected malignancy should be investigated by ultrasound/CT and fine needle aspiration cytology. Imaging is undertaken using ^{99m}Tc-pertechnetate which is trapped by the thyroid by the same transporter mechanism as iodine, but unlike iodine, is not organified. ^{123}I is more sensitive and specific for the investigation of congenital hypothyroidism.

Indications

- Characterisation of thyrotoxicosis—diffuse toxic goitre (Graves' disease), toxic multinodular goitre (Plummer's disease).
- Solitary autonomous nodule.
- Acute thyroiditis.

Patient preparation

Thyroxine and iodine rich preparations, e.g. iodine supplements, contrast media, amiodarone will block tracer uptake by the thyroid for up to 9 months. T4 should be withdrawn for 6 weeks; T3 for 2 weeks. Anti-thyroid drugs can be continued.

Procedure

Inject ^{99m}Tc-pertechnetate IV. Image after 15–30min. Include anterior thorax views if retrosternal extension is suspected. Neck palpation essential to assess function in discrete thyroid nodules. ^{123}I may be administered either orally or IV. Imaging is carried out at 2h.

Results

- Uptake reflects function of the thyroid iodine trap.
- Diffuse ↑ uptake in Graves' disease.
- Heterogeneous uptake with suppressed background activity indicates toxic multinodular change.
- Solitary autonomous nodules show intense increased uptake with complete suppression of the remainder of the gland.
- Acute thyroiditis is characterised by absent tracer uptake.

Interpretation

Sensitive and specific for hyperthyroidism.

Advantages

Simple, cheap and non-invasive. Essential to planning therapy in hyper-thyroidism.

Pitfalls

Anatomical definition inferior to ultrasound, CT etc. Superseded by ultra-sound guided FNA for diagnosis of thyroid mass lesions.

(a)

(b)

Fig. 14.7 Thyroid scintigraphy: (a) in Graves' disease and (b) in toxic multi-nodular goitre.

Parathyroid scintigraphy

Background
Hyperparathyroidism may be primary, i.e. functioning adenoma; secondary—where there is hypocalcaemia from chronic lowering of serum calcium, e.g. renal insufficiency; or tertiary, i.e. hypersecretion of PTH in the presence of either normal or elevated levels of calcium. Nuclear medicine is of value in localising parathyroid adenomas, particularly following previous surgery.

Indications
Localisation of parathyroid adenoma in proven hyperparathyroidism.

Patient preparation
Withdraw thyroxine or iodine containing compounds (*cf.* thyroid imaging).

Procedure
3 different techniques are available:
1. ^{123}I iodide IV followed by ^{99m}Tc sestamibi, *or*
2. ^{99m}Tc sestamibi IV 5min and 4h delayed images, *or*
3. ^{99m}Tc pertechnetate followed by ^{201}thallous chloride.

Image anterior neck and mediastinum after each administration.

Results
Normal thyroid concentrates ^{123}I, ^{99m}Tc pertechnetate, ^{99m}Tc sestamibi and ^{210}Tl whereas parathyroid only concentrates ^{99m}Tc sestamibi and ^{201}Tl.

Computer assisted image subtraction [(thyroid + parathyroid) − thyroid] identifies abnormal parathyroid tissue.

Interpretation
Parathyroid adenoma shown as hyperfunctioning nodule(s).

Advantages
Good when other imaging fails, particularly ectopic adenomas and after unsuccessful neck exploration.

Pitfalls
Multinodular thyroid prevents subtraction analysis. False −ves in multiple parathyroid adenomata or hyperplasia. Many surgeons still prefer intra-operative blue dye.

Fig. 14.8 Parathyroid scintigraphy showing images obtained with both ^{123}I and ^{99m}Tc sestamibi.

MIBG (meta iodobenzylguanidine) imaging

Background

Neuroendocrine tumours are rare. Symptoms reflect hormone hyper-secretion but intermittent secretory patterns can result in false negative screening tests e.g. 24h urine collections. MIBG is concentrated by adrenergic tissue via the noradrenaline reuptake mechanism. Virtually all phaeochromocytomas and neuroblastomas will be demonstrated using ^{123}I-mIBG scintigraphy. The sensitivity for other neuroendocrine tumours is variable. High dose ^{131}I-MIBG therapy is a useful treatment for MIBG +ve neuroendocrine tumours.

Indications

- Localisation, staging and response monitoring of neuroectodermal tumours.
- Phaeochromocytoma (imaging investigation of choice).
- Neuroblastoma.
- Carcinoid tumours.
- Medullary thyroid cancer.

Patient preparation

- Multiple known and theoretical drug interactions. *Stop for >48h:*
  - Antidepressants: tricyclics, tetracyclics, MAOIs, serotonin reuptake inhibitors.
  - Phenothiazines.
  - Labetolol*.
  - L-dopa, dopamine agonists.
  - Sympathomimetics—including OTC nasal decongestants.
- Block thyroid—potassium iodate/iodide; perchlorate.

*No interaction with any other α or β blocker or antihypertensive.

Procedure

Inject ^{123}I MIBG slowly IV with blood pressure monitoring. Image posterior abdomen at 5min to identify renal outlines, then whole body imaging at 18–24h. Tomographic imaging may improve tumour localisation—not always required.

Results

Physiological uptake at 24h in salivary glands, myocardium, liver and normal adrenals with gut and renal excretion.

Interpretation

- Intense ↑ uptake in phaeochromocytomas, with suppressed activity in the contralateral, normal adrenal and myocardium. Whole body imaging identifies extra adrenal and metastatic disease.
- Diffuse bone marrow uptake common in stage IV neuroblastoma.

Advantages

Sensitive, non-invasive tumour localisation pre-operatively excludes multi-focal and extra-adrenal tumours. Non-invasive treatment response monitoring in neuroblastoma—avoids sampling errors compared with bone marrow biopsy.

Pitfalls

Drug interactions causing false −ve results. Dilated renal pelvis sometimes confused with tumour uptake. Check with 5min renal image if in doubt.

Anterior

Posterior

(a)

(b)

Fig. 14.9 ^{123}I-MIBG scan: (a) right intra-adrenal phaeochromocytoma; (b) whole body scan—right intra-adrenal phaeochromocytoma. Excludes multifocal, ectopic and malignant tumour. **(Colour plate 9.)**

Somatostatin receptor scintigraphy

Background

Somatostatin receptor (SSR) imaging identifies neuroendocrine tumours including gastroenteropancreatic tumours e.g. carcinoids, gastrinomas, insulinomas. Many other common neoplasms also express surface somatostatin receptors. Somatostatin analogues, e.g. octreotide, bind to cell surface somatostatin receptors. Radiolabelled SSR analogues demonstrate receptor positive disease. Sub-centimetre (i.e. below the limits of cross-sectional radiology) hyperfunctioning primary tumours can be detected. High-dose radiolabelled SSR therapy is used to treat multi-site disease.

Indications

Localise and stage neuroendocrine tumours (NETs), e.g. carcinoid, insulinoma, gastrinoma, phaeochromocytoma, and medullary thyroid cancer.

Patient preparation

None. Prophylactic laxatives at time of radiopharmaceutical administration accelerate gut clearance and improve image quality.

Procedure

Inject ^{111}Indium labelled SSR analogue (octreotide or lanreotide) IV. Whole body gamma camera imaging at 24 ± 48h, with tomography if necessary.

Results

Normal uptake in thyroid, liver, spleen, kidneys and RE system with gut and renal excretion.

Interpretation

↑ uptake in tumours expressing surface somatostatin receptors. Tomography improves detection of small pancreatic and intra hepatic tumours.

Advantages

Tumour uptake predicts symptom response to somatostatin analogue therapy. Image co-registration with CT or MRI improves localisation of occult pancreatic NETs.

Pitfalls

Interpretation often hindered by gut excretion.

Fig. 14.10 Whole body ¹¹¹In-octreotide scan showing neuroectodermal tumour with hepatic metastases. (**Colour plate 10**.)

Radioiodine thyroid cancer imaging

Background

The primary treatment for thyroid carcinoma is total thyroidectomy with lymph node dissection, depending on tumour stage. Radioactive iodine is administered postoperatively to ablate the thyroid remnant. Thyroglobulin (Tg) can then be used as a tumour marker—Tg is undetectable in the absence of functioning thyroid tissue. Rising Tg following ^{131}I ablation indicates recurrence. If Tg rises, a diagnostic ^{131}I imaging study localises the site of relapse and assess the feasibility of further radio iodine therapy. The sensitivity of imaging is increased by recombinant TSH stimulation.

Indications

Routine differentiated follicular thyroid cancer follow up, after surgery and ^{131}I thyroid remnant ablation.

Patient preparation

Need high TSH drive to stimulate ^{131}I uptake—stop T3/T4 replacement for minimum 2 (T3) or 6 weeks (T4) or give recombinant TSH. Avoid iodine administration, IV contrast media, amiodarone (cf. thyroid imaging).

Procedure

Give ^{131}I sodium iodide PO/IV. Obtain blood samples for Tg and TSH at the time of ^{131}I administration. Whole body gamma camera imaging 2–5d later.

Results

Physiological uptake in salivary glands. Occasional stomach and GI retention. Renal excretion.

Interpretation

Abnormal uptake indicates functioning thyroid metastasis. Anatomical markers improve localisation.

Advantages

Detects residual tumour and identifies patients likely to benefit from ^{131}I therapy.

Pitfalls

False −ves without significant TSH drive—aim for TSH >50mU/L; undifferentiated and papillary tumours may be ^{131}I negative.

Fig. 14.11 Anterior whole body ^{131}I image showing local tumour recurrence in the thyroid bed and mediastinum.

Sentinel node imaging

Background
Regional lymph node dissection is performed for cancer staging, to determine the need for adjuvant therapy. Lymphatic drainage can be demonstrated by radiolabelled colloid imaging which identifies the first or 'sentinel' draining node. Staging based on the excision and histological examination of this node for evidence of metastasis is as reliable as that obtained from block dissection and avoids the morbidity of extended lymph node dissection.

Indications
Pre-operative assessment in breast cancer and melanoma. May have applications in head and neck, vulval and penile cancer staging.

Patient preparation
None. Usually undertaken within 24h of planned surgery.

Procedure
Intradermal, subcutaneous or intratumoural injection of ^{99m}Tc labelled nanocolloid. Gamma camera imaging of draining lymph nodes to identify sentinel node. Where surgery is undertaken within 24h, an intraoperative gamma probe can be used to identify the sentinel node for staging excision biopsy.

Results
Sentinel node usually identifiable 15min to 2h post-injection, depending on the primary tumour location and injection technique used.

Interpretation
The sentinel node is the first lymph node identified on gamma imaging or the node with the highest radioactive count rate using the gamma probe.

Advantages
Accurate sentinel node identification avoids block node dissection, where this is undertaken solely for tumour staging.

Pitfalls
May fail if local lymphatic channels have been disrupted by previous surgery.

Fig. 14.12 ^{99m}Tc-nanocolloid sentinel node study—anterior thorax, right arm abducted. Peri-tumoural, subcutaneous injection right breast and sentinel node (arrow). (**Colour plate 11**.)

Scintimammography

Breast cancer diagnosis relies on accurate localization (ultrasound ± mammography) and tissue biopsy (fine needle aspirate (FNA) or core biopsy). Where mammography is non-diagnostic MRI, CT or ^{18}FDG PET/CT are useful. Nuclear medicine scintimammography is as sensitive but more specific than MRI and mammography in palpable lesions.

Indications
Investigation of suspicious breast lesions, in difficult-to-interpret mammograms, e.g. dense or lumpy breast tissue, calcification, breast implants, previous surgery.

Patient preparation
None.

Procedure
1. ^{99m}Tc-sestamibi administered IV ideally into contralateral foot, with early (5–10min) imaging post-injection.
2. Patient is imaged prone, with breast fully dependent, with prone and lateral views of each breast, to include axillae.

Results
Normal distribution of ^{99m}Tc-sestamibi is to the myocardium, liver and occasionally thyroid.

Interpretation
Focal accumulation in breast and/or axilla implies the presence of tumour. Findings should be interpreted in conjunction with other tests.

Advantages
Can demonstrate multifocal, multicentric disease, both ipsilateral and contralateral axillary spread. May be used to identify most suitable site for guided biopsy.

Pitfalls
Not reliable in small (<1cm) lesions; extravasation of injection in upper limbs may result in false-positive axillary uptake.

Pitfalls
Poor injection technique will lead to errors in analysis. The camera and supporting software require high count rate capability and the technique require expertise in data analysis to ensure reliable, reproducible results. Close liaison with referring clinician is essential to maximise value of the investigation.

Buscombe J, Hill J, Parbhoo S. (1998) *Scintimammography. A Guide to Good Practice*. Gibbs Associates Ltd.; Murray IPC, Ell PJ (eds). (1994) *Nuclear Medicine in Clinical Diagnosis and Treatment*. Chapter 101 (Vol 2). Churchill Livingstone.

Positron emission tomography (PET)

PET is developing rapidly. Tomographic PET images are acquired using a dedicated PET scanner after administration of positron emitting radiopharmaceuticals. Spatial resolution (5–7mm) is significantly superior to conventional nuclear medicine imaging.

PET images biologically important molecules such as radiolabelled water, ammonia, amino acids or glucose derivatives—the glucose analogue ^{18}F-fluorodeoxyglucose (^{18}FDG) is used for most clinical PET studies, particularly in oncology. Malignant cells have both a higher glycolytic rate and overexpression of membrane glucose transporters leading to high ^{18}FDG uptake compared to normal tissues. ^{18}FDG is trapped within metabolically active cells so that abnormalities are detected by metabolic differences rather than anatomical size i.e. inherently more sensitive than structure based imaging.

The main indications for PET imaging are in oncology where ^{18}FDG PET is used for diagnosis, staging and monitoring treatment response. Low grade uptake occurs in granulomatous disease, inflammation and sepsis.

PET allows radioactive concentrations within tissues to be measured accurately so that physiological processes can be expressed in absolute units. The standardised uptake value (SUV) measures the concentration of tracer within a tumour compared to the injected activity, normalised to body weight. Serial SUV measurements allow ^{18}FDG uptake to be followed as a marker of treatment response and may be of prognostic value.

Other major applications include nuclear cardiology, where patterns of myocardial ^{18}FDG uptake are used to detect myocardial hibernation. In neurosciences, PET remains a largely research tool for the investigation of movement disorders, dementia and degenerative disease.

Other tracers that are available for clinical use include ^{11}C methionine, measuring tumour amino acid transport and protein synthesis and $H_2^{15}O$ water for blood flow measurements. Future developments will include labelled thymidine analogues to measure proliferation, hypoxic markers and tracers capable of detecting apoptosis and angiogenesis.

The main limitation of PET imaging in oncology is limited anatomical definition. To improve attenuation correction and tomographic localisation, PET imaging is usually combined with low dose CT. The combination of functional and anatomical data in fused images significantly improves the sensitivity and specificity of imaging. Future developments may involve combined PET/magnetic resonance imaging.

Indications

- Tumour diagnosis—solitary pulmonary nodule characterisation; location of carcinoma of unknown primary origin.
- Tumour staging—non small cell lung cancer; lymphoma; oesophageal cancer; colorectal cancer; head and neck cancer; melanoma.
- Response assessment/relapse detection—as above.

Patient preparation
- Cellular ^{18}FDG uptake is glucose-dependent.
  - Non-diabetic patients—6h fast.
  - Aim for blood glucose <7mmol/L.
  - Insulin-dependent diabetic patients—allow normal diet and insulin.
  - Avoid hyperglycaemia—use sliding scale if necessary or defer investigation.
- Patients should be rested—to avoid skeletal muscle uptake.
- Diazepam administration 5mg PO reduces physiological brown fat uptake in young patients.
- Patients with head and neck cancer should be silent during injection and until completion of imaging to prevent vocal chord uptake.

Procedure
- ^{18}FDG injected IV supine in restful surroundings.
- Whole body or half body (base of skull to proximal femora) imaging undertaken 60–90min post-injection.

Results
The normal distribution of ^{18}FDG is to the brain and myocardium with gastrointestinal and renal excretion.

0 deg

Fig. 14.13 Normal ^{18}FDG PET scan—coronal tomogram.

Interpretation
Abnormal uptake should be correlated with cross-sectional imaging for precise anatomical localisation. SUV (see *above*) measurement helpful in serial studies.

Advantages
- Discriminates between viable and necrotic/scar tissue where a residual mass may persist on anatomical imaging post-therapy.
- Non-invasive, whole body, 3D imaging.

Pitfalls

- Sensitivity lower in more indolent tumours—lung carcinoid, alveolar cell carcinoma, neuroendocrine tumours, depending on proliferative index and, occasionally, in pancreatic tumours.
- Limited availability—specialist centres only.
- Relatively expensive.

Fig. 14.14 ^{18}FDG PET scan—non-small cell lung cancer right lung. Whole body coronal.

Fig. 14.15 ^{18}FDG PET scan—transaxial views showing CT (top left) correlation with PET (top right). The image fusion is shown bottom left. (**Colour plate** 12.)

Fig. 14.16 ¹⁸FDG PET scan—non-Hodgkin's lymphoma. Whole body coronal view of patient pre-treatment showing extensive FDG avid adenopathy.

Fig. 14.17 ¹⁸FDG PET scan—non-Hodgkin's lymphoma. Post-treatment showing complete metabolic response.

Myocardial perfusion imaging: MPI

Background

MPI reflects regional blood flow during stress (increased demand) and at rest providing prognostically significant information which, both in isolation and in conjunction with coronary angiography, can be used to optimise patient management.[1]

Originally performed using ^{210}thallous chloride but now based on ^{99m}Tc labelled tracers—MIBI (methoxy-isobutylisonitrile) or tetrofosmin. Exercise or pharmacological stress are used to challenge coronary artery reserve. Exercise is performed by treadmill or bicycle, while pharmacological stressors are either adenosine/dipyridamole infusion, which increases coronary artery blood flow by vasodilatation, or dobutamine infusion with both inotropic and chronotropic activity.

Indications

Ischaemic heart disease

1. Pre-angiography

- When conventional stress testing fails, e.g. bundle branch block.
- Left ventricular hypertrophy.
- Atypical chest pain.
- Recurrent chest pain post-intervention. Good prognostic indicator.

2. Post-angiography

- Assess functional significance of known stenoses.
- Identify critical vascular territory for intervention.

Patient preparation

- Stop β-blockers 24h prior to stress study.
- Sometimes helpful to withdraw all anti-anginal medication.
- Assess optimal stress technique for individual patient, i.e. exercise or pharmacological.
- Attach 12-lead ECG.
- Insert IV cannula.
- Check baseline blood pressure.

Procedure

2-part investigation comparing myocardial perfusion during stress and at rest

Stress test

- Treadmill or bicycle exercise to >85% maximum predicted heart rate or adenosine 140μg/kg/min IVI for 6min—sometimes with submaximal exercise **or**,
  Dobutamine 5–40μg/kg/min in 5μg/kg/min increments over 16min
- Inject radiopharmaceutical (^{201}thallous chloride, ^{99m}Tc-MIBI (methoxy-isobutylisonitrile) or ^{99m}Tc-tetrofosmin) at peak stress.
- Tomographic imaging immediately (^{201}Tl) or 15–60min post-injection (^{99m}Tc compounds).

Rest study
- 2nd radiopharmaceutical injection under resting conditions.
- Tomographic imaging as before.

Results

Myocardial uptake reflects radiopharmaceutical delivery and myocyte function.

Interpretation

Infarction causes matched perfusion defects during stress and rest. Inducible ischaemia creates a perfusion defect at stress which re-perfuses at rest = reversible ischaemia. The severity, extent and number of reversible defects are prognostically significant. A normal MPI study implies risk of an adverse cardiac event <0.5% per annum.

Advantages

Non-invasive; relatively inexpensive compared with angiography.

Pitfalls

Less sensitive in multiple small vessel coronary disease—e.g. diabetes mellitus. Sensitivity depends on stress test quality.

Fig. 14.18 Normal myocardial perfusion scan. (**Colour plate 13.**)

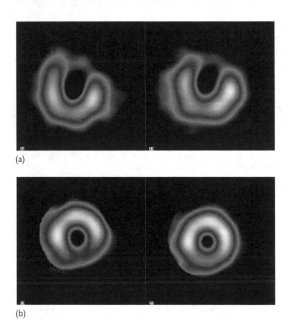

(a)

(b)

Fig. 14.19 Myocardial perfusion scan: (a) in fixed perfusion loss (anterolateral infarction) and (b) in inferior stress-induced (reversible) ischaemia. (**Colour plate 14**.)

1 Kaul S, Lilly DR, Gascho JA *et al.* (1988) Prognostic utility of the exercise thallium-201 test in ambulatory patients with chest pain: comparison with cardiac catheterization. *Circulation* **77**, 745–748.

Radionuclide ventriculography: MUGA scans

Background
Increasingly replaced by transthoracic echocardiography (TTE), trans-oesophageal echocardiography (TOE) and contrast ventriculography at time of cardiac catheterisation. MUGA scans are less operator-dependent than either TTE or TOE which may be important if serial assessment is required. The cardiac blood pool is imaged dynamically after injection of radiolabelled red blood cells. From this, wall motion, synchronicity of ventricular contraction and ejection fraction are measured. The estimated ejection fraction is unreliable in the presence of dysrhythmias—the acquisition requires a relatively regular heart rate.

Indications
- LV ejection fraction measurement, e.g. unechogenic patients.
- Monitor anthracycline cardiotoxicity.

Patient preparation
None.

Procedure
Radiolabel red cells (*in vivo* or *in vitro*) using ^{99m}Tc pertechnetate. Image patient supine in anterior and left anterior oblique projections. Camera acquisition gated to cardiac cycle. Imaging sometimes combined with low impact exercise/pharmacologic stress to assess cardiac reserve.

Results
Visual image of 300–400 summated cardiac cycles. Computer generated images used to assess regional wall motion and synchronous contraction. Computer generated ejection fraction calculation. Normal EF 60–70%, ↓ with age.

Interpretation
EF used to monitor treatment response in cardiac failure, cardiomyopathy.

Advantages
Good for serial measurement during anthracycline chemotherapy. Reliable in unechogenic subjects.

Disadvantage
High radiation dose—echocardiography preferable in most patients.

Pitfalls
Cardiac dysrrhythmias interfere with gating e.g. atrial fibrillation.

Fig. 14.20 Computer-generated ejection fraction 40%.

(a)

(b)

(c)

(d)

Fig. 14.21 MUGA scan showing (a) LV regions of interest at end diastole and (b) end systole for ejection fraction calculation; (c) amplitude image showing relative anteroseptal hypokinesis but (d) synchronous LV contraction. (**Colour plate 15**.)

Radionuclide first pass cardiac studies

Background
Nuclear medicine can assess simple shunts e.g. left-to-right shunts (ventricular and atrial septal defects) but has no place in bidirectional shunting or multiple sources of pulmonary blood flow (e.g. patent ductus arteriosus). First pass studies quantify shunt severity both pre- and postsurgical correction. Complementary to cardiac catheterisation and colour Doppler flow echocardiography. Dynamic imaging of a small bolus of IV radioactivity, usually ^{99m}Tc-DTPA (diethylenetriaminepenta acetic acid) outlines cardiac venous return, pulmonary circulation, left heart and the systemic circulation. Largely superseded by angiography and MRI.

Indications
Measurement of simple left-to-right cardiac shunts.

Patient preparation
None.

Procedure
1. ^{99m}Tc-diethylene-triamine-penta-acetic acid (DTPA) administered IV as a bolus into a right antecubital vein with shoulder abducted.
2. Images are obtained immediately, as a dynamic acquisition over 60sec.

Results
Normal circulation will demonstrate sequential appearance of right heart, pulmonary outflow tract, lungs, left heart and aorta.

Interpretation
Variation in the normal sequence implies cardiac shunting. Interpretation must be performed in conjunction with definitive knowledge of patient's anatomy, e.g. echocardiography with Doppler colour flow.

Advantages
Relatively non-invasive technique for serial follow-up of congenital heart disease. Mathematical analysis of the data allows quantification of shunt size, important for consideration and timing of corrective surgery.

Lung scan: ventilation/perfusion imaging

Background
One of the most widely requested nuclear medicine studies. Sensitivity and specificity reduced in coexisting lung disease, when CTPA (computerised tomographic pulmonary angiography) is more useful. All patients should have had a chest radiograph within 24h to aid V/Q interpretation and exclude other causes of pleuritic chest pain and hypoxia, e.g pneumothorax.

Lung perfusion shown by injection of tiny ^{99m}Tc particles which are trapped by the pulmonary capillary bed. Ventilation shown using radio-labelled gases or aerosols.

Indications
- Suspected pulmonary embolism.
- Pre-operative lung function assessment.

Patient preparation
None. Relative contraindication in right left intracardiac shunts; caution in severe pulmonary hypertension.

Procedure
- Lie patient supine and inject ^{99m}Tc macroaggregates or albumin IV.
- Obtain gamma camera perfusion images in 4 views.
- Ventilation images are obtained in same projections by continuous breathing of ^{81m}Kr gas (same day) or using ^{99m}Tc aerosol or ^{133}xenon gas (separate day).

Results
Homogeneous, matched ventilation and perfusion patterns.

Interpretation
Four abnormal patterns recognised
1. Segmental perfusion loss with preserved ventilation—pulmonary embolism.
2. Segmental matched perfusion and ventilation loss—pulmonary infarction/infection.
3. Segmental/subsegmental ventilation loss with preserved perfusion—infection.
4. Non-segmental, patchy, matched perfusion and ventilation loss—COPD.

Advantages
Quick, non-invasive. Normal scan virtually excludes PE.

Pitfalls
Specificity reduced in underlying lung disease—COPD, asthma giving indeterminate results. False +ves with tumour, bullae, vasculitides, fibrotic lung disease and old, unresolved PE.

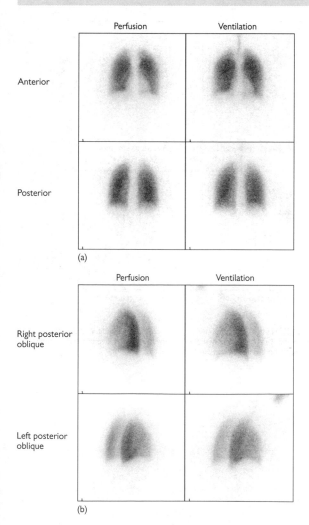

Fig. 14.22 Normal lung V/Q images.

(1990) Value of the ventilation/perfusion scan in acute pulmonary embolism. Results of the prospective investigation of pulmonary embolism diagnosis (PIOPED). The PIOPED Investigators. *JAMA* **263**, 2753–2759.

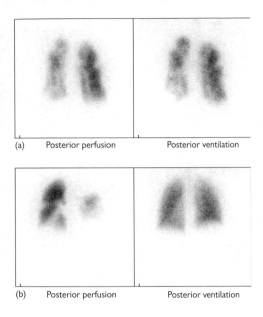

(a) Posterior perfusion   Posterior ventilation

(b) Posterior perfusion   Posterior ventilation

Fig. 14.23 Lung scans: (a) showing matched, non-segmental V/Q defects in COPD; and (b) showing segmental V/Q mismatch—extensive bilateral pulmonary thromboembolism and unmatched perfusion loss.

Lung shunt studies

Background
Largely research procedure.

Indications
Suspected pulmonary A-V shunting.

Patient preparation
None.

Procedure
Inject ^{99m}Tc-nanocolloid IV. Gamma camera lung, abdomen and head imaging. Calculate relative uptake in lungs, kidneys and brain. Express as fraction of cardiac output to quantify shunt fraction.

Results
Kidneys and brain not normally visible on lung perfusion imaging.

Interpretation
Abnormal extrapulmonary activity implies degree of shunting. Intensity of uptake rises with shunt severity.

Advantages
Non-invasive, quantitative. Can be used to monitor response to intervention.

Pitfalls
Injection extravasation invalidates shunt calculation.

Lung permeability studies

Background
Altered alveolar permeability affects gas exchange—also shown by lung transfer factor measurement.

Indications
- *Pneumocystis carinii* (PCP) infection—rapid screening in high risk patients with normal CXR.
- Monitor treatment response in cryptogenic fibrosing alveolitis.

Patient preparation
None.

Procedure
Patient breathes ^{99m}Tc-DTPA aerosol. Gamma camera images of thorax over 1h. Computer data analysis generates lung clearance curves reflecting integrity of alveolar cell barrier.

Results
Clearance curves used to calculate permeability index. Individual results compared with centre defined normal range.

Interpretation
Accelerated clearance in PCP which ↓ with successful treatment.

Advantages
Non-invasive. Allows rapid PCP diagnosis.

Pitfalls
Non-specific, e.g. accelerated clearance in smokers.

Lymphoscintigraphy

Background
Lymphoedema can be congenital or acquired. The lymphatic system normally drains subcutaneous tissues → local lymphatic channels and regional nodes. Lymphatic channels can be imaged using radiolabelled colloid particles (see *Sentinel node imaging* p750).

Indication
Unexplained limb swelling, e.g. lymphatic hypoplasia.

Patient preparation
None.

Procedure
^{99m}Tc-colloid injection subcutaneously into finger or toe webspace on affected and contralateral limb. Regional gamma camera imaging at 10min intervals over next hour.

Results
Normally rapid clearance via lymphatic channels to regional nodes.

Interpretation
Slow clearance and failed regional node uptake in hypoplastic systems or metastatic regional node infiltration, depending on clinical context.

Advantages
Much easier than conventional (contrast) lymphography—avoids lymphatic channel cannulation.

Pitfalls
Lymphatic drainage may be disrupted by surgery or radiotherapy.

Feet/ankles   Pelvis/abdomen

Fig. 14.24 Normal lymphoscintograms.

Static cortical renography: DMSA imaging

Background

Dimercaptosuccinic acid (DMSA) is concentrated by the proximal convoluted tubules in the renal cortex. ^{99m}Tc-DMSA provides good definition of functioning renal parenchyma. It should be used in conjunction with anatomical imaging, e.g. ultrasonography, to differentiate between scarring, cysts or calculi.

Indications

- Urinary tract infection: 'gold standard' for renal scarring.
- Measurement of relative renal function.
- Renal duplication assessment.
- Ectopic kidney localisation.
- Renal trauma.
- Renal vein thrombosis.
- Pre-biopsy.

Patient preparation

None: but avoid dehydration.

Procedure

^{99m}Tc-DMSA (dimercaptosuccinic acid) injected IV. Static anterior, posterior and posterior oblique images acquired 2–4h later.

Results

Visual image evaluation, assessing integrity of cortical outlines for scarring. Quantitative computer image analysis is used to measure relative renal function, i.e. the contribution of each kidney to overall GFR.

Interpretation

Cortical scars distort renal outline. Duplication may result in nonfunctioning upper moiety, usually due to obstruction, or scarred lower moiety, secondary to vesicoureteric reflux. Relative renal function is usually 50:50 ± 5%.

Advantages

Sensitive for renal scarring; superior to ultrasound. Non-invasive.

Pitfalls

False +ves during or immediately after acute pyelonephritis—may give cortical defects that do not progress to scarring. Splenic impression at left upper pole may be mistaken for scarring.

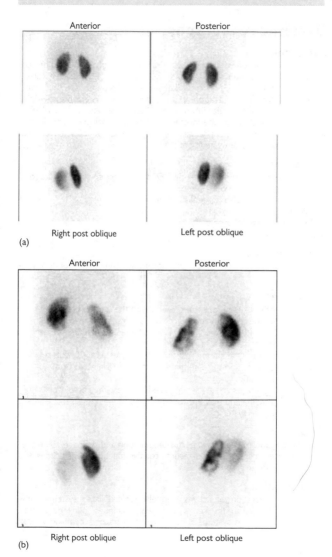

Fig. 14.25 DMSA static renogram: (a) normal, and (b) showing extensive bilateral cortical scarring.

Dynamic renography

Background

Nuclear medicine offers unique 'real time' imaging of renal function, i.e. visualisation of uptake, drainage and bladder emptying. Available radio-pharmaceuticals: ^{99m}Tc-DTPA (diethylenetriaminepenta acetic acid), cleared by glomerular filtration, and ^{99m}Tc-MAG-3 (trimercaptoacetylgly-cine), cleared by glomerular filtration and tubular secretion. ^{99m}Tc-MAG-3 preferred particularly in the presence of renal impairment and in the immature kidney. ^{99m}Tc-DTPA reserved for assessment of acute tubular necrosis, post transplant viability etc.

Indications

- Assessment of renal drainage—discrimination between renal dilatation and outflow obstruction.
- Measurement of relative renal function.
- Loin pain.
- Post-pyeloplasty follow-up.
- Renal artery stenosis (see *next section*).

Patient preparation

Good hydration essential. Empty bladder immediately before undertaking study.

Procedure

1. Position patient supine or seated erect, with the camera behind.
2. Obtain good peripheral venous access. Bolus radiopharmaceutical injection ^{99m}Tc-MAG-3 or ^{99m}Tc-DTPA followed by 10–20mL saline flush.
3. Image immediately acquiring real time dynamic data for 20–30min.
4. Diuretic administration is essential to distinguish dilatation from outflow obstruction.
5. Post-voiding images are always required to assess the completeness of bladder emptying and may improve drainage of the upper renal tracts in high pressure systems.

Results

Visual inspection of renal size, perfusion, function and drainage. Quantitative computer image analysis measures relative function, transit times and generates drainage graphs.

Interpretation

Uptake and excretion of activity normally rapid. Dilated systems show progressive pooling in the renal pelvis which empties following diuretic challenge. Obstructed systems show progressive tracer accumulation with no diuretic response, often associated with ? function on the affected side.

Advantages

Sensitive, non-invasive, quantitative renal function assessment. Anatomical Imaging, e.g. IVU, better for renal morphology, stones, etc.

Pitfalls

Movement artefact, chronic renal failure and dehydration reduce data reliability. Renal drainage may be gravity dependent—always complete study with an erect image. Drainage curves invalidated by radiopharmaceutical extravasation.

5min
(a)

20min

20min
(b)

60min

Fig. 14.26 Dynamic renogram posterior images: (a) normal, showing an early parenchymal image and later symmetrical excretion with bladder filling; (b) outflow obstruction: early image shows left hydronephrosis secondary to pelviureteric junction obstruction, with poor drainage at 60min.

Captopril renography

Background

Renal artery stenosis is a rare (<2%) cause of hypertension. Suspected in young adults presenting with hypertension, usually due to fibromuscular dysplasia. In patients >50 years, the most common cause is atherosclerosis. Perfusion pressure is maintained by angiotensin II in renal artery stenosis. Captopril is an angiotensin converting enzyme inhibitor (ACEI) which blocks the conversion of angiotensin I to angiotensin II. Captopril reduces perfusion pressure leading to fall in relative function and delayed tracer uptake on affected side. Captopril administration is contraindicated in the presence of a solitary kidney.

Indications

Diagnosis of renal artery stenosis (especially fibromuscular dysplasia) and prediction of response to revascularisation.

Patient preparation

Well-hydrated. Baseline blood pressure. IV access. Stop ACE inhibitors for 48h prior to test.

Procedure

- Perform standard dynamic renogram.
- Repeat renogram 1h after oral captopril 25mg single dose PO.
- Monitor blood pressure—beware hypotension.

Results

Quantitative evaluation of R:L renal function and time to peak activity in each kidney.

Interpretation

RAS due to fibromuscular dysplasia—fall in relative renal function and delayed time to peak renal activity >10 minutes.

Advantages

Distinguishes generalised atherosclerosis (often poor blood pressure outcome following angioplasty) from fibromuscular hyperplasia (good angioplasty response).

Pitfalls

- ↓ reliability in the presence of renal impairment.
- Severe hypotension.

Gastrointestinal bleeding: labelled red cell imaging

Background

The source of gastrointestinal blood loss is usually identified by GI endoscopy but may be difficult to localise. Labelled red cell studies are useful when there is evidence of ongoing bleeding (typically falling Hb of 1g/L/day). The patient must be actively bleeding at the time of the study. Time-consuming investigation, with serial imaging beyond 24h often performed.

Indications

Localise source of active GI haemorrhage when other techniques (e.g. endoscopy or angiography) have failed.

Patient preparation

No recent contrast barium studies. Fasting during first 2h of imaging.

Procedure

Label red cells (*in vitro* or *in vivo*) using ^{99m}Tc-pertechnetate. Abdominal gamma camera blood pool imaging immediately and at intervals for up to 36h post-injection or until bleeding source is identified.

Results

Activity normally restricted to vascular compartment.

Interpretation

Any activity in gut lumen implies active haemorrhage. Serial images helpful.

Advantages

More sensitive and less invasive than angiography for intermittent bleeding.

Pitfalls

- Poor red cell label—degrades image quality.
- Limits of detection—0.5mL/min blood loss.

30min

2h

6h

Fig. 14.27 Anterior abdominal images showing increasing red cell haemorrhage into the distal ileum.

Gastric emptying studies

Background
The diagnosis of dysfunctional gastric emptying can be difficult. In children, delayed gastric emptying may contribute to gastro-oesophageal reflux. In adults, both gastric stasis and 'dumping' syndromes occur, sometimes following previous surgery. Imaging following ingestion of radiolabelled solids or liquids demonstrates timing and pattern of gastric emptying.

Indications
Altered GI motility—delayed or accelerated gastric emptying.

Patient preparation
Starve for 4h. Stop drugs likely to influence GI motility, e.g. domperidone, metoclopramide.

Procedure
Milk study
- Give radiolabelled milk drink orally.
- Image anterior abdomen immediately and at 10min intervals for 1h. Generate computer derived clearance curves to calculate emptying half time.
- Delayed thoracic image helpful to exclude lung aspiration if clearance significantly delayed.

Dual isotope method
- Give ^{99m}Tc-labelled standard meal with ^{111}In-labelled water.
- Anterior abdomen gamma camera imaging as before using dual isotope settings.
- Generate solid and liquid phase clearance curves.

Results
Normal gastric emptying half time (milk = 20min). Normal range for solids is centre-specific, depending on standard meal composition.

Interpretation
Visual image evaluation and half time calculation.

Advantages
Non-invasive and quantitative.

Pitfalls
Vomiting during study invalidates emptying time calculations.

10min

20min

60min

Fig. 14.28 Normal gastric emptying study: Anterior images showing clearance of ^{99m}Tc labelled milk into the proximal small intestine.

Meckel's scan: ectopic gastric mucosa localisation

Background
Meckel's diverticulum is the commonest congenital anomaly of the GI tract, occurring in ~2% of the population. <10% contain ectopic gastric mucosa, which may bleed, but diverticuli can also cause obstruction or become inflamed. Typically childhood presentation. Nuclear medicine provides a straightforward imaging technique which targets gastric mucosal cells which normally take up ^{99m}Tc-pertechnetate.

Indications
Unexplained abdominal pain or GI haemorrhage—after endoscopy/contrast radiology.

Patient preparation
- Starve for 4h.
- H_2 antagonist administration may improve specificity.
- No recent barium studies.

Procedure
Inject ^{99m}Tc pertechnetate IV. Immediate and serial abdominal imaging over 1h.

Results
Normal uptake in gastric mucosa.

Interpretation
Focal abnormal uptake appearing at the same time as the stomach implies ectopic gastric mucosa (Meckel's diverticulum) or, occasionally, duplication cyst. Commonest site—RIF.

Advantages
Non-invasive.

Pitfalls
False +ves due to activity in renal tract—lateral images usually help.

Hepatobiliary scintigraphy

Background

Amino-diacetic acid (IDA) compounds are cleared from the circulation by the hepatocytes and secreted into the bile in the same way as bilirubin. ^{99m}Tc-labelled IDA compounds show biliary excretion through the biliary tree and gallbladder → duodenum. Useful in acute/chronic acalculous cholecystitis and to diagnose biliary atresia.

Indications

- Acute cholecystitis.
- Trauma.
- Post-operative leak detection.
- Bile duct/stent patency.
- Gallbladder emptying.
- Bile reflux.
- Neonatal biliary atresia.

Patient preparation

- *Adults*: starve for 6h.
- *Neonates*: phenobarbitone 5mg/kg/d PO for 3d prior to study (enzyme induction).

Procedure

- *Adults*: IV injection ^{99m}Tc-labelled iminodiacetic acid complex (IDA). Gamma camera imaging over 1h.
- *Neonates*: IV injection ^{99m}Tc-IDA. Immediate dynamic imaging for 5min then serial static images for up to 36h, or until activity reaches small bowel lumen.

Results

Gallbladder and biliary tree normally shown with tracer excretion via common bile duct into duodenum by 30min post-injection. Cholecystokinin 0.5unit/kg IV sometimes administered to stimulate gallbladder emptying.

Interpretation

- Acute cholecystitis: absent gallbladder.
- Obstruction, leak or reflux assessed visually.
- Neonates: passage of activity into gut lumen excludes biliary atresia.
- Quantification of T0 to T10min images improves specificity for atresia diagnosis.

Advantages

Non-invasive. Straightforward pattern recognition.

Pitfalls

Delayed IDA excretion in severe jaundice: bilirubin >300µmol/L.

Splenunculus detection: heat-damaged red cell imaging

Background

Splenectomy may be indicated in haemolytic syndromes and in refractory haemorrhagic tendencies (e.g. ITP) if associated with hypersplenic thrombocytopenia. Remnant splenic tissue or 'splenunculi' can give rise to recurrent thrombocytopenia—difficult to detect on anatomical imaging. As the spleen removes abnormal red cells from the circulating blood pool, radiolabelled heat damaged red cells can be used to localise ectopic splenic tissue.

Indications

Recurrent thrombocytopenia post-splenectomy.

Patient preparation

None.

Procedure

- Obtain venous blood sample.
- Separate red cells and radiolabel using ^{99m}Tc-pertechnetate.
- Heat to 39.5°C for 30min.
- Cool and reinject IV.
- Image anterior abdomen 30min later.

Results & interpretation

Damaged red cells taken up by splenic remnants.

Advantages

Investigation of choice for splenunculus detection.

Pitfalls

Enlarged left lobe of liver may obscure small splenic remnant.

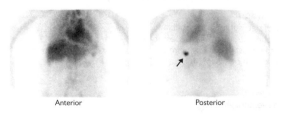

Anterior   Posterior

Fig. 14.29 Post-splenectomy. Intense uptake in splenunculus lying in splenic bed.

Hepatosplenic scintigraphy

Background
Largely superseded by ultrasonography and cross-sectional imaging. Maps reticuloendothelial tissue within the liver (Kupffer cells) and spleen, to identify space occupying lesions and confirm the presence or absence of functioning splenic tissue.

Indications
Liver space occupying lesions—now largely replaced by ultrasound, CT or MRI.

Patient preparation
None.

Procedure
^{99m}Tc-colloid injected IV. Abdominal gamma camera images 30min post-injection.

Results
Normal, homogeneous liver and spleen uptake.

Interpretation
Focal ↓ uptake in space occupying lesions. ↑ spleen and bone activity in portal hypertension. Focal ↑ uptake in caudate lobe pathognomonic of Budd–Chiari syndrome.

Advantages
Cheap.

Pitfalls
Non-specific. Largely superseded by anatomical imaging.

Labelled leucocyte imaging

Background

Localisation and assessment of acute or chronic infection/inflammation can be difficult. Nuclear medicine techniques show inflammation but do not differentiate infective from non-infective causes. Radiolabelled leucocytes are injected and imaged. The normal distribution includes liver and spleen making peri-diaphragmatic collections difficult to identify. Delayed imaging useful in chronic low grade infection, e.g. osteomyelitis, where cell migration to the site of inflammation is slow.

Indications

- Sepsis localisation.
- Inflammatory bowel disease to determine disease activity, extent, severity.

Patient preparation

None. Avoid recent barium contrast radiology.

Procedure

1. Obtain 40–60mL blood sample.
2. Separate white cell layer and radiolabel *in vitro* using ^{99m}Tc exametazine (HMPAO) or ^{111}In oxine.
3. Reinject labelled cells IV.
4. Image 1 and 3h later (inflammatory bowel disease) or 2, 4 and 24h for intra-abdominal sepsis/osteomyelitis.

Results

Physiological uptake in reticuloendothelial system. Variable GI and renal excretion, depending on radiopharmaceutical used.

Interpretation

Focal ↑ uptake indicates sepsis. Diffuse ↑ gut uptake reflects extent and activity of inflammatory bowel disease.

Advantages

Very sensitive in inflammatory bowel disease. Non-invasive, useful in sick patients, e.g. acute exacerbation of inflammatory bowel disease.

Pitfalls

- *False −ves*: leucopenia and poor white cell label, perihepatic and perisplenic collections obscured by normal liver and spleen uptake.
- *False +ves*: physiological gut and renal activity.
- Damaged white cells during labelling causing lung sequestration.
- ^{99m}Tc-exametazine (HMPAO) preferred for routine imaging and inflammatory bowel disease—lower radiation dose and earlier result than ^{111}In-oxine label.
- Reserve ^{111}In-oxine for low grade bone sepsis localisation.

(a)   (b)

Fig. 14.30 Labelled leucocyte imaging: (a) normal, and (b) acute inflammatory bowel disease—intense uptake in small and large bowel loops (Crohn's disease).

Gallium scintigraphy

Background

Previously used to diagnose and monitor sarcoid and lymphoma but increasingly superseded by [18]FDG PET (see *previous section*) and cross-sectional imaging. Sometimes useful in 'pyrexia of unknown origin', PUO, e.g. immunocompromised patient where there is a suspicion of *Pneumocystis carinii* infection cf. lung permeability studies.

Indications

- PUO and infection localisation, especially in AIDS.
- Lymphoma follow-up.
- Sarcoidosis follow-up.

Patient preparation

None.

Procedure

- Inject ^{67}Ga-citrate IV. Gamma camera imaging at 48–96h with tomography.
- Non-specific gut retention reduced by laxative administration.

Results

Normal uptake in lacrimal glands, nasal mucosa, blood pool, liver, spleen, testes, female perineum, breast.

Interpretation

- Focal lymph node uptake in lymphoma and sarcoid distinguishes active disease from post-therapy scarring/fibrosis.
- In AIDS, ↑ lung uptake indicates infection—PCP, CMV, mycobacterium—chest radiograph correlation essential.
- ↑ activity in inflammatory bowel disease and focal sepsis; largely superseded by WBC imaging.

Advantages

Excellent, non-invasive marker of disease activity in lymphoma—but likely to be superseded by [18]FDG.

Pitfalls

Poor specificity. High radiation dose often difficult to justify when alternative techniques available.

Dacroscintigraphy

Background
Epiphora may arise from excessive tear production or inadequate drainage due to lower lid ectropion or nasolacrimal obstruction i.e. nasal puncti, lacrimal sac, nasolacrimal ducts. Straightforward technique to assess function of the nasolacrimal apparatus.

Indications
Epiphora.

Patient preparation
None.

Procedure
1–2 drops ^{99m}Tc-labelled DTPA or pertechnetate instilled into outer canthus of each eye. Immediate dynamic gamma camera imaging for 20min with delayed static scans as required.

Results
Normal rapid radiopharmaceutical clearance through nasolacrimal apparatus.

Interpretation
Delayed clearance implies obstruction—level of dysfunction usually identified, i.e. punctum, lacrimal sac, nasolacrimal duct.

Advantages
Non-invasive. Avoids nasolacrimal duct cannulation (*cf.* dacrocystography).

Pitfalls
Obstructed systems result in excess radiolabelled tears on cheek altering drainage times.

Right   Left

Fig. 14.31 Dacroscintigram (lacrimal drainage) showing normal lacrimal drainage on the right and, on the left, obstructed drainage at the proximal nasolacrimal duct.

Glomerular filtration rate measurement

Background
In many instances, GFR estimation from creatinine clearance (CC) is adequate, but accurate measurement is essential in renal impairment or to monitor nephrotoxic drug therapy. Glomerular compensation prevents early renal damage detection by CC measurements—60% of filtration activity can be lost before CC falls.

Indications
Accurate GFR to monitor renal failure, cytotoxic chemotherapy, immunosuppression, e.g. cyclosporin.

Patient preparation
Well-hydrated.

Procedure
- IV injection ^{51}Cr-EDTA or ^{99m}Tc-DTPA.
- Venous sampling 2 and 4h later.
- Count plasma sample radioactivity in gamma counter. Correct for height and weight.

Results
Normal GFR = 125mL/min (age-dependent).

Interpretation
↓ values in CRF.

Advantages
More reliable and reproducible than CC—avoids need for urine collection.

Pitfalls
Accuracy depends on good injection technique—avoid any extravasation. Unreliable results in severe peripheral oedema.

Urea breath test

Background

Helicobacter pylori infection is associated with duodenal ulceration. Eradication therapy reduces ulcer recurrence. *H. pylori* produces urease which converts labelled urea → labelled CO_2, detected in breath samples.

Indications

Helicobacter pylori detection—diagnosis and confirmation of eradication.

Patient preparation

Stop antibiotics, H_2 antagonists, proton pump inhibitors for 2–4 weeks.

Procedure

- Patient swallows urea drink labelled with ^{13}carbon (stable isotope) or ^{14}carbon (radioactive isotope).
- Breath samples (CO_2) collected over next 30min.
- Labelled CO_2 measured by mass spectroscopy (^{13}C) or liquid scintillation counting (^{14}C).

Results

Normal range varies according to local protocol.

Interpretation

↑ Exhaled CO_2 levels imply abnormal urea breakdown by urease-producing bacteria in stomach, e.g. *H. pylori*.

Advantages

- Very sensitive marker of active *H. pylori* infection (*cf.* serology).
- Non-invasive (*cf.* endoscopy) and avoids sampling errors.
- Good for non-invasive monitoring of recurrent symptoms.

Pitfalls

Occasional false +ves in oral *H. pylori* infection.

B$_{12}$ absorption studies

Background
Vitamin B$_{12}$ deficiency is of insidious onset and causes a megaloblastic anaemia and peripheral neuropathy. Dietary sources are meat and dairy products, with total body stores sufficient for at least 3 years. B$_{12}$ is absorbed in the terminal ileum as a B$_{12}$–intrinsic factor (IF) complex, IF from gastric parietal cell. B$_{12}$ deficiency occurs after terminal ileal resection, gastrectomy, autoimmune pernicious anaemia. B$_{12}$ absorption can be measured using radiolabelled B$_{12}$.

Indications
B$_{12}$ malabsorption; pernicious anaemia.

Patient preparation
Investigate before initiating B$_{12}$ therapy where possible. Otherwise, avoid B$_{12}$ supplements for 1 month prior to investigation.

Procedure
2 techniques available:
1. Administer ^{57}cobalt-B$_{12}$ PO. Measure isotope retention 7d later using whole body counter.
2. Give 1mg IM B$_{12}$ then ^{57}cobalt-B$_{12}$ PO.
   Collect all urine for 24h. Measure urinary ^{57}cobalt-B$_{12}$ excretion.

If abnormal
Repeat study using ^{57}cobalt-B$_{12}$ + IF 2 weeks later.

Results
Whole body retention method:

Table 14.1 B$_{12}$ absorption test results

Retention normally >50%:
Ratio ^{57}cobalt-B$_{12}$ + IF/^{57}cobalt-B$_{12}$ retention <1.8
Urine excretion method:
24h ^{57}cobalt-B$_{12}$ excretion normally >14–40%
Ratio ^{57}cobalt-B$_{12}$ + IF/^{57}cobalt-B$_{12}$ excretion 0.7–1.2

Interpretation
- ↓ ^{57}Co and ^{58}Co levels indicate B$_{12}$ malabsorption.
- Intrinsic factor corrects B$_{12}$ absorption in pernicious anaemia i.e. Ratio ^{57}cobalt-B$_{12}$ + IF/^{57}cobalt-B$_{12}$ retention rises.

Advantages
Non-invasive. Only available technique.

Pitfalls
Urine excretion method—incomplete urine collection invalidates result. Severe GI atrophy—may invalidate IF response.

Ferrokinetic studies

Background
Iron is an essential component of erythropoiesis. Most iron disorders are deficiency states due to inadequate dietary intake or excess loss, e.g. chronic peptic ulcer disease. Uptake and transport problems, recycling or storage failures are rare but may require correction with parenteral iron. Formal iron metabolism studies useful where abnormal iron metabolism is suspected.

Indications
- Unexplained, refractory anaemia.
- Abnormal iron metabolism.

Patient preparation
None.

Procedure
1. Inject ^{59}Fe labelled transferrin IV.
2. Measure activity over liver, spleen, sacrum and heart using gamma probe daily for 14d.
3. Measure blood ^{59}Fe clearance daily for 14d.
4. Calculate plasma iron clearance, plasma iron turnover (µmol/L/d) and iron utilisation.
5. Organ ^{59}Fe uptake/clearance curve identifies extramedullary haemopoiesis.

Results
- Normal plasma iron clearance half time = 60–120min.
- Normal iron utilisation at 14 days = 80%.
- Normal iron turnover = 70–140µmol/L/d.

Interpretation
- Haemolysis—↑ plasma iron turnover, utilisation and marrow activity.
- Myelofibrosis—↑ splenic uptake compared with marrow.
- Aplasia—prolonged plasma iron clearance, low utilisation and hepatic accumulation.

Advantages
Only technique available for iron metabolism.

Pitfalls
Lengthy and labour-intensive. Consistent probe positioning essential for accurate organ uptake curves.

Red cell survival studies

Background
Although infrequently performed, provides evidence of abnormal red cell survival and localises sites of red cell destruction. The investigation is prolonged, with initial *in vitro* red cell labelling and daily activity measurements over target organs—spleen, liver and heart for 14 days.

Indications
- Haemolytic anaemia (to confirm ↓ RBC survival, i.e. active haemolysis).
- Localise abnormal red cell sequestration.
- Predict response to splenectomy.

Patient preparation
None. Avoid blood transfusion during study.

Procedure
1. Label patient's red cells with ^{51}Cr chromate.
2. Reinject cells and measure blood activity over 14d using gamma counter.
3. Measure activity over liver, spleen and heart using gamma probe daily for 14d.

Results
- Normal red cell half-life >24d.
- Equal fall in heart, liver and spleen counts with time.

Interpretation
Short red cell life confirms abnormal destruction. Ratio of counts in liver: spleen indicates site of red cell destruction.

Advantages
Only available technique.

Pitfalls
Lengthy and labour-intensive. Sensitivity reduced by blood transfusion during 14d measurement period. Consistent probe positioning essential for accurate organ sequestration curves.

Red cell volume/plasma volume measurement

Background
Polycythaemia is suspected when haemoglobin and haematocrit are raised. Routine laboratory screening does not differentiate true polycythaemia, i.e. elevated red cell mass, from apparent, stress or pseudopolycythaemia, i.e. reduced plasma volume. Radiolabelled red cells can be used to measure red cell mass. Plasma volume can be calculated from the haematocrit or measured independently using radiolabelled serum.

Indications
Polycythaemia, to distinguish between true polycythaemia (↑ RBC mass) from apparent polycythaemia (↓ plasma volume).

Patient preparation
Avoid recent therapeutic venesection. Less sensitive in patients already receiving myelosuppressive therapy.

Procedure
1. Obtain 10mL venous blood.
2. Separate plasma and red cells.
3. Radiolabel red cells using ^{99m}Tc or ^{51}Cr. Label plasma (if required) using ^{125}I-albumin.
4. Reinject radiolabelled blood.
5. Obtain venous samples at 15 and 30min.
6. Count activity in blood samples compared with known standards using gamma counter to establish plasma and red cell volumes.

Results
Compare measured red cell mass and plasma volume with predicted values for height and weight.

Interpretation
Distinguish relative polycythaemia (due to ↓ plasma volume) from genuine elevation of red cell mass.

Advantages
Only technique available.

Pitfalls
Recent venesection or myelosuppressive therapy reduces test reliability. Plasma volume measurement unreliable in severe peripheral oedema.

Bile salt deconjugation studies

Background
Bile salts are synthesised and stored in the liver and are essential for adequate gastrointestinal absorption. They are excreted into the gut as conjugated, water soluble bile salts and recycled by the enterohepatic circulation with terminal ileal reabsorption. Bile salt deconjugation products are insoluble and cannot enter the enterohepatic circulation, leading to bile salt malabsorption. Bacterial overgrowth after small bowel surgery, or terminal ileal disease can ↑ deconjugation.

^{14}C-labelled synthetic bile acid, glycocholine, is administered PO. Rapid transit into the large bowel will result in breakdown of the label by the normal large bowel flora and a rise in detected exhaled $^{14}CO_2$. Small bowel bacterial overgrowth, e.g. due to a 'blind loop', will also result in increased liberation of $^{14}CO_2$.

Indications
- Bacterial overgrowth.
- Bile salt malabsorption.

Patient preparation
- Starve overnight.
- Avoid antibiotics for one month before study.

Procedure
1. Give oral ^{14}C-labelled glycocholic acid in water.
2. Count $^{14}CO_2$ activity in breath samples over 6h using beta liquid scintillation counter.

Results
Glycocholate is deconjugated into ^{14}C glycine and cholic acid by small intestine bacteria releasing expired $^{14}CO_2$. Correct result for age-related variations in endogenous $^{14}CO_2$ production.

Interpretation
↑ $^{14}CO_2$ levels imply bacterial colonisation or bile salt malabsorption.

Advantages
Accurate. Only available test.

Pitfalls
False −ves (unusual).

Index

Notes: Page numbers in **bold** indicate the main discussion of a topic. Subjects are indexed in their unabbreviated form: a list of abbreviations appears on pp. xiii–xxi.

A

abdominal distension 4–5
abdominal pain 6–7
abdominal x-ray (AXR) 354, **668–71**, 684
  iron toxicity 623
absorption tests 454
acetaminophen (paracetamol) poisoning 628–32
acetylcholine receptor antibodies (ACRAb) 317
acid–base balance, assessment of 578–80
acromegaly 116
activated partial thromboplastin time (APTT) 245, 247
acute myocardial infarction 176
acute phase proteins 296–7
adam (MDA) 614–15
Addison's disease 146
adrenal antibodies 314
adrenal failure 144–6
airway hyperresponsiveness test 472–3
alanine transaminase (ALT) 461
albumin 461
albumin/IgG clearance 575
alcoholic ketoacidosis 183
alkaline phosphatase (ALP) **461**, 642
allergic disease 319
  drug allergy testing 322
  mast cell tryptase 322
  RAST tests 321
  skin prick tests 320
alteration of behaviour 7–8
alteration in bowel habit 8–9
amenorrhoea 148–9
American Academy of Allergy, Asthma and Immunology 325

American Association of Clinical Endocrinologists 109
American College of Radiology 724
American Diabetic Association 176
amiodarone 161
ammonium chloride loading test 581
amphetamines 614–15
amyloidosis 298
anabolic steroids screen 365
anaemia 9–11
  dimorphic 640
  haemolytic
    acquired 240–1
    hereditary 228
    investigation of 220
  investigation 453
  iron deficiency 210–12
  macrocytic 640
  microcytic hypochromic 640
  rheumatology 640
anaphylaxis 11
angioedema 11–12
angiography **526–7**, 708
  cerebral 718
  CT 531
  magnetic resonance 388, 532, **698**
  urinary tract 685
anion gap 579–80
  acidosis 183
  ethylene glycol, ethanol and methanol poisoning 620
anorectal manometry 460
anorexia 12–13
anti-adrenal antibodies 146
antibiotic plasma concentration monitoring 364
antibiotic sensitivity of bacteria 336–7
antibodies
  adrenal 314
  anti-GAD **313**, 317

anti-neutrophil cytoplasmic (ANCA) 318
  renal medicine 604
  rheumatology 644
diagnostic 555–7
double-stranded DNA (ds-DNA) 307
endomysial (EMA) 315
to extractable nuclear antigens (ENA) 307–8
gastric parietal cell (GPC) 311
gliadin 315
insulin 313
insulin-receptor 313
intrinsic factor 311
islet cell (ICA) 313
paraneoplastic 556–7
prognostic 555–7
rheumatology 643–4
to Saccharomyces cerevisiae (ASCA) 450
tissue transglutaminase (tTG) 315
antibody deficiency in adults 291–2
antibody tests 341–3
anticonvulsants 615–16
antidepressants, tricyclic 635
anti-DNA antibody 643
anti-GAD antibodies **313**, 317
anti-ganglioside antibodies 317
anti-GBM disease 318–19
antigen tests 344
antiglobulin test 264
anti-M2 antibodies 309
anti-mitochondrial antibodies (AMA) 309
anti-neuronal antibodies 317
antineutrophil antibody tests 268
anti-neutrophil cytoplasmic antibodies (ANCA) 318
  renal medicine 604
  rheumatology 644

anti-nuclear antibodies
(ANA), patterns of 306
antinuclear factor 643
antiphospholipid antibodies
(ACL) **309**, 644
antiplatelet antibody tests
268
antithrombin (AT) 253
anti-TSH receptor antibody
testing 163
anti-Yo antibodies 317
anuria 13–14
anxiety states 7
aortic dimensions, normal
414
aortic disease 414–16
aortic regurgitation 408–9
aortic stenosis 407–8
aortography 526
appendicectomy 555
arch angiography 526
ARMS PCR technique 238
arrhythmias 71
arterial blood gases
in poisoned patient 612
carbon monoxide 617
cyanide 618
iron 623
salicylate 633
theophylline 634
tricyclic antidepressants
635
sampling 474–5
arthritis
infective 39
rheumatoid 304
particle agglutination
test (RAPA) 643
arthrocentesis 646
arthroscopy 646
ascending urethro-
graphy 685
ascites 4
ascitic fluid, investigations of
468–9
aspartate transaminase
(AST) 461
aspirin poisoning 633
asplenia 292
ataxia 14–16
atrial septal defects 415
atrophic thyroiditis 160
autoantibodies
in autoimmune hepatitis
310–11
in connective tissue
disease 645
and neurological disease
317
autoantibody screen **305–6**,
309–10, 311
autoimmune adrenalitis 146

autoimmune hepatitis,
autoantibodies in
310–11
autoimmune polyglandular
syndromes 314
autoimmune skin diseases
316
autoimmunity 304

B

backache, post-LP 521
bacterial antibody tests 343
bacterial antigen tests 344
bacterial contamination of
blood products 262, **264**
bacterial culture techniques
335–7
bacterial overgrowth tests
455–6
barium enema 682–3
barium follow-through
451–2
barium meal 676–7
barium studies 672–3
barium swallow 674–5
Bartter's syndrome 140
basal plasma ACTH 146
behavioural alterations 7–8
Bence Jones proteins 294
detection and quantitation
576
immunological tests
602, 603
benzodiazepine overdose
616
bicarbonate infusion test
582
bile salt deconjugation
studies 798
bile salt malabsorption 454
biliary system drainage 710
bilirubin 461
jaundice **58**, 59
serum 224
biochemical markers
558–9
biochemical tests 558
infectious and tropical
diseases 358–9
rheumatology 642–3
biochemistry, normal
ranges *inside front cover*
biopsy
infectious and tropical
diseases 360–3
liver 466–7
neurology 553–5
percutaneous 710
renal 596–8
transiliac bone 601–2
tuberculosis 369

bladder stones,
investigations 594–6
bleeding disorder,
suspected 90–1
bleeding time 242
blindness 98–9
blood clotting studies 614
blood films
infectious and tropical
diseases 352
parasites 206–7
peripheral 202–3
vitamin B_{12} and folate
status 213–14
white cell morphology
208
blood gases, arterial
in poisoned patient 612
carbon monoxide 617
cyanide 618
iron 623
salicylate 633
theophylline 634
tricyclic antidepressants
635
sampling 474–5
blood glucose
diabetes mellitus 172
self-testing by patient
179–80
iron toxicity 623
blood lead concentration
624
blood lithium concentration
624
blood markers 555–7
blood methaemoglobin
concentration 625–6
blood opioid concentration
626–7
blood pressure
grading 52
hypertension 52–3
endocrine 132–9
essential 132
'white coat' 132
monitoring, cocaine
overdose 617
blood products, bacterial
contamination of
262, **264**
blood samples, error
minimisation xxiv
blood tests, toxicology 608
cocaine 617
blood transfusion 260–1
bacterial contamination of
blood products
262, **264**
HLA-related issues 277
reactions 261–3
body mass index (BMI) 68

bone, renal bone disease 600–2
bone biochemistry, markers of 600–1
bone marrow
  biopsy 555
  examination **254–5**, 352
  pancytopenia 72
  parasites in 206–7
  scintigraphy 732
bone scan 730–1
bone scintigraphy 730–1
bony trauma imaging, basic principles 704
bowel habit, alteration in 8–9
bradycardia **16–17**, 418
brain receptor imaging 736–7, plate 8
brainstem auditory evoked potentials **547–8**, 549
brainstem biopsy 554
brainstem death testing, poisoning and overdose 611
branched chain DNA (bDNA) 351
breast imaging 688–9
  scintimammography 752
breathlessness 17–18
British Diabetic Association 176
British Institute of Radiology 724
broad-complex tachycardias 94
bronchoalveolar lavage (BAL) 362
bronchoscopy
  fibreoptic 484–5
  infectious and tropical diseases 362
  video 484–5
Bruce protocol, exercise testing 425
bruising 18–19
bullous pemphigoid 316
buscopan, barium studies enema 682

C

C1 esterase inhibitor 300–1
calcium excretion 595, 596
calf swelling 19–20
caloric testing, neurootology 564
captopril renography 778
carbamazepine toxicity 615
carbohydrate antigen 19-9 (CA 19-9) 450–1

carbohydrate malabsorption tests 454
^{14}C fat breath test 454
^{14}C-glycoholic acid test 455–6
carbon monoxide poisoning 616–17
carboxyhaemoglobin (COHb) poisoning 616
carboxyhaemoglobinaemia 28
carcinoembryonic antigen (CEA) 450
carcinoid syndrome, testing for 457
carcinoid tumours 458, plate 5
  testing for 457
cardiac catheterisation 380–2
cardiac chamber abnormalities, causes 403–4
cardiac CT **386–9**, 393
cardiac dimensions, normal values 403
cardiac enlargement 664
cardiac enzymes, cocaine overdose 617
cardiac magnetic resonance 386–93
cardiac markers of myocardial necrosis 384–5
cardiac masses, echocardiography 413–14
cardiac rhythm, ECG 418–19
cardiac volumetric imaging 386–93
cardiology **379–437**
  infectious and tropical diseases 364
cartilage, imaging 704
Casoni test 364
casts, urine microscopy 593–4
cellular casts, urine microscopy 593
cellular function assays 323–4
cellulose acetate, haemoglobin electrophoresis 232
central cyanosis 28–9
central motor conduction time 550
central nervous system (CNS) infections 543–4
cerebellar ataxia 14–15
cerebral angiography 718
cerebral blood flow imaging 734–5, plate 7
cerebrospinal fluid (CSF)
  constituents, normal values 521

  infectious and tropical diseases 360
  lumbar puncture 518–23
  pressure measurement 519
  shunt patency 738–9
cerebrovascular accident (CVA)
  completed 91
  diabetes mellitus 176
  neuroradiology 718
  suspected 91–2
cervical spine, imaging 704
Charcot's triad 369
chest pain 20–2
chest x-ray (CXR) 656–60
  infectious and tropical diseases 354
cholangiography 680–1
cholinesterase 627
chorionic villus sampling (CVS) 272
chromatography 610–11
chromosome abnormalities 270–5
chromosome anatomy 273
chymotrypsin 456
cine sequences, MRI **387**, 390–1
citrate agar, haemoglobin electrophoresis 232
citrate excretion 595
clubbing 23
coagulation studies 352
cocaine overdose 617
Cockroft and Gault formula 568
cold agglutinins 352
colonic polypectomy 441
colonoscopy 683
  flexible 440, 441, **444**
colour Doppler echocardiography 396, **398**, plate 1
coma **24–5**, 544
combined anterior pituitary function testing 189
complement, rheumatology 644
complement breakdown products 303
complement components, serum 300
complete blood count (CBC) 198
  see also full blood count
completed stroke 91
compound motor action potential (CMAP) 535–6
computed tomography (CT) 530–1, **694–7**
  cardiac **386–9**, 393
  infectious and tropical diseases 354–5

computed tomography (continued)
  rheumatology 649
  role 652
  thorax 666–7
  urinary tract 685
confusional states **26**, 544
congenital heart disease 414–15
constipation 27–8
constrictive pericarditis 413
continuous wave (CW) Doppler echocardiography 397, **398**, plate 3
contrast echocardiography 399
contrast nephropathy 598
conversion table, mass and molar units 636
Coombs' test 264
Courvoisier's law 369
cranial CT 530–1
C-reactive protein (CRP) **296–7**, 641–2
cryofibrinogen 295
cryoglobulinaemia 603
cryoglobulins **294–5**, 603–4
crystals, urine microscopy 594
culture/sputum cytology 504–5
culture techniques 335–9
Cushing's syndrome 69, **126–31**
cyanide poisoning 618
cyanosis 28–9
cystatin C 570
cystine excretion, renal or bladder stones 595
cystometry 551
cytochemistry tests 256–7
cytogenetics 270–1
  haematological malignancies 274–5
  prenatal diagnosis 272–3
  when to do it 560

D

dacroscintigraphy 791
D-dimers **246**, 352
deep aspiration specimens 360–3
deep duodenal/jejunal aspiration 455
deep vein thrombosis (DVT) 19
delayed contrast agent imaging, MRI **388**, 391
delayed puberty 156–7
delayed transfusion reaction 263
delirium, acute 7

dementia 7
  EEGs 544
dental radiography 354
dermatitis herpetiformis 316
dermatological tests 364–5
  skin biopsy 362–3
  skin prick tests 320
desferrioxamine test 601
desmopressin D-arginyl vasopressin (DDAVP)
  diagnostic trial of 191
  polyuria/polydipsia 120
dexamethasone-suppressed CRH test 191, **192**
  hypercortisolism 127
dexamethasone suppression test
  high dose 128, **192–3**
  low dose 127, **191–2**
DEXA scan 647
diabetes insipidus 118–21
diabetes mellitus (DM) 172–6
  emergencies 182–3
  monitoring control 179–81
  potential diagnostic difficulties 177–8
Diabetes UK 176
diabetic keto-acidosis (DKA) 182–3
diabetic nephropathy 574
diagnostic antibodies 555–7
diagnostic imaging, rheumatology 648–9
diagnostic pleural aspiration 476–7
diarrhoea 29–30
  infectious and tropical diseases 370–1
  investigation algorithm 453
diethylcarbamazine (DEC) test 364
digital radiology 654
digital subtraction angiography (DSA) 708
digoxin toxicity 619–20
dilute Russell viper venom test (dRVVT) 309
dimercaptosuccinic acid (DMSA) imaging 774–5
dimorphic anaemia 640
direct antiglobulin test (DAT) 264
disseminated intravascular coagulation (DIC) 248–9
distal acidification, tests of 581–2
distal motor latency (DML) 535
dizziness 30–2

dobutamine stress echocardiography 404–5
Doppler echocardiography 398
Doppler ultrasound **690**, 692, plate 6
double-stranded DNA antibodies (ds-DNA) 307
driving
  dizziness/syncope 32
  first fit 37
drug allergy testing 322
Duke Treadmill Score 426
dynamic renography 776–7
dysarthria 32–3
dyspepsia 448
dysphagia 33–4
dysphasia 32
dyspnoea 17–18

E

early-onset type 2 diabetes 178
echocardiography 405–16
  abnormalities, causes of 403–4
  imaging modalities 394–9, plates 1–3
  normal values for cardiac dimensions 403
  possible results 403
  principle 394
  regional wall abnormalities 404
  stress 404–5
  transthoracic and transoesophageal 399–402
  2-D 395, **398**
ecstasy 614
ectopic gastric mucosa localisation 784
edrophonium test 552
Eisenmenger's syndrome 28
elastase 456
elbow, ossification centres 723
electrocardiogram (ECG) 416–20
  poisoning and overdose
    amphetamines 614
    carbon monoxide 617
    cocaine 617
    cyanide 618
    digoxin 619
    tricyclic antidepressants 635
electrocardiographic monitoring 420–3

electroencephalography
(EEG) 539
abnormalities 541–2
in epilepsy 542–3
infectious and tropical
diseases 365
invasive techniques 545
normal 540–1
using 542–4
electromyography (EMG)
537–8
infectious and tropical
diseases 365
rheumatology 647
sphincter disturbance 551
electrophoresis
Bence Jones proteins
294
haemoglobin **231–2**, 353
IgD 292–3
Elsworth-Howard test 168
embolic phenomena 56–7
embolisation, therapeutic
708
endocarditis 367
endocrine autoantibodies
314
endocrine hypertension
132–9
endocrinology and metabo-
lism **107–94**
guiding principles of investigation 108–10
endomysial (EMA)
antibodies 315
endoscopic retrograde
cholangiopancreato-
graphy (ERCP) 354, 440,
441, **445**, 680
endoscopic ultrasound
(EUS) 446
endoscopy **440–7**, 451,
plates 4–5
endovascular repair of
abdominal aortic
aneurysms 711
enteroclysis 451, **678**
enteroscopy 443–4
eosinophilia 641
epidemiology of infectious
diseases 329–31
epilepsy
EEGs in 542–3
temporal lobe 8
epiphyseal plate fractures
723
Epstein–Barr virus (EBV)
281
Epworth test/Epworth
sleepiness scale (ESS)
478–9
errors, minimising xxiv

erythrocyte sedimentation
rate (ESR) **216**, 296
infectious and tropical
diseases 352
rheumatology 641
erythroenzymopathies,
specialised assays 285
erythropoietin (Epo) assay
266
essential hypertension 52
ethanol poisoning 620–2
ethylene glycol poisoning
620–1, 622
European Federation of
Immunological Societies
325
event monitors **421**, 422
evoked potentials or
responses (EPs or ERs)
546–9
exercise testing
cardiology 423–6
and myocardial
perfusion imaging
428, 429
ischaemic forearm
exercise test 558–9
respiratory medicine
480–1
exhaled nitric oxide 482
external loop recorders
421, 422
extractable nuclear antigens
(ENA) antibodies
307–8, 644

F

facial pain 34
factor H 303
factor I 303
faecal antigen test 448
faecal calciprotectin 450
faecal fat test, 3-day 454
faecal incontinence 53–4
faecal occult blood 449
faecal testing, pancreatic
exocrine function 456
Fairley test 591
familial benign hypocalciuric
hypercalcaemia
(FBHH/FHH) 166
fasting plasma glucose
(FPG) 174
fatigue 95
fat malabsorption tests 454
fat microscopy 454
febrile transfusion
reactions 263
ferritin 210
infectious and tropical
diseases 352–3

rheumatology 642
ferrokinetic studies 795
fetal haemoglobin (HbF),
estimation of 236
α-fetoprotein 450
fever of unknown origin (FUO
or PUO) 35, **366–75**
fibreoptic bronchoscopy
484–5
fibrin degradation products
352
fine needle aspirate (FNA)
361
first fit 36–7
first pass contrast agent
imaging, MRI **387–8**,
392
fit, first 36–7
'fitness to fly' assessment
486–7
flash-evoked visual evoked
potentials 546
'flatbush' diabetes 178
flatus 4–5
flexible sigmoidoscopy and
colonoscopy 440, 441,
444
flowmetry 551
flow volume loops 488–9
fluorescence *in situ* hybridisation (FISH) 282–3
flying, fitness assessment
486–7
focal cerebral dysfunction,
use of EEGs in 543
folate status, assessment of
213–15
fractional phosphate
excretion 577
fractional sodium excretion
587
fractional tubular reabsorption of phosphate (TRP)
577
fractional urate excretion 578
Friedewald formula 184
frontal lobe syndrome 7
fructosamine 181
full blood count (FBC) 198
paediatric normal ranges
inside back cover
poisoning and overdose
614
iron 623
functional magnetic
resonance imaging
(FMRI) 528, **532**
functional residual capacity
(FRC) **506**, 508
fungal antibody tests 343
fungal antigen tests 344
fungal culture techniques 339

G

galactomannan 339
galactorrhoea 38, **152–3**
gallium scintigraphy 790
gamma camera scanning 528
gas–liquid chromatography (GLC) 610–11
gastric emptying 460, **782–3**
gastric parietal cell (GPC) antibodies 311
gastroenterology **439–69**
gastrointestinal bleeding, labelled red cell imaging 780–1
gastrointestinal physiology 459–60
gastrointestinal tract investigations 356–7
genetic risk factors 562
genetic tests 560–2
genotypic assays 339
Gitelman's syndrome 140
glandular fever 218
Glasgow Coma Scale (GCS) 24
gliadin antibodies 315
glomerular filtration rate (GFR)
  kidney function, estimation of 568–9
  measurement **570–2**, 792
glucagon, barium studies 673
glucose
  blood
    diabetes mellitus **172**, 179–80
    iron toxicity 623
  urine dipstick testing 589
glucose 6-phosphate dehydrogenase (G6PD) deficiency 285
  infectious and tropical diseases 353
γ-glutamyl transpeptidase (γGT) 461
glycaemia 175
glycaemic control, laboratory assessment of 180–1
glycated haemoglobin 180–1
L-glycerate 595
glycollate 595
glycolytic defects 285
glycosuria 172
  self-testing by patient 179
goitre **161**, 162
Goodpasture's syndrome 318–19
gout 39
granular casts, urine microscopy 593

Graves' disease 160, **161**, 162, 163
growth hormone
  deficiency 112–14
  excess 116
gynaecomastia 40–1
  endocrinology 152, **155**

H

haematemesis 41
haematocrit 200
haematology **196–285**
  infectious and tropical diseases 352–3
  normal ranges inside front cover
  rheumatological investigations 640–1
  specialised assays 284–5
haematuria 42
  renal imaging 599
  urine microscopy 592–3
haemodialysis
  lithium poisoning 625
  toxicological analysis 608
haemoglobin (Hb)
  abnormalities 231
  analysis 231–3
  concentration **199**, 353
  electrophoresis **231–2**, 353
  fetal (HbF), estimation of 236
  neonatal screening 235
  plasma 226
  rheumatological investigations 640
  sickle (HbS), investigation of 234–5
  specialised assays 284
  unstable, testing for 237
  urine dipstick testing 588–9
haemoglobin A₂ (α₂β₂), estimation of 235
haemoglobin H bodies (β₄) 236
Haemoglobinopathy Reference Laboratory **238**, 284
haemolysis
  general tests of 220–1
  screen 353
haemolytic anaemias
  acquired 240–1
  hereditary 228
  investigation of 220
haemolytic complement 302
haemolytic-uraemic syndrome (HUS) 303

haemoptysis 42–3
haemorrhage, post-LP 521
haemosiderin 210, **224–5**
haemosiderinuria 225
haemostasis, normal ranges inside back cover
hair sampling 362
Ham's acid lysis test 241
hands
  radiology 716–17
  wasting of small muscles 99–100
haptoglobins, serum 223–4
Hashimoto's disease **160**, 163
headache 43–4
  following LP 520–1
  meningitic illness 371–3
Heaf test 364
heart, radiograph 658–60
heart disease, congenital 14–15
heart rate 417–18
heart sounds and murmurs 45–9
heat-damaged red cell imaging 786
Heinz bodies 236–7
Helicobacter pylori, tests for 448–9
helminthic antibody tests 343
helminthic antigen tests 344
hepatitis
  autoantibodies in autoimmune 310–11
  hepatitis A (HAV) 462
  hepatitis B (HBV) 340–1, 462
  hepatitis C (HCV) 361, **462**
  hepatitis E (HEV) 462
hepatobiliary scintigraphy 785
hepatomegaly 50
hepatosplenic scintigraphy 787
herniation, post-LP 521
heroin overdose 626–7
herpes gestationis 316
herpes zoster 51
high dose dexamethasone suppression test 128, **192–3**
high-performance liquid chromatography (HPLC)
  haemoglobin electrophoresis 232–3
  toxicology **610**, 611
high resolution CT (HRCT) **666**, 667
hirsutism 150–1

histamic challenge test 472–3
histoplasmin test 364
HIV 351
Holter monitors 421
Hughes' syndrome 309
human leucocyte antigen B27 (HLA B27) 644–5
human leucocyte antigen (HLA) (tissue) typing 276–7
hyaline casts, urine microscopy 593
hybridisation with nucleic acid probes 351
hydrogen breath tests 455
hyperaldosteronism 132, **133–8**
hypercalcaemia 166–7
hypercholesterolaemia 184, **185**, 186
hypercortisolism (Cushing's syndrome) 69, **126–31**
hypergammaglobulinaemia 289
hyperkalaemia **142**, 582, 583–4, 585
hyperlipidaemia 51–2, **184–7**
hyperliproteinaemias 186
hyperosmolar non-ketotic (HONK) syndrome 182
hyperparathyroidism hypercalcaemia 166–7
hypocalcaemia 170
hyperprolactinaemia 38, **152–3**
hyperpyrexia 614
hypertension 52–3
endocrine 132–9
essential 132
'white coat' 132
hyperthyroidism **161–3**, 165
hypertriglyceridaemia 184, **185**, 186
hypertrophic pulmonary osteoarthropathy (HPOA) 23
hyperuricaemia 39
hypoadrenalism 122, **144–6**
hyperkalaemia 142
hypothyroidism 164
hypocalcaemia 168–70
hypocalciuria 166
hypocomplementaemia 604
hypogammaglobulinaemia 288–9
hypogonadism, male 154
hypogonadotrophic hypogonadism 154
hypokalaemia **140–1**, 582, 584–5
hypomagnesaemia 170

hyponatraemia 122–4
hypophosphataemia differential diagnosis 576
osteomalacia 169
hypopigmentation 86
hypopituitarism 112–14
hypothalamic dysfunction 112
obesity 69
hypothyroidism endocrinology 163–5
obesity 69

I

ileal conduits, obtaining urine samples from 590
immune complexes 302–3
immunoassays 610
immunoblotting 562
immunocytochemistry 562
immunofixation Bence Jones proteins 294
IgD 292–3
immunoglobulins **288–9**, 602–3
IgD 292–3
IgE 319
RAST tests 321
IgG subclasses 290–2
liver function testing 461–2
immunohaematology 268
immunological tests in renal medicine 602–4
immunology **287–325**
infectious and tropical diseases 358
normal ranges inside front cover
rheumatology 643–5
websites 325
immunophenotyping 269–70
impaired fasting glucose (IFG) 173, **174**
impaired glucose tolerance (IGT) 173, **174**
implantable loop recorders (ILRs) **421**, 422–3
impotence 154
incontinence faecal 53–4
urinary 54–5
indigestion 55–6
indirect antiglobulin test (IAT) 264
indwelling catheter urine specimens 591
infection, post-LP 521
infectious diseases **327–76**
infective arthritis 39
infective endocarditis echocardiography 412
signs 56–7

inferior petrosal sinus sampling (IPSS) 128
infertility 150
inflammatory bowel disease (IBD) 450
inflammatory markers 641–2
'in–out' catheter urine specimens 590
in situ hybridisation 282–3
inspiratory capacity 506
inspiratory reserve volume 506
insulin antibodies 313
insulinoma 69
insulin-receptor antibodies 313
insulin tolerance test (insulin stress test) 144, **188–9**
intermenstrual bleeding 148
international normalised ratio (INR) **628**, 629
intestinal transit studies 460
intravascular contrast agents, managing adverse reactions to 722
intravenous urogram (IVU) **684**, 685
intrinsic factor antibodies 311
inulin clearance **570**, 572
iodine 161
iron status, assessment of 210–12
iron toxicity 622–3
irregular pulse 57–8
ischaemic forearm exercise test (ischaemic lactate test) 558–9
islet cell antibodies (ICA) 313
isoelectric focusing (IEF), haemoglobin electrophoresis 232
IVP 354

J

jaundice **58–9**, 369–70
Jod–Basedow effect 161
joint pain/swelling 59–60
jugular venous pulse (JVP) 60–1
J wave, ECG 420

K

Kallman's syndrome 154
kaolin cephalin clotting time (KCCT) 245

karyotyping 271
  haematological
    malignancies 274–5
  prenatal 272–3
ketones, urine dipstick tests
    589
ketonuria 179
kidney disease, classification
    of 570–2
kidney function, estimation
    of 568–9
Kleihauer test 265

L

labelled leucocyte imaging
    788–9
labelled red cell imaging
    780–1
lactic acidosis (LA) 182–3
lactose-hydrogen test 454
lactose tolerance test 454
Lambert–Eaton myasthenic
    syndrome 317
lamotrigine toxicity 615
laparoscopic liver biopsy 467
lead poisoning 624
left ventricular diastolic
    function 405
leg, red painful swollen
    lower 374–5
leucocyte esterases and
    nitrites 589
leucocyturia 593
leukaemia
  cytochemistry tests 256–7
  cytogenetics 274–5
  immunophenotyping
    269–70
libido, loss of 154
Liddle's syndrome 138
ligase chain reaction (LCR)
    350
lithium toxicity 624–5
liver disease, investigation
    of 462
  algorithm 464
liver investigations
  amphetamines 614
  biopsy 360–1, **466–7**
  non-invasive 461–4
lobar collapse, patterns of
    662–3
localisation tests, urine
    culture 591
loin pain 62
long (depot) ACTH test
    193–4
  adrenal failure 146
low dose dexamethasone
    suppression test 127,
    191–2

lumbar spine, imaging 705
lumbar puncture (LP) 365,
    518–23
lung biopsy 362
lung disease 660
lung permeability studies
    771
lung scan 766–8
lung shunt studies 770
lymphadenopathy 63–4
lymph node sampling 361
lymphocyte function tests
    324
lymphocyte surface markers
    323–4
lymphocytosis 641
lymphoma 275
lymphopenia 641
lymphoscintigraphy 772–3
lytic complement function
    tests 302

M

macrocytic anaemia 640
macrophage function 324
macroprolactin 152
magnetic resonance an-
    giography (MRA) 388,
    532, **698**
magnetic resonance cholan-
    giopancreatography
    (MRCP) 354, 445, **680–1**
magnetic resonance imaging
    (MRI) 532–3, **698–703**
  breast 688–9
  cardiac 386–93
  functional (FMRI) 528,
    532
  infectious and tropical
    diseases 354
  rheumatology 649
  role 652
  sphincter disturbance 551
  urinary tract 685
malabsorption tests 454
malaria 369
  culture 339
  geographical distribution
    330
mammography 688
Mantoux test 364
mass and molar units,
    conversion factors 636
massive splenomegaly 87
mast cell tryptase 322
maturity onset diabetes of
    the young (MODY)
    177–8
maximum expiratory flow-
    volume curve 488
Mazzotti test 364

MDA (adam) 614–15
MDEA 614–15
MDMA (ecstasy) 614–15
mean cell haemoglobin
    (MCH) 200
mean cell haemoglobin
    concentration
    (MCHC) 200
mean cell volume (MCV)
    199, 353
Meckel's diverticulum 453
Meckel's scan 784
mediastinum, radiograph
    568–60
medicolegal issues, poison-
    ing and overdose 610
meningeal biopsy 554
meningitic illness 371–3
menorrhagia 148
metabolic acidosis 612
metabolic alkalosis 612
meta iodobenzylguanidine
    (MIBG) imaging 744–5,
    plate 9
methacholine challenge test
    472–3
methaemoglobinaemia
  cyanosis 28–9
  poisoning and overdose
    625–6
methanol poisoning
    620–1, 622
metoclopramide, barium
    studies 673
metryapone test
    128–9, 144
microalbuminuria 575
microcytic hypochromic
    anaemia 640
β_2-microglobulin 295
microcytic hypochromic
    anaemia 640
β_2-microglobulin 295
microorganisms, urine
    microscopy 593
micturating cystourethro-
    gram (MCUG) 685
micturition, urgency of 96
mid-stream urine sample,
    obtaining a 590
migraine 43
mineralocorticoid defi-
    ciency, isolated 142
mineralocorticoid excess
    136, **138**
minimum inhibitory concen-
    tration (MIC) 336–7
minimum inhibitory concen-
    tration (MIC) 336–7
mitral regurgitation 409–10
mitral stenosis 409
M-mode echocardiography
    396, **398**
  normal values 403
Modification of Diet in
    Renal Disease (MDRD)
    formulae 568–9

Modified Bruce protocol, exercise testing 425
molar units and mass, conversion factors 636
Molecular Absorbance Recirculating Systems (MARS) 608
molecular cytogenetics 274
molecular diagnostics 350–1
molecular genetics 560–2
monoclonal antibodies (MoAbs) 269
monoclonal antibody immobilisation of platelet antigens (MAIPA) 268
monophonic wheeze 101
Monospot test **218**, 353
motor conduction velocity 534–5
motor unit potentials (MUPs) 538
movement disorders 15
MUGA scans 762–3, *plate 15*
multiple sclerosis 718
multiple sleep latency test 545
myasthenia gravis 79
myelin associated glycoprotein associated antibodies (MAG) 317
myelography 527
myocardial necrosis, cardiac markers of 384–5
myocardial perfusion imaging (MPI) **428–31**, 758–60, *plates 13–14*
myoglobin 614
myoglobinuria 634

N

narcotics screen 365
narrow-complex tachycardias 93
National Academy of Clinical Biochemistry **109**, 163, 164
National Cholesterol Education Programme 186
National Haemoglobinopathy Reference Laboratory **238**, 284
National Radiological Protection Board 724
nausea 64–5
neck stiffness 66
neonatal haemoglobin screening 235

nephrolithiasis 599
nephrotic syndrome 574
nerve biopsy 553–4
nerve conduction studies 365, **534–6**
neuroendocrine tumours MIBG imaging 744–5
testing for 457–8, *plate 5*
neurological disease autoantibodies 317
gliadin antibodies 315
neurological investigation of sphincter disturbance 551
neurology **517–65**
infectious and tropical diseases 365
neuro-otology 564–5
brainstem auditory evoked responses **547–8**, 549
neuroradiology 718–19
ultrasound 525
neutropenia immunohaematology 268
rheumatology 641
neutrophil alkaline phosphatase (NAP) 258–9
neutrophil function 324
neutrophilia 641
Nijmegen questionnaire 490–1
nitric oxide, exhaled 482
NK cell function 325
normal values xxii
adult *inside front cover*
paediatric *inside back cover*
normoglycaemia 173, **174**
nuclear magnetic resonance (NMR) imaging 532–3
nuclear medicine **727–98**
rheumatology 649
small bowel pathology 452–3
nucleic acid sequence-based amplification (NASBA) 351
nystagmus 66–7

O

obesity 68–9
hypercortisolism 126–31
obstructive uropathy 600
oesophageal manometry 459–60
oesophagogastroduodenoscopy (OGD) 440, 441, **442**
Helicobacter pylori 448–9
oligoclonal bands (OCBs) 555

oligomenorrhoea 148
oliguria 70
open lung biopsy 362
ophthalmology 365
opioid poisoning 626–7
oral glucose tolerance test (OGTT) 173, **175**, 176
organ donation 611
organophosphorus insecticides 627–8
osmolal gap 620–1
osmotic fragility test 228
osteomalacia 168, **169**
overdose and poisoning **607–36**
general principles 608–9
oxalate crystals, ethylene glycol, ethanol and methanol poisoning 621
oxalate excretion 595

P

PABA 457
packed cell volume (PCV) 200
palpitations 71
pancreatic exocrine function tests 456–7
pancreatic tumours, hormone-secreting 457–8
pancreolauryl test 457
pancytopenia 72
paracetamol poisoning 628–32
screening 627
paraesthesiae 72–4
paraneoplastic antibodies 556–7
paraproteins 602–3
parasites on the blood film and marrow 206–7
parathyroid hormone (PTH) 600
parathyroid scintigraphy 742–3
partial thromboplastin time with kaolin (PTTK) 245
pattern-evoked visual evoked potentials **546**, 548
Paul–Bunnell test **218**, 353
peak flow charts 492–4
PEG placement 440, **441**
pelvis, radiology 706–7
pemphigus 316
Pendred's syndrome 163
percutaneous biopsy 710
liver 467
percutaneous drainage 710

percutaneous transhepatic cholangiogram (PTC) 445, **680**
pericardial disease 413
pericardial effusion 413
perinuclear antineutrophil cytoplasmic antibodies (pANCA) 450
peripheral blood film 202–3
peripheral CRH test 129
peripheral cyanosis 28
peripheral neuropathy 74
paraesthesiae 73
peripheral oedema 75
petechiae 76
pH
  monitoring, gastro-enterology 459
  urine dipstick testing 588
phaeochromocytoma 132, **138–9**
phenotypic assays 339
phenytoin toxicity 615–16
phosphate excretion, fractional 577
phosphate reabsorption, assessment of 576–7
photophobia 371–3
picture archiving and communication systems (PACS) 654
pituitary dysfunction 112–14
plasma alanine and aspartate aminotransferases 628–9
plasma antidepressants concentration 635
plasma bicarbonate 578
plasma chloride 578, **579**
plasma digoxin concentration 619
plasma ethanol concentration 621
plasma haemoglobin 226
plasma potassium 582–4
plasma salicylate concentration 633
plasma theophylline concentrations 634
plasma viscosity (PV) 217
plasma volume measurement 797
platelet adhesion 250
platelet aggregation 250–1
platelet clumping 201
platelet count **201**, 250
rheumatology 641
platelet distribution width (PDW) 201
platelet function tests 250–1

platelet immunofluorescence tests (PIFT) 268
platelet morphology 250
platelet release 251
plethora 76–7
pleural aspiration, diagnostic 476–7
pleural disease 362
pleural needle biopsy 496–7
pneumonic illness 371
poisoning and overdose **607–36**
  general principles 608–9
polycythaemia 76, **77**
polydipsia 118–21
polyglandular syndromes, autoimmune 314
polymerase chain reaction (PCR) **280–2**, 350
polyphonic wheeze 101
polysomnography **498–9**, 545
polyuria 77–8
  endocrinology 118–21
porphyrias 285
positron emission tomography (PET) 528–9, **754–7**, plate 12
  infectious and tropical diseases 355
  rheumatology 649
potomania 123
precocious puberty 158
pregnancy
  cytogenetics 271, 272–3
  diabetes mellitus 180
  hyperthyroidism 162
  hypothyroidism 164
  nuclear medicine 728
PR interval, ECG 419
prognostic antibodies 555–7
prolactin, asymptomatic raised 152
prosthetic heart valves 412
protein C 253
protein S 253
proteins, urine dipstick testing 589
proteinuria
  assessment of 574–6
  postural 575
  tubular 575
prothrombin time (PT) **244**, 247, 461
  paracetamol poisoning **628**, 629
protozoal antibody tests 343
protozoal antigen tests 344
protozoal culture techniques 339
pruritis 78

pseudo-gout 39
pseudohyperkalaemia 582–3
pseudohypoaldosteronism 142
pseudohypokalaemia 584
pseudohyponatraemia **122**, 124
pseudohypoparathyroidism **168**, 170
pseudopseudohypoparathyroidism 168
pseudo-seizures 37
psychogenic limb weakness 550
psychosis 8
ptosis 79
puberty
  delayed 156–7
  precocious 158
pulmonary angiography 708
pulmonary disease 28
pulmonary embolism 80
pulmonary function tests 365
pulmonary hypertension 405–7
pulmonary regurgitation 412
pulmonary stenosis 411–12
pulse, jugular venous (JVP) 60–1
pulse character 81
pulse irregularities 57–8
pulse oximetry 500
pulse wave (PW) Doppler echocardiography 397, **398**, plate 2
pure-tone audiometry 564
Purkinje cell antibodies 317
purpura 82
P wave, ECG 419
pyrexia of unknown origin (PUO or FUO) 35, **366–75**

Q

QRS axis, ECG 419
QRS complex, ECG 419
QT interval, ECG 420
Quelling reaction 336
Q waves, ECG 419

R

radiofrequency ablation 711–12
radioiodine thyroid cancer imaging 748–9
radiolabelled ^{14}C fat breath test 454
radiolabelled ^{14}C-glycocholic acid test 455–6

radiolabelled white cell scintigraphy 452
Radiological Society of North America 724
radiology **652–724**
  abbreviations 722
  digital 654
  infectious and tropical diseases 354–5
  Internet resources 724
  interventional 710–14
  renal or bladder stones 594
  rheumatology 648
  role 652–3
  small bowel pathology 451–2
radionuclide first pass cardiac studies 764
radionuclide imaging 428–31
radionuclide scanning 355, **528–9**
radionuclide studies
  kidney disease, classification of 571
  for Meckel's diverticulum 453
radionuclide ventriculography (RNV) 432–3, **762–3**, *plate 15*
rapid urease test, *Helicobacter pylori* 448–9
RAST tests 321
reagent test strips, DM 172–3
rectal biopsy 555
recurrent thrombosis 82–3
red cell count (RCC) 199
red cell distribution width (RDW) 200
red blood cells
  enzyme assays 230
  membrane disorders **228–9**, 285
  morphology 204–5
  parameters **199–200**, 353
  survival studies 796
  volume measurement 797
red painful swollen lower leg 374–5
reference ranges xxii
  adult *inside front cover*
  paediatric *inside back cover*
reflux nephropathy 599–600
regional wall motion and abnormalities 404
renal artery stenosis
  hypertension 132, **133**
  imaging 599

renal biopsy 596–8
renal bone disease 600–2
renal disease, progressive 574
renal failure 586–7
renal function 642
renal imaging 598–600
renal impairment 599
renal medicine **567–604**
  immunological tests 602–4
renal stones, investigations 594–6
renal transplant dysfunction 600
renal tubular acidosis 142
renal tubular function, assessment of 576–8
renin, high levels of 133
renography
  captopril 778
  dynamic 776–7
  static cortical 774–5
residual volume (RV) **506**, 507, 508
respiratory acidosis 612
respiratory alkalosis 612
respiratory medicine **471–514**
respiratory samples 362
restriction fragment length polymorphisms (RFLP) 351
reticulocyte count 353
reticulocytes 222–3
reticuloendothelial system 732
retinal haemorrhage 83–4
retrograde pyelography 685
Rhesus haemolytic disease of the newborn 265
rheumatoid arthritis 304
  particle agglutination test (RAPA) 643
rheumatoid factor (RF) **304**, 643
rheumatological investigations 640–1
rheumatology **639–50**
rhonchi 101–2
right atrial pressure, estimation of 407
right heart function 405
right to left shunts 28
rigors 84
Royal College of Physicians 109
Royal College of Radiologists 724

S

salicylate poisoning 633
Salter Harris classification of epiphyseal plate fractures 723
Schick test 364–5
Schumm's test 226–7
scintigraphy 728
  bone 730–1
  bone marrow 732–3
  gallium 790
  hepatobiliary 785
  hepatosplenic 787
  parathyroid 742–3
  radiolabelled white cell 452
  somatostatin receptor 746–7, *plate 10*
  thyroid 740–1
scintimammography 752
secretin test 456
^{75}selenium homotaurocholate (SeHCAT) scan 454
sensitivity of tests xxiii
sensory ataxia 14
sensory conduction velocity 534
sensory evoked potentials or responses 546–7
sensory nerve action potential (SNAP) 534
sentinel node imaging 750–1, *plate 11*
sequencing, molecular diagnostics 351
serology 340–3
  Helicobacter pylori 448
  inflammatory bowel disease 450
  liver investigations 461
  small bowel pathology 451
serum aluminium 601
serum amyloid A (SAA) 296
serum bactericidal test (sbt) 337
serum bilirubin 224
serum bone alkaline phosphatase 601
serum calcium 642
serum complement components 300
serum creatine kinase 614
  theophylline toxicity 634
serum creatinine 568–9
serum electrophoresis for paraproteins 602–3
serum ferritin 642
serum free light chains 294

serum haptoglobins 223–4
serum immunoglobulins
    288–9
    IgD 292–3
    IgG subclasses 290–2
serum iron concentrations
    622–3
serum lactate 618
serum phosphate 601
serum total alkaline
    phosphatase 601
serum urea 570
shell vial spin amplification
    cultures 339
short ACTH (synacthen)
    test 122, 142, **144**
short stature **84–5**, 158
sick cell syndrome 123
sickle cell disease, molecu-
    lar diagnosis of 235
sickle haemoglobin (HbS),
    investigation of 234–5
sickling test 353
sigmoidoscopy, flexible
    440, 441, **444**
silhouette sign 662
single fibre electro-
    myography 538
single photon emission
    computed tomography
    (SPECT) **528–9**, 649
sinus arrhythmia 57
sinus tachycardia 93
skeletal muscle biopsy
    553
skeletal survey, renal bone
    disease 601
skin biopsy **362–3**, 554
skin diseases, autoimmune
    316
skin pigmentation 86
skin prick tests
    allergy 320
    respiratory medicine 501
skin snips 362–3
skin tests 364–5
skull x-ray (SXR) 524, **720–1**
small bowel enema 451, **678**
small bowel pathology,
    investigations for 451–3
small intestine, radiology
    678–9
sodium amytal test 546
sodium excretion
    fractional 587
    renal or bladder stones
    595
sodium wasting and
    retaining states 587
somatosensory evoked
    potentials **547**, 549

somatostatin receptor
    (SSR) scintigraphy
    746–7, *plate 10*
Southern blotting 278–9
specific gravity, urine
    dipstick testing 588
specificity of tests xxiii
specimen collection 346–8
spectrophotometry 610
spherocytosis, hereditary
    (HS) 228–9
sphincter disturbance,
    neurological
    investigation of 551
sphincter of Oddi
    manometry 460
spinal imaging 704–5
spine, computed
    tomography of 531
spirometry 502–3
splenomegaly 87
splenunculus detection 786
spondylolisthesis 705
sputum microscopy 504–5
sputum tests 362
Stamey–Mears test 591
static cortical renography
    774–5
static lung volumes 506–8
steatorrhoea 58
stiff man syndrome 177
stone analysis 594–5
stress echocardiography
    404–5
stridor 88–9
stroke (CVA)
    completed 91
    diabetes mellitus 176
    neuroradiology 718
    suspected 91–2
ST segment, ECG 419
sulphaemoglobinaemia 28
suprapubic aspiration of
    urine 590
suspected bleeding disorder
    90–1
suspected epilepsy 542–3
suspected nephrolithiasis 599
suspected stroke 91–2
Swan–Ganz catheterisation
    434–5
sweating 92–3
sweat test 510–11
syncope 30–2
syndrome of inappropriate
    ADH (SIADH)
    122–4, 587
systemic lupus erythe-
    matosus (SLE) 308
Syva Emit antidepressant
    assay 610

T

T1 weighted images, MRI
    387
T3 tests 160
T4 tests 160
    hypothyroidism 164
tachycardia **93–4**, 418
temporal (giant cell)
    arteritis (TA) 99
temporal lobe epilepsy 8
Tensilon® test 552
'tension' headache 43
testicular failure 154
testosterone
    raised 150–1
    reduced 154
thalassaemias
    haemoglobin abnormali-
    ties 231
    investigation of possible
    234
    molecular tests for
    diagnosis 238
    specialised assays 238,
    284
theophylline poisoning 634
thin layer chromatography
    (TLC) 610
thoracic spine, imaging 705
thoracoscopy, medical
    512–13
thorax, CT of the 666–7
thrombin clotting time
    (TCT) **246**, 247
thrombocytopenia 76
    immunohaematology 268
    infectious and tropical
    diseases 353
    rheumatology 641
thrombophilia screening
    82–3, **252**
thrombosis, recurrent
    82–3
thyroid autoantibodies 160
thyroid cancer, radioiodine
    imaging 748–9
thyroid disease 312
    GPC antibodies 311
thyroid eye disease
    (Graves' disease) 160,
    161, 162, 163
thyroid function testing
    160, 161
thyroiditis
    hyperthyroidism 161
    hyopthyroidism 163
thyroid microsomal
    antibodies 312
thyroid peroxidase
    antibodies 312

thyroid scintigraphy 740–1
thyroid-stimulating
  hormone (TSH) tests
  160, 164, 165
thyroid storm 162
thyrotoxicosis **161–3**, 165
tidal volume 506
tilt table testing 436–7
Tine test 364
tinnitus 94–5
tiredness 95
tissue transglutaminase
  (tTG) antibodies 315
tissue typing 276–7
tonsillar biopsy 555
total lung capacity (TLC)
  506, 507, 508
toxic-metabolic encephalo-
  pathies, use of EEGs
  in 544
toxicology
  blood and urine tests 608
  medicolegal issues 610
  methods 610–11
  sample requirements
    608–10
  see also poisoning and
    overdose
transcranial magnetic
  stimulation (TMS) 550
transcription-mediated
  amplification (TMA)
  350–1
transfer factor 514
transferrin 210
  receptor (TfR) 210
transferrin/IgG clearance
  575–6
transient ischaemic attacks
  (TIA) 91
transiliac bone biopsy
  601–2
transjugular intrahepatic
  portosystemic stent
  shunt (TIPS) 710
transjugular liver biopsy
  467
transoesophageal echocardiography (TOE) 399–402
transthoracic echocardi-
  ography (TTE) 399–402
transtubular potassium
  gradient (TTKG) 585
tricuspid regurgitation 411
tricuspid stenosis 410
tricyclic antidepressants
  635
tropical diseases **327–76**
tuberculosis 364, **368–9**
tubular maximum for
  phosphate reabsorption
  (TmP/GFR) 577

tubular reabsorption of
  phosphate (TRP), frac-
  tional 577
tubular urate handling,
  assessment of 577–8
tumour markers 450–1
T wave, ECG 420
'two glass test' 590

U

UK Haemoglobinopathy
  Reference Laboratory
  238, 284
ultrasound 690–2, plate 6
  breast **688**, 689
  cholangiography 680
  infectious and tropical
    diseases 355
  neurology 525–6
  rheumatology 648–9
  role 652
  urinary tract 685
unstable haemoglobins,
  testing for 237
urate excretion, fractional
  578
urea, serum 570
urea breath test 448, **793**
urethritis 374
urgency of micturition 96
uric acid 643
urinary acidification,
  assessment of 581–2
urinary haemosiderin
  224–5
urinary 5-hydroxyindole
  acetic acid (5HIAA) 457
urinary incontinence 54–5
urinary light chains 576
urinary phosphate, renal or
  bladder stones 596
urinary system, drainage of
  the 710
urinary tract, radiology of
  the 684–6
urine chloride measure-
  ments 585–6
urine culture 590–2
urine markers 555–7
urine microscopy **591–4**,
  621
urine potassium measure-
  ments 584–5
urine sodium concentration
  586–7
urine testing
  by diabetic patients 179
  dipstick **588–9**, 614
  rheumatology 643
  'spot' 595
  toxicology 608

amphetamines 615
cocaine 617
urobilin 224
urobilinogen 224
urodynamics 551
urticaria 96–7
  with angioedema 12
U wave, ECG 420

V

valproate toxicity 615
valvular heart disease 407
variable health parameters,
  factors affecting **xxii**, xxiv
vascular catheterisation 708
vascular intervention,
  radiology 708–9
vasculitic syndromes 318–19
vasculitis 97–8
velocity encoded imaging,
  MRI 388
venography, magnetic
  resonance 532
ventilation/perfusion
  imaging 766–8
ventricular septal defects 415
vesicular rashes 375
vestibular ataxia 14
video bronchoscopy 484–5
viral antibody tests 342
viral antigen tests 344
viral culture techniques
  337–9
viral haemorrhagic fever
  (VHF) 373
virilisation 150
visual evoked potentials
  (VEPs) **546–7**, 548
visual loss 98–9
vital capacity (VC) **506**, 507
vitamin B_{12} absorption
  studies 794–5
vitamin B_{12} status,
  assessment of
  213–15, 353
vitamin D deficiency
  168, **169**

W

Wada test 546
waist girth 68
waist to hip ratio 68
wasting of small hand
  muscles 99–100
water deprivation test
  190–1
waxy broad casts, urine
  microscopy 594
weight loss 100–1
wheeze 101–2

white blood cells (WBCs)
201
differential white
cell count in
peripheral blood
352
morphology 208–9
white cell casts, urine
microscopy 593
white cell count,
rheumatology 640–1

white cell scintigraphy,
radiolabelled 452
whole body
plethysmography
506–8
wireless capsule endoscopy
(WCE) 446–7
Wolff–Chaikoff effect
161
World Health Organisation
(WHO) 176

X

x-rays 654
abdominal (AXR) 354,
623, **668–71**, 684
chest (CXR) 354, **656–60**
infectious and tropical
diseases 354
rheumatology 648
skull 524, **720–1**
D-xylose tolerance test 454